Acute Medicine

Acute Medicine:
Lecture Notes

Edited by Glenn Matfin
MSc (Oxon), MB ChB, FRCPE

Former Chief of Medicine, University of California, San Francisco (UCSF)
Fresno, USA; Valley Medical Foundation Endowed Chair in Medicine,
UCSF Fresno, USA; Vice-Chair of Medicine and Professor of Clinical
Medicine, UCSF School of Medicine, San Francisco, USA

WILEY Blackwell

Registered Offices
John Wiley & Sons, Inc., 111 River Street, Hoboken, NJ 07030, USA
John Wiley & Sons Ltd, The Atrium, Southern Gate, Chichester, West Sussex, PO19 8SQ, UK

For details of our global editorial offices, customer services, and more information about Wiley products visit us at www.wiley.com.

Wiley also publishes its books in a variety of electronic formats and by print-on-demand. Some content that appears in standard print versions of this book may not be available in other formats.

Library of Congress Cataloging-in-Publication Data applied for
Paperback ISBN: 9781119672852

Cover Design: Wiley
Cover Image: © vm/Getty Images

Set in 8.5/11pt UtopiaStd by Straive, Pondicherry, India
Printed and bound by CPI Group (UK) Ltd, Croydon, CR0 4YY

C9781119672852_160424

Contents

Preface, vii

Contributors, ix

Section One: General Aspects of Acute Medicine, 1

1 Introduction to Acute Medicine, 3
   Glenn Matfin and Nick Murch

2 Clinical reasoning in Acute Medicine, 12
   Glenn Matfin

3 Generic capabilities relevant to Acute Medicine, 22
   Glenn Matfin

4 Safe prescribing in Acute Medicine, 40
   Glenn Matfin

5 The acutely unwell patient, 50
   Glenn Matfin

6 Resuscitation, 65
   James Piper and Glenn Matfin

7 Enhanced and critical care Acute Medicine, 86
   Glenn Matfin

8 Acute medicine in the ambulatory care setting, 100
   Glenn Matfin

9 Acute medicine in the home, 104
   Daniel Lasserson

10 Effective discharge planning, 107
   Glenn Matfin

11 Point-of-care ultrasound in Acute Medicine, 113
   Rasha Buhumaid

12 Putting it all together – managing the acute medical take, 138
   James Piper

Section Two: Acute Medicine in Special Populations, 145

13 Older persons, 147
   Glenn Matfin and Howell Jones

14 Perioperative medicine, 160
   Robert Grange, Joshua Griffiths and David Shipway

15 The obstetric woman in the acute setting, 176
   Siara Teelucksingh, Emma Page and Anita Banerjee

16 Adolescents and young adults, 194
   Glenn Matfin

17 People with learning disabilities, 197
   Glenn Matfin

18 Inclusion health, 201
   Glenn Matfin

19 Lesbian, gay, bisexual, transgender, queer or questioning, and others (LGBTQ+), 209
   Howell Jones and Glenn Matfin

20 People living with HIV, 215
   Nadia Ahmed and Robert Miller

21 The poisoned patient, 221
   Glenn Matfin

22 Alcohol, drugs and substance abuse, 230
   Nick Murch

23 People with diabetes and other hormonal disorders, 245
   Glenn Matfin

24 People with neurological disorders, 299
   Hani Ben Amer

25 People with mental health issues, 335
   James Bolton

26 Acute oncology, 351
   Glenn Matfin

Section Three: Common Presentations in Acute Medicine, 365

27 Common presentations in Acute Medicine, 367
   Glenn Matfin and Aya Akhras

Index, 432

Preface

Acute Medicine (or Acute Internal Medicine) is the specialty concerned with the initial assessment, investigation, diagnosis and management of adult patients with urgent medical needs. The challenge for Acute Medicine is to provide a range of high-quality services to a heterogeneous group of patients across the acute care setting (e.g. ambulatory, inpatient, home). Acute Medicine was formally recognised as a specialty with defined training programmes in 2009.

Despite its relative youth as a specialty, most physician trainees now receive much of their training in the care of acutely unwell medical patients while working in the Acute Medicine service. Acute Medicine has been described as the powerhouse of undergraduate and postgraduate generalist training. Despite this recognition, most Acute Medicine textbooks are designed to be used either as an encyclopaedic resource or 'cook-book' style approach. The aim of *Lecture Notes: Acute Medicine* is to outline the *principles* of Acute Medicine (i.e. who, what, when, where and why). Therefore, this brand-new title in the renowned *Lecture Notes* series is relevant to medical students, physicians, mid-level clinicians and other members of the multidisciplinary team involved in Acute Medicine provision.

The contents of the book are completely up to date and reflect the newly developed Acute Internal Medicine curriculum introduced in August 2022. The proposed curriculum changes aim to produce doctors with the generic professional and specialty-specific capabilities needed to manage patients presenting with a wide range of medical symptoms and conditions. This book is divided into three sections. Section One covers general aspects of Acute Medicine care. Section Two focuses on special populations of patients presenting to Acute Medicine. Section Three focuses on common presentations in Acute Medicine.

I would like to acknowledge the tremendous effort and generosity of my co-authors. I also owe special thanks to the reader. Your commitment to delivering excellent patient care, while maintaining (and even expanding) your knowledge using resources like this book, is to be applauded – it is not easy! Your feedback is always welcome.

Glenn Matfin, Editor

Contributors

Nadia Ahmed
Consultant HIV and Sexual Health Physician,
Central and North West London NHS Foundation
Trust,
London, UK

Aya Akhras
Clinical Research Fellow in Gastroenterology,
Mayo Clinic,
Rochester, USA

Anita Banerjee
Obstetric Physician,
Diabetes and Endocrinology and General Internal
Medicine Consultant,
Guy's and St Thomas' NHS Foundation Trust,
London, UK;
Honorary Reader in Obstetric Medicine,
King's College London, UK

Hani Ben Amer
Professor of Neurology,
Mohammed Bin Rashid University of Medicine and
Health Sciences,
Dubai, UAE

James Bolton
Consultant in Liaison Psychiatry,
Epsom and St Helier University Hospitals NHS Trust,
Carshalton, UK

Rasha Buhumaid
Assistant Professor of Emergency Medicine,
Mohammed Bin Rashid University of Medicine and
Health Sciences, Dubai, UAE

Robert Grange
Senior Clinical Fellow in Perioperative Geriatric
Medicine and Geriatric Trauma,
North Bristol NHS Trust,
Bristol, UK

Joshua Griffiths
Physician Associate in Perioperative Geriatric
Medicine and Geriatric Trauma,
North Bristol NHS Trust,
Bristol, UK

Howell Jones
Academic Clinical Fellow and Specialist Registrar in
Geriatric and General Internal Medicine,
Royal Free Hospital,
London, UK

Daniel Lasserson
Professor of Acute Ambulatory Care,
Warwick Medical School,
Warwick, UK;
Clinical Lead, Acute Hospital at Home,
Department of Geratology/AGM,
Oxford University Hospitals NHS Foundation Trust,
Oxford, UK

Glenn Matfin
Chief of Medicine,
University of California,
San Francisco (UCSF) Fresno;
Professor of Clinical Medicine, UCSF,
Fresno and San Francisco, USA

Robert Miller
Honorary Consultant Physician,
Central and North West London,
Royal Free and UCL Hospitals,
London, UK

Nick Murch
Consultant Physician in Acute Medicine,
Royal Free Hospital, London;
Honorary Clinical Associate Professor,
UCL Medical School,
London, UK;
President-elect, Society for Acute Medicine, UK

Emma Page
Physician Associate in Emergency Medicine,
Guy's and St Thomas' NHS Foundation Trust,
London, UK;
Lead Physician Associate Ambassador for London,
Health Education England, UK

James Piper
Senior Fellow in Emergency Medicine and
Education, Sussex University Hospitals, Brighton,
UK; Clinical Lecturer in Acute Medicine, UCL
Medical School, London, UK

David Shipway
Consultant Physician and Perioperative Geriatrician, North Bristol NHS Trust, Bristol, UK; Honorary Senior Clinical Lecturer, University of Bristol, Bristol, UK

Siara Teelucksingh
Obstetric Medicine and Education Fellow, Registrar in Acute and General Internal Medicine, Guy's and St Thomas' NHS Foundation Trust, London, UK

Section One

General Aspects of Acute Medicine

Introduction to Acute Medicine

Glenn Matfin and Nick Murch

 KEY POINTS

- Acute Medicine (or Acute Internal Medicine) is the specialty concerned with the initial assessment, investigation, diagnosis and management of adult patients with urgent medical needs.
- There is a broad spectrum of clinical work within the specialty, including the immediate management of life-threatening medical emergencies, the initial treatment (generally first 48–72 hours) of all presenting general medical ailments, and the provision of ambulatory care. More recently, acute medical care within the patient's home via telemedicine, Hospital at Home service and 'virtual wards' has also been implemented.
- The delivery of Acute and Internal Medicine care is dependent on the close working and interrelationship between members of the multidisciplinary team.
- Most physician trainees now receive much of their training in the care of acutely unwell medical patients while working in the Acute Medicine service.
- As Acute Medicine is an evolving specialty, and many acute medical services have a varied configuration and staffing model, the role of the Acute Medicine clinician varies across the UK.

Introduction

Acute Medicine (or Acute Internal Medicine) is the specialty concerned with the immediate and early specialist initial assessment, investigation, diagnosis and management of adult patients requiring urgent or emergency care for one or more of a wide range of medical conditions.

Acute Medicine evolved to provide patients suffering from a wide range of medical conditions who present to, or from within, hospitals requiring urgent or emergency management with the best quality care, in the right environment. These patients are often treated on distinct wards called acute medical units (AMUs) and patient care is generally led by consultant physicians, trained or with an interest in Acute Medicine. A patient admitted to the AMU will receive care that will include the necessary investigations and management required until the patient is discharged,

---

Acute Medicine: Lecture Notes, First Edition. Edited by Glenn Matfin.
© 2023 John Wiley & Sons Ltd. Published 2023 by John Wiley & Sons Ltd.

transferred downstream to an internal medicine or specialty ward, or escalated to a higher level of care.

Acute Medicine and AMUs are relatively new innovations aimed at improving care given to patients with acute medical illness. Acute Internal Medicine was formally recognised as a specialty with defined training programmes in 2009, having previously been a subspecialty of General Medicine (now known as Internal Medicine) since 2003. The creation of Acute Medicine as a specialty has been a success in improving NHS urgent and emergency care provision.

Despite its relative youth, the specialty of Acute Medicine has good support and advocacy from clinical professional bodies, such as Royal Colleges and the Society of Acute Medicine (SAM). This organisation and specialisation mean that most physician trainees now receive much of their training in the care of acutely unwell medical patients while working in the Acute Medicine service.

There is a broad spectrum of clinical work within the specialty, including the immediate management of life-threatening medical emergencies, the initial treatment (generally the first 48–72 hours) of all presenting general medical ailments, and the provision of ambulatory care. AMUs may be co-located with the emergency department (ED) and same-day emergency care (SDEC) areas. More recently, acute medical care within the patient's home via telemedicine, Hospital at Home service and 'virtual wards' has also been implemented.

Given the variety of patient presentations to Acute Medicine services, medical specialty in-reach or co-location with cardiology, medicine for care of the older person, stroke medicine and respiratory medicine is common. Ready availability of advice and management pathways from the other medical specialties is also critical. Some of this workload is performed by Acute Medicine physicians with subspecialty expertise. As well as medical specialties, Acute Medicine services need to work closely with other disciplines, for example surgical specialties, obstetrics and gynaecology, and psychiatry. Access to higher level care is also important – Acute Medicine specialists work closely with colleagues in high-dependency, intensive care and coronary care units. There has been a trend to having higher level of care provided on AMUs in enhanced care areas.

It is imperative to explore ways of incentivising doctors to work in the most challenging and in-demand areas of medicine, such as Acute Medicine. The rapid growth of hospitalists in the USA is a good example of attracting clinicians to an area of unmet clinical need. Bob Wachter (Chair, Department of Medicine, University of California,

San Francisco) coined the term 'hospitalist' in 1996, more than 25 years ago. In naming a physician whose practice is dedicated to caring for a patient during the entirety of their hospital stay, he and his esteemed colleague (Lee Goldman) started a new movement. Hospitalists usually care for all medical inpatients and, in some organisations, every single inpatient, 24 hours a day, seven days a week. Hospitalists now number more than 50 000 in the USA and are more numerous than any subspecialty of Internal Medicine (the largest of which is cardiology with 22 000 physicians).

Hospital Medicine and Acute Medicine share a lot in common, both having core expertise in managing the clinical problems of acutely ill, hospitalised patients. However, the key lesson for the continued growth of Acute Medicine lies not in hospitalism as a suggested model of care, but in the process of how it became so successful – right leadership, financial impetus, workforce capacity and buy-in from other hospital specialties (e.g. offering co-management service, especially perioperative care).

As Acute Medicine is an evolving specialty, and many acute medical services have a varied configuration and staffing model, the role of the Acute Medicine clinician varies across the UK. However, it is critical that there is a multiprofessional approach to providing all the relevant knowledge and skills that the acutely ill medical patient may require.

The roles of the Acute Medicine physician include the following.

- Stabilise acutely ill patients, and then either discharge or transfer these individuals, when stable and if required, to the most appropriate acute care setting for their needs.
- Minimise length of stay by delivering safe and effective care for short-stay patients.
- Fully differentiate the presenting complaint or problem.
- Risk-stratify the cause of admission (i.e. 'assess to admit') to determine the best place for ongoing care and management (e.g. ambulatory, inpatient, home).
- Improve hospital patient flow, including reducing ED overcrowding.
- Provide leadership and guidance for the medical acute take.

In the UK, there is a shift from the terms *General Medicine* or *General Internal Medicine* to the more commonly used international term of *Internal Medicine*. Internal Medicine is the specialty that encompasses the care, investigation, diagnosis and management of *all* medical needs, including acute medical problems, of both inpatients and outpatients.

Where is acute medical care administered?

The challenge for Acute Medicine is to provide a range of high-quality services to a heterogeneous group of patients across the acute care setting. In time-sensitive conditions where early intervention is paramount – such as sepsis, diabetic ketoacidosis and acute kidney injury – Acute Medicine clinicians can make a real difference to outcomes for patients.

In addition to the assessment and admission of adult patients, Acute Medicine clinicians also have an important role in developing services to enable the safe delivery of care in ambulatory and home settings (Figure 1.1). Many patients previously admitted to hospital for investigation or treatment of conditions such as deep vein thrombosis, pulmonary embolism and cellulitis can now be treated safely as outpatients with the help of Acute Medicine-led SDEC services and follow-up clinics. Rapid-access ('hot') medical clinics also allow unwell patients access to specialist clinicians and rapid diagnostics without admission to hospital. Acute medical care within the patient's

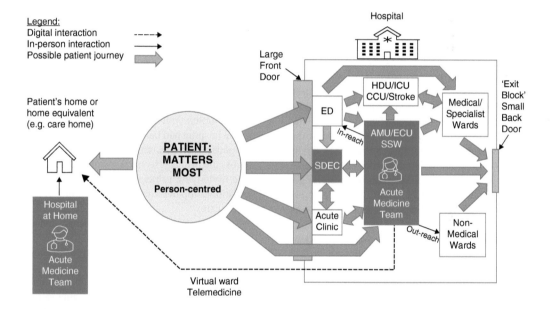

Figure 1.1 Changing landscape of Acute Medicine services. The circle in the middle of the figure represents the patient – who should be at the centre of all we do (i.e. person-centred care). The solid blue arrows represent the different directions of travel of possible patient journeys throughout the acute medical care setting. The solid orange boxes represent the major bases for the Acute Medicine team. On the left side of the figure, the patient can be managed by the Acute Medicine team at home, either in person by the Hospital at Home team or digitally via the virtual ward or telemedicine. On the right side, patients traditionally entered the hospital 'front door' – the point of arrival/entry to hospital – via the emergency department (ED). However, this leads to ED crowding. Front-door reconfiguration measures to reduce ED crowding and hospital admission include patients attending ambulatory care, such as acute clinics (e.g. rapid-access 'hot' specialty clinics) or same-day emergency care (SDEC). Alternatively, patients can be admitted directly to the acute medical unit (AMU) or short-stay ward (SSW). Acute medical patients needing more enhanced care can be managed in the Acute Medicine enhanced care unit (ECU) or transferred to critical care – high-dependency unit (HDU)/intensive care unit (ICU), coronary care unit (CCU) or stroke unit. The Acute Medicine service also offers specialty in-reach to ED and out-reach to the non-medical wards. The hospital 'back door' is depicted smaller than the front door in the illustration, which represents the functional reality that it is more challenging to discharge patients back home or into the community. This 'exit block' leads to overall hospital crowding (patient flow 'gridlocked') and unnecessarily increases length of stay.

home via telemedicine, Hospital at Home service and 'virtual wards' is rapidly evolving.

Acute care hub

The Royal College of Physicians (RCP) Future Hospital Commission describes the hospital footprint of acute medical services across five areas, termed the 'acute care hub' (see Figure 1.1).

- AMU
- Short-stay ward (SSW)
- Ambulatory emergency care (AEC)/SDEC
- Emergency department
- Enhanced care/Critical care

Acute Medicine in the in-hospital setting

- AMUs - defined by the RCP as 'a dedicated facility within a hospital that acts as the focus for acute medical care for patients who have presented as medical emergencies to hospital'. AMUs, as a base for the practice of Acute Medicine, have become integral to the care pathway of most patients who require hospital-based acute medical care in the UK. AMUs provide the initial treatment (generally first 48–72 hours) of all presenting Internal Medicine ailments. Those patients requiring longer hospital stays beyond 72 hours should be transferred to Internal Medicine or specialist medicine beds.
- SSW – bed base providing targeted care for patients requiring brief hospitalisation (estimated date of discharge of less than 72 hours) and dischargeable as soon as clinical conditions are resolved. Short-stay beds are based within the AMU or co-located with AMU in a separate ward-based environment.
- Frailty service – in-reach or embedded within AMU/SSW/SDEC and typically led by a geriatrician. This service may also provide emergency perioperative medical care (e.g. frail patient with fractured neck of femur).
- Enhanced care beds – enhanced care takes place in a ward setting (usually AMU) but provides ready access to the critical care team through established communication links. It is a pragmatic approach to reducing the risk of patients falling into a service gap: patients who would benefit from higher levels of monitoring or interventions than expected on a routine ward, but who do not require admission to critical care.

- Specialist out-reach – Acute Medicine outreach provides urgent and emergency acute care for the hospital, in collaboration with the critical care team. This can be as part of a *medical emergency team*.
- Acute Medicine in-reach to ED.
  - Review acutely unwell medical patients waiting for a bed in AMU or SSW.
  - Work collaboratively with the ED team to identify patients who attend ED and can be: 1. sent to AEC (SDEC); 2. referred to a rapid-access clinic or telemedicine; 3. referred to Hospital at Home or virtual ward service; 4. discharged back to the care of their GP; and 5. discharged home.

Acute Medicine in the ambulatory setting

- AEC/SDEC – AEC provides patients with the traditional aspects of acute medical care but avoids hospital admission.
  - The RCP defines AEC as 'clinical care which may include diagnosis, observation, treatment and rehabilitation, not provided within the traditional hospital bed base or within the traditional outpatient services, and that can be provided across the primary/secondary care interface'.
  - The underlying principle of AEC is to convert traditional inpatient care into same-day emergency care.
  - Acute and Internal Medicine teams deliver SDEC in AEC units.
- Acute care clinics – there are several types of acute care clinics.
  - Rapid-access ('hot') clinics are for patients accessing specialty care and usually offer same-day appointments. Can also be triaged or managed via telemedicine.
  - Early-discharge clinics are for patients who do not need to remain in hospital but where early follow-up is best served by their discharging team as opposed to their GP. These clinics may be part of the SDEC services.

Acute Medicine in the community

Interface Medicine: managing patients with undifferentiated illness who are at an interface between primary and secondary acute care.

- Hospital at Home – innovative care model that provides hospital-level care for acute conditions that would normally require an acute hospital bed, in a patient's home for a short episode through a multidisciplinary healthcare team.
- Virtual wards – observe and manage patients in their home supported with technological innovations that will enable monitoring of a person's vital signs and well-being through phone calls or other virtual technology from a team of clinicians, as well as patient monitoring apps.
- Telemedicine (remote) services.

Scope of Acute Medicine care – what are the common presentations or conditions?

The range of clinical problems encountered in Acute Medicine is very wide, which gives the work a great deal of variability. Examples of common Acute Medicine presentations and conditions are outlined in Table 1.1.

Challenges in Acute Medicine

There is a crisis in acute medical care for multifarious reasons.

- Medical emergencies are the most frequent cause of unplanned hospital admission, and place considerable demands on acute healthcare services (Box 1.1). In the Getting It Right First Time (GIRFT) Acute Medicine national report (2022), approximately 92% of the inpatients on medical wards had been admitted as an emergency, and most of these were admitted via the AMU. This has led to rising acute medical admissions with increased bed occupancy levels and hospital crowding. During times of increased pressure, such as the perennial winter period or waves of the recent COVID-19 pandemic, increased unplanned admissions also negatively impact the delivery of elective services.
- Increasing numbers of older, frailer patients with complex, high-acuity illnesses. Frailty defines the

Table 1.1 Common Acute Medicine presentations and conditions (not including COVID-19)

Abdominal pain
Acute back pain
Acute confusion (delirium)
Acute kidney injury (AKI)/chronic kidney disease (CKD)
Blackout/collapse
Breathlessness
Chest pain
Cough
Diarrhoea
Dizziness
Falls
Fever
Fits/seizure
Haematemesis and melaena
Headache
Hyperglycaemia
Jaundice
Lethargy
Limb pain and swelling
Nausea and vomiting
Palliative and end-of-life care
Palpitations
Poisoning
Rash
Weakness and paralysis

Box 1.1 NHS England and SAM (2022) 'six to help fix' areas to improve in-hospital flow

- Protect SDEC capacity and function.
- Diagnostics should be provided on the basis of clinical need, but areas such as AMU, SDEC and ED must have the same level of access in terms of availability, priority and reporting times.
- Ward rounds and handover. Twice-daily review on the AMU, seven days per week. Internal medical/specialty wards – daily ward and board round on weekdays and board round with targeted patient reviews at weekends.
- Workforce optimisation.
- Access to Acute Medicine. Develop services to enable direct access, ensuring clinical conversations are used to direct patients to the most appropriate service/areas to meet their clinical needs.
- Specialties and in-reach. It must be recognised that medical patients who present as an emergency admission are the responsibility of *all relevant* specialties working within the hospital.

group of older people who are at highest risk of adverse outcomes, such as falls, disability, admission to hospital or the need for long-term care. Nearly two-thirds of patients admitted to hospital are over 65 years old and around 25% of these patients have a diagnosis of dementia (with more than a third of people living in care homes having this diagnosis).

- Multimorbidity. One in three patients admitted now has five or more health conditions compared to one in 10 a decade ago.
- Systemic failures of care, with lack of candour when things go wrong.
- Poor patient experience.
- Existence of racial, social and healthcare disparities.
- People who live in areas of higher than average deprivation are more likely to be admitted to hospital and to spend longer in hospital. This is independent of social class, educational level and behavioural factors.
- Alcohol and substance abuse. The UK continues to have high numbers of alcohol- and drug-related deaths, as well as associated morbidity. In addition, the COVID-19 pandemic has had a detrimental impact. For example, alcohol consumption has shifted more towards at-home, late-night drinking – and frequently alone. Drug decriminalisation, drugs consumption rooms, managing risky drug use behaviour and addressing the social determinants such as deprivation are all on-going debates and challenges.
- Unwarranted clinical variation – defined as 'variation that cannot be explained by the condition or the preference of the patient; it is variation that can only be explained by differences in health system performance'. Unwarranted clinical variation in NHS practice has long been accepted as a barrier to quality care.
- Healthcare workforce crisis. Healthcare is experiencing a global workforce crisis, with the World Health Organization projecting that an additional 40 million health workers will be needed by 2030. Approximately 13% of the total UK workforce is employed in the health and care sector. However, NHS currently has *130 000* vacancies. For example, 52% of advertised consultant posts were unfilled in 2021, with three quarters of these remaining unfilled due to having no applicants.
  - Poor workforce planning has resulted in inadequate numbers of medical, nursing and other healthcare professionals.
  - In addition, the current healthcare workforce is suffering from growing pressures with increased risk of burnout leading to physical and emotional exhaustion and drop in productivity. Working in depleted teams, facing daunting backlogs in patient care, and treating people with more advanced disease have become commonplace.
  - Workforce safety has also been a growing concern. In the context of COVID-19, persistent abuse and violence towards NHS doctors by patients and public compound the emotional toll on staff, damages morale and threatens patient safety.
  - All these factors have led to a potential mass exodus – '*the great resignation*'.
- Social and primary care crisis.
- Medical trainees are also under increased pressure and there is evidence that they do not get the mentorship or training that they deserve because of increasing demands on senior staff and the impact of the COVID-19 pandemic.
- Constant reconfiguration in health and social care delivery and legislation.
- Ever increasing costs of health and social care in a time of austerity and/or financial instability. Lack of modernisation of the NHS estate, rising energy costs, and cost-of-living challenges all impact negatively on healthcare provision.
- Overcomplex, slow, non-integrated digital health systems (e.g. electronic health records and electronic prescribing).
- The climate emergency is a health crisis. Climate change has worldwide effects on health, including Acute Medicine provision: heat waves (defined as ≥2 days of unusually hot weather) are increasing in frequency and intensity and can lead to heat-related illness; hypothermia (energy insecurity and fuel poverty); extreme weather events (e.g. floods); poor air quality and pollution (e.g. asthma); food insecurity (e.g. malnutrition and obesity); water insecurity and safety; vector distribution and ecology (e.g. mosquitoes, ticks); and social factors (e.g. increased risk of displacement).

Impact of COVID-19 on health and social care

COVID-19 has highlighted major issues in the capacity and resilience of the health and care system. Urgent and emergency care services remain under huge pressure with concerns regarding overcrowding, delays in patient care, exhausted staff with a worrying picture of rising burnout and unsustainable workloads exacerbated by the COVID-19 pandemic (e.g. staff sickness, isolation and long-COVID). Staff remaining in work suffer 'left behind syndrome', where pressure to do more with less is even greater. Sustained moral distress (i.e. 'the psychological unease generated where professionals identify an ethically correct action to take but are constrained in their ability to take that action') leading to moral injury and impaired function or longer term psychological harm have also been common during the COVID-19 pandemic.

Opportunities in Acute Medicine

Academy of Medical Royal Colleges 'Fixing the NHS' report (2022) highlighted some of the key healthcare delivery challenges and solutions: Expanding workforce numbers; Improving patient access to care across all settings; Reforming social care; Embracing new ways of working; Grasping the digital agenda; Valuing our staff; Modernising the NHS estate; Revitalising primary care; Greater focus on prevention and tackling health disparities; Making better use of resources and ensuring there is adequate investment.

A new model of care for hospitals of the future has been proposed. The first principle is that of putting patients first (i.e. patient-centred). Patients should be treated with compassion and dignity. They should be involved in decisions on their condition and treatment (i.e. shared decision making), considering social and cultural norms, especially for multiethnic populations (i.e. cultural distinction).

There should be a medical division led by a chief of medicine (like the current practice in the USA) as the senior doctor responsible for making sure working practices facilitate collaborative, patient-centred working and that teams work together toward common goals and in the best interest of patients. Therefore, *effective leadership* is essential.

Patient safety is critical and having an open culture of providing safe care can help. Having real-time 'root cause analysis' ('huddle') when things do go wrong is desirable to prevent further occurrences. A duty of candour when problems arise is needed. Seven-day care is important too and there should be cover 24 hours a day, seven days a week; this should be across the multidisciplinary team, with nurses, pharmacists, discharge teams and radiology services, for example, required seven days per week so not just clinicians working in isolation.

Patient care should cross the boundaries of primary, secondary, postacute and social care with care pathways designed for each of the morbidities that a patient experiences. In this regard, as in all, *effective communication* is key.

There are important consequences of this and one is that there need to be more doctors trained and engaged in *generalist* medicine (including Acute Internal Medicine and Internal Medicine). This does not mean that specialist care is less important or less prioritised. This will remain essential and, indeed, the degree of expertise available in the specialties is ever increasing. Postgraduate medical education in the UK (i.e. 'Shape of Training') is trying to redirect toward more patient-focused, generalist training, and with more flexibility of career structure. It is also important to increase the number of medical and nursing students. Undergraduate medical education is also evolving, with greater focus on generalist training. Acute Medicine has been described as the powerhouse of undergraduate and postgraduate generalist training.

Healthcare workers are the cornerstone of health systems. Focusing on the 'three Rs' of the workforce – recruitment, retention and returners – is critical. In these challenging times, it is more important than ever to have working environments that are supportive, inclusive and safe. We need to:

- improve staff well-being by ensuring employers 'get the basics right', including providing facilities for rest (e.g. after night shifts), spaces to carry out non-clinical work, and easily accessible hot food and drink so staff can keep refreshed during their shifts
- ensure that job planning at all levels facilitates flexible training and working
- facilitate improved work–life balance which can be enhanced by the sessional basis of Acute Medicine clinical work, which lends itself to less than full-time working (improved rostering and use of shifts), and annualised job plans for consultants. It is important to incentivise senior doctors to continue working in our NHS.

The focus on *retention* must be matched by a commitment to sustainable *recruitment*. This includes both developing the next generation of UK-trained talent and *ethical* international recruitment (more than a third of doctors registered in the UK gained their primary medical qualification overseas). Overseas doctors, who continue to be an essential part of the workforce mix, must be given the tools they need to thrive (such as the new NHS standardised induction programme). Diversity, equity and inclusion (DEI) and antiracism in healthcare are top priorities in all our work. Promoting innovative models of medical staffing including nurse practitioners, physician associates and other mid-level clinicians is important.

Digital health encompasses the use of technologies such as telemedicine, smartphone apps, wearables and artificial intelligence to deliver healthcare. These digital solutions have rapidly evolved during the COVID-19 pandemic and have the potential to improve patient outcomes and efficiency of care, which can further enhance safer patient care.

Health equity means that everybody should have the opportunity to lead the healthiest life possible. This requires removing obstacles to health such as poverty, discrimination and their consequences. Greater focus on prevention is also critical.

The world has changed due to COVID-19. This will undoubtedly influence all aspects of health and social care delivery for the foreseeable future. An appropriate legacy would be for co-operative working across hospital specialties to be retained. The additional skills obtained by many medical, nursing and allied health professionals need to be usefully retained, such as in enhanced care provision.

Realistic medicine

Realistic medicine recognises that a 'one size fits all' approach to health and social care is not the most effective path for the patient or the NHS.

- Shared decision making.
- Providing a personalised (individualised, patient-centred) approach to care.
- Reducing harmful and wasteful care caused by both overprovision and underprovision of care.
- Reduce unwarranted clinical variation.
- Managing risk better.
- Become improvers and innovators.

Getting It Right First Time (GIRFT)

> GIRFT is a national programme designed to improve medical care within the NHS by reducing unwarranted variations. By tackling variations in the way services are delivered across the NHS, and by sharing best practice between trusts, GIRFT identifies changes that will help improve care and patient outcomes, as well as delivering efficiencies, such as the reduction of unnecessary procedures, and cost savings.

The GIRFT Acute Medicine national report (2022) had 19 recommendations aiming to help trusts across England standardise patient care, and to introduce measures to help care for an increasingly older population (Box 1.2).

Training in Acute Medicine

The range of clinical problems encountered in Acute Medicine is very wide, which enables trainees to become experts in diagnosis, investigation and management across multiple disciplines (see Table 1.1). The practice of Acute Medicine requires the generic and specialty knowledge, psychomotor skills and professional attitudes to manage patients presenting with a wide range of medical symptoms and conditions. It involves particular emphasis on diagnostic reasoning, managing uncertainty, dealing with co-morbidities, and recognising when another specialty opinion or care is required. Doctors in training will learn in a variety of settings using a range of methods, including workplace-based experiential learning, formal postgraduate teaching and simulation-based education.

There is also significant overlap between Acute (Internal) Medicine and Internal Medicine training.

Internal Medicine stage 1 training (2019)

Internal Medicine stage 1 (IM stage 1) will form the first stage of specialty training for most doctors training in physicianly specialties. The purpose of the IM stage 1 curriculum is to produce doctors with the generic professional and clinical capabilities needed to manage patients presenting with a wide range of general medical symptoms and conditions. They will be entrusted to undertake the role of the medical registrar in NHS district general and teaching hospitals and qualified to apply for higher specialist training.

IM stage 1 will normally be a three-year programme that will include mandatory training in geriatric medicine, intensive care, outpatients and ambulatory care. The scope of Internal Medicine requires diagnostic reasoning and the ability to manage uncertainty, deal with co-morbidities and recognise when specialty opinion or care is required. There will be a critical progression point at the end of the second year (IMY2) to ensure trainees have the required capabilities and are entrusted to 'step up' to the medical registrar role in IMY3. For most, the trainee will be entrusted to manage the acute unselected medical take and manage the deteriorating patient with indirect supervision in IMY3.

At completion of IM stage 1, trainees will be required to meet all curriculum requirements, including passing the summative 'high-stakes' assessment – Membership of the RCP diploma examination – by the time of completion.

Box 1.2 GIRFT Acute Medicine national report (2022) recommendations

Acute medical units (AMU)

Ensure the acute medical pathway is adequately resourced to manage the projected patient need in a safe, effective and efficient manner, 24/7.

Ensure there is seven-day access to medical specialties and services for all patient needs.

Ensure that there is cross-trust consistency in the use of acronyms when referring to acute and general medicine services (i.e. at least 30 different names are being used across England for the units that care for acute medical patients when they are first admitted to hospital: the AMU).

Ensure that the AMU is sited appropriately in relation to other parts of acute care hub.

Ensure the AMU is appropriately resourced in regard to time and space to train all healthcare staff in both acute patient care and the use of relevant equipment.

Ensure the AMU is resourced with the appropriate space and equipment to manage unstable medical patients (e.g. enhanced care unit interventions such as non-invasive ventilation, use of vasopressors).

Ensure there are systems in place to track patients and ensure good communication between staff, including handover and referral.

Act to improve and repeatedly monitor processes of patient care in the AMU.

Same-day emergency care (SDEC)

Ensure the SDEC pathway is adequately resourced to manage the projected demand in a safe, effective and efficient manner, including prompt access to diagnostic and specialist services.

Patient pathways

Ensure that evidence-based pathways are used optimally within trusts.

Ensure admission and readmission data is routinely and accurately recorded and monitored, and used to inform the provision of safe, effective and efficient pathways.

Ensure that the outcomes for sentinel conditions (e.g. chest pain, headache, pneumonia) are regularly monitored to identify any deterioration in performance and provide feedback to medical teams.

Ensure that patients presenting with sepsis are identified accurately and treated safely, efficiently and effectively.

Activity data and clinical coding

Ensure physicians and clinical coders improve the accuracy of data collection and ensure that all coding is undertaken consistently.

Ensure that services are provided in a cost-effective and efficient way.

Workforce planning

Ensure the workforce reflects the requirements of the Acute Medicine and Internal Medicine service.

Acute (Internal) Medicine curriculum (2022)

Training in Acute Medicine will take trainees who have completed IM stage 1 (or equivalent) to the level at which they have the capabilities required to acquire a certificate of completion of training (CCT) in Acute Medicine and are thereby deemed capable of working as independent practitioners in this specialty. All trainees will undertake Acute Medicine training alongside training in stage 2 of IM.

The purpose of the Acute Medicine curriculum is to produce doctors with the generic professional and specialty-specific capabilities needed to manage patients presenting with a wide range of medical symptoms and conditions. Acute Medicine training will be a four-year programme in combination with IM stage 2 training. The programme will include mandatory training placements in geriatric medicine, intensive care, respiratory medicine and cardiology, in addition to dedicated training on AMUs and SDEC units.

Training in Acute Medicine produces clinicians who are comfortable managing a wide range of medical conditions, with a particular focus on risk assessment and ambulatory management. Critical care competencies form part of the programme and Acute Medicine trained clinicians will be able to manage critically unwell patients in conjunction with critical care teams. Acute Medicine trained clinicians will be able to understand the importance of flow through acute services and also the integration of these services within the wider healthcare community. There will be a critical progression point at the end of the training programme to ensure trainees have the required capabilities and are entrusted to undertake the role of the Acute Medicine consultant.

2

Clinical reasoning in Acute Medicine

Glenn Matfin

 KEY POINTS

- Clinical reasoning describes the thinking and decision-making processes associated with clinical practice.
- Clinical reasoning promotes safe and effective patient care.
- The barometer of failed clinical reasoning is diagnostic failure.
- Diagnostic errors – failures to establish an accurate and timely explanation of a patient's health problem or to communicate that explanation to the patient – harm patients worldwide.
- Metacognition (thinking about one's thinking), slowing down and reflection on action may help decrease some diagnostic errors.

Introduction

Diagnostic accuracy is an important component of clinical excellence. Expert clinicians make a medical diagnosis through a process of hypothesis generation and hypothesis testing. Diagnostic excellence involves making a correct and timely diagnosis using the fewest resources while maximising patient experience and managing uncertainty.

An accurate and timely diagnosis is of paramount importance for Acute Medicine patients. Diagnosis is the process of integrating a patient's symptoms, signs and investigations to categorise the underlying illness and guide treatment. This complex categorisation task is driven by mental models (e.g. *illness scripts* and *diagnostic schemas*) that reside in long-term memory. Through education and experience, clinicians form illness scripts that encapsulate their knowledge of specific conditions (e.g. community-acquired pneumonia, asthma, heart failure) and develop diagnostic schemas that structure their approach to a specific health problem (e.g. diagnostic approach to hyponatraemia, such as categorising into hypovolaemic, euvolaemic and hypervolaemic hypotonic hyponatraemia). This cognitive process intersects with systems, teamwork and social factors that can enhance or reduce diagnostic accuracy. Diagnosis is often a dynamic longitudinal process in which patients' clinical features evolve, multiple interactions with the healthcare system occur, and additional information surfaces.

However, diagnostic reasoning is only a portion of the task of clinical reasoning. Clinical reasoning describes the thinking and decision-making processes associated with clinical practice (Figure 2.1).

Clinical reasoning is the process wherein clinicians:

- collect cues (i.e. gather data from history, physical examination and health records)
- process information (i.e. interpret data) using critical thinking (metacognition)
- come to an understanding of a patient problem (i.e. working diagnosis)

Acute Medicine: Lecture Notes, First Edition. Edited by Glenn Matfin.
© 2023 John Wiley & Sons Ltd. Published 2023 by John Wiley & Sons Ltd.

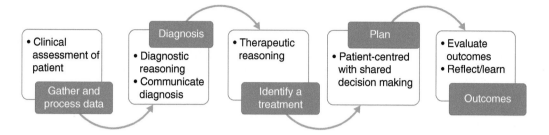

Figure 2.1 Clinical reasoning overview.

- plan and implement evidence-based interventions (i.e. diagnostic tests and treatment)
- communicate the diagnosis
- evaluate outcomes
- reflect on and learn from the process (such as understanding the role of cognitive biases and human factors).

Clinical reasoning overview

1 Process translation of the patient's story (i.e. data) into precise *medical terms*. For example, days becomes 'acute'; shortness of breath becomes 'dyspnoea'.
2 Establish the *database* – gathering data from history, physical examination and other medical documentation.
3 Generate a *problem list* (i.e. a simple list of a patient's medical and social problems that 'encourages doctors to think holistically about their patients and means that minor problems are less likely to be forgotten').
4 Create a *problem representation* related to the major presenting complaint(s). This is a 'one-sentence' summary (a 'tweet') that highlights the defining features of a case.
5 Effective problem representation allows clinicians to summarise their thoughts and then *hypothesis generate* a provisional *differential diagnosis* (i.e. list of plausible explanations for a patient's presentation) using techniques such as pattern recognition, mnemonics and/or diagnostic schema.
6 Once a prioritised differential diagnosis is created, *first*:

- consider *red flags* – clinical features that may implicate serious pathology
- *rule out worst-case scenarios (ROWS)* – conditions that are both common and can deteriorate rapidly and/or cause fatality.
7 Clinicians store and recall knowledge as diseases, conditions, or syndromes – *'illness scripts'* – that are connected to problem representations. Compare and contrast *key* and *differentiating features* (such as MUST HAVE features – without which the disease cannot be diagnosed – and REJECTING features – if present, this diagnosis cannot be made) of the patient's problem representation with illness scripts related to diseases, conditions or syndromes included in the differential diagnosis. Consider *most likely* and *least likely* diagnoses.
8 Perform *diagnostic testing* to help confirm ('rule in') or eliminate ('rule out') various illnesses (i.e. investigative diagnostic reasoning). Monitor trends (if data available) and try and be systematic in approach. For example, if you are considering 'Could it be an acute coronary syndrome?', check the troponin level to 'rule out' the diagnosis. The decision about which potential diagnoses to investigate initially depends on probability (i.e. starting with the *most likely* ones), as well as on the severity and acuity of a potential diagnosis (i.e. common *'ROWS'* first).
9 Refine the differential diagnosis iteratively as more information on history, examination and diagnostic tests becomes available, leading to a *working* or *final diagnosis*.
10 *Communicate* diagnosis to patient/carer.
11 *Therapeutic reasoning* with *patient-centred, shared decision making* to define best management plan.
12 *Reflection* and *evaluation of outcomes*.

Diagnostic schemas are mental flowcharts or algorithms that allow clinicians to systematically approach a clinical problem such as anaemia, organised into a logical framework by clinically meaningful variables such as size of the red blood cells – i.e. microcytic, normocytic or macrocytic. In a schema, the clinician is asked to go through a series of prioritised steps where at each step the presence or absence of practically any symptom, observation, laboratory or radiograph is determined. Based on the presence or absence of the finding, a subsequent step is solved (with a shorter list of potential diagnostic entities).

Gathering data

History

The single modality contributing most to clinical diagnosis is the history.

The aphorism 'A careful history will lead to the diagnosis 80% of the time' depends on context. For example, physical examination and investigations may be of higher importance when assessing an unconscious patient. Clinical context determines the relative utility of history, examination, imaging and laboratory tests, and, in general, as diagnostic classification becomes more refined, clinical information becomes proportionately less important. However, at first presentation in primary or secondary care, core clinical information remains central to primary diagnosis and the appropriate selection of subsequent supporting diagnostic tests.

Physical examination

In an era where time is a scarce commodity and technology seems to dominate Acute Medicine, we are in danger of neglecting the value of the physical examination. This has been further compounded by the recent impact of the COVID-19 pandemic on bedside medicine which has limited patient contact time, clinical teaching and assessment, plus the detrimental effects of wearing personal protective equipment on eliciting clinical signs. Despite this, physical examination remains important (Box 2.1).

The acquisition of all bedside skills requires *deliberate* practice, directly observed by trainers who provide immediate formative feedback, and clear standards of competence (e.g. milestones) against which to assess learners.

Effective problem representation

The problem representation helps clinicians summarise their thoughts and then generate a differential diagnosis (Table 2.1). By summarising the most salient features and minimising distractors, effective

---

Box 2.1 Physical examination contributes to diagnosis

- Prognosis and ongoing care. For example, efficacy of treatment is commonly judged based on clinical findings, such as symptoms and signs of fluid retention and elevated filling pressures in a heart failure patient.
- Patient safety. If you don't do the physical examination, you will make mistakes.
- Patient contact. The physical examination takes you to the bedside – that's where the patient is. More than 50% of US trainee time is spent administering to the representation of the patient on a computer screen (the 'i-patient') rather than the patient themselves. Point-of-care ultrasound (POCUS) as needed - complements exam.
- Teaching observation. Sir William Osler's famous aphorism 'The whole art of medicine is in observation' remains just as relevant today.
- Teaching clinical reasoning. Information-gathering skills must be taught at the bedside. Simulation supports the acquisition of clinical skills but should be seen as complementary. Learning physical examination in the presence of the patient teaches many other skills, such as communication, rapport building, professionalism and, perhaps most importantly, how to navigate uncertainty.
- Reducing overinvestigation. Effective physical examination should increase diagnostic accuracy, improve patient–physician relationships, reduce unnecessary testing and decrease the overall cost of care.

Table 2.1 **Effective problem representation**

A thorough problem representation should initially answer **three questions**.

1 **Who is the patient?**
   What type of person gets this disease and what are the risk factors (*epidemiological risk factors*)?
   - *Pertinent demographics*: age, gender, ethnicity
   - *Risk factors*: other conditions such as diabetes, hypertension, smoking, alcohol, family history
   - *Exposures*: travel, occupation, activities (e.g. sexual, drugs of abuse, hobbies), pets, infectious contacts

2 **What is the temporal pattern of illness?**
   How does this disease present with respect to time?
   Length – definition varies but typically:
   - *Hyperacute* - instantaneous
   - *Acute* – few days
   - *Subacute* – few weeks
   - *Chronic* – few months
   Tempo –
   - *Constant* – e.g. stable, worsening, resolving
   - *Pattern* – e.g. intermittent, 'waxing and waning' (e.g. delirium)

3 **What is the clinical syndrome?**
   Those features that allow you to distinguish between diseases that may present with the same syndrome.
   - *Key symptoms and signs*
   - *Differentiating features*

Case 2.1 **Example of effective problem representation**

Case presentation
- 42-year-old male presents to emergency department with abrupt onset continuous anterior chest pain.
- 2 hours ago, felt crushing central chest pain. Worse with exertion, shooting down to his arm and up to his jaw. He is unable to take his breath.
- Construction worker, smoker, type 2 diabetes (T2DM).
- His father died aged 43 due to 'heart problem' (i.e. likely positive family history).
- Examination: patient distressed; in pain; with profuse sweating; restless and dyspnoeic.

What is your problem representation or 'one-liner'?

A thorough problem representation should initially answer **three questions**.
1 **Who is the patient?**
   'Middle-aged male smoker with T2DM and Family History of cardiac disease. . .
2 **What is the temporal pattern of illness?**
   . . .presents with hyperacute constant . . .
3 **What is the clinical syndrome?**
   crushing central chest pain, present at rest and aggravated by exertion, radiating to arm and jaw and associated with dyspnoea, diaphoresis and agitation'

problem representations reduce cognitive load and facilitate clinical problem solving.

A well-formed problem representation ('one-liner') facilitates clinical reasoning and serves as the backbone for how clinicians communicate with one another (Case 2.1). A problem representation should be updated iteratively as the clinician gathers data (including diagnostic test results) throughout a patient encounter.

An effective problem representation includes the following.

- Includes discriminating features and often excludes non-specific ones (e.g. malaise, which doesn't often narrow differential diagnosis) or irrelevant information (e.g. patient's inguinal hernia is unlikely to be related to their exertional chest pain).
- Uses 'semantic qualifiers' which are abstract, often binary terms that help narrow or specify the meaning of a symptom, sign, pathological process or

Box 2.2 **Examples of semantic qualifiers**

- '45-year-old': *middle-aged*
- 'Last night and started all of a sudden': *hyperacute*
- 'I have had problems like this before': *recurrent*
- 'It always happens on my left side': *unilateral*
- 'The pain kept me up all night and was 10/10': *severe*

disease to help sort through and organise patient information (Box 2.2). Semantic qualifiers add specificity and allow one to compare/contrast (e.g. *acute* versus *chronic; monoarticular* versus *polyarticular; painful* versus *painless*).

Illness scripts

The initial problem representation activates illness scripts of potential diagnoses. Illness scripts are organised mental summaries of a clinician's structured knowledge of diseases (Box 2.3). Illness script knowledge should include a general sense of the base rates of diseases (e.g. in adult patients presenting with dyspnoea, the most common causes include asthma, chronic obstructive pulmonary disease, pneumonia and heart failure).

For the patient in Case 2.1 presenting with chest pain, an illness script for acute coronary syndrome (ACS) may be appropriate (Table 2.2).

Illness scripts are built by starting with textbook or classic cases and then refining based on experiential and further learning (*chunking* is the term used for adding new clinical information to the existing illness script, which enables experts to

> **Box 2.3 Illness scripts**
>
> Classically, the components of a thorough illness script include clinically relevant information (i.e. same three categories as in problem representation, plus additional information).
> - **Problem representation**
>   - Who: Who gets it? Risk factors?
>   - When: Temporal pattern of illness?
>   - What: What is the clinical syndrome?
> - **Pathophysiology**
>   - Why: Known derangements in bodily processes (e.g. anatomy, physiology, immunology, pathology, genetics, biochemistry); and environmental contributors (e.g. microbiological, toxins, pharmacology).
> - **Principles of management (*management script*)**
>   - Diagnostic testing.
>   - Treatment.

Table 2.2 Generating illness scripts – example for acute coronary syndrome (ACS)

Features	Illness script of ACS
Epidemiological risk factors	• Middle-aged/elderly • Postmenopausal female – women represent majority of patients with ACS ≥75 years old • Personal history of cardiovascular disease • Family history of cardiovascular disease • Ethnic predisposition • Smoking • Metabolic syndrome: obesity, diabetes, hypertension, lipid abnormalities
Pathophysiology	• Coronary artery disease – atherosclerotic obstruction or plaque rupture leading to ischaemia or infarction of myocardium
Time course/pattern	• Hyperacute/acute onset • Constant – stable, worsening or improving; intermittent
Symptoms and signs	• Central, substernal crushing pain/pressure • Radiating jaw/shoulder • Relieved rest/nitrates (e.g. glyceryl trinitrate) • Aggravated by activity and exercise
Diagnostics	• Electrocardiogram • Troponins • Cardiac catheterisation • Coronary computed tomography angiography
Treatment	• Analgesia (and antiemetics) • Medical, e.g. dual antiplatelet agents, antithrombin agents, beta-blockers, angiotensin-converting enzyme (ACE) inhibitor, statins and other lipid-lowering therapy as needed • Percutaneous coronary intervention (PCI) with drug-eluting stents • Thrombolysis • Coronary artery bypass grafting • Cardiac rehabilitation

increase the availability of working memory to solve problems while minimising cognitive loading). The experiential knowledge base of an experienced clinician is analogous to a large filing cabinet filled with many exemplars (i.e. memories of specific patients with unique features), filed according to diagnostic category.

Rule out worst-case scenarios (ROWS)

Effective problem representation allows clinicians to summarise their thoughts and then *hypothesis generate* a provisional *differential diagnosis* using techniques such as pattern recognition, mnemonics and/or diagnostic schema. Once a differential diagnosis is created, *first* consider *red flags* and *rule out worst-case scenarios* (ROWS). ROWS are conditions that are both common and can deteriorate rapidly and/or cause fatality. Possible examples of ROWS for the patient in Case 2.1 with chest pain are shown in Figure 2.2.

Prioritised differential diagnosis

> Through a comparison process (conscious and/or subconscious), the clinician develops a prioritised differential diagnosis based on the degree of match between the patient's problem representation and their illness scripts for relevant diseases, conditions or syndromes.

Key and *differentiating features* are those features that allow you to distinguish between diseases that may present with the same syndrome (e.g. chest pain, polyuria, breathlessness, headache). Subsets (not present in all conditions) include:

- MUST HAVE features – without these, the disease can't be diagnosed. For example, patients with myxoedema coma must have *altered* mental status
- REJECTING features – if present, this diagnosis cannot be made. For example, chest pain that can be *localised* with one finger is incompatible with a diagnosis of ACS.

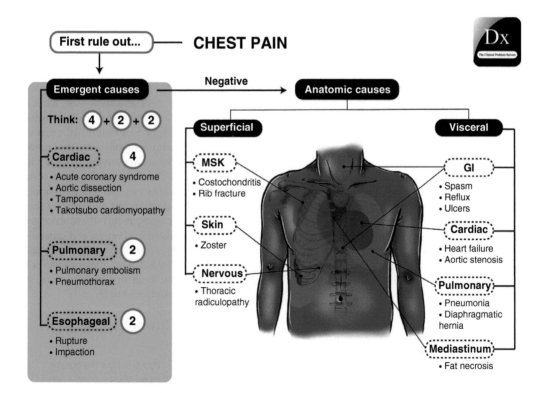

Figure 2.2 First, rule out worst-case scenarios (ROWS) for people presenting with chest pain, prior to considering the wider differential diagnosis based on an anatomical diagnostic schema approach in this example. Source: With Permission of Clinical Problem Solvers.

Acute Chest Pain	Epidemiological Risk Factors	Symptoms and Signs	Time course/ pattern	Pathophysiology	Diagnostics	Treatment
Most Likely Coronary artery disease	Middle-Late age Family history Smoking Type 2 diabetes Lipids Ethnicities	Central, substernal pain/ pressure, rediating jaw/ shoulder, relieved GTN/rest	Hyperacute/ Acute	Coronary artery disease– obstruction or plaque rupture leads to ischaemia or infarction	Electrocardiogram Troponins Cardiac catheter	Analgesia Medical treatment Percutaneous coronary intervention (PCI) Thrombolysis CABG
ROWS Acute aortic dissection	Hypertension Pregnancy Bicuspid aortic valve Coarctation	Severe, 'tearing' pain radiating to back Pulse and BP discrepancy +/- aortic regurgitation	Hyperacute/ Acute	Intimal tear leads to blood dissecting aorta media Stanford Type A or Type B	Echocardiogram CT - Angiogram MR - Angiogram Invasive angiography	Analgesia Medical treatment including BP control Surgery
Least likely Herpes zoster	Older age, immunosuppression	Acute neuropathic pain, dermatomal distribution, followed by rash	Acute/ Subacute	Reactivation of latent varicella zoster virus	Classic appearance of rash on exam, Tzanck smear, test antigen or DNA testing	Analgesia Antiviral treatment Prevention-vaccine

Figure 2.3 Examples of illness scripts relevant to conditions that can cause chest pain and can be considered for Case 2.1. They are listed as *Most Likely*, *ROWS* and *Least Likely* diagnoses. The prioritised differential diagnosis will be based on the degree of match between the patient's problem representation and pertinent illness scripts. For example, compare and contrast the patient's symptoms and signs with stereotyped ones highlighted within the red box to assess the degree of match.

Compare and contrast *key* and *differentiating features* of the patient's problem representation and illness scripts related to diseases, conditions or syndromes included in the differential diagnosis, considering *most likely*, *ROWS* and *least likely* diagnoses (example for the patient in Case 2.1 with chest pain is illustrated in Figure 2.3). If important information in the script is missing, the clinician seeks out that information from the patient. If the patient's clinical findings match with the clinician's illness script, the script is retained for continued consideration.

Summary statement

Once the clinician is satisfied that enough information is known to put forth a probable diagnostic hypothesis, the summary statement is the articulation (verbal or written) of the patient's clinical problem, based on data acquisition and synthesis. The summary statement frames discussion of the leading diagnostic hypotheses (e.g. clinical reasoning argument) during a case presentation with justification for the leading diagnosis and other plausible or 'ROWS' diagnoses.

> A succinct problem representation connected to a short list of two or three diagnostic possibilities should be encouraged. This shorter differential diagnosis can give learners more time to explain which discriminating findings lead to the prioritisation of the leading diagnosis over other less likely diagnoses.

Decision making

> Decision making underpins all aspects of clinical and professional behaviour and is one of the most common activities in which we engage.

Diagnosis reflects the clinician's knowledge, clinical acumen (i.e. instinct or astuteness) and problem-solving skills. The distinguishing feature of the master diagnostician is the ability to mobilise and use knowledge from past experience. In everyday practice, clinicians use expert skills to arrive at a diagnosis, often taking advantage of various mental shortcuts under conditions of uncertainty known as *heuristics* (e.g. rule of thumb, intuitive judgement). These strategies are highly efficient, relatively effortless and generally accurate, but they are *not infallible* (when they fail, they are called *cognitive biases* or 'thinking failures'). Cognitive biases result from our brain's efforts to simplify the complex world we live in.

Dual process theory

> Dual process theory describes how the human brain has two distinct types of processes when it comes to decision making.
> - System 1 (or type 1) thinking – intuitive, quick, automatic and effortless. Dependent on pattern

recognition – the near-instantaneous recognition that all (or almost all) components of a known disease are present.
- System 2 (or type 2) thinking – analytical, slow, deliberate and effortful.

other distractions). As you can imagine, most clinical encounters do not occur under these idealised circumstances (e.g. human factors such as HALT: **H**ungry, **A**ngry, **L**ate, **T**ired). The major cause of *rationality failure* (i.e. making an incorrect decision) is vulnerability to *cognitive bias*.

Clinicians often use both non-analytic (System 1; fast) and analytic (System 2; slow) thinking. We will often switch back and forth as a means of cross-checking decision-making processes, depending on the situation. Most expert clinicians use this two-pass diagnostic approach (i.e. double-check) which is compatible with dual process theory (Figure 2.4): initial impression (System 1) combined with a more analytic approach (System 2). Diagnosticians typically have between three and five diagnoses in mind within seconds to minutes after starting a diagnostic encounter.

Rational decision making

The best calibrated decisions are described as 'rational' – they come from a blend of System 1 and System 2 decisions.

Rationality in this context means the best possible decision given the available evidence and the prevailing conditions. This assumes you are well slept, well rested, well fed, and can give your undivided attention (i.e. no cognitive overloading such as multitasking or

Diagnostic error

Medical error was the third leading cause of death in the USA prior to COVID-19. Diagnostic error (or failure) is a common cause of medical error and occurs in ~10–15% of medical inpatients.

The World Health Organization and the National Academy of Medicine (USA) have identified measuring and reducing diagnostic error as a patient safety priority.

- Diagnostic error has been defined as a diagnosis that is missed, wrong or delayed.
- Patient consequences range from no harm ('near miss') to severe harm and death. It is estimated that 30% of avoidable medical deaths in the UK are related to missed diagnosis.
- Cognitive and system-related factors are the most cited contributing causes to diagnostic error.
  - Individual failure (75%). Errors in reasoning are the most common example of individual failure leading to diagnostic errors. This occurs when available data is not processed correctly under

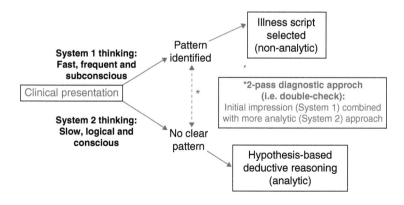

Figure 2.4 The interplay between System 1 and System 2 thinking in the diagnostic process.

conditions of complexity, uncertainty and pressure of time (i.e. *cognitive bias* or 'thinking failures'). Diagnostic errors related to incomplete knowledge base and/or inadequate experience are less common causes.
  o System failures (25%).

More than 150 types of cognitive biases exist – the most common examples include premature closure (acceptance of a diagnosis before it has been fully verified), framing (e.g. how the patient is 'framed' during the referral process) and anchoring (tendency to fixate on first impressions as predictors of specific diagnosis, leading the practitioner to anchor on an incorrect diagnosis).

Diagnostic error prevention

Metacognition (thinking about one's thinking), slowing down and reflection on action may help decrease some diagnostic errors (debiasing). Clinical algorithms, guidelines, protocols and checklists may all help in supporting decision making as they ensure that important issues have been considered, especially under conditions of complexity, stress and/or fatigue.

System 2 thinking cannot make up for gaps in knowledge, inexperience or deficits in clinical skills (e.g. physical examination). However, experience and effective learning can help to prevent cognitive bias.

Strategies for achieving diagnostic excellence and reducing diagnostic error

Take 2 – Think, Do **framework**

This framework supports accurate diagnostic decision making in complex clinical environments. It is designed to improve awareness and recognition of the potential for diagnostic errors across a broad clinical arena, and reduce the morbidity and mortality associated with wrong, missed or delayed diagnoses. The framework consists of three components.

- *Take 2*
  o Take 2 minutes to deliberate on the diagnosis; this still allows quick progression of care in more straightforward cases and promotes a quick reflection for each clinical presentation (e.g. consider differential diagnosis, red flags, ROWS, uncertainty, identify when something doesn't fit).
- *Think*
  o Provides clinicians with insight into clinical situations in which it may be appropriate to think twice and take a closer look (incorrect decision due to human cognitive processing factors, e.g. HALT; system factors, e.g. workload pressures; or patient factors, e.g. communication challenges with person with learning disabilities or delirium).
  o Identifies specific patient journey checkpoints that are ideal opportunities (heightened awareness) to review the working diagnosis (e.g. things aren't going as planned, deteriorating patient, expected treatment response is not occurring, handover, patient or carer concern related to correct diagnosis).
- *Do*
  o Do something to take a closer look and challenge the diagnosis. Provides the strategies that enable clinicians to take action and work through the presenting problem in a different way to identify alternative possibilities (e.g. seek help from more senior colleague).

Approaches to reducing diagnostic errors include the following.

1 Seek feedback on diagnostic decisions. Formative feedback – 'no-stakes' feedback for learning – is crucial for learning in clinical settings. Clinicians can integrate diagnostic performance feedback into their day-to-day work.
2 Consider bias (Box 2.4).
3 Make diagnosis a team sport. Leveraging the expertise of a diagnostic team can help reduce errors. This is a major departure from the classic physician-centred approach. Interprofessional huddles, where the hierarchy between physicians and other health professionals is flattened, can be effective forums to synthesise all diagnostic information and hypotheses. Simply stating that 'this is a tough case' can prime metacognition (i.e. 'thinking aloud') amongst team members and other colleagues.

4 Foster critical thinking. Critical thinking skills can help clinicians optimise their acquisition and interpretation of data throughout the diagnostic process.

5 Performing a *cognitive autopsy* following the recognition of diagnostic error is a self-reflection process which encourages reflective learning, the development of insight and a change in clinical cognition that reduces the likelihood of the error being repeated. These findings can be shared with team members in forums such as morbidity and mortality meetings.

Clinical reasoning in the acutely unwell patient

For medical emergencies, the traditional path to diagnosis (i.e. history, physical examination and investigation) is modified and integrated with the standard Airway, Breathing, Circulation, Disability, and Exposure (ABCDE) approach. Diagnostic synthesis and the ABCDE approach should be viewed as complementary and simultaneous processes (Figure 2.5). Depending on the acuity of the clinical presentation, targeted history and physical examination may be performed together.

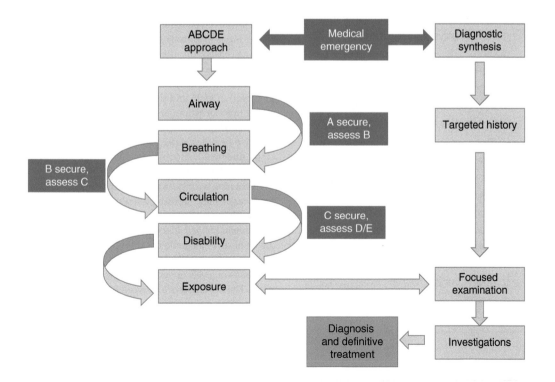

Figure 2.5 Clinical reasoning in the acutely unwell patient.

3

Generic capabilities relevant to Acute Medicine

Glenn Matfin

 KEY POINTS

- The Acute (Internal) Medicine capabilities in practice (CiPs) describe the professional tasks or work within the scope of Acute Medicine.
- The Acute (Internal) Medicine training programme has six generic CiPs that cover the universal requirements of all doctors. These generic capabilities (such as communication skills, professionalism, patient safety, quality improvement, research and teaching) are needed for safe, effective and high-quality medical care.
- By the end of the Acute (Internal) Medicine training programme, trainees should be able to demonstrate that they have independently performed all tasks and documented an adequate level of entrustment. At this point, the trainee has the required capabilities and is *entrusted* to undertake the role of Acute Medicine consultant.

Introduction

One of the major goals of undergraduate and post-graduate medical training is to assure that required clinical competencies – knowledge, psychomotor skills and attitudes (KSA) – have been attained. Many trainee doctors often lack the necessary KSA to care for patients independently and feel unprepared for more advanced postgraduate medical training.

This is one of the major drivers for reforming medical training based on the application of entrustable professional activities (EPAs) and milestones across the continuum of clinical practice. EPAs were first proposed in 2005 and describe the everyday professional tasks or work ('activities') within the scope of being a doctor. Trust is a central concept for safe and effective healthcare. Patients must trust their physicians, and healthcare providers must trust each other in a highly interdependent healthcare system.

In teaching settings, supervisors decide when and for what tasks they entrust trainees to assume clinical responsibilities. EPAs are acts that require *trust*; *professional*-life *activities* (tasks) of doctors. Milestones are an observable marker of an individual's ability, (i.e. KSA and other abilities) compared against narrative standards of levels of performance for a given competency. The key difference between EPAs and milestones is that EPAs are the tasks or activities that must be

Acute Medicine: Lecture Notes, First Edition. Edited by Glenn Matfin.
© 2023 John Wiley & Sons Ltd. Published 2023 by John Wiley & Sons Ltd.

accomplished in everyday clinical practice (e.g. measuring a person's blood pressure, completing a discharge summary), whereas milestones are the abilities of the individual to perform those specific tasks along a developmental continuum (i.e. novice to expert).

> Entrustment is defined as trustworthiness in applying KSA in performance of an EPA. To be 'trustworthy', doctors must consistently demonstrate attributes such as conscientiousness, knowledge of their own limits and help-seeking behaviour (discernment), and truthfulness.

Entrustable professional activities

> An EPA is a unit of professional practice that can be fully entrusted to a trainee once they have demonstrated the necessary competence to execute this activity unsupervised.

Entrustable professional activities are:
- *entrustable* – they can be *entrusted* (i.e. assigning the responsibility for doing something to someone else)

- *professional* – relating to or characteristic of a profession (i.e. being a doctor)
- *activities* – a 'unit' signifies a discrete task (e.g. taking a history, performing a physical examination, providing a differential diagnosis, communicating with a patient, communicating with a colleague, prescribing an antibiotic) or bundle of tasks (e.g. managing an unselected acute medical take).

Entrustable professional activities bridge the gap between theoretical competencies (i.e. descriptors of doctors – 'good interpersonal skills' are person descriptors) and practical clinical work (e.g. 'managing the cardiac arrest team' is a work descriptor). EPAs are designed to be developmental – they go from smaller tasks to bigger tasks as trainees progress through stages of training.

In the UK, EPAs are termed 'capabilities in practice' (CiPs). The Acute (Internal) Medicine CiPs describe the professional tasks or work within the scope of Acute Medicine. Each CiP has a set of descriptors (milestones) associated with that activity or task. The purpose of the descriptors is to help determine the level of each trainee's current ability to perform a series of clinical tasks in the workplace (i.e. EPAs and CiPs are types of workplace-based assessment).

The iconic Miller's pyramid (Figure 3.1), proposed in 1989, characterises four levels of assessment in medical education (i.e. 'knows,' 'knows how,' 'shows how' and 'does'). Real-life clinical

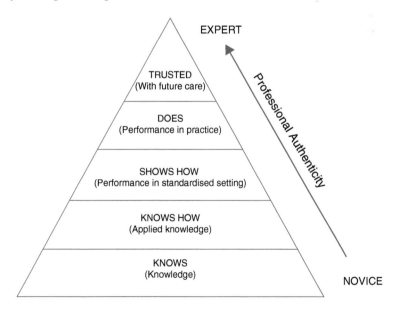

Figure 3.1 Miller's pyramid (extended). A new fifth level ('trusted') reflects the process for awarding a learner an attestation of completion of training, such as the Certificate of Completion of Training in Acute Medicine, that provides permission to act unsupervised.

practice is the most authentic training environment. This has led to the use of EPAs (CiPs) as a framework of assessment and the related *entrustment* decision making for clinical responsibilities at designated levels of supervision of learners (e.g. direct, indirect, no supervision). By the end of the Acute Medicine training programme, trainees should be able to demonstrate that they have independently performed all tasks and documented an adequate level of entrustment. At this point, trainees have the required capabilities and are *entrusted* to undertake the role of the Acute Medicine consultant. This has led to a proposal to add the level 'trusted' to the apex of Miller's pyramid (see Figure 3.1).

Generic capabilities in practice

The Acute (Internal) Medicine training programme has six generic CiPs that cover the universal requirements of all doctors as described in the General Medical Council's Good Medical Practice (GMP) and the Generic Professional Capabilities (GPC) framework. These resources detail the essential generic capabilities needed for safe, effective and high-quality medical care in the UK (Table 3.1).

Before we describe the generic CiPs in more detail, it is important to appreciate that these core generic competencies (as well as all aspects of doctoring) are negatively impacted by three overarching themes:

- lack of diversity, equity, and inclusion (DEI).
- racism.
- clinician burnout.

Table 3.1 **Generic capabilities in practice (CiPs)**

1 Able to successfully function within National Health Service (NHS) organisational and management systems.

2 Able to deal with ethical and legal issues related to clinical practice.

3 Communicates effectively and is able to share decision making, while maintaining appropriate situational awareness, professional behaviour and professional judgement.

4 Is focused on patient safety and delivers effective quality improvement in patient care.

5 Carrying out research and managing data appropriately.

6 Acting as a clinical teacher and clinical supervisor.

Diversity, equity and inclusion

> Clinicians need to provide safe, equitable, high-quality, respectful care to an increasingly diverse population of people, in a manner aligned with the elicited goals of those individuals and their families.

Healthcare organisations have a growing responsibility to improve DEI efforts not only for their employees, but also to better serve patients and their families.

- *Diversity* – understanding the background of employees and patients being served, including culture, gender, sexual orientation, religious beliefs and socioeconomic status (Figure 3.2). Diversifying the medical workforce by encouraging people underrepresented in medicine to apply and train in medicine is critical to reducing healthcare disparity and improving patient outcomes. Community engagement and partnership are also important.
- *Equity* – the process by which resources are distributed according to need. Equity is *fairness*.

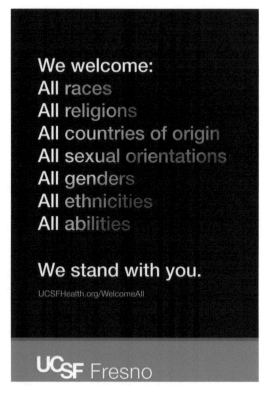

Figure 3.2 Diversity matters.

Equality is a state/outcome that is the same among different groups of people. Equality is *sameness*.

- *Inclusion* – deliberate action to create a welcoming and respectful environment for all on our team and those whom we serve.

Implicit (or unconscious) bias refers to the unconscious prejudice individuals might feel about another group or person.

- Implicit bias can lead to subtle, intentional and unintentional behaviours that communicate some sort of bias (microaggressions).
- The personal histories that clinicians and patients bring to each encounter play a significant role in implicit bias.
- Implicit bias can interfere with clinical assessment, decision making and provider–patient relationships such that the health goals that the provider and patient are seeking are compromised.
- Implicit bias is a major contributor to healthcare disparities.
- To attain healthcare equity, we must become aware of our implicit bias and develop ways to decrease this.

Race in medicine

Health inequalities are widening in many high-income countries and have been thrown into focus by the COVID-19 pandemic.

Health inequity is pervasive across race, gender, age and income, but is especially apparent along lines of race. Ethnic inequalities in access to, experiences of and outcomes of healthcare are longstanding problems in the NHS. Similar problems occur in the USA. For example, the COVID-19 pandemic was the third leading cause of death in the USA in 2020. COVID-19 generally hit people of colour harder, a pattern experts trace back to historical disparities in income, poor housing (i.e. 'redlining'), unemployment, geography, medical access and educational attainment that contribute to social exclusion and disadvantage. Non-COVID health outcomes have also worsened. For example, a 2022 review in the UK found that ethnic minority women's experiences of poor communication and discrimination during interactions with healthcare staff may explain some of the stark inequalities observed in maternal health outcomes. Healthcare may therefore be less safe for some patients than others.

The concept of race was constructed as a tool to categorise people with the purpose of validating racism. Put simply, racism refers to the prioritisation of people who are considered white and the devaluation, exploitation and exclusion of people racialised as non-white. Racism occurs in various forms.

- Implicit bias.
- Individual racism.
- Institutional racism – describes how the 'representation and organisations of races' are insidiously embedded in societal institutions and projects (e.g. political, economic, educational) that, together, compound and reinforce inequitable access and barriers to opportunities and resources.
- Structural racism – describes how these institutions combine across history and present-day reality to create systems that negatively impact communities of colour.
- Race-conscious medicine – recurring themes throughout medicine include the view of race as an innate biological variable (biomedical) predictive of health when in fact it is socially constructed (biosocial), with health consequences that are largely biological manifestations of structural racism.
  - For example, the UK National Institute for Health and Care Excellence (NICE) recently recommended that doctors no longer adjust for race when estimating glomerular filtration rate because it contributed to inequalities such as inappropriate treatments and delays in access to care (e.g. specialists and transplant waitlist).

Anti-racism seeks to promote equity and colour consciousness, rather than equality and colour blindness. Anti-racism and anti-oppression are the purposeful action taken against racist behaviours, systemic racism and the oppression of marginalised groups.

How do we tackle these inequalities? First, by using appropriate terminology. Collation of ethnicities into broad groupings may mask inequality within them.

For example, considering black, Asian and minority ethnic (so-called 'BAME') communities as one group stops us from tailoring services according to evidence of risk; rates of diabetes are substantially increased among south Asian people in the UK, while rates of myeloma and cancers of the prostate, stomach and liver are increased among black people.

> We must improve cultural literacy across society and particularly in healthcare. From board to ward, our workforce must reflect the diversity of the population it serves, with staff that look like our patients and understand their language and culture.

Clinician burnout

Burnout is important for both clinicians and patients. A key component of burnout is depletion, which is characterised by feeling physically and emotionally drained. Burnout can adversely affect a clinician's professionalism and 'sense of calling'. It has been linked to alcohol misuse, the breakdown of personal relationships, depression and suicide. It can have an adverse effect on patient quality of care.

Burnout has been the topic of much interest in the context of an increasingly busy NHS. Nearly one in four doctors in training in the UK and one in five trainers said they felt burnt out to a high or very high degree because of their work. This situation has been greatly exacerbated by the impact of the COVID-19 pandemic on mental health and work–life balance. Furthermore, burnout can translate into 'burn away'. Many are reducing hours or taking early retirement.

Resilience is the ability to adapt well and recover quickly from stress, adversity, trauma or tragedy. To ensure better resilience, well-being and motivation at work, and to minimise workplace stress, people have three core work needs (ABC), and all three must be met.

- *A Autonomy/control* – the need to have control over our work lives, and to act consistently with our work and life values.
- *B Belonging* – the need to be connected to, cared for and caring of others around us in the workplace and to feel valued, respected and supported.
- *C Competence* – the need to experience effectiveness and deliver valued outcomes, such as high-quality care.

> Time management is important too.
> - Do the right things – know what your job consists of and the demarcation of duties.
> - Do things right. Get it right first time – know what is being asked and timeline. Prioritise.
> - Know who can make your life easier. Delegate when possible. Extended team-based care can help reduce administrative tasks.

NHS organisational and management systems

> Around 1.6 million people work for the NHS in the UK. Approximately half have a clinical role, either patient facing or in laboratories or other clinical services. Every 24 hours more than a million people come into contact with the NHS.

The NHS is the UK Government-funded healthcare system. It was set up so that everybody shared the burden of paying for health services. The NHS is a complex system with regular devolved national adjustments to priority and policy. Consequently, most doctors do not fully understand the various structures within the NHS, how it is funded, how it is regulated and commissioned, how it works and who is responsible for what. As an individual working or training within the NHS, it is important to have a grasp of the NHS 'big picture'. This includes the structure and organisation of the health service and system, including the independent sector and the wider health and social care landscape. However, your major focus should be on providing the best patient-centred care for your patients within your local healthcare system, and its relationship to and interaction with social care.

The *Triple Aim* is a useful framework that describes a 'value-based' care approach to optimising health system performance through the simultaneous pursuit of three dimensions.

- *Better health* – excellent patient outcomes and quality.
- *Better care* – excellent patient experience.
- *Better value* – reasonable costs (cost-effective).

This needs to be matched by triple integration, removing the boundaries between mental and physical health, primary and specialist services, health and social care.

The NHS is under tremendous pressure: health inequalities are widening, waiting times for hospital treatment are lengthening, access to primary care is becoming more difficult, the stock of ill health in the population is increasing and we are at the limits of affordability. The model of care that has evolved since the NHS was created in 1948 has to change.

Management and leadership in healthcare

Effective leadership and management are central to the success of the NHS, and the role of managers should be celebrated and not undermined. Leadership in the NHS is needed from the 'board to the ward' and involves clinicians as well as managers.

Effective clinical management and leadership are vital for ensuring that health services run effectively and efficiently, that all members of the heathcare team work well together, and that patient care and safety are improved.

Management matters. Without it, nothing happens. Management can be concisely summarised as 'getting the job done'. Managers are concerned with planning, budgeting, organising, staffing, controlling and problem solving. Effective management ensures that systems are set up and working safely and efficiently. Management is focused on ensuring that everyone in the team is clear on their role and contributing towards the common task.

In comparison, leadership is focused on developing and communicating a vision for the future and defining a strategy to get there. Leadership involves setting priorities and establishing direction of travel (organisation's vision), aligning people, motivating and inspiring.

Why does leadership matter?

- Leaders make improvements in service and outcomes.
- Leaders promote professional cultures that support teamwork, continuous improvement and patient engagement.
- High performance requires distributed leadership, including clinical champions. Effective leadership

for improvement requires engaging doctors to participate in redesign efforts and to build support for these activities among their colleagues.

Leadership styles

Leadership theory provides us with many models and approaches. Most clinicians have a portfolio of leadership styles which are adaptable depending on setting. For example, an Acute Medicine consultant may demonstrate the following leadership styles within any given day.

- *Democratic* – 85–90% of time. Engaging and motivating others whilst working collaboratively as part of the acute medical unit (AMU) multidisciplinary team (MDT). This involves working together, sharing responsibility for problem solving and decision making.
- *Authoritative (autocratic)* – 5–10% of time. Considered useful in emergency situations as the leader makes (all) decisions, such as managing a complex patient's acute medical emergency care.
- *Transformational* – 5% of time. For example, trying to 'sell' a shared vision to colleagues for a new electronic prescribing system that will add value and improve patient safety over time, but will be disruptive and time-consuming for all during the initial planning and implementation phase.

Numerous official reports on NHS healthcare scandals repeatedly expose failures in leadership, teamwork and listening to patients. The Francis Report (2013) highlighted a culture of not listening to patients (i.e. not being patient centred). Francis also warned that the NHS was facing an 'existential crisis'. The Ockenden Report (2022) once again exposes common problems underlying health service scandals: failures in leadership and teamwork, failure to follow clinical guidelines, failure to learn and improve, and a failure to listen to patients.

Ethical and legal issues related to clinical practice

An understanding of the relationship between ethics, the law, personal beliefs and professional guidance will help you to become a more effective and mindful doctor. There are differences between legal and ethical standards. Whilst legal standards are set by governmental laws, ethical standards do not necessarily have a legal basis. Ethical standards are primarily based on human principles of *right* and *wrong*.

Ethics

> Ethical issues and dilemmas form part of everyday clinical practice. Making ethical decisions often leads us into 'grey areas'. For the everyday clinician, the law and professional guidance remain the appropriate points of reference.

Key ethical principles applied to medicine include the following.

- *Autonomy* – the right of patients to make decisions about their own medical care without their healthcare provider trying to overinfluence the decision. A patient's independence is traditionally the highest priority in medical ethics. Expressing respect for patient autonomy means acknowledging that patients who have decision-making capacity have the right to make decisions regarding their care, even when their decisions contradict their clinicians' recommendations.
- *Beneficence (doing good)* – the obligation of clinicians to act for the benefit of the patient.
- *Non-maleficence (doing no harm)* – the clinician has a duty to do no harm nor allow harm to be caused to a patient through neglect. Any consideration of beneficence is likely, therefore, to involve an examination of non-maleficence.
- *Justice* – the principle that when weighing up if something is ethical or not, we have to think about whether it is compatible with the law and the patient's rights, and if it is fair and balanced.

The law and direct clinical care

> Doctors must be aware of their legal responsibilities and be able to apply in practice any legislative requirements relevant to their jurisdiction of practice.

Common key legal issues relating to the role of the doctor include consent, confidentiality, capacity, access to treatment, standards of care, end-of-life care, certifying death and research.

- *Consent* – any intervention which carries a risk or which constitutes an invasion of privacy would meet the legal requirement for consent. Informed consent means providing a patient with an in-depth understanding of the risks and benefits of a treatment or intervention. You should know the limits of your own competence in obtaining consent and seek senior advice if necessary.
- *Patient confidentiality* – a confidential relationship between healthcare professionals and their patients is essential. Confidentiality helps create a setting of trust in which a patient can share their private feelings and personal history, enabling a clinician to form a diagnosis. All NHS staff need to be aware of their responsibilities for safeguarding confidentiality and preserving information security.

> The law is constantly being reviewed and modified. It is important to keep up to date with the law as it relates to medical practice. Always seek early senior advice and MDT input if in doubt.

Communication and professionalism

> Communication is about how doctors and patients interact with each other in the search for mutual understanding and shared solutions to problems.

Good communication between doctor and patient forms the basis for excellent patient care and the clinical consultation lies at the heart of medical practice. Patients perceive communication skills as an integral aspect of medical professionalism. Good doctor–patient communication will positively influence the patient's perception of the physician. In contrast, communication problems between doctors and patients are often the root cause of patient complaints. It is important to be aware that certain situations can be especially challenging for effective communication, such as end-of-life discussions, breaking bad news, dealing with a person with learning disabilities, dealing with a difficult colleague, or interacting with an agitated and potentially violent person (e.g. patient, carer or family member). Under these circumstances, it may be best to have a colleague with you (e.g. nurse) or seek expert advice. If the discussion goes badly, make sure you record accurately what occurred and inform your consultant. Saying sorry for any miscommunication is important too.

Communication

> Due to the complex nature of medical practice, doctors must develop high levels of communication skills. Communication skills in medicine include interaction between doctor and patient, between colleagues and with other healthcare professionals.

Patients prefer clinicians who are warm and compassionate, listen to their patients and ask relevant questions. Shared decision making is widely accepted as a core feature of good healthcare and is an important part of patient-centred care. It requires a collaborative relationship between patient and healthcare provider. It involves informing the patient of their options, prioritising the patient's wishes and respecting the patient's *ideas* (what the patient thinks is wrong), *concerns* (what the patients fears is wrong) and *expectations* (ICE).

Communication in healthcare is a more complicated landscape than previously due to the use of rapidly evolving digital technologies and changes in the way we interact with patients and colleagues. In addition, as communication now seemingly occurs 24/7, it may also feel harder than ever to carve out 'no-contact' times with patients and colleagues alike. This can be a factor in clinician burnout. Effective communication skills and etiquette are now needed for face-to-face interactions (e.g. real or virtual via telemedicine), written patient records, telephone consultations, and electronic written media like emails and texts. It is important to remember that these diverse multifaceted communication channels with patients and colleagues need capturing in the patient record, and that patient confidentiality must still be maintained.

Effective team communication

Effective team communication is vital for safe clinical care. The situation, background, assessment, recommendation and readback (SBARR) system of communication is a structured way to communicate about a patient with another healthcare professional and increases the amount of relevant information being communicated in a shorter time. Examples of when SBARR should be used include:

- escalating a sick patient
- referring to a different specialty/profession
- formal handover to hospital at night.

Errors at the time of transition (also known as handoff errors) are among the most common errors in healthcare. Handover is the system by which the responsibility for immediate and ongoing care is transferred between healthcare professionals. Failure in handover is a major preventable cause of patient harm and is principally due to the human factors of poor communication and systemic error. These can lead to inefficiencies, repetitions, delayed decisions, repeated investigations, incorrect diagnoses, incorrect treatment and poor communication with the patient. A good handover ensures that changes in clinical teams are not detrimental to the quality of healthcare and improves communications between all members of the healthcare team, and those with the patient and their family. Always make sure that patients have continuity of care.

During everyday clinical work, you must be very careful with informal (curbside) consults (i.e. a colleague asking for your input on a case that you are not officially involved in during a chance meeting in the corridor or elsewhere) as opposed to formal consultations. Formal consultation is preferred in general, but needs to balance patient safety and provider workload. What is an appropriate curbside consultation? The Goldilocks of curbside consultation:

- not too simple – can be easily looked up
- not too complicated – requires nuanced clinical judgement, data interpretation, reading the literature
- just right – hypothetical, factual question.

Learning communication skills

Effective communication is a product of appropriate KSA that can be taught, learned and assessed. Effective communication skills involve both:

- non-verbal skills (e.g. reflective listening, eye contact, posture, gesture)
- verbal skills (e.g. use open-ended questions effectively, use closed questions appropriately, interim summaries avoiding jargon, and empathy).

Several models of communication for clinical practice have been described. They are generally similar,

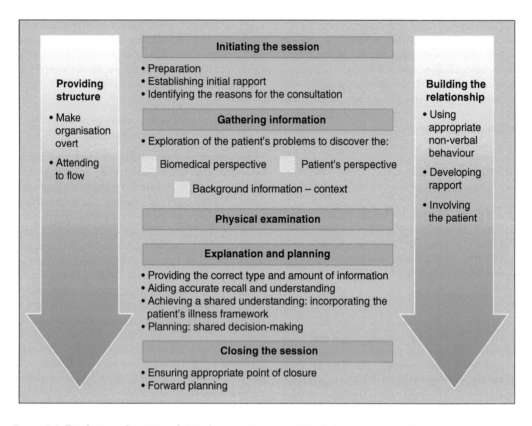

Figure 3.3 The Calgary–Cambridge Guide. Source: Kurtz et al. 2005 / with permission of Taylor & Francis.

and all emphasise the importance of patient-centred interview methods. The Calgary–Cambridge approach has become well established as a generic guide to consultations (Figure 3.3). The basic elements of a successful consultation are as follows.

- Sequential in the consultation.
  - Initiating the session. Preparation, establishing initial rapport and identifying the reasons for the consultation.
  - Gathering information. An accurate clinical history provides about 80% of the information required to make a diagnosis.
  - Explanation and planning. This includes shared decision making.
  - Closing the session. This allows the doctor to summarise and clarify the plans that have been agreed and what the next steps will be and any contingency plans (e.g. safety-netting advice is aimed at protecting patients from harm by empowering appropriate health-seeking behaviours in patients with undifferentiated

disease and those at risk of deterioration or developing a serious complication).

- Throughout the consultation.
  - Organisation. Allows a flexible but ordered and logical process to occur within an appropriate timeframe.
  - Building the relationship.

Clinical documentation

Documenting accurately is an important part of communication (Box 3.1).

Professionalism

Doctors must always demonstrate appropriate personal and professional values and behaviours. This is implicit during their duty of care to patients. However, it also includes a wide range of other professional responsibilities, such as acting as an employee, educator, scientist and scholar.

> ## Box 3.1 Clinical documentation
>
> - Date, time and sign every entry.
> - Write your name and role as a heading and the names and roles of all others present at the encounter.
> - Make entries immediately or as soon as possible after care is given. This ensures that all other team members are aware of any changes to a patient's condition or management plan.
> - Be legible.
> - Be thorough, accurate and objective.
> - Maintain a professional tone.
> - Only use approved abbreviations, if you must, but it is better to use no abbreviations at all to avoid confusion.
> - If the note is not electronic, sign off with time and your full details.
> - Addenda. If an addendum is made, this should also be verbally communicated to other teams and nursing staff. Sign off any addenda with the time and your full details.
> - Mistakes. If a mistake is made, correct it with a single strikethrough. Follow that by clearly signing and dating the correction.

- What is professionalism? Professionals (doctor) do their best to give the best to their clients (patients). The principle of primacy of patient welfare is based on a dedication to serving the interest of the patient.
- Why bother about professionalism in medical practice? The doctor–patient relationship is between two *very* unequal partners. . . on a matter that concerns life and death. This is implicit in the Hippocratic Oath (500 BC).
  - Professionalism is associated with improved medical outcomes.
  - Unprofessional behaviour is associated with adverse medical outcomes.
- Professionalism is the basis of medicine's contract with society (Physician Charter 2002). It demands placing the interests of patients above those of the physician, setting and maintaining standards of competence and integrity, and providing expert advice to society on matters of health. Essential to this contract is public trust in physicians, which depends on the integrity of both individual physicians and the whole profession.
- The '10 commitments' of medical professionalism: 1. Competence; 2. Appropriate relationship with patient; 3. Improving quality of care; 4. Maintain trust by avoiding conflict(s) of interest; 5. Professional responsibilities; 6. Honesty with patients; 7. Patient confidentiality; 8. Just distribution of finite resources; 9. Scientific knowledge; 10. Improving access to care.
- Lack of professionalism (examples) – abuse of power (e.g. abuse while interacting with patients and/or colleagues); arrogance (i.e. offensive display of superiority and self-importance); greed; misrepresentation (e.g. lying); impairment (e.g. alcohol or substance abuse preventing discharge of duties); lack of conscientiousness (i.e. failure to fulfil professional responsibilities); and conflicts in interest.

Patient safety and quality improvement

In England, the NHS is 'organising itself around a single definition of quality': care that is effective, safe and provides as positive an experience as possible by being caring, responsive and patient centred. This definition also states that care should be well led, sustainable and equitable. Clinical governance ensures that this quality is maintained to a high standard.

To improve the quality of healthcare, we must have several factors in place.

- Effective leadership for improvement.
- Creating governance arrangements and processes to identify quality issues that require investigation and improvement.
- Giving everyone a voice and bringing staff, patients, carers and the public together to improve and redesign the way that care is provided.
- Sharing expertise and helping to spread the adoption and adaptation of best practices (e.g. 'Getting It Right First Time' [GIRFT] is a national programme designed to improve medical care within the NHS by reducing unwarranted variations).

Doctors must demonstrate that they can participate in and promote activity to improve the quality and safety of patient care and clinical outcomes. It is also critical that doctors raise and escalate concerns where there is an issue with patient safety or quality of care without fear of retribution ('whistleblowing').

Patient safety

> Patient safety is a priority in clinical practice. It aims to prevent and reduce risks, errors and harm that occur to patients during provision of healthcare.

Although patient safety has improved steadily, harm remains a substantial global challenge. Additionally, safety needs to be ensured not only in hospitals but also across the continuum of care. Safety is one of the key questions that the Care Quality Commission (CQC) asks of all health and social care services.

An *adverse event* is an unintended injury caused by the healthcare system.

- A patient safety incident (or error) refers to an unintended event caused by the healthcare system which may or may not have led to harm (e.g. physical or psychological) and includes 'near misses'.
- Medical errors are acts of *commission* (doing something wrong) or *omission* (failing to do the right thing) leading to an undesirable outcome or significant potential for such an outcome.

Historically, the approach to medical errors was to blame the provider delivering care to the patient. The current approach to patient safety replaces 'the blame and shame game' with *systems thinking* – a paradigm that acknowledges the human condition – namely, that *humans err* – and concludes that safety depends on creating systems that anticipate errors and either prevent or catch them before they cause harm.

James Reason's 'Swiss cheese model' is the dominant paradigm for understanding the relationship between active ('sharp end') errors and latent ('blunt end') errors; it is important to resist the temptation to focus solely on the former and neglect the latter (Figure 3.4). He argued that many errors committed by individuals had their roots in 'upstream' influences. Reason's model holds that all complex organisations harbour many 'latent errors', unsafe conditions that are, in essence, mistakes waiting to happen. This alone is not enough to cause harm. Just as Swiss cheese has holes at different places and angles, different aspects of medical care may have weaknesses. When the holes line up, mistakes are more likely to happen. You can decrease the risk of harm if you shrink the 'size' of the holes or add more layers of protection.

A variety of strategies should be employed to create safer systems, including simplification, standardisation, building in redundancies and cross-checks (e.g. checklists), improving teamwork and communication, and learning from past mistakes (e.g. morbidity and mortality meetings, 'root cause' analyses). Finally, there is increasing appreciation of the importance of a

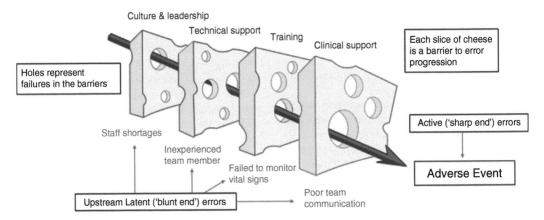

Figure 3.4 An example to show how the generic Swiss cheese model can lead to adverse events. Source: Adapted from Seshia et al. J Eval Clin Practice 2018; 24:187–197.

well-trained, well-staffed and well-rested workforce in delivering safe care.

Human factors is the study of how we adapt our behaviour to minimise patient safety incidents. This includes *situational awareness* (knowing what is going on around you and being alert to potential problems) and *effective team communication* (e.g. using SBARR) and *dynamics* (i.e. team-based care). Doctors must also recognise and work within their limits of personal competence. If you feel uncomfortable or out of your depth, escalate and seek senior advice and/or interprofessional support.

Clinical risk management

Health services are inherently risky. Common patient safety problems include medication errors, procedural complications, diagnostic errors and hospital-acquired infections (always wash your hands or use antiseptic gel; not just good advice for times of COVID-19 – it helps to protect your patients and can prevent you getting ill).

Clinical risk management is concerned with improving the safety of healthcare by:

- identifying the circumstances that put patients at risk of harm
- reducing risks by implementing risk systems (e.g. checklists).

Thorough risk assessments and reporting of patient safety incidents and near misses are the main ways in which an organisation can learn and change. Never events are serious, largely preventable patient safety incidents that should not occur if the available preventive measures have been implemented (e.g. incorrect route of medication administration, transfusion of ABO incompatible blood components).

A duty of candour and saying sorry are required when problems arise. An incident report (Datix) should be lodged.

Patient safety incidents are experienced disproportionately by marginalised patient groups, further exacerbating health inequalities.

Quality improvement

Improving the quality of care and support that patients, carers and the public experience is at the heart of health and social care. To do this effectively, we must make sure we measure and monitor quality of care, ensuring we maintain the current quality of care as we implement actions that will improve it (i.e. quality improvement).

Quality improvement is about giving the people closest to issues affecting care quality the time, permission, skills and resources they need to solve them. It involves a systematic and co-ordinated approach to solving a problem using specific methods and tools with the aim of bringing about a measurable improvement. Through quality improvement, there is the potential to create a healthcare service capable of ensuring 'no needless deaths; no needless pain or suffering; no helplessness in those served or serving; no unwanted waiting; no waste; and no one left out'.

What is quality? There is no single accepted definition of quality in health and social care but there is acknowledgement that it has different dimensions.

- *Safe* – avoiding harm from care that is intended to help people.
- *Timely* – reducing waits and sometimes harmful delays.
- *Effective* – providing services based on evidence and which produce a clear benefit.
- *Efficient* – avoiding waste.
- *Patient centred* – establishing a partnership between practitioners and patients to ensure that care respects patients' needs and preferences.
- *Equitable* – providing care that does not vary in quality because of patient characteristics.

Quality improvement models

Quality improvement is the continual actions undertaken to improve outcomes for patients and to develop the workforce that supports them using systematic methods. The two key elements are 'continual' and 'systematic'. There are many accepted care improvement methods, such as Lean, PDSA (Plan, Do, Study, Act), and audit.

- Lean emphasises the patient's central position to all activities and aims to eliminate or reduce activities that do not add value to the patient.

- An audit involves measurement of the effectiveness of healthcare against agreed and proven standards for high quality and taking action to bring practice in line with these standards so as to improve the quality of care and health outcomes. It looks at how you care for patients and seeing if it can be done better. The audit cycle provides a structured way of ensuring that all steps in the process are addressed (i.e. 1. identifying a problem; 2. defining standards/criteria; 3. collecting data; 4. analysis; 5. implementing change; and 6. re-audit).

The choice of method for an improvement activity is less important than choosing one that takes a systematic approach. Doctors should be familiar with the design and implementation of quality improvement projects (QIPs) or interventions that improve clinical effectiveness, patient safety and patient experience.

Model for improvement

The model for improvement was designed to provide a framework for developing, testing and implementing changes that lead to improvement. The framework includes three key questions to ask before embarking on a change programme, supported by a process for testing change ideas using PDSA cycles (Figure 3.5).

1 What are we trying to accomplish? Clear goals that focus on problems that cause concern for patients and staff.
2 How will we know if a change is an improvement? What can we measure that will change if the system is improved? How can we obtain this data? What is the best way to display the data we collect so that we can decide whether we are improving the system and whether the improvement is sustainable?
3 What changes can we make that will result in improvement?

Carrying out research and managing data appropriately

Keeping up to date is a core life-long requirement of doctors. However, millions of medical articles are published each year and patients benefit from only a tiny fraction of this new clinical information. It is important that doctors have appropriate knowledge of research methods, including qualitative (non-numeric data, i.e. ordinal – ordered in some way such as mild, moderate and severe) and quantitative (numeric data) approaches to scientific enquiry, in order to differentiate well-run studies from those with errors.

Errors in clinical studies lead to results that are misleading and conclusions that are wrong. Interventions and treatments may appear more promising or less beneficial than they are. Errors in studies can happen either by chance or through mistakes in design or interpretation. There are two types of common errors in studies.

- *Bias* – describes an error (at any stage of the study) that was not due to chance, and therefore it cannot be measured or controlled for statistically. Researchers will try to reduce bias as much as possible.
- *Confounding* – literally means 'confusion of effects'. Confounding is a problem if a variable is different between two groups and affects the outcome being studied. For example, does coffee cause cardiovascular disease (CVD)? Smoking may be more common in people who drink coffee and can cause CVD – so it could be a potential confounding factor if there are more smokers in the coffee group compared with controls. Confounders cannot be removed from a study but can be accounted for in the statistical analysis.

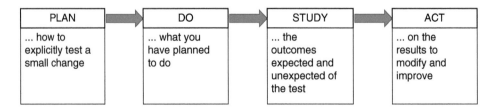

Figure 3.5 Plan, Do, Study, Act (PDSA) cycles.

Evidence-based medicine

How do we filter the scientific evidence to best benefit patients? Evidence-based medicine (also known as evidence-based practice) describes the process of practising medicine based on combining the best research evidence with clinical expertise and patient values to achieve the best possible management.

Evidence-based medicine (EBM) has five key steps (Table 3.2).

Research

Why do we need the critical appraisal step in EBM? There could be conflicting results from clinical studies, in part because real-life medicine does not reflect the restrictive environment of clinical studies.

- *Efficacy* describes the impact of interventions under optimal (trial) conditions.
- *Effectiveness* describes the impact of interventions under ordinary (clinical) conditions.

Critical appraisal seeks to answer the following questions.

- Does the research have *internal validity* (i.e. it reflects true results based on study design and methodology)?
- Does the research have *external validity* (i.e. to what extent can results be generalised to a wider population)?

The concept of *'hierarchy of evidence'* (level of evidence) is used to demonstrate how reliable a study is by starting with the most robust at the top and then working downwards (Figure 3.6). However, both observational (no intervention) and experimental (interventional) studies can be regarded as complementary approaches to EBM as part of the *'network of evidence'*, because they bring different information to light (e.g. observational studies are generally bigger and more generalisable and consequently are especially useful for signalling safety events).

Types of clinical studies

The type of *clinical question* determines the type of *study*.

- Observational studies.
  - Descriptive – report what has been observed in a sample (e.g. survey, case report, case series).
  - Analytical – report the similarities and differences observed between two or more samples (e.g. case–control study, cohort study, cross-sectional survey).

Table 3.2 Evidence-based medicine – the five steps		
1	**Question**	Formulate an answerable question
		The **PICO** tool is often used for precise, specific question building
		• **P**atient (or **P**roblem) – How would you describe or define your patient group?
		• **I**ntervention (or exposure) – Describe the intervention you are studying.
		• **C**omparison – What is the main comparative group?
		• **O**utcome – What outcome are you interested in?
		Example:
		P: COVID-19; I: Drug A; C: Drug B; O: Improved in-hospital survival
		Question: In COVID-19, does drug A, compared to drug B, improve in-hospital survival?
2	**Evidence**	Search for the best evidence
3	**Critical appraisal**	Evaluate the evidence – relevance; validity; impact (size of the benefit); applicability
4	**Application**	Apply the results, combining with clinical expertise and patient circumstances
5	**Implementation and monitoring**	Implement and monitor the process

Hierarchy of research methodologies is based on premise that different study* designs differ in ability to predict what will happen to patients in real life

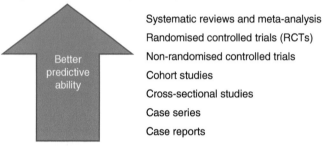

Systematic reviews and meta-analysis

Randomised controlled trials (RCTs)

Non-randomised controlled trials

Cohort studies

Cross-sectional studies

Case series

Case reports

*Not all studies using same design are of equal quality

Figure 3.6 Evidence-based medicine – the hierarchy of evidence.

- Experimental studies.
  - o Researcher intervenes in some way with the experimental group and reports any differences between this group and a control group in whom no intervention or a different intervention was offered (e.g. cross-over trial, randomised controlled trial).
  - o Randomisation is the preferred way of assigning participants to control and intervention groups. Simplistically, each patient has an equal chance of being assigned to either group. Avoids randomisation bias.
  - o Comparator – used to show superiority (better than), equivalence (same as) or non-inferiority (no worse than) between new and other intervention.
    - Placebo controlled – effect of intervention is compared to effect of placebo. Patients have a chance of receiving the placebo during the trial, and therefore do not receive effective treatment (although they may have additional background therapies, as well as 'escape' therapy available should their condition acutely deteriorate). Researchers must have genuine uncertainty about the superiority of the new treatment (i.e. clinical 'equipoise').
    - Active controlled – effect of intervention is compared to effect of an active reference intervention (e.g. current 'gold standard' treatment).

- Appropriate and well-defined population.
- Ethics and consent – it is imperative that all investigators in clinical research follow guidelines on ethical conduct and consent for research.
- An adequate sample size based on a clinically important outcome difference between treatment groups (e.g. in a diabetes study, a reduction in glycosylated haemoglobin of 0.4% (~5 mmol/mol) or more in the interventional group compared to comparator).
  - o Power of study – probability of detecting a difference in the study if one really exists.
- Concurrent control group (i.e. active or placebo).
- Randomised/blinded assignment of subjects.
- Standardisation/optimisation of treatment regimens, measures, procedures, etc.
- Appropriate statistical methods defined *a priori*.
  - o Statistical significance level – if p-value is <0.05, a real difference exists.
- Clinically meaningful and well-characterised endpoints.
  - o Is there a difference? Effect size and confidence intervals.
  - o Is the effect real? Statistical significance (i.e. p-value).
  - o Are the results *clinically significant*? Effect size, cost, adverse effects, mode of administration are all important considerations. Are other effective therapies available (unmet need)?

Evaluation of clinical studies

When comparing the results of various clinical studies (e.g. as part of EBM or when participating at a journal club), it is important to consider the essential elements of a study.

- What is the clinical study question? Each clinical trial requires a primary question.
- Appropriate study design (including duration) and treatment structure.

Sometimes the results of several studies or all available evidence are combined and re-evaluated.

- Meta-analysis – combines the results of *several* studies and produces a quantitative assessment. More powerful estimates of true effect size than derived in single study

- Systematic review – attempts to access and review systematically *all* the pertinent articles in the field.

To undertake effective meta-analysis and systematic reviews, *all* trial results (negative or positive) should be published – this remains an ongoing challenge.

Using data to improve care

Collecting and understanding data is central to patient safety and quality improvement, as without information and data, a clinician has little to draw on to answer two fundamental questions.
- How am I and my team doing?
- What can we do to improve?

For individual clinicians and teams, the most meaningful information is qualitative (non-numerical) information about the outcomes of care and quantitative information about the process of care. Examples include:

1 learning from clinical incidents and complaints – complaints and clinical incident reports can be a rich source of learning for clinicians about the quality and safety of their service
2 using feedback from staff, colleagues and patients (including multisource feedback)
3 understanding morbidity and mortality data.

Data may also be collected for research (to test hypotheses about treatments and processes) and for judgement (accountability to others).

Acting as a clinical teacher and clinical supervisor

Pedagogy is the theory of learning. The pillars of education are innovation, relevance and quality. The educational process has three core elements – curriculum, trainee and teacher.

Key areas of education include the following.
- What should be learned or taught (outcomes)?
- How should training be organised (curriculum – everything that happens in the educational program)?
- How do trainees learn most effectively (teaching and learning methods)?
- How should assessment be carried out (workplace-based assessment is most authentic for doctors)?

Clinicians as teachers

Good teachers facilitate learning. All doctors have a responsibility to teach and need to invest time in developing the skills to do so. Ultimately, medical trainees' success hinges on their ability to *doctor*.

It is important that Acute Medicine consultants and trainees deliver high-quality, innovative teaching and learning experiences to medical students, colleagues and other healthcare professionals. Being a good role model helps but purposeful preparation is key. A range of strategies can be used to engage learners and develop their thinking (Box 3.2). For effective teaching, meeting learners where they are, or applying specific techniques that target the learner's level of clinical experience, is essential.

Most consultants need additional skills in teaching and learner assessment, and this can occur via various instructional techniques as part of continuing (life-long) professional development (CPD), including

Box 3.2 Aspects of the most effective learning

- Trainee centred
- Active learning – as opposed to passive
- Individualised – own pace and choice of modalities
- Effective feedback – timely, specific and constructive
- Self-directed learning
- Experiential – 'real-life' with early patient contact
- Application of knowledge occurs
- Systematic – although much teaching is opportunistic, especially in the clinical setting
- Relevant

faculty development. Teaching can also occur 'peer to peer', such as between medical trainees. As healthcare is undertaken by multidisciplinary teams, learning should also be with and from other members of the interprofessional team.

Challenges to effective clinical teaching

One of the major reasons stated for lack of teaching in the clinical setting is *time pressure*. Several tools can be used by preceptors to opportunistically teach in small bite-sized chunks, within literally *minutes*. Examples include the One-Minute Preceptor and SNAPPS (Figure 3.7).

> Patients in modern healthcare frequently transition from one clinician to another (e.g. shift work), between wards, and from one specialty to another. This is common practice in Acute and Internal Medicine. These transitions can interrupt the natural feedback loop on the iterative clinical reasoning process and observation of natural history of (un)common disorders, limiting the opportunity to learn from clinical practice. Teachers should encourage learners to keep track of and follow up on patients' outcomes as an important learning strategy to improve clinical diagnostic reasoning and patient care.

Assessment

'Assessment drives learning'. Multiple assessment modalities are required to have a better judgement of attainment of clinical competencies (see Figure 3.1). Types of assessment include formative and summative.

- Formative.
  - ○ Assessment *for* learning.
  - ○ Requires effective and detailed feedback.

- Summative.
  - ○ Assessment *of* learning at a given time.
  - ○ Usually 'high stakes' (e.g. contributes to progression criteria).

Workplace-based assessments

Direct observation of learners in the authentic clinical environment is critical. Workplace-based assessments (WPBAs) are an essential part of any assessment system, alongside traditional 'high-stakes' examinations. WPBAs are generally formative, and should be clinically relevant, real-life and feasible. Examples of WPBAs include the following.

- Mini-clinical evaluation exercise (Mini-CEX) – example of an observed clinical encounter. The assessor observes a trainee interacting with a patient around a focused clinical task.
- Case-based discussion (CbD) – structured interview of specific aspects of a case.
- Direct observation of procedural skills (DOPs) – evaluation of procedural skills of trainees within a workplace setting.
- EPAs (CiPs) – acts that require *Trust*; *Professional-life activities* (tasks) of doctors.

'Bedside' assessment by the clinical supervisor (and approved and trained designates) using various WPBA tools during each work placement, and review of a longitudinal comprehensive e-portfolio (i.e. programmatic assessment), including log book of activity in the workplace and simulation lab, and clerkship reports encompassing professionalism, commitment, participation in learning, teaching of others, colleague views and global assessment, will allow early identification of weaknesses and permit remediation throughout the rotation. Clinical supervisors also make judgements with members of the extended clinical team about how much help (co-activity) or supervision a medical trainee needs (i.e. *level of entrustment*).

S	N	A	P	P	S
Summarise briefly the history and findings	Narrow the differential to two or three relevant possibilities	Analyse the differential comparing and contrasting the possibilities	Probe the preceptor by asking questions about uncertainties, difficulties, or alternative approaches	Plan management for the patient's medical issues	Select a case-related issue for self-directed learning

Figure 3.7 SNAPPS: a six-step learner-centred approach to clinical education.

Other evidence-based educational strategies and assessments will be utilised during Internal Medicine and Acute Medicine training, such as the 'high-stakes' exam – Membership of the Royal College of Physicians (MRCP) diploma.

> Workplace-based assessments (observational tools frequently constructed to align with EPAs) can be used to assess *moment-in-time* clinical reasoning and other important elements of doctoring.

Other training roles and responsibilities

Acute Medicine consultants can act as clinical supervisors to doctors in earlier stages of training. Clinical supervisors are defined as 'a trainer who is selected and appropriately trained to be responsible for overseeing a specified trainee's clinical work and providing constructive feedback during a training placement'.

Acute Medicine doctors can also be involved in:

- *mentoring* – a dynamic, collaborative relationship focused on career and professional development. The traditional 'dyad' model pairing a senior mentor with a junior mentee is most effective. Highly structured with clear goals
- *coaching* – more task orientated, focused on teaching specific tasks or skills.

> Simple experience is not sufficient for the development (or maintenance) of expertise in the medical trainee. A long period of immersion in activities involving effortful practice of skill, often under the direction of a coach or mentor, is needed to develop and maintain expertise (i.e. *deliberate practice*). Maximising quality of clinical experiences requires learners to reflect on their performance to identify gaps in their knowledge and diagnostic skills and develop goals and strategies to fill the gaps.

4

Safe prescribing in Acute Medicine

Glenn Matfin

 KEY POINTS

- Rational prescribing describes a logical approach that includes making a (differential) diagnosis, estimating prognosis, establishing the goals of therapy, selecting the most appropriate treatment, and monitoring the effects of that treatment.
- The decision to prescribe or deprescribe a drug always involves a judgement of the balance between therapeutic risks of an adverse outcome versus the potential benefits.
- Medication safety is an important aspect of clinical risk management and includes both adverse drug reactions (ADRs) and medication errors.
- An ADR is 'any untoward medical occurrence associated with the normal use of the drug (dose and indication) for which there is a causal link between the drug and harm caused'.
- ADRs are common and cause excess morbidity and mortality. In the USA, ADRs are the fourth leading cause of death among hospitalised patients (prior to the COVID-19 pandemic). The percentage of hospital admissions due to ADRs in the UK has been estimated to be as high ~20% in older persons.
- While it is impossible to remember all potentially life-threatening 'drug–drug' interactions, a prescriber should strive to check prescriptions during medicine reconciliation and all new prescriptions should be considered for potential interactions.
- A medication error is any patient safety incident where there has been an error in the process of prescribing, preparing, dispensing, administering, monitoring or providing advice on medicines.
- More than 200 million medication errors occur every year in England.

Introduction

Prescribing is the most important tool used by physicians to cure illness, relieve symptoms and prevent future disease.

Prescribing is a complex intellectual task (i.e. therapeutic reasoning) that requires diagnostic skills, knowledge of common medicines, understanding of the principles of clinical pharmacology, communication skills, and the ability to make decisions based on judgements of potential benefit and risks, having considered the available evidence and specific factors

Acute Medicine: Lecture Notes, First Edition. Edited by Glenn Matfin.
© 2023 John Wiley & Sons Ltd. Published 2023 by John Wiley & Sons Ltd.

relating to the patient and condition(s) being treated. Unfortunately, the selection of a medicine and dosage regimen is sometimes suboptimal, leading to poor patient outcomes such as treatment failure and avoidable adverse reactions.

The UK Government published a review evaluating overprescribing in England (2021). It revealed how NHS spending on medicines increased sharply from £13bn in 2010–11 to £18.2bn in 2017–18. Over 1 billion prescription items were dispensed in primary care alone, with an estimated 10% being 'overprescribed' – that is, not needed or wanted by the patient, potentially more harmful than beneficial, or having more appropriate alternatives. The negative consequences for patients are clear: a fifth of hospital admissions among adults over 65 are the result of adverse effects of prescribed drugs.

Clinicians are responsible for both commencing and stopping medications. Deprescribing, 'the process of withdrawal of an inappropriate medication, supervised by a healthcare professional with the goal of managing polypharmacy (i.e. commonly defined as the use of five or more medications daily by an individual) and improving outcomes', is a relatively new concept in healthcare. The decision to prescribe or deprescribe a drug always involves a judgement of the balance between therapeutic risks of an adverse outcome versus the potential benefits. For excellent 'patient-centred care', a truly informed therapeutic decision between prescriber and patient (i.e. 'shared decision making') requires:

- consideration of both treatment risks and benefits
- many other treatment factors (e.g. costs, dose frequency, route of administration).

Rational prescribing

Rational prescribing describes a logical approach that includes making a (differential) diagnosis, estimating prognosis, establishing the goals of therapy, selecting the most appropriate treatment, and monitoring the effects of that treatment.

Rational prescribing in the acute care setting is more challenging due to the high turnover of predominantly elderly, high-acuity frail patients with altered physiology, polypharmacy, multimorbidity, cognitive impairment and communication difficulties. Acute Medicine patients may also lack continuity of care,

due to being moved around different wards because of hospital crowding. In addition, many patients are managed as medical outliers (i.e. medical patients within the surgical or non-medical bed base), where ward staff may not be as familiar with medical therapies. This can lead to issues with medicines reconciliation, monitoring treatment effects and discharge medications. All these various patient, drug and system factors can lead to adverse outcomes.

This situation has been compounded by the COVID-19 pandemic. For example, communication with patients has been limited due to concerns about viral transmissibility, and negatively impacted by personal protective equipment (PPE) and respiratory interventions (e.g. non-invasive positive pressure respiratory support). Medicines reconciliation has been difficult due to these communication challenges, as well as lack of access to patient carers, care homes, GPs and community pharmacists. The use of largely experimental therapies for the treatment of COVID-19 (often as part of a clinical trial) has often led to unexpected adverse effects, 'drug–drug' interactions and therapeutic failure. More recently, patients are rationing their use of vital medicines to save on prescription charges.

Medication safety

Medication safety can be related to the following factors.

- Adverse drug reaction (ADR): 'any untoward medical occurrence associated with the normal use of the drug (dose and indication) for which there is a causal link between the drug and harm caused'.
- Medication error: any patient safety incident where there has been an error in the process of prescribing, preparing, dispensing, administering, monitoring or providing advice on medicines.
- Poor prescribing is one of the greatest causes of iatrogenic harm. Harm occurs when prescribers make irrational, inappropriate and ineffective choices of medications, underprescribe, overprescribe, write faulty prescriptions, and fail to alter therapy when needed.

Medication safety is an important aspect of clinical risk management. Clinical risk management is concerned with improving the safety of healthcare by:

- identifying the circumstances and opportunities that put patients at risk of harm then acting to prevent or control those risks (e.g. using national or local guidelines on appropriate and safe prescribing).

Pharmacovigilance

> Medication (or drug) safety is known as pharmacovigilance: clinical science that includes objectives of surveillance, evaluation and signalling of undesirable effects of pharmaceutical products used for medical therapy.

Pharmacovigilance focuses heavily on ADRs. However, medication errors such as overdose, misuse and abuse of a drug as well as drug exposure during pregnancy and breastfeeding are also of interest because they may result in harm.

> Adverse drug event (ADE) is a term used by some authorities to combine all drug exposures that can result in *harm*: 'Harm caused by *appropriate* (i.e. ADR) or *inappropriate* use of a drug'.

Major signals of medication safety

Derived from the following sources.

- Clinical trials.
- 'Real-world' clinical practice – spontaneous reporting, e.g. Yellow Card scheme in the UK.
- Case reports, case series.
- 'Big data' from large databases (e.g. healthcare administrations).
- 'Record linkage' – clinical events linked with prescription.
- Previous experience of drug class – e.g. angiotensin-converting enzyme (ACE) inhibitors causing cough.

Pharmacovigilance definitions

- Side-effect.
  - Any unintended effect on a patient, whether beneficial, neutral or harmful, of a pharmaceutical product at doses used in humans, related to the pharmacological properties of the drug (e.g. bradycardia with beta-blockers; tremor with salbutamol; pink urine with rifampicin).
  - The term 'side-effect' is often used interchangeably with ADR, although the former usually

implies an effect that is less harmful, is predictable and may not require discontinuation of therapy (e.g. ankle oedema with vasodilators).

- ADR.
  - Response to a drug (or investigational product) that is noxious and unintended, occurring at doses normally used in humans (i.e. for prophylaxis, diagnosis or therapy of disease), e.g. oral/vaginal thrush with broad-spectrum antibiotics, throbbing headache with sublingual glyceryl trinitrate (recognised side-effect, but 'throbbing' is noxious).
  - An ADR will usually require the drug to be discontinued or the dose reduced, or 'drug–drug' or 'drug–environment' interaction(s) modified.
  - ADR definition (harm caused by appropriate use of drug at normal doses) excludes harm caused by *inappropriate use* of a drug such as therapeutic failures (drug didn't work), overdose, drug misuse, non-adherence and medication errors.
- Serious ADRs (SADR) cause *serious harm*. SADRs are those that:
  - are fatal
  - are life-threatening
  - cause hospitalisation (generally >24 hours)
  - result in persistent or major disability or incapacity
  - require intervention to prevent permanent damage
  - cause congenital defect.
- Drug toxicity.
  - Drug toxicity is any harmful or toxic effect caused by a drug in a patient.
  - Drug toxicity can present as an ADR.
  - There are many types of adverse drug effects, such as gastrointestinal effects, organ toxicity, carcinogenesis, teratogenesis and immunological reactions.
- Drug allergy.
  - Harmful immunological reaction directly or indirectly caused by a medicine, e.g. toxic epidermal necrolysis from carbamazepine, anaphylaxis caused by penicillin, various severe immune-related adverse events (irAEs) have been reported with immune checkpoint inhibitors.
  - Most feared form of drug allergy is anaphylaxis – swelling of the airways, wheeze, hypotension, tachycardia and urticaria within minutes of exposure. Non-serious drug rashes are much more common.
  - Non-immunological ADRs are often incorrectly labelled 'drug allergy'.
  - Unnecessarily labelling patients as 'allergic' to a drug can be harmful and deny them best

treatment. For example, 1 in 10 Americans are labelled 'penicillin allergic', yet only 1 in 100 is reckoned to be at risk of acute reaction. In order to document penicillin allergy more accurately, check and document the nature of the reaction: mild = rash; moderate to severe = angioedema, swollen tongue, anaphylaxis.

- A detailed history can help clinicians decide if readministration is safe, although specialist tests and referral may be necessary.

Adverse drug reactions

- ADRs are underreported in most countries. It is estimated only 1–10% are ever reported.
- ADRs are a common cause of increased morbidity and mortality.
  - USA: fourth leading cause of death among hospitalised patients (prior to the COVID-19 pandemic).
  - UK: ADRs are thought to occur in 10–20% of hospital inpatients. The percentage of hospital admissions due to ADRs in the UK could be as high as 20% in patients over 65 years of age.
- Thirty percent to 60% ADRs are preventable.

Risk factors for ADRs

Patient factors

- Older person, e.g. frailty and low physiological reserve.
- Gender, e.g. ACE inhibitor-induced cough more common in women.
- Polypharmacy, e.g. 'drug–drug' interactions.
- Hypersensitivity/allergy, e.g. beta-lactam antibiotics.
- Diseases altering:
  - pharmacokinetics (PK) – *what the body does to the drug*, e.g. hepatic dysfunction, acute kidney injury (AKI) and/or chronic kidney disease (CKD) can all alter PK
  - pharmacodynamic responses (PD) – *what the drug does to the body*, e.g. hypoglycaemia more common with hypoglycaemic agents such as sulfonylureas or insulin in patients with AKI and/or CKD (example of 'drug–disease' interaction). Hypoglycaemia occurs because the drug may accumulate in these states (i.e. sulfonylureas not eliminated) or the injected exogenous or secreted endogenous insulin is not cleared by the kidneys.

> **Box 4.1 Stevens–Johnson syndrome and toxic epidermal necrolysis related to medications**
>
> - Allopurinol therapy (gout treatment) – in patients with HLA-B*5801 allele.
> - Carbamazepine therapy (epilepsy treatment) – in patients with HLA*1502 allele.
>   - Both above alleles are common in Han Chinese, Thai and other Asians. At-risk population should be screened for the allele *before* treatment.
> - Abacivir therapy (protease inhibitor) – in patients with HLA-B*5701 allele. Patients with the HLA-B*5701 allele must not be treated, so testing before treatment is *mandatory* for *all* patients.

- Adherence problems, e.g. polypharmacy, cognitive impairment.
- Genetic predisposition, e.g. serious T-cell-mediated cutaneous ADRs (SCARs), including Stevens–Johnson syndrome and toxic epidermal necrolysis secondary to certain medications (Box 4.1).

Drug factors

- Steep dose–response curve, e.g. insulin, theophylline.
- Low therapeutic index, e.g. digoxin, cytotoxic drugs.

Prescriber factors

- Inadequate understanding of the principles of clinical pharmacology and therapeutics.
- Inadequate knowledge of the prescribed drug(s) and other agents taken, e.g. over-the-counter (OTC) or internet-derived drugs, and herbal therapies.
- Taking an ineffective drug history.
- Inadequate instructions and warnings provided to patients.
- Inadequate monitoring arrangements planned.

'Drug–environment'

- Photosensitivity, e.g. tetracycline.
- Food, e.g. decreased absorption of thyroxine and bisphosphonates when taken with food.

Drugs that are common causes of ADRs

Drugs that are commonly associated with ADRs are listed in Table 4.1.

Table 4.1 Drugs that are common causes of ADRs. Top four drug classes commonly causing serious ADRs in USA marked with *

Drug or drug class	Common ADRs
Angiotensin-converting (ACE) enzyme inhibitors Angiotensin receptor blockers	Acute kidney injury (AKI)/chronic kidney disease (CKD) Hyperkalaemia Cough with ACE inhibitors
Antibiotics*	Diarrhoea ('antibiotic-associated') Torsades de pointes due to QT prolongation (e.g. macrolides)
Anticoagulants*	Bleeding
Antipsychotics	Falls Sedation Confusion
Aspirin	Gastrotoxicity (dyspepsia, gastrointestinal bleeding) Other bleeding (e.g. haemorrhagic stroke)
Benzodiazepines	Drowsiness Falls
Calcium channel blockers	Ankle oedema Constipation
Checkpoint inhibitors	Autoimmune dermatological, endocrine, respiratory, gastrointestinal and rheumatological adverse effects
Digoxin	Nausea and anorexia Bradycardia
Diuretics	Dehydration Electrolyte disturbance (hypokalaemia, hyponatraemia) Hypotension AKI
Insulin and insulin secretagogues*	Hypoglycaemia
Non-steroidal anti-inflammatory drugs	Gastrotoxicity (dyspepsia, gastrointestinal bleeding) AKI/CKD
Opioid analgesics*	Nausea and vomiting Confusion Constipation Respiratory depression
Statins	Myalgia Rhabdomyolysis

Classification of ADRs

Adverse drug reactions have traditionally been classified into two major groups: type A and type B.

Type A ('augmented') ADRs

- 85–90% of all ADRs.
- Predictable from the known PD effects of the drug (i.e. frequently called 'side-effects'), are dose dependent, common (detected early in drug development) and usually mild.

- For example, constipation caused by opioids; hypotension caused by antihypertensives.

Type B ('bizarre') ADRs

- Not predictable, not obviously dose dependent in the therapeutic range, and are rare (usually remain undiscovered until the drug is marketed) and often severe.
- Patients who experience type B reactions are generally 'hypersusceptible' because of:
  - unpredictable genetic/immunological factors (e.g. anaphylaxis caused by penicillin)

o other factors (e.g. fulminant acute liver failure with the discontinued antidiabetic drug troglitazone occurred in 1 in 60 000 patients. SADR due partly to molecular design of drug).

Other ADR types

- Type C ('chronic') ADRs – adverse effects that only occur with prolonged treatment, e.g. iatrogenic Cushing syndrome with chronic prednisolone treatment.
- Type D ('delayed') ADRs – adverse effects that occur remotely after treatment, e.g. second cancers many years after chemotherapy.
- Type E ('end of treatment') ADRs – adverse effects that occur after suddenly stopping drug, e.g. worsening angina after stopping beta-blocker, acute adrenal crisis after suddenly stopping long-term glucocorticoid therapy.

DoTS classification system for ADRs

(Table 4.2)

Table 4.2 DoTS classification system for ADRs

Category	Example
Dose	
Below therapeutic dose	Anaphylaxis with penicillin
In the therapeutic dose range	Nausea with morphine
At high doses	Hepatotoxicity with paracetamol (acetaminophen)
Timing	
With the first dose	Anaphylaxis with penicillin
Early stages of treatment	Hyponatraemia with diuretics
On stopping treatment	Benzodiazepine withdrawal syndrome
Significantly delayed	Osteoporosis with glucocorticoids
Susceptibility	See risk factors for ADRs (see earlier text section)

How do you know it is an ADR?

TREND analysis of suspected ADRs.

- **T**emporal relationship. What is the time interval between the start of drug therapy and the reaction?
- **R**echallenge. What happens when the patient is rechallenged with the drug?
- **E**xclusion. Have other drugs been excluded?
- **N**ovelty. Has the reaction been reported before?
- **D**echallenge. Does the reaction improve when the drug is withdrawn or the dose reduced?

Management options for ADRs

Prevention is always preferred. Engaging in reducing a patient's medication burden (i.e. deprescribing) is a common aspect of modern clinical practice. Medications that were once deemed appropriate may become less effective or even harmful, potentially causing ADRs. Also consider the following factors.

- Careful medication and OTC history.
- Key role of pharmacists – especially for elderly patients, special populations (e.g. transplant, people with HIV), but also inpatient setting.
- Electronic prescribing systems – give 'alerts' regarding:
  o patient factors such as renal function, weight
  o potential 'drug–drug' interactions, e.g. aspirin and anticoagulant co-prescription.
- Risk evaluation and mitigation strategies (REMS) – for example, bisphosphonates (osteoporosis, oncology, severe hypercalcaemia treatment) can cause:
  o osteonecrosis of the jaw – must get dental check and treatment (e.g. tooth extraction) prior to starting high-dose therapy (e.g. oncology patients)
  o severe oesophagitis – must sit upright for 30 minutes after taking oral formulation to reduce oesophagitis risk.
- Warnings – if a significant ADR is uncovered, drug regulators (e.g. UK Medicines and Healthcare products Regulatory Agency) can require that the relevant summary of product characteristics adds appropriate warnings (e.g. black triangle warning which alerts healthcare professionals to serious ADRs).
- Drug withdrawal – drug is withdrawn from the market due to safety concerns.
- Precision (stratified) medicine – patients stratified according to who might benefit from treatment and who are more predisposed to harm based on presence or absence of various biomarkers. A pharmacogenomic approach, where genetic variation informs choice of drug and dose, can facilitate greater precision in prescribing and an increasingly personalised approach to drug therapy (Figure 4.1). It has the potential to improve patient outcomes by increasing the efficacy of

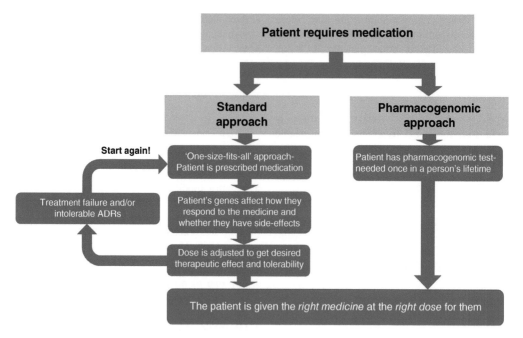

Figure 4.1 Pharmacogenomic approach to prescribing.

medicines and decreasing ADRs. This is associated with reducing the number of preventable health conditions and deaths, as well as costs to the NHS.

- Many reactions with minor symptoms and no sinister consequence require no specific treatment and are accepted as the price to be paid for the benefits of therapy.
- Discontinue the offending agent if:
  o it can be safely stopped
  o event is life-threatening or intolerable
  o there is a reasonable alternative therapy
  o continuing the medication will further exacerbate the patient's condition.
- Continue the medication (modified as needed) if:
  o it is medically necessary
  o there is no reasonable alternative
  o the problem is mild and will resolve with time.
- Consider desensitisation if drug allergy (e.g. insulin or penicillin allergy).
- Consider rechallenge if the drug is important (not if serious ADR). Examples of ADRs where it is reasonable to consider rechallenge include the following.
  o Flushing with acetylcysteine infusion – slow infusion rate.
  o Oral candida infection with glucocorticoid inhalers – rinse mouth after dosing and consider use of a spacer.

- Administer appropriate emergency treatment and supportive care (e.g. C-ABCDE) for serious ADRs.
- Consider antidote – for example, vitamin K for warfarin-related international normalised ratio (INR) in excess of treatment targets or bleeding.
- Specific treatments – e.g. chemotherapy-related neutropenia, consider granulocyte-colony stimulating factors (GCSF).

Medication errors

Medication errors are the third most prevalent source of reported patient safety incidents (i.e. 'any unintended or unexpected incident, which could have or did lead to harm for one or more patients receiving NHS care') in England. Medication errors are any patient safety incident where there has been an error in the process of prescribing, preparing, dispensing, administering, monitoring or providing advice on medicines. These patient safety incidents can be divided into two categories.

- Errors of *commission* – this includes, for example, wrong medicine or wrong dose.
- Errors of *omission* – this group includes, for example, omitted dose or a failure to monitor, such as INR for anticoagulant therapy treated with warfarin.

The harms caused by medication errors have been recognised as a global issue, amid increasingly complex healthcare needs and the introduction of many new medicines. More than 200 million medication errors are made every year in England, the avoidable consequences of which cost the NHS upwards of £100 million and more than 1700 lives every year. Most of the resulting deaths (80%) are caused by gastrointestinal bleeds from non-steroidal anti-inflammatories (NSAIDs), aspirin or warfarin. Around 1 in 5 medication errors are made in hospitals.

Errors are made at every stage of the process, with over half made at the point of administration (with a third of these due to errors of omission) and around 1 in 5 made during prescribing. Dispensing accounts for ~15% of the total.

The most common reasons for errors include failure to communicate drug orders, illegible handwriting, wrong drug selection chosen from a drop-down menu, confusion over similarly named drugs, confusion over similar packaging between products, or errors involving dosing units or weight. Nearly 75% of medication errors have been attributed to distraction. A prevalent cause of medication errors is distortions. The majority of distortions may originate from poor writing, misunderstood symbols, use of abbreviations or improper translation.

Acute Medicine best practice approach to safe prescribing

- The first principle is that of putting patients first (i.e. patient-centred care).
- Patients should be involved in deciding their treatment regimen when appropriate (i.e. shared decision making).
- 'Prescribing' is used to describe many related activities, including:
  - supplying prescription-only medicines
  - prescribing medicines, devices, dressings and activities, such as exercise
  - advising patients on the purchase of OTC medicines and other remedies.
- Adhere to the General Medical Council's Good Medical Practice in prescribing and managing medicines and devices (2021).
  - The clinician is responsible for the prescriptions that they sign.
  - You must only prescribe medicine when you have adequate knowledge of your patient's health.
  - You must be satisfied that the medicine serves your patient's need.
- The ward pharmacist is a key member of the acute medical care multidisciplinary team. Pharmacists have an important role in:
  - medicines reconciliation
  - checking prescriptions
  - medication review – 'a structured, critical examination of a patient's medicines with the objective of reaching an agreement with the patient about treatment, optimising the impact of medicines, minimising the number of medication-related problems and reducing waste'
  - checking technique of drug delivery (e.g. inhalers)
  - making sure that drug supplies (or acceptable substitutes) are available on the ward in a timely fashion
  - facilitating discharge medications
  - patient education.
- Always use national or local guidelines on appropriate and safe prescribing.
- Check and update drug allergy status, confirm with the patient or carers before prescribing, dispensing or administering *any* drug. If penicillin allergy is reported, consult microbiology as needed.
- Approach every prescription with caution. Give your undivided attention (i.e. minimise cognitive overloading such as multitasking or other distractions).
  - Always check the patient's age and body weight to ensure that the dose administered is correct.
  - Always check current renal and liver function.
  - Review list of medications and OTC agents for possible interactions, especially if on cytochrome P450 inducers and inhibitors.
  - Make sure the drug is given by the correct route.
  - Make sure of the correct dose and units.
- If unsure about the drug or the dose, speak to the pharmacist or senior colleague.
- If emergency drugs need administering – such as antibiotics within one hour if suspected sepsis – it is not enough to write it up. Check availability of the drug on the ward, and check that nurses understand the urgency of giving the drug to the patient.
- Remain alert and seek help for high-risk medications. Double-check the dosing and frequency of all *high-alert* medications.
  - Antibiotics.
  - Anticoagulants (if on warfarin, monitor INR and adjust dose).
  - NSAIDs.
  - Antiplatelet agents.

Box 4.2 Medication errors with insulin

- About 10% of prescriptions in UK hospitals have errors. In comparison, insulin prescribing errors in this setting occur in ~30–50%.
- This has important negative health consequences, because insulin is a potent drug with a narrow therapeutic window.
- Examples of insulin errors.
  - Insulin not written up.
  - Name of insulin incorrect.
  - Type of insulin incorrect (e.g. rapid- or long-acting insulin).
  - Insulin given/prescribed at wrong time.
  - Number (dose) unclear.
  - Units abbreviated to 'u' or written unclearly.
  - Insulin not signed – either when prescribed or when (if) given.

Box 4.3 STOPP/START and updated Beers criteria to review medications in older people

- STOPP (Screening Tool of Older Persons' Prescriptions)/START (Screening Tool to Alert to Right Treatment) are criteria used as a tool for clinicians to review potentially inappropriate medications in older adults.
- The American Geriatrics Society (AGS) Updated Beers Criteria (2019).
  1 Potentially inappropriate medications in older adults.
  2 Potentially inappropriate medications to avoid in older adults with certain conditions.
  3 Medications to be used with considerable caution in older adults.
  4 Medication combinations that may lead to harmful interactions.
  5 List of medications that should be avoided or dosed differently for those with poor renal function.

  - Diuretics.
  - Opiates.
  - Hypoglycaemic agents – insulin (Box 4.2) and sulfonylureas.
- Remain alert and seek help for prescribing in *high-risk* patients.
  - Pregnant patients.
  - Transplant and immunosuppressed patients. Always consult the transplant service before making medication changes. Dedicated transplant pharmacists are invaluable.
  - Patients on biological therapies.
  - People with HIV.
  - Patients with alcohol and substance abuse.
  - People in clinical trials.
  - Palliative care and end-of-life patients.
  - Patients on insulin or glucocorticoids – don't omit unless on senior advice as there is a risk of acute decompensation (i.e. hyperglycemia and acute adrenal crisis respectively).
  - Ramadan – managing acute and chronic conditions during the Islamic month of Ramadan can be challenging, especially as many patients may prioritise fasting over health concerns. Make shared decisions about whether to fast, and safe options for administration of medicines. Seek specialist input for patients taking diabetes treatments (risk of hypoglycaemia), undergoing oncological treatment (risk of dehydration) and other specialist medications.
  - Older people – stopping potentially inappropriate medications has been shown to result in cognitive improvement, fewer falls and a positive change in a patient's global health, with no

evidence of increased mortality. Guides exist to support patients and clinicians; for example, the STOPP/ START guidelines or Beers criteria have made progress in aiding clinicians in deprescribing decision making (Box 4.3).

- The Department of Health has recommended the wider use of electronic prescribing (e-prescribing) to reduce the risk of medication errors. Electronic prescribing systems with clinical decision support can check automatically for allergies, dose errors and drug–drug and drug–disease interactions and provide immediate warning and guidance, allowing the prescriber to make appropriate changes before a prescription is finalised.
- If not using electronic prescribing – beware illegible writing.
  - Write down the precise dosage.
  - Avoid abbreviations.
- Monitor selected therapeutic drug levels at the appropriate time points and in relation to dosing.
- Witness tablet taking. Some patients presenting with very high blood pressure or hyperglycaemia despite being on several antihypertensive or antihyperglycaemic agents, respectively, may be due to poor treatment adherence. Witnessing tablet taking and monitoring response is a reasonable way to avoid unnecessary treatment escalation or overinvestigation.
- Some ADRs occur within minutes of administration, whereas others can present years after treatment. The dose of the drug, time since starting

treatment, and potential susceptibility (i.e. DoTS) of the patient can help determine if ADRs enter the differential diagnosis.

- Report suspected serious or unusual ADRs to the national medicines regulator; you don't have to be certain in order to report.

Antimicrobial stewardship (AMS)

> NICE AMS guideline definition – 'an organisational or healthcare system-wide approach to promoting and monitoring judicious use of antimicrobials to preserve their future effectiveness'.

Antibiotic therapy is often started empirically to provide initial control of a presumed infection of unknown cause. Local cumulative antibiograms can determine which empiric antibiotics are most appropriate for patients with common infections.

The four goals of AMS are as follows.

1 Improve patient outcomes with effective treatment or prevention of infection.

2 Improve patient safety (e.g. *Clostridioides difficile*).
3 Reduce resistance.
4 Reduce healthcare costs.

Adhere to the 'Start smart' approach.

- *Do not start* antibiotics in the absence of evidence of bacterial infection.
- Then *focus* with clinical review and decision at 48 hours – check microbiology cultures, make and document decision.

1 STOP antibiotic(s) if there is no evidence of infection.
2 IV/oral switch: temperature has been <38 °C for 48 hours or more; oral foods/fluids are tolerated; there is no unexplained tachycardia; there is no evidence of impaired absorption; it is not a condition such as endocarditis or meningitis, for example, in which extra high tissue antibiotic concentrations are essential; and a suitable oral formulation is available.
3 Change to narrow (or broader) spectrum antibiotic.
4 Continue and review after 24 hours.
5 Consider outpatient parenteral antibiotic therapy (OPAT).

5

The acutely unwell patient

Glenn Matfin

 KEY POINTS

- Acute medical emergencies are those illnesses that can cause organ failures and death within minutes to hours of their presentation.
- Medical emergencies may present with little warning; however, most in-hospital cardiac arrests and patients prior to intensive care unit admission are predictable and preventable.
- Despite the widespread use of early warning scores and rapid response teams (such as medical emergency teams), there remain problems with the early recognition and management of sick patients in hospital.
- Acutely ill patients require rapid but careful assessment. Resuscitation is about recognising and effectively intervening when patients have seriously abnormal vital signs.
- Effective, early management of acute medical emergencies requires prompt recognition, immediate correction of life-threatening physiological abnormalities, the methodical application of the Control of obvious problem – Airway, Breathing, Circulation, Disability, and Exposure (C-ABCDE) approach, and rapid diagnosis and treatment of the underlying condition.
- Always inform the senior resident doctor about any seriously ill patient.

Introduction

> Acute medical emergencies are those illnesses that can cause organ failures and death within minutes to hours of their presentation.

Acute medical emergencies may present with little warning; however, most in-hospital cardiac arrests and those patients prior to admission to critical care are predictable and preventable. Affected patients are usually distressed, frightened and often unco-operative. Episodes can occur in any hospital location, and therefore the ability of available staff to deal with them may vary considerably. Given these circumstances, it is unsurprising that patient management errors occur, resulting in failures of care and often poor outcomes.

Despite the widespread use of early warning scores and rapid response teams (such as medical emergency teams), deficiencies in the recognition of ill patients have been identified for many years and the care of the acutely ill hospitalised patient presents ongoing problems for healthcare services. Deficiencies are often related to poor management of simple aspects of acute care – those involving the patient's airway, breathing and circulation, oxygen therapy, fluid balance and monitoring.

Acutely ill patients require rapid but careful assessment. Working out how ill the patient is and what needs to happen to them next underpins the effective,

Acute Medicine: Lecture Notes, First Edition. Edited by Glenn Matfin.
© 2023 John Wiley & Sons Ltd. Published 2023 by John Wiley & Sons Ltd.

safe management of all adult medical emergencies. Resuscitation is about recognising and effectively intervening when patients have seriously abnormal vital signs. Effective, early management of acute medical emergencies requires prompt recognition, immediate correction of life-threatening physiological abnormalities, the methodical application of the Control of obvious problem – Airway, Breathing, Circulation, Disability, and Exposure (C-ABCDE) approach, and rapid diagnosis and treatment of the underlying condition.

Illness severity assessment informs four key decisions.

1 What level and speed of intervention are required?

2 Is senior help required immediately, and, if so, whom?

3 Where should the patient be looked after?

4 What co-morbidities are present?

Recognition of medical emergencies

Medical emergencies are usually recognised by clinical signs of severe cardiorespiratory or neurological insufficiency.

- Tachypnoea (respiratory rate >20/min) – often the first adverse sign seen in acute illness.
- Tachycardia (heart rate >100/min).
- Hypotension (systolic blood pressure <90 mmHg).
- Altered level of consciousness (e.g. confusion, restlessness) – most common cause of compromised airway in healthcare setting.

Serious physiological deterioration, most frequently tachypnoea, hypotension and an altered level of consciousness as detected by the Glasgow Coma Scale (GCS), is documented in 60–80% of patients 4–6 hours *prior* to cardiac arrest, death or intensive care unit (ICU) admission. The most common abnormalities before cardiac arrest are:

- hypoxaemia – partial pressure of arterial oxygen (PaO_2) <8 kPa (60 mmHg) defines respiratory failure
- increased respiratory rate
- hypotension leading to hypoperfusion with an accompanying metabolic acidosis and tissue hypoxia.

If these abnormalities are left untreated, a downward physiological spiral ensues. With time, these abnormalities may become resistant to treatment with fluids and drugs. Therefore, early action is vital.

Although the underlying diagnosis may initially be elusive, the clinical signs that accompany a medical emergency are readily identified (i.e. signs of sympathetic activation; signs of hypoperfusion; and signs of organ failure) and include tachycardia or bradycardia; hypotension; cold peripheries; oliguria; cyanosis; tachypnoea or bradypnoea; seizures; agitation; confusion; and coma (Box 5.1).

These clinical findings are usually detected by simple, bedside observations, such as pulse, blood pressure (BP), respiratory rate, peripheral oxygen saturations, temperature and conscious level.

Box 5.1 Medical emergency – possible clinical findings

- Skin: mottled; sweaty; cyanosis; warm and vasodilated or cold peripheries.
- Neurological: agitation; confusion; depressed level of consciousness; seizures; localising signs.
- Respiratory: stridor; grunting; drooling; use of accessory muscles; tracheal tug; intercostal indrawing; nasal flaring; respiratory rate >25 breaths/minute or <8 breaths/minute; audible wheeze or silent chest.
- Cardiovascular: capillary refill time >2 seconds; pulse >130 beats/minute or <50 beats/minute; low-volume pulse; absent peripheral pulses; systolic blood pressure <90 mmHg; mean arterial pressure (MAP) <70 mmHg; postural hypotension; urine output <0.5 ml/kg/h or anuria.

Early warning scores

Think: Do they need specialist/critical care input NOW?

If the answer is yes, get help immediately.

Early warning scores provide a physiological 'track and trigger' system to efficiently identify and respond to patients who present with or develop acute illness and to assess and manage using a C-ABCDE approach.

- In the UK, these bedside observations have been used to develop a National Early Warning Score (NEWS2). It is a decision support tool that

Table 5.1 UK National Early Warning Score (NEWS2)

Physiological parameter	3	2	1	0	1	2	3
Respiratory rate (per minute)	≤8		9–11	12–20		21–24	≥25
SpO$_2$ Scale 1 (%)	≤91	92–93	94–95	≥96			
SpO$_2$ Scale 2 (%)	≤83	84–85	86–87	88–92 (≥93 on air)	93–94 on oxygen	95–96 on oxygen	≥97 on oxygen
Air or oxygen?		Oxygen		Air			
Systolic BP (mmHg)	≤90	91–100	101–110	111–219			≥220
Pulse (per minute)	≤40		41–50	51–90	91–110	111–130	≥131
Consciousness				Alert			CVPU
Temperature (°C)	≤35.0		35.1–36.0	36.1–38.0	38.1–39.0	≥39.1	

CVPU = confused, responds to voice, responds to pain, unresponsive.
Use SpO$_2$ Scale 2 if target saturations are 88–92% for patients with known Type 2 respiratory failure.

complements clinical judgement and provides a method for prioritising clinical care. NEWS2 is derived by aggregating points assigned to increasing deviations from the normal range, in each observation (Table 5.1). This score is linked to a graded response strategy, such that acutely ill patients who score highly trigger immediate review by an appropriately trained, rapid-response team (usually the patient's own team or the critical care outreach team).

- There is evidence that the introduction of aggregate weighting scoring systems (e.g. NEWS2) improves survival and reduces unplanned ICU admissions and cardiac arrests.
- Over recent years, rapid-response systems have been adopted by hospitals worldwide as the default mechanism for the recognition and immediate management of deteriorating patients and medical emergencies.

Clinical risk and response

Each NEWS2 observation has a score. The total score determines the potential clinical risk and what should happen next. Higher scores also mandate closer monitoring.

- Total score 0–4: low risk, ward-based response.
- Score 3 in any single parameter: low–medium risk, urgent ward-based response.
- Total score 5–6: medium risk, urgent response by a team with competence in the assessment and

management of acutely ill patients and in recognising when the escalation to a critical care team is appropriate.

- Total score 7 or more: high risk, urgent response by a team which must include staff with critical care skills, including airway management.

Deficiencies in early warning scores

- Although intuitively sensible, deficiencies in rapid-response systems include the fact that observations may not be reliably taken and scores miscalculated. Moreover, the sensitivity and specificity of the NEWS2 as a test for acute illness will be affected by patient-specific factors such as age, drug therapy and co-morbidity. For example, a severe gastrointestinal (GI) bleed may not cause a high NEWS2 score in a previously hypertensive patient treated with beta-blockers because BP and pulse rate may remain in the 'normal range' despite significant hypovolaemia. Recognition of the emergency nature of these sorts of presentations remains dependent on a high degree of clinical suspicion informed by clinical experience.
- COVID-19 patients – NEWS2 is commonly lower than severity of illness would imply. Tachypnoea is much less prominent than in other critical illness – the respiratory rate is less than you would expect for degree of respiratory failure and may be falsely reassuring.

- In addition, certain clinical *red flag* scenarios (i.e. collections of symptoms and signs suggestive of clinical risk to the patient) are not necessarily associated with altered physiology. Failure to recognise the significance of these scenarios can have serious adverse clinical consequences for the patient. Here are some examples.

  - Cardiac chest pain at rest lasting longer than 20 minutes.
  - Headache of dramatically sudden onset.
  - Cauda equina syndrome.

Immediate assessment of the deteriorating patient

> If you are called to a sick patient, GO AND SEE THEM. Ensure proper use of personal protective equipment (PPE), depending on context. Five seconds ('five second rule') critically looking at the patient will tell you more than 10 minutes on the phone.

Care must be escalated for patients with persistent abnormalities (or their ceilings of care defined). They must not be allowed to progress to cardiopulmonary arrest or have delayed ICU admissions – 'failure to rescue'. Conversely, when a patient's NEWS2 falls, it may be appropriate to reduce the frequency of clinical monitoring.

Once alerted to a medical emergency, the challenge for the responsible clinician is to make the diagnosis while providing supportive care, so that effective treatment can be administered. These activities may best be co-ordinated using a C-ABCDE approach.

- *C – Control of obvious problem*: for example, if the patient has ventricular tachycardia on the monitor or significant blood loss is apparent, immediate action is required.
- *A and B – Airway and Breathing*: by introducing yourself and saying hello, you can rapidly assess the airway, breathing difficulties and conscious level. If the patient is talking, A is clear and B isn't dire. A rapid targeted history should be obtained while the initial assessment is undertaken. Breathing should be assessed with a targeted respiratory examination. Oxygen saturations and arterial blood gas (ABG) should be checked early.

- *C – Circulation*: a targeted cardiovascular examination should include heart rate and rhythm, BP, jugular venous pressure, evidence of bleeding, signs of shock and abnormal heart sounds. The carotid pulse should be palpated in the collapsed or unconscious patient, but peripheral pulses should also be checked in conscious patients.
- *D – Disability*: conscious level should be assessed using the GCS and/or the Alert, Confusion, responsive to Voice, Pain or Unresponsive (ACVPU) tool. Check pupil size and reactivity. A brief neurological examination looking for focal signs should be performed. Capillary blood glucose should always be measured to exclude hypoglycaemia or severe hyperglycaemia.
- *E – Exposure (Examination), Evidence and Explanation.*
  - 'Exposure' indicates the need for targeted clinical examination of the remaining body systems, particularly the abdomen and lower limbs.
  - 'Evidence' may be gathered via a collateral history from other healthcare professionals or family members, recent investigations, prescriptions or monitoring charts.
  - 'Explanation', reassurance and analgesia are integral parts of acute care. Always keep the patient, family and relevant others informed about progress.
- *Do not move on* without treating an abnormality. For example, there is no point in doing an ABG on a patient with an airway obstruction.
- Make or confirm escalation and ceiling (level) of care decisions now (ICU and cardiopulmonary resuscitation), not later.
- Independent of their presenting complaint, many seriously ill patients become systemically unwell as a complication of infection. Sepsis should therefore be considered in any patient with an abnormal NEWS2 score, and it is essential that clinicians are familiar with the criteria for its diagnosis. Early antimicrobial therapy can improve survival.
- You should call a senior colleague now if you have not done so already.

Application of this approach at the bedside requires that the senior clinician organises available staff into an effective team. This leadership role is crucial to achieving good outcomes. Crisis resource management (CRM) has been defined as: 'the ability to translate the knowledge of what needs to be done into effective treatment activity in the complex and real world of medical treatment'. It is important that clinicians managing medical emergencies are familiar with CRM principles and adhere to them whenever possible.

Situational awareness is a concept that summarises some of the important factors in assessing patient acuity and responding appropriately in a timely fashion. Simply, it is being alert and maintaining a knowledge of what is happening around you. Three key concepts describe situational awareness: perception of the situation, understanding the meaning of the perception, and rapidly predicting the outcome of the situation. A multifaceted educational approach (including simulation) may improve clinician situational awareness in Acute Medicine.

The C-ABCDE approach

It is axiomatic that outcomes from medical emergencies are improved by early diagnosis and treatment. For example, prompt reperfusion can reduce infarct size and prolong life in myocardial infarction and stroke, while early, effective antibiotics improve survival in septic shock. However, before a diagnosis is reached, these patients may die from severe physiological disturbances, such as hypoxaemia and shock.

- The C-ABCDE approach can be seen as a mechanism to preserve life, while a diagnosis is sought so that definitive treatment can be administered.

- The process starts at the bedside with a preliminary assessment of the patient's general condition; this swift assessment focuses on the presence of clinical signs associated with life-threatening cardiorespiratory and/or neurological insufficiency (see Box 5.1).
- Much of this preliminary assessment can be completed by observation of the patient, inspection of the clinical observation charts and brief discussion with the bedside nurse.
- At the conclusion of this assessment, it may be obvious that the patient is moribund or 'peri-arrest' and that the 'cardiac arrest' or 'rapid-response team' (or similar such as medical emergency team) should be called.
- Real-time continuous monitoring is invaluable in the acutely ill.
- Effective team communication is vital for safe clinical care. The situation, background, assessment, recommendation and readback (SBARR) system of communication has been recommended by the UK's Patient Safety First campaign for referring acutely ill patients (Table 5.2). It is a structured way to communicate with another healthcare professional about a patient and increases the amount of relevant information being communicated in a shorter time.
- Regardless of the hospital communication system in place, once an emergency is recognised, assistance should be requested immediately. It is rarely

---

Table 5.2 Situation, background, assessment, recommendation and readback (SBARR) communication tool

Situation: Identify yourself (name, role, location); person you are speaking to and patient. State reason for call and urgency:

> *Example: My name is Dr Smart, I am the House Officer (Resident) on Ward 6. Are you the on-call critical care clinician? I am with Mrs Smith, a 65-year-old lady, who is in extremis with oxygen saturations of 78%.*

Background: Briefly relate history – date of admission, diagnosis and current management:

> *Example: Mrs Smith is a previously well lady who was admitted one week ago, following a stroke, for which she is undergoing rehabilitation.*

Assessment: State your working diagnosis:

> *Example: I think Mrs Smith has respiratory failure secondary to a severe hospital-acquired pneumonia.*

Recommendation: State the request:

> *Example: I think Mrs Smith is likely to need endotracheal intubation and mechanical ventilation. Please attend the ward immediately.*

Readback: The listener should summarise what they think you have said and what they are going to do now.

the case that these situations can be effectively managed by a single practitioner.

- At this juncture, the team (or individual clinician awaiting the arrival of assistance) should establish basic monitoring (e.g. electrocardiogram, pulse oximetry, BP), and calmly and methodically work through the C-ABCDE approach, correcting life-threatening physiological disturbances as they are discovered. Other measures should be performed as clinically indicated.

Selecting the appropriate location for ongoing management

Following initial or ongoing assessments and the delivery of any immediate treatment, the newly admitted or established patient's subsequent inpatient care should be on a ward that has facilities appropriate to their clinical condition (i.e. 'right patient – right bed').

Airway assessment and management

> Causes of airway obstruction:
> - Airway oedema (e.g. angioedema, anaphylaxis)
> - Blood
> - Decreased conscious level and loss of protective reflexes
> - Foreign body
> - Mass – malignancy (e.g. anaplastic thyroid cancer)
> - Secretions
> - Vomit

Treating acute upper airway obstruction (UAO) in the clinical setting is complicated and requires managing a sometimes chaotic environment, understanding the potentially multiple causes of disease (e.g. infectious, inflammatory, traumatic, mechanical and iatrogenic), and having the technical ability to quickly secure a challenging airway.

Upper airway obstruction must be diagnosed and treated quickly; complete obstruction will lead to cardiac arrest within minutes, while partial obstruction can impair ventilation and cause hypoxaemia. UAO may be recognised by impaired or absent speech; stridor; grunting; drooling; severe respiratory distress; paradoxical chest wall movement ('see-saw'

movements); prominent neck veins; facial swelling; and absent breath sounds. In general terms, the aim of management is to provide a secure, patent airway but specific therapy will be determined by the underlying cause.

- When the diagnosis is obvious, interventions to clear and support the airway can proceed immediately. For example, oral-pharyngeal inspection and removal of an easily accessible foreign body or application of simple, airway-opening-manoeuvres, such as a chin-lift or jaw-thrust, for coma.
- When the diagnosis is unclear, manipulation of the airway and insertion of airway adjuncts should be avoided as these interventions may precipitate complete UAO, for example, in the setting of epiglottitis.
- Generally, if conscious, patients with UAO should be allowed to assume the position in which they find it most comfortable to breathe. Forcing these patients into the recovery or supine position can precipitate cardiac arrest.
- All patients with UAO should be assessed by an anaesthetist as endotracheal intubation is frequently required to definitively secure the airway.
- Occasionally, the airway can only be secured by a surgical technique such as cricothyroidotomy or tracheostomy.
- Computed tomography (CT) of the neck and chest and/or flexible bronchoscopy may be required for diagnosis of the underlying cause of the UAO, but for safety, the airway should be secured prior to these investigations being undertaken.

Breathing assessment and management

Once the airway is deemed to be safe or secured, then breathing should be assessed for signs of respiratory insufficiency (see Box 5.1). As you assess breathing, targeted examination of the chest is appropriate. Auscultation is important both diagnostically and as a means to assess response to treatment; bronchial breath sounds may help confirm the diagnosis of pneumonia, while the detection of breath sounds following drainage of a pneumothorax suggests that the lung has reinflated. The work of breathing and pattern may also be informative.

Peripheral oxygen saturations should be routinely measured in all patients with respiratory distress and hypoxaemia rapidly corrected. The concentration of oxygen the patient breathes in is determined by the type of mask as well as the flow from the wall and the breathing pattern. By using a fixed performance system (Venturi), you can gauge the percentage much more accurately. A wide variety of oxygen delivery devices are available.

- In the setting of acute illness, the most appropriate device to use is a non-rebreathing facemask with reservoir and one-way valve. When connected to wall oxygen at a flow rate of 15 l/min, this device may provide an inspired oxygen concentration (FiO_2) of up to 90%.
- High-flow nasal oxygen therapy is increasingly being used postoperatively, and in ward-based and critical care areas. For example, it has been widely used in hospitalised COVID-19 patients, although it can be associated with aerosol generation with a potential risk for nosocomial COVID-19 infection. A number of commercial devices are available and provide high gas flow rates (up to 60 l/min) of blended gas up to 100% oxygen. Gases are warmed and humidified to increase patient comfort and compliance, and the high flow rates generate a small degree of positive end-expiratory pressure (PEEP).
- ABG should always be checked early to assess oxygenation, ventilation (partial pressure of arterial carbon dioxide, $PaCO_2$) and metabolic state (bicarbonate and base deficit). Always record the FiO_2 (oxygen concentration).
- Oxygen therapy should be adjusted in the light of ABGs: oxygen requirements may increase or decrease as time passes.

Expert consensus guidance suggests that in the setting of critical illness, oxygen saturation targets should generally be 94–98%. In some patients with chronic obstructive pulmonary disease (COPD) and carbon dioxide retention, supplemental oxygen therapy is associated with worsening hypercapnia (i.e. $PaCO_2$ >6.5 kPa [50 mmHg]) and type 2 respiratory failure. In patients with chronic respiratory failure, start with a 28% Venturi mask and titrate oxygen therapy to ABG. In these patients, inspired oxygen should be titrated to achieve saturations of 88–92%, and non-invasive ventilation (NIV) considered.

Mechanical ventilation should be considered for those patients with reversible disease and persistent failure of oxygenation and/or ventilation (i.e. carbon dioxide clearance). NIV is particularly indicated in patients with COPD and respiratory acidosis (pH 7.25–7.35), and hypercapnic respiratory failure secondary to chest wall deformity or neuromuscular disease. It is also useful in congestive heart failure. It is important to recognise when a patient is failing on NIV and requires intubation and invasive mechanical ventilation, as delayed intubation in this setting is associated with worse outcomes. Generally, invasive ventilation (i.e. tracheal intubation) is indicated in those patients with respiratory failure and impaired consciousness or copious pulmonary secretions.

Circulatory assessment and management

Once appropriate steps have been taken to address any breathing difficulties, attention should be directed to the assessment and management of circulatory insufficiency (see Box 5.1).

- As you assess circulation, targeted examination of the heart is appropriate.
- Intravenous (IV) access is often difficult in sick patients.
- The gauge of cannula needed is dictated by the required use.
  - Large-bore cannulae are required for volume resuscitation. Ideally, insert two large-bore (at least 16 gauge grey) cannulae, one in each arm, in the severely hypovolaemic patient.
  - An 18 gauge green cannula is usually adequate for drug administration.
- Consider intraosseous access.
- The femoral vein offers an excellent route for large-bore access.
- Central venous catheters are used for:
  - central venous pressure measurements
  - delivering irritant or vasoactive drugs (e.g. inotropes and vasopressors)
  - patients with difficult peripheral venous access.
- If there is major blood loss, speak to the laboratory and blood transfusion service; you may need coagulation factors as well as blood. Consider activating the Massive Haemorrhage protocol. Call senior help.
- Use pressure infusors and blood warmers for rapid, high-volume fluid resuscitation.
- Machine-derived cuff BP is inaccurate at extremes of BP and in tachycardias (especially atrial fibrillation). Manual sphygmomanometer BP is more accurate in hypotension.
- In severe hypotension which is not readily corrected with fluid, early consideration should be given to arterial line insertion and vasoactive drug therapy: GET HELP.

Acute or chronic fluid loss is usually followed by peripheral vasoconstriction and a compensatory tachycardia in order to preserve perfusion of vital organs. There is a wide spectrum in the ability of patients to compensate for fluid loss; unsurprisingly, young, fit patients can compensate for greater fluid losses than older patients, particularly those with significant cardiovascular co-morbidity. Typically, after 30–40% of circulating volume has been lost, decompensation occurs, manifested by marked hypotension and multiorgan dysfunction, characteristic of shock.

Treatment of shock requires the restoration of an effective circulating blood volume to reverse decompensation and restore organ perfusion. This process depends on diagnosis of the underlying condition, so that specific therapies can be administered. A useful *aide-mémoire* for the differential diagnosis of shock is to classify this condition into four groups according to the main mechanism of decompensation.

1 Hypovolaemia.
2 Cardiogenic.
3 Obstructive (e.g. pulmonary embolism, cardiac tamponade).
4 Distributive (e.g. sepsis, anaphylaxis).

In the setting of infection, patients with septic shock can be clinically identified by a vasopressor requirement to maintain a MAP of 65 mmHg or greater and serum lactate level greater than 2 mmol/l in the absence of hypovolaemia.

As always, accurate history is the most important determinant of the diagnosis; physical examination, aside from confirming the presence of a shock state, may be less rewarding, particularly in advanced disease.

Patients with shock require urgent resuscitation, but shock subtypes (noted above) necessitate specific investigations and treatment. A useful mnemonic to describe the important components of treatment is the **VIP** rule.

- **V**entilate (oxygen administration).
- **I**nfuse (fluid resuscitation).
- **P**ump (administration of vasoactive agents).

Generally, patients with shock require IV fluid resuscitation; a caveat to this are those patients with pulmonary oedema as gas exchange may deteriorate in these individuals. If there is diagnostic uncertainty, a fluid challenge can be helpful in identifying those patients who are likely to be fluid responsive. The aim of a fluid challenge is to produce an increase in cardiac output by a small but rapid increase in intravascular volume and then to assess the response by a repeated bedside examination. The fluid challenge technique thus evaluates the balance between the benefit – increase in oxygen delivery to the tissues – and the risk – increased oedema formation. The fluid challenge can be delivered by administering 250–500 ml of IV fluid over 10 minutes; hypovolaemic patients will show an improvement in their BP and pulse rate without excessive increase in filling pressures (e.g. central venous pressure).

There has been considerable debate in the literature as to the optimal resuscitation fluid. Over the years, a variety of fluids, including crystalloids, colloids and human albumin solutions, have been used and a number of problems identified. Current evidence would seem to support the use of balanced electrolyte solutions, such as Ringer's lactate or Hartmann's solution, as appropriate first-line resuscitation fluids.

Regardless of the type of resuscitation fluid selected, frequent patient reassessment against relevant clinical endpoints such as peripheral perfusion, pulse, BP and urine output is essential so that therapy can be titrated, and inadvertent fluid and electrolyte overload can be averted (fluid overload is associated with worse outcomes).

Hyperlactataemia (>1.5 mmol/l) is also typically present in acute circulatory failure and can be monitored. Vasoactive drugs (inotropes/vasopressors) may be necessary if BP and cardiac output remain low; these patients need to be transferred to the ICU for further management.

Blood transfusions

> Blood transfusion is the transfer of blood or blood components (e.g. red cells, platelets, fresh frozen plasma and cryoprecipitate) from one person (the donor) into the bloodstream of another (the recipient).

Stored whole blood has a haematocrit of 40% but plasma, platelets and other components are removed, leaving concentrated red cells with a haematocrit of 60% (i.e. packed red cells). Using packed red cells decreases the risk of fluid overload.

The following are indications for blood transfusion.

- To restore intravascular volume in haemorrhage.
- To restore oxygen-carrying capacity.

Administering blood carries a risk and uses a valuable resource. Apart from haemorrhage, blood transfusion is generally not indicated with a haemoglobin (Hgb) above 70 g/l (although slightly higher thresholds may be preferred in certain conditions such as acute coronary syndrome). A restrictive transfusion strategy is recommended in the UK with a trigger for transfusion

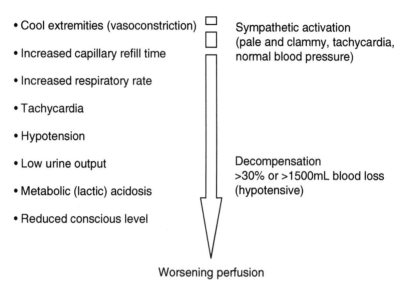

Figure 5.1 Responses to increasing hypovolaemia in bleeding.

when the Hgb drops below 70 g/l, and Hgb target of 70–90 g/l after transfusion.

Generally, one unit of packed red cells increases Hgb levels by 10 g/l (or 3% haematocrit).

- Consider one unit of packed red cells for anaemic adults who have no active bleeding.
- Consent is needed for transfusion.
- Both group and save and cross-match are needed for transfusion.
- Recheck Hgb levels and clinically assess following each single-unit transfusion.
- If the patient has suspected acute transfusion reaction, STOP transfusion immediately and check that the right patient is getting the right blood. Recheck ABCDE, give oxygen and get senior help immediately. Follow standard protocol.

The early recognition of major blood loss and the institution of effective actions are vital if hypovolaemic shock and its consequences are to be avoided (Figure 5.1). One such action is the rapid provision of blood and blood components. This complex process is termed Massive Haemorrhage protocol (generic example in Figure 5.2). The blood bank must be informed using the trigger phrase to activate the massive blood loss protocol: 'I want to trigger the massive blood loss protocol' or similar. In serious haemorrhage, there are different types of blood available.

- Negative blood is immediately available.
- Type-specific blood (group and rhesus state only).
- Fully cross-matched blood.

The risks of transfusion decrease with more specific matching. Severe transfusion reactions are rare but can occur with only small amounts of blood and death occurs in 1 in 100 000–400 000 transfusions. The leading causes are haemolysis, transfusion-related acute lung injury (TRALI) and transfusion-associated circulatory overload (TACO). Complications of blood transfusion are shown in Box 5.2.

Active bleeding

With active bleeding, it is always important to consider and manage the underlying cause or aggravating factors (usually medications) such as the following.

- Peptic ulcer or varices causing GI bleeding.
- Acquired bleeding disorder due to anticoagulants, including antiplatelet agents (Box 5.3).
- Thrombocytopenia – must be evaluated according to platelet count and clinical setting. First, review blood film and confirm platelet deficiency. Review history (especially medications, including recent heparin exposure) and evidence of bleeding (e.g. mucocutaneous and easy bruising). Mechanisms leading to thrombocytopenia are:
  o a failure of platelet production by the megakaryocytes (e.g. marrow infiltration, chemotherapy)
  o a shortened lifespan of the platelets (e.g. idiopathic thrombocytopenic purpura, heparin-induced thrombocytopenia)
  o increased pooling of platelets in an enlarged spleen.
- Coagulation factor deficiency or inhibitor.

Transfusion Management of Massive Haemorrhage in Adults

Insert local arrangements:
Activation Tel Number(s)

• Emergency O red cells
- location of supply:

* **Time to receive at this clinical area:**
• Group specific red cells

• XM red cells

Transfusion lab ☎

Consultant Haematologist ☎

Patient bleeding / collapses
Ongoing severe bleeding eg: 150 mls/min and Clinical shock
Administer Tranexamic Acid – esp in trauma and ideally within 1 hour
(1g bolus followed by 1g infusion over 8 hours)

Activate Massive Haemorrhage Pathway

Call for help
'Massive Haemorrhage, Location, Specialty'
Alert emergency response team (including
blood transfusion laboratory, portering/
transport staff)
Consultant involvement essential

RESUSCITATE
Airway
Breathing
Circulation

Take bloods and send to lab:
XM, FBC, PT, APTT, fibrinogen, U+E, Ca^{2+}
NPT: ABG, TEG/ROTEM if available
and
Order Massive Haemorrhage Pack 1

Red cells*	4 units
FFP	4 units

(*Emergency O blood, group specific blood,
XM blood depending on availability)

Continuous cardiac monitoring

Prevent Hypothermia
Use fluid warming device
Used forced air warming blanket

STOP THE BLEEDING

Give MHP 1

Reassess
Suspected continuing haemorrhage
requiring further transfusion
Take bloods and send to lab:
FBC, PT, APTT, fibrinogen, U+E, Ca^{2+}
NPT: ABG, TEG/ROTEM if available

Consider 10 mls Calcium
chloride 10% over 10 mins

2 packs cryoprecipitate if
fibrinogen < 1.5g/L or as guided
by TEG/ROTEM (< 2g/L for
obstetric haemorrhage)

Haemorrhage Control
Direct pressure/tourniquet if
appropriate
Stabilise fractures
Surgical intervention – consider
damage control surgery
Interventional radiology
Endoscopic techniques

Haemostatic Drugs

Vit K and Prothrombin complex concentrate for warfarinised
patients and
Other haemostatic agents and reversal of new anticoagulants:
discuss with Consultant
Haematologist

Cell salvage_if available and appropriate
Consider ratios of other
components:
1 unit of red cells = c.250 mls
salvaged blood

Aims for therapy
Aim for:

Hb	80-100g/L
Platelets	>75 × 10^9/L
PT ratio	< 1.5
APTT ratio	<1.5
Fibrinogen	>1.5g/L
Ca^{2+}	>1 mmol/L
Temp	>36°C
pH	>7.35(on ABG)

Monitor for hyperkalaemia

Order Massive Haemorrhage Pack 2

Red cells	4 units
FFP	4 units
Platelets	1 dose (ATD)

and subsequently
request Cryoprecipitate 2 packs
if fibrinogen <1.5g/l or according to TEG/
ROTEM (<2g/l for obstetric haemorrhage)

Give MHP 2

Once MHP 2 administered, repeat bloods:
FBC, PT, APTT, fibrinogen, U+E,
NPT: ABG, TEG/ROTEM if available
To inform further blood component
requesting

STAND DOWN
Inform lab
Return unused
components
Complete
documentation
Including audit
proforma

Thromboprophylaxis should be considered when patient stable

ABG–Arterial Blood Gas	APTT–Activated partial thromboplastin time	ATD-Adult Therapeutic Dose
FFP-Fresh Frozen plasma	MHP–Massive Haemorrhage Pack	NPT–Near Patient Testing
PT-Prothrombin Time	TEG/ROTEM-Thromboelastography	XM-Crossmatch

Figure 5.2 Generic Massive Haemorrhage protocol highlighting the complex, rapid and interprofessional response to major haemorrhage. Generally, do not aim for *normal BP*: SBP ~70 mmHg or MAP ~50 mmHg is probably adequate during active haemorrhage (if BP is too high, this can cause a blood clot to dislodge and exacerbate bleeding).

Box 5.2 Complications of blood transfusion

Immunological

- Haemolysis (haemolytic transfusion reaction – usually present with fever, flank pain, hypotension, haemoglobinaemia and haemoglobinuria. Delayed haemolytic reaction can occur 1–2 weeks after transfusion.
- Allergic reactions (e.g. urticaria, fever).
- Anaphylaxis.
- Transfusion-related acute lung injury (TRALI) – occurs within six hours.

Infective

- Rarely, red cells can become contaminated with bacteria during storage.
- UK blood is screened for hepatitis B, C and E, HIV, human T-cell lymphotropic virus (HTLV) and syphilis. Variant Creutzfeldt–Jakob disease (vCJD) is extremely rare. Other infections may be transmitted (e.g. cytomegalovirus).

Massive blood transfusion has particular problems.

- Thrombocytopenia.
- Coagulopathy.
- Hypothermia (packed red cells stored at 4 °C).
- Hypocalcaemia (citrate used to prevent clotting chelates calcium. Keep free (ionized) calcium >1 mmol/l).
- Hyperkalaemia.
- Metabolic acidosis followed by metabolic alkalosis (due to citrate which metabolises to bicarbonate).
- Transfusion-associated circulatory overload (TACO) – occurs within 12 hours; differentiate from TRALI by presence of pulmonary oedema, echocardiogram, NT-pro BNP (brain natriuretic peptide) and response to diuretic.
- Acute respiratory distress syndrome.
- Impaired oxygen delivery for 24 hours due to left shift of O_2 dissociation curve in stored blood.

Box 5.3 Bleeding related to anticoagulants

Consider antidote – for example, anticoagulant reversal principles – '**HASHTI**'.

Hold further doses.

Antidote:

- Vitamin K and other blood coagulation factors for warfarin-related bleeding.
- Idarucizumab (monoclonal antibody) is used to reverse the anticoagulant effects of dabigatran.
- Andexanetalfa (recombinant, inactive human factor Xa analogue) that non-specifically binds factor Xa inhibitors (e.g. apixaban, edoxaban and rivaroxaban).

Supportive treatment – volume resuscitation, haemodynamic support.

Haemostatic measures – e.g. antifibrinolytics (such as tranexamic acid).

Transfusion: red blood cells; fresh frozen plasma; prothrombin complex concentrates.

Investigate source of bleeding.

Check a full blood count (FBC), blood film and coagulation screen (including fibrinogen level). Check renal and liver function. Other investigations and management will be determined by the clinical context. Seek expert advice from a haematologist.

Thrombocytopenia may be associated with thrombosis, bleeding or both.

Typical platelet count associated with excess bleeding (highly variable):

- $<50 \times 10^9$/l: excessive bleeding seen after surgery or trauma
- $<20 \times 10^9$/l: spontaneous bleeding is common (e.g. melaena, haematemesis and haematuria).
- $<10 \times 10^9$/l: spontaneous bleeding is usual.

Aside from the actively bleeding patient, rare but life-threatening causes of thrombocytopenia must be identified early as they require urgent treatment. These include thrombotic thrombocytopenic purpura (mortality of over 90% if untreated), disseminated intravascular coagulation, suspicion of new acute promyelocytic leukaemia, and COVID-19 vaccine-induced prothrombotic immune thrombocytopenia.

Disability assessment and management

Neurological dysfunction is frequently implicated in medical emergencies and is either due to primary neurological disease or arises because of non-neurological illnesses. For example, coma (i.e. defined as a persisting state of deep unconsciousness) may arise due to intracerebral haemorrhage, severe hypoglycaemia, severe hyponatraemia or severe circulatory shock (Box 5.4). In patients <40 years of age, poisoning is the most common cause of a reduced conscious level not due to trauma, and in those >60, it is stroke.

Disability refers to emergency neurological assessment and management and starts with a basic assessment of level of consciousness. A reduction in conscious level should prompt an urgent assessment of the patient, a search for the likely cause and an evaluation of the risk of airway loss.

The ACVPU and GCS are two systems that standardise the assessment of consciousness. ACVPU is simple to remember and apply.

- A = the patient is **a**lert.
- C = **c**onfusion.
- V = the patient only responds to **v**oice.
- P = the patient only responds to **p**ain (recommended painful stimuli are supraorbital pressure or trapezius pinch).
- U = the patient is **u**nresponsive.

Box 5.4 Causes of coma; *aide-mémoire*
IF SOMNOLENT

Infection

Fits

Stroke

Overdose: alcohol, tricyclic antidepressants, benzodiazepines

Metabolic: uraemia, hepatic encephalopathy, hyponatraemia, hypernatraemia

Neoplasm: primary or secondary brain tumours

Oxygen deficiency: post cardiac arrest, near drowning

Low temperature; **L**ow blood pressure

Endocrine: hypoglycaemia, hyperglycaemia, hypopituitarism, hypothyroidism, hypercalcaemia, Addison disease

Narcotics

Trauma

The GCS provides a more detailed description of consciousness in terms of eye opening, verbal response and motor response. Document all three components accurately with best eye, best verbal and best motor responses. GCS can also be summarised using an aggregate numerical score ranging from 3, deeply unconscious, to 15, alert and co-operative. Serial GCS recordings can plot improvement or deterioration. An individual patient is best described using the physical response as well as the numerical score. On the GCS, a patient is arbitrarily defined as being in a coma if they can perform no better than eye opening to pain (E2), incomprehensible sounds (V2) and withdraw to a painful stimulus (M4).

It is not possible to define a total score below which a patient is unlikely to be able to protect the airway (from aspiration or obstruction), Generally, if the GCS is <8/15, or if the patient only responds to pain, or is unresponsive on the ACVPU scale, their ability to maintain a patent airway might be impaired. This can cause partial airway obstruction, reduced ventilation and an increased vulnerability to pulmonary aspiration. Adherence to the C-ABCDE approach should ensure that the airway is secured in these patients (see section on Airway above).

There is a wide differential diagnosis for coma and its evaluation requires a comprehensive history, general physical examination and neurological assessment including brain CT scan, electroencephalogram (EEG) and lumbar puncture (LP) if clinically indicated.

Exposure (Examination), Evidence and Explanation

The C-ABCDE approach concludes with Exposure, which is a prompt to complete a full physical examination. At this stage, life-threatening abnormalities have been addressed and the patient is better able to tolerate and co-operate with the demands of the examination. Evidence may also be gathered. Explanation, reassurance and analgesia are integral parts of acute care. Always keep the patient, family and relevant others informed about progress.

Definitive diagnosis and treatment

For medical emergencies, the traditional path to diagnosis (i.e. history, physical examination and investigation) is modified and integrated with the standard C-ABCDE approach. Diagnostic synthesis and the C-ABCDE approach should be viewed as complementary and simultaneous processes. Depending on the acuity of clinical presentation, targeted history and physical examination may be performed together (see Figure 2.5).

History

The patient should not be needlessly exhausted by detailed interrogation; much of the relevant history can be gleaned from medical records, nursing staff or relatives. However, it is important to enquire as to the presence and characteristics of any pain as not only is this a cardinal diagnostic symptom but it will need to be relieved.

It is likely that clinicians will use both System 1 non-analytical (pattern recognition) and System 2 analytical methods in formulating a diagnosis. This process has been termed iterative diagnosis and is prone to well-recognised cognitive errors (biases). Diagnostic errors usually arise because of overreliance on pattern recognition and intuition rather than analytical reasoning. Diagnostic uncertainty should be managed by mental reversion to a highly analytical approach, rigorously analysing available data against diagnostic hypotheses. In the setting of severe shock, the *aide-mémoire* (i.e. hypovolaemia, cardiogenic, obstructive or distributive) provides the full range of diagnostic possibilities against which available clinical data can be analysed.

Physical examination

Physical examination is completed at the conclusion of the C-ABCDE approach and is focused on those systems which are likely to be diagnostically helpful. For example, a comprehensive abdominal examination is essential in a patient with suspected peritonitis and shock but not necessarily immediately required in a patient with an acute myocardial infarction. Similarly, in a person with confusion or decreased conscious level, a thorough general medical examination, looking for clues such as needle tracks indicating drug abuse, rashes, fever and focal signs of infection, including neck stiffness or evidence of head injury, is indicated.

The physical examination should be modified to minimise patient exertion and the deleterious effects of repositioning. It is important to note that breathing difficulties and hypoxaemia are exacerbated by movement from the semi-recumbent to supine position, particularly in obese patients.

Investigations

These are guided by diagnostic impressions but basic blood tests such as ABG or venous blood gas, FBC, clotting screen (where indicated), urea, creatinine, electrolytes, lactate, blood glucose, C-reactive protein (CRP), COVID-19 testing, procalcitonin and blood cultures are usually helpful. Consider sending blood for group and save and cross-matching. Toxicology screen may also be warranted depending on context.

Markers of severe illness include the following.

- Metabolic (lactic) acidosis – one prospective study reported an 83% mortality in patients with a blood lactate of >5 mmol/l. Base deficit can be followed as a guide to response to treatment (i.e. the more negative, the more chance the patient will die, <-5 to -10 sick; and severely ill patients typically base deficit -10 and below).
- High or low white cell count (especially neutropenia or lymphopenia).
- Low platelet count (early sign of inflammation or infection).
- High creatinine – can also measure urea-to-creatinine ratio (usually ~1:10):
  o higher in dehydration or GI bleed.
  o lower in rhabdomyolysis.
- High CRP – trends may be more important.
- COVID-19 infection.
  o In addition to the above biomarkers, fibrinogen, D-dimer, ferritin, BNP, troponin and hyperglycaemia are all markers of severe COVID-19 infection.

Other bedside investigations such as electrocardiogram (ECG), plain radiology (especially chest X-ray), point-of-care ultrasound (POCUS) and echocardiography may be diagnostic.

It may be necessary to transfer patients for other tests such as CT scanning. In these circumstances, patients should be stabilised (as much as possible), and the transfers undertaken by suitably trained personnel. It is important to consider the risks and benefits of all investigations, as overinvestigation may delay definitive treatment.

Acid–base disorder

The human body is continually producing acid as a by-product of metabolism. But it must also maintain a narrow pH range, necessary for normal enzyme activity and other chemical reactions needed for homeostasis.

Normal blood pH is 7.35–7.45 and this is maintained by the following mechanisms.

- Intracellular and extracellular buffers – substance that resists pH change by absorbing or releasing hydrogen ions (H^+) when acid or base is added to it.
- Excretory functions of the:
  - kidneys – mainly excrete H^+ by reabsorbing bicarbonate (HCO_3) which in turn combines to form carbonic acid (H_2CO_3) and continually breaks down to form carbon dioxide (CO_2) and water
  - lungs – CO_2 produced by above reaction is expired.

Acid–base definitions are as follows.

- Acidosis – low pH (<7.35); H^+ >45 nmol/l.
- Alkalosis – high pH (>7.45); H^+ <35 nmol/l.
- Compensation – normal acid–base balance is a normal pH plus a normal $PaCO_2$ (4.6–6 kPa [35–45 mmHg]) and normal bicarbonate (22–26 mmol/l). Compensation has occurred when there is a normal pH but the bicarbonate and $PaCO_2$ are abnormal.
- Base excess – this measures how much extra acid or base is in the system because of a *metabolic* problem. It is calculated by measuring the amount of strong acid that must be added to a sample to produce a pH of 7.4. A minus figure means the sample is already acidotic so no acid had to be added. A plus figure means the sample is alkalotic and acid had to be added. The normal range is –2 to +2. A minus base excess (i.e. <-2 indicates metabolic acidosis) is often termed a 'base deficit'. A positive base excess (i.e. >+2) indicates a metabolic alkalosis.

Acid–base disturbances occur when there is a problem with the following.

- Lungs.
  - Decreased alveolar ventilation (CO_2 build-up) leads to *respiratory acidosis*.
  - Increased alveolar ventilation (CO_2 decreased) leads to *respiratory alkalosis*.
- Renal: a problem with renal function (a deficiency of HCO_3) leads to *metabolic acidosis*.
- An overwhelming acid (i.e. *metabolic acidosis*) or base load (i.e. *metabolic alkalosis*) which the body cannot handle.

When interpreting an ABG report, always consider the clinical context; an abnormal pH indicates the primary acid–base problem; the body never overcompensates; and mixed acid–base disturbances are common in clinical practice (Box 5.5).

Box 5.5 A general approach to follow when interpreting an ABG result is listed below

- Acidosis or alkalosis? Look at the pH first.
- Metabolic or respiratory? Look at the $PaCO_2$ (i.e. is it >6 kPa [45 mmHg] – hypercarbia, or <4.6 kPa [35 mmHg]?) and the standard bicarbonate (i.e. is it <22 mmol/l – metabolic acidosis, or >26 mmol/l – metabolic alkalosis?) or base excess to see whether this is a respiratory or a metabolic problem, or both.
- Is the disturbance compensated? For example, in a metabolic acidosis, you would expect the $PaCO_2$ to be low. If the $PaCO_2$ is normal, this indicates a 'hidden' respiratory acidosis as well.
- Check or calculate the anion gap if there is a metabolic acidosis.
  - Anion gap = serum sodium – (chloride + HCO_3).
  - A normal anion gap is <12 mmol/l.
  - High anion gap (>12 mmol/l) implies excess unmeasured plasma anions, which may be the cause of metabolic acidosis.

ABG analysis can be performed quickly and gives the following useful information.

- A measure of oxygenation (PaO_2).
- A measure of ventilation ($PaCO_2$).
- A measure of perfusion (standard HCO_3 or base excess).

In other words, a measure of A, B, and C – which is why it is an extremely useful test in the management of a critically ill patient.

Treatment

Generally, medical emergencies will be managed in an emergency department, acute medical unit (AMU) or equivalent, specialist and general medical wards, ambulatory acute medical services, as well as more advanced step-up facilities such as enhanced care beds, high-dependency unit (HDU) or ICU.

Many therapies, such as blood and blood products, drugs (e.g. antimicrobials, antiplatelet agents, analgesics, diuretics), and, of course, oxygen and IV fluid should be given at the bedside prior to transfer to HDU/ICU if required. International guidelines recommend the administration of broad-spectrum antibiotics within one hour of recognising sepsis or septic shock. Definitive management of this condition may require surgical, source control (e.g. drainage of an abscess or resection of ischaemic bowel).

Intensive care unit admission is indicated for patients who require organ support, most commonly mechanical ventilation, and close nursing observation. The decision to admit a patient to the ICU is informed primarily by clinical factors, such as the potential reversibility of the illness, and the wishes of the patient or their surrogates.

Medical emergencies should not be confused with the natural process of dying. The distinction is not always straightforward, but where there is clear evidence of terminal illness, such as advanced cancer, the treatment imperatives are comfort and dignity, not aggressive resuscitation.

For elderly frail people, take a holistic approach and use the Clinical Frailty Scale (CFS) when appropriate to assess baseline health and to assist with critical care decision making, given its ease of use and rapid assessment. The CFS uses a nine-item scale ranging from more fit and managing well (1–3), those living with mild/moderate frailty (4–6), to those living with more advanced frailty (7–8), and terminally ill patients (9). Use of this scale is based on patient mobility, function and cognition from two weeks prior to presentation. Preventing unnecessary harm to the patient and unnecessary use of resources are important. Symptomatic care may be more appropriate than escalation of support.

Assessment and reassessment

Assess response to treatment by continuous clinical observation, repeated assessment of A, B, C and D (conscious level) as above with uninterrupted monitoring of ECG and oxygen saturation. POCUS may also be useful for diagnosis and monitoring response to treatment. Reassess regularly to see the effects of intervention, or to spot deterioration.

If the patient is not improving, consider the following.

- Is the diagnosis correct?
- Is the diagnosis complete?
- Is there more than one diagnosis?
- Are they so ill that help is needed now?
- Is there an unrecognised problem or diagnosis?

6

Resuscitation

James Piper and Glenn Matfin

 KEY POINTS

- Cardiorespiratory arrest is rapidly fatal without resuscitation.
- Cardiopulmonary resuscitation (CPR) is an emergency procedure performed during a cardiac arrest to re-establish circulation and breathing. CPR is performed to keep a patient alive until a reversible cause can be treated, and advanced emergency care provided.
- A great deal of attention and training is focused on saving life *after* cardiac arrest.
- Having systems in place such as the national early warning scores (NEWS2) to identify patients with adverse signs *prior* to arrest is paramount.
- Delivering effective resuscitation and managing the deteriorating patient are requisite skills for a clinician involved in Acute Medicine.
- Clinicians should keep up to date with competencies in resuscitation and attend accredited courses.

arrest to re-establish circulation and breathing. CPR is performed to keep a patient alive until a reversible cause can be treated, and advanced emergency care provided.

A great deal of attention and training is focussed on saving life *after* cardiac arrest but most in-hospital cardiac arrests are predictable and preventable. Recognising and managing acutely ill patients is critical – the patient's airway, breathing and circulation, oxygen therapy, fluid balance and monitoring. Having systems in place such as the national early warning scores 2 (NEWS2) to identify patients with adverse signs *prior* to arrest is paramount; 70–80% of patients who have cardiac arrest in hospital display adverse signs prior to collapse.

Resuscitation is therefore not only about CPR. It is about recognising and effectively treating patients in reversible physiological decline. Once these patients are identified, hospital-based healthcare professionals, including Acute Medicine and critical care outreach teams, can provide rapid review and help stabilise a patient's peri-arrest.

Peri-arrest

There is increasing recognition that patients who have a cardiac arrest have premonitory signs. The use of early warning scores (e.g. NEWS2) should support escalation of care to appropriate decision makers to facilitate acute care or indeed identify that escalation would be inappropriate. Clinicians should empower all staff to call for help when they identify a patient at risk of physiological deterioration. This includes calls based on clinical concern, rather than solely on NEWS2 scores.

Introduction

When we think about 'resuscitation', we usually have cardiopulmonary resuscitation (CPR) in mind. CPR is an emergency procedure performed during a cardiac

Acute Medicine: Lecture Notes, First Edition. Edited by Glenn Matfin.
© 2023 John Wiley & Sons Ltd. Published 2023 by John Wiley & Sons Ltd.

Peri-arrest arrhythmias

The assessment and treatment of all arrhythmias address the condition of the patient (stable versus unstable) and the nature of the arrhythmia.

Life-threatening features in an unstable patient include the following.

- *Shock* – appreciated as hypotension (e.g. systolic blood pressure <90 mmHg) and symptoms of increased sympathetic activity and reduced cerebral blood flow.
- *Syncope* – because of reduced cerebral blood flow.
- *Severe heart failure* – manifested by pulmonary oedema (failure of the left ventricle) and/or raised jugular venous pressure (failure of the right ventricle).
- *Myocardial ischaemia* – may present with chest pain (angina) or may occur without pain as an isolated finding on the 12-lead electrocardiogram (silent ischaemia).

Peri-arrest arrhythmias: tachycardia

Electrical cardioversion is the preferred treatment for tachyarrhythmia in the unstable patient displaying potentially life-threatening adverse signs (Figure 6.1). Conscious patients require anaesthesia or sedation, before attempting synchronised cardioversion. To convert atrial or ventricular tachyarrhythmias, the shock must be synchronised to occur with the R-wave of the electrocardiogram (ECG).

- For atrial fibrillation (AF): an initial synchronised shock at maximum defibrillator output rather than an escalating approach is a reasonable strategy based on current data.
- For atrial flutter and paroxysmal supraventricular tachycardia:
  - give an initial shock of 70–120 J
  - give subsequent shocks using stepwise increases in energy.
- For ventricular tachycardia (VT) with a pulse:
  - use energy levels of 120–150 J for the initial shock
  - consider stepwise increases if the first shock fails to achieve sinus rhythm.

If cardioversion fails to restore sinus rhythm and the patient remains unstable, give amiodarone 300 mg intravenously (IV) over 10–20 minutes (or procainamide 10–15 mg/kg over 20 minutes) and reattempt electrical cardioversion. The loading dose of amiodarone can be followed by an infusion of 900 mg over 24 hours.

If the patient with tachycardia is stable (no life-threatening adverse signs or symptoms) and is not deteriorating, pharmacological treatment may be possible.

Consider amiodarone for acute heart rate control in AF patients with haemodynamic instability and severely reduced left ventricular ejection fraction (LVEF). For patients with LVEF <40%, consider the smallest dose of beta-blocker to achieve a heart rate less than 110/min. Add digoxin if necessary.

Peri-arrest arrhythmias: bradycardia

If bradycardia is accompanied by life-threatening adverse signs, give atropine 500 mcg IV (or intraosseous, IO) and, if necessary, repeat every 3–5 minutes to a total of 3 mg. If treatment with atropine is ineffective, consider second-line drugs (Figure 6.2).

Consider pacing in patients who are unstable, with symptomatic bradycardia refractory to drug therapies. If transcutaneous pacing is ineffective, consider transvenous pacing.

Peri-arrest: anaphylaxis

> Anaphylaxis is a potentially life-threatening allergic reaction. Recognise anaphylaxis based on:
> - sudden onset and rapid progression of symptoms
> - airway and/or breathing and/or circulation problems
> - skin and/or mucosal changes (flushing, urticaria, angioedema) – but these may be absent in up to 20% of cases.

The diagnosis of anaphylaxis is not always obvious (Figure 6.3). It can be supported if a patient has been exposed to an allergen known to affect them. Treat life-threatening features, using the Airway, Breathing, Circulation, Disability, Exposure (ABCDE) approach. Adrenaline is the first-line treatment for anaphylaxis. Give intramuscular (IM) adrenaline early (in the anterolateral thigh) for A/B/C problems. A single dose of IM adrenaline is well tolerated and poses minimal risk to an individual having an allergic reaction. If in doubt, give IM adrenaline. Repeat IM adrenaline after 5 minutes if A/B/C problems persist. For those patients with refractory anaphylaxis, consult Figure 6.4.

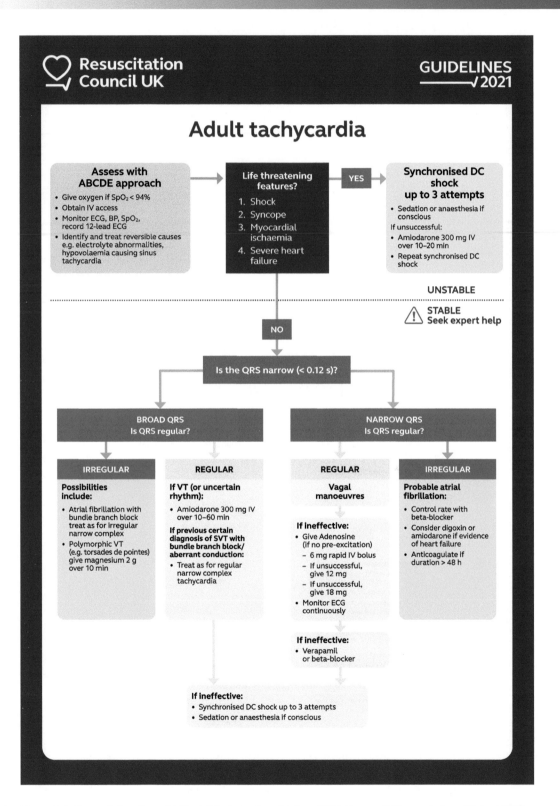

Figure 6.1 Resuscitation Council UK adult tachycardia guidelines 2021. Source: With permission of Resuscitation Council (UK)

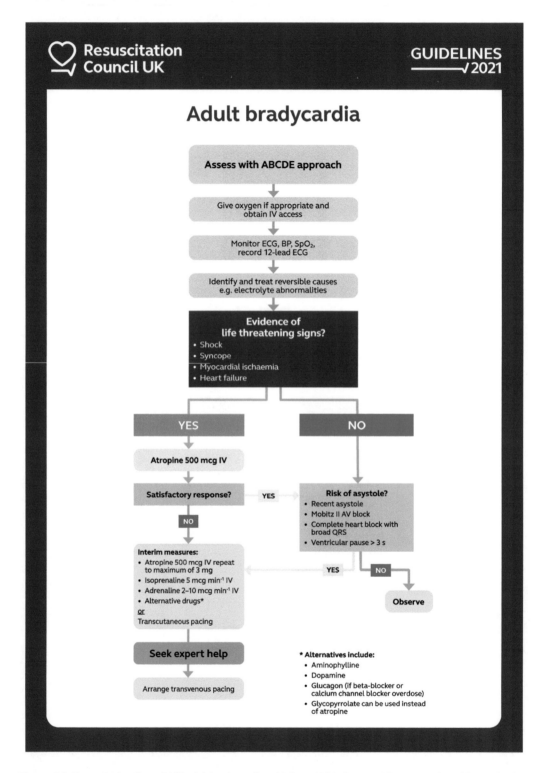

Figure 6.2 Resuscitation Council UK adult bradycardia guidelines 2021. Source: With permission of Resuscitation Council (UK)

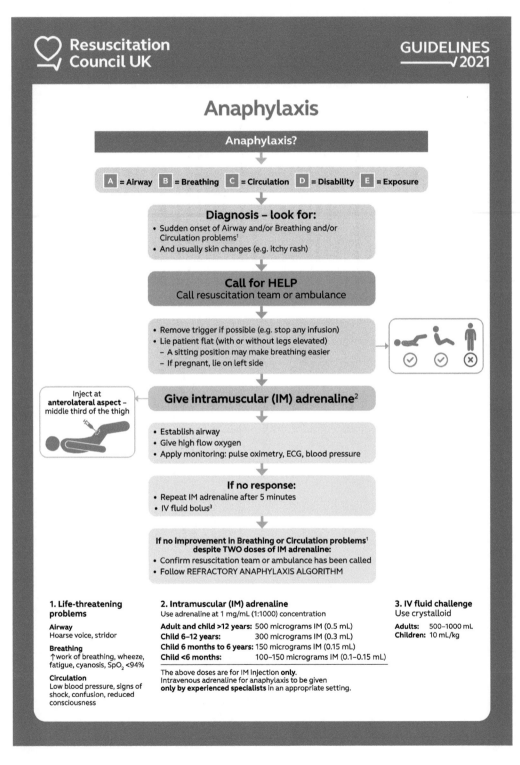

Figure 6.3 Resuscitation Council UK anaphylaxis guidelines 2021. Source: With permission of Resuscitation Council (UK)

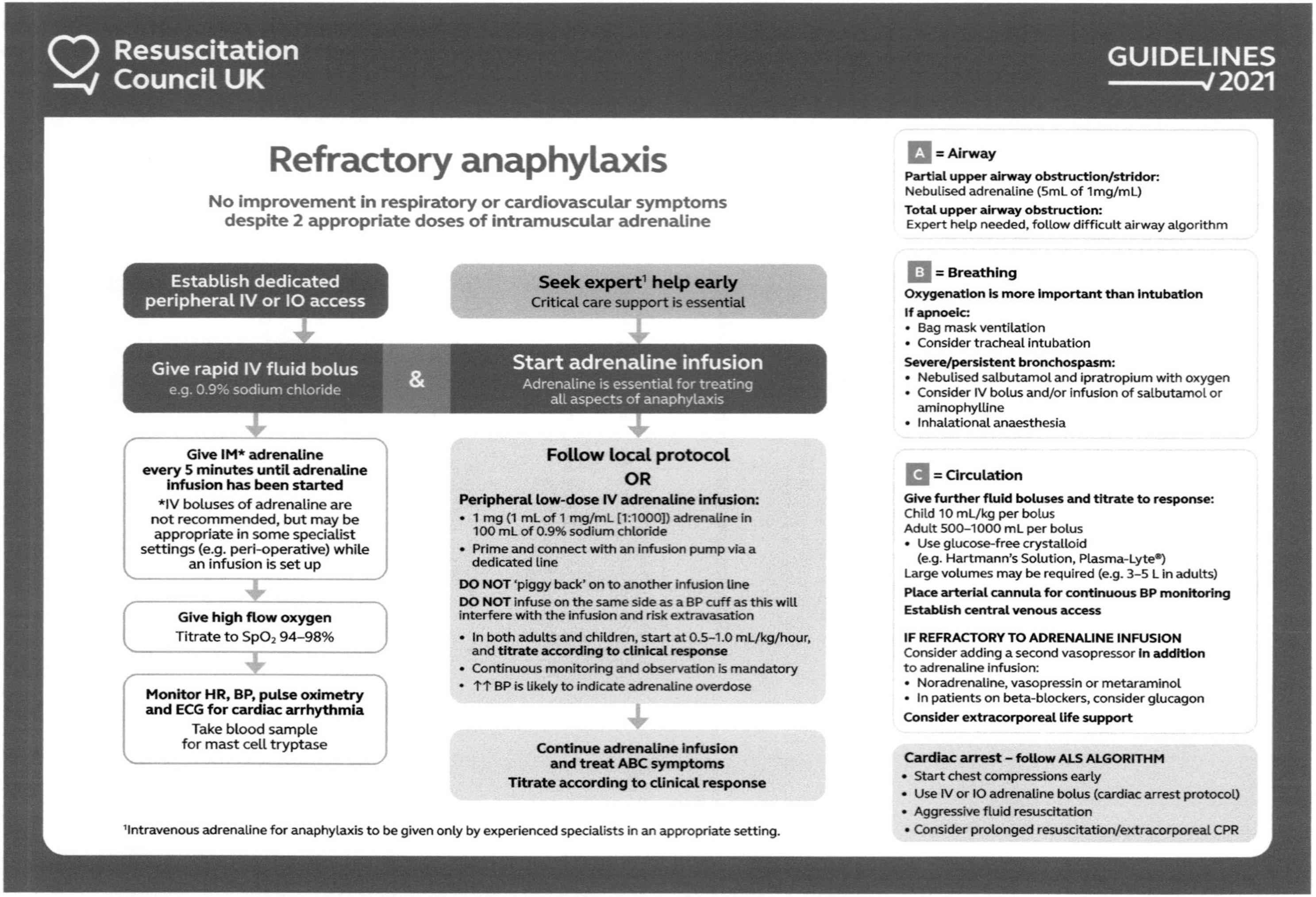

Figure 6.4 Resuscitation Council UK refractory anaphylaxis guidelines 2021. Source: With permission of Resuscitation Council (UK)

Follow the National Institute for Health and Care Excellence (NICE) guideline for the assessment and referral of patients suspected to have had anaphylaxis.

- All patients need appropriate follow-up – refer to a specialist clinic for allergy assessment.
- Offer patients (or, if appropriate, their parent and/or carer) an appropriate adrenaline injector as an interim measure before the specialist allergy assessment (unless the reaction was drug induced).
- Patients prescribed adrenaline auto-injectors (and/or their parents/carers) must receive training in their use, and have an emergency management or action plan.
- Anaphylaxis reactions should be reported to the UK Anaphylaxis Registry by contacting anaphylaxis.registry@imperial.ac.uk.

Peri-arrest: sepsis

- *Sepsis*: life-threatening organ dysfunction caused by a dysregulated host response to infection.
- *Septic shock*: a subset of sepsis in which profound circulatory (shock), cellular, and metabolic abnormalities occur.

Follow the Surviving Sepsis (or Sepsis Six) guidelines for the initial resuscitation of sepsis and septic shock.

- Measure lactate level.
- Obtain blood cultures prior to administration of antibiotics.
- Administer broad-spectrum antibiotics.
- Begin rapid administration of 30 ml/kg crystalloid for hypotension or a lactate ≥4 mmol/l.
- Apply vasopressors if the patient is hypotensive during or after fluid resuscitation to maintain mean arterial pressure (MAP) ≥65 mmHg.

Estimating MAP.
- Double the diastolic blood pressure (DBP) and add the sum to the systolic blood pressure (SBP). Then divide total by 3.
- Most people need a MAP of ≥60 mmHg to ensure adequate blood flow to vital organs, such as the heart, brain and kidneys.

Cardiac arrest

Cardiac arrest is the abrupt loss of heart function.

Epidemiology of out-of-hospital cardiac arrest (OHCA)

- NHS Ambulance Services attempt resuscitation in approximately 30 000 people each year.
- 80% of OHCAs are due to a primary cardiac cause such as myocardial infarction.
- Bystander CPR is attempted in 70% cases, but public access defibrillators are reported as being used in <10%. This lack of use is of concern since the initial cardiac arrest rhythm is shockable in up to 25% cases and early, successful defibrillation can significantly improve chance of survival and reduce neurological sequalae.
- A return of spontaneous circulation (ROSC) is achieved in approximately 30% of attempted resuscitations.
- Currently less than 10% of OHCA arrests survive to discharge.

There is evidence of health inequalities in the incidence of cardiac arrest, bystander CPR and distribution of public access defibrillators. Deprived areas and areas with a greater proportion of residents from minority ethnic backgrounds have a higher incidence of cardiac arrest, lower incidence of bystander CPR and less availability of public access defibrillators.

Epidemiology of in-hospital cardiac arrest (IHCA)

- Most cardiac arrests (85%) occur on wards and in patients admitted to hospital for medical reasons.
- The initial rhythm is shockable in ~17% of cardiac arrests, pulseless electrical activity (PEA) 52%, asystole 20% and the remainder are unknown or undetermined.
- ROSC is achieved in half (53%) of those treated by a hospital's resuscitation team for IHCA.
- A quarter (23.6%) of those treated by a hospital's resuscitation team for IHCA survive to hospital discharge.

Epidemiology of post resuscitation care

- One in ten patients admitted to critical care and requiring invasive mechanical ventilation had sustained a cardiac arrest prior to admission.
- The average length of stay in critical care is 4–6 days and in hospital 14–21 days.
- One in ten (OHCA) and one in 25 (IHCA) of those admitted to critical care go on to gift organs for transplantation.
- Approximately half of those admitted to critical care following OHCA survive to hospital discharge whilst one-third of those admitted to critical care following IHCA survive to hospital discharge.
- Two-thirds of patients who survive are discharged home.

Basic Life Support (BLS)

The BLS algorithm should be implemented until advanced support and resources arrive (Figure 6.5). CPR should be commenced in any unresponsive person with absent or abnormal breathing. Agonal breathing should be considered a sign of cardiac arrest.

> What are high-quality chest compressions?
> - Starting chest compressions as soon as possible.
> - Compressions that occur on the lower third of the sternum ('the centre of the chest').
> - Compressions to a depth of at least 5 cm but not more than 6 cm.
> - Compressions at a rate of 100–120/min with as few interruptions as possible.
> - Allowing the chest to recoil completely after each compression – do not lean on the chest.
> - Chest compressions on a firm surface whenever feasible.

Rescue breaths should be performed after 30 compressions in a ratio of 30:2. The performance of rescue breaths should be balanced against the risk of vomit/blood in the airway and transmission of infectious diseases. If in doubt, give continuous chest compressions.

An automated external defibrillator (AED) is part of the BLS algorithm, and their use should be encouraged. Whilst automated, it is important to ensure correct pad position (underneath the right shoulder and laterally in the ECG V4–V6 position), safety maintained, and instructions followed carefully. Do not delay defibrillation to provide additional CPR once the defibrillator is ready. Do not continue chest compression during shock delivery.

> Advanced Life Support (ALS) should start as soon as possible.

Advanced Life Support (ALS)

> Maintaining personal and patient safety during resuscitation is important. Ensure that it is safe to approach the patient. Check for and remove hazards. During the COVID-19 pandemic, all inpatients must be considered as potentially positive – don appropriate level of personal protective equipment (PPE) and take care during aerosol-generating procedures (e.g. chest compressions and advanced airway procedures).

Adult in-hospital resuscitation

Adults who are found collapsed or who are acutely unwell in the hospital setting should be managed as per adult in-hospital resuscitation guidelines (Figure 6.6).

Cardiac arrest

Hospital systems should aim to recognise cardiac arrest, start CPR immediately and defibrillate rapidly (if shockable rhythm) in less than three minutes (Figure 6.7). Hospitals should use a standard 'cardiac arrest call' telephone number (2222).

Hospital resuscitation team members should immediately respond to IHCA. They should follow the Resuscitation UK Adult Advanced Life Support guidelines 2021 (Figure 6.8).

Rhythm recognition and defibrillation

Continue CPR while a defibrillator is retrieved and pads applied. Give a shock as early as possible when

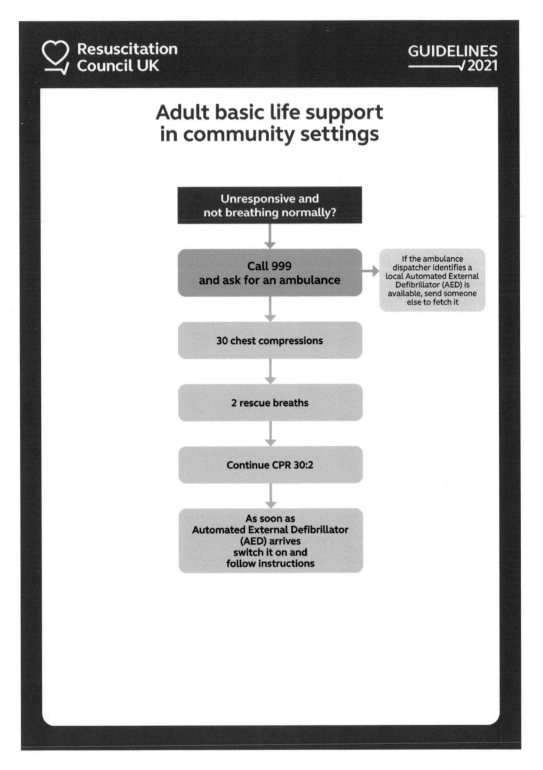

Figure 6.5 Resuscitation UK Adult Basic Life Support guideline 2021. Source: With permission of Resuscitation Council (UK)

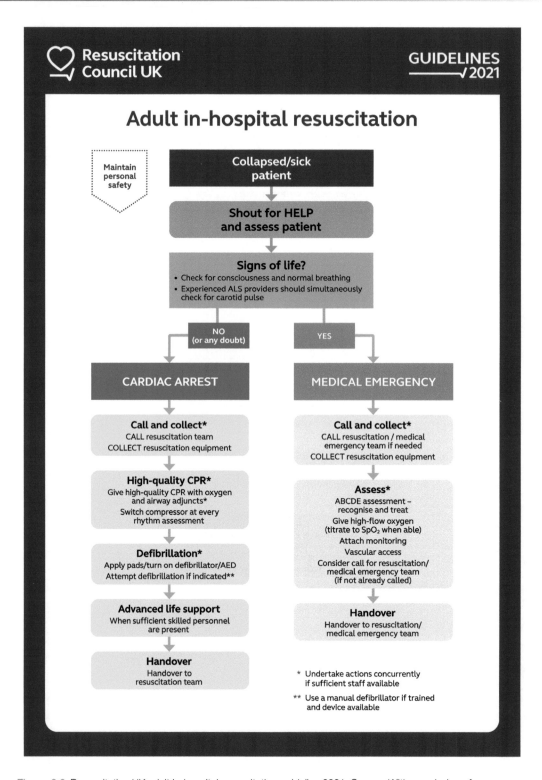

Figure 6.6 Resuscitation UK adult in-hospital resuscitation guideline 2021. Source: With permission of Resuscitation Council (UK)

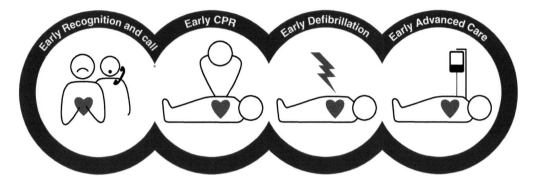

Figure 6.7 The chain of survival.

ventricular fibrillation (VF, Figure 6.9) or pulseless VT (pVT, Figure 6.10) is identified.

Anterolateral pad position is the position of choice for initial pad placement. Ensure that the lateral pad is positioned correctly (midaxillary line, level with the V6 ECG electrode position), i.e. below the armpit. In patients with an implantable device, place the pad >8 cm away from the device, or use an alternative pad position. Also consider an alternative pad position when the patient is in the prone position (biaxillary), or in a refractory shockable rhythm.

Use single shocks where indicated, followed by a two-minute cycle of chest compressions. The use of up to three-stacked shocks may be considered only if initial VF/pVT occurs during a witnessed, monitored cardiac arrest with a defibrillator immediately available (e.g. during cardiac catheterisation or in a high-dependency area). In the absence of any clear evidence for the optimal initial and subsequent energy levels, any energy level within the range 120–360 J is acceptable for the initial shock, followed by a fixed or escalating strategy up to the maximum output of the defibrillator.

> Deliver shocks with minimal interruption to chest compression and minimise the preshock and postshock pause. This is achieved by continuing chest compressions during defibrillator charging, delivering defibrillation with an interruption in chest compressions of less than five seconds and then immediately resuming chest compressions. Immediately resume chest compressions after shock delivery.

Airway and ventilation

> 'Pure' respiratory arrest – cessation of breathing with persisting effective cardiac activity – may complicate respiratory diseases such as asthma, exacerbations of chronic obstructive pulmonary disease, airways obstruction, neuromuscular disease and respiratory depressants such as opiates.

Airway and ventilation in a cardiac arrest.

- During CPR, start with basic airway techniques and progress stepwise according to the skills of the rescuer until effective ventilation is achieved.
- If an advanced airway is required, only rescuers with a high tracheal intubation success rate should use tracheal intubation.
- The expert consensus is that a high success rate is over 95% within two attempts at intubation.
- Aim for less than a five-second interruption in chest compression for tracheal intubation.
- Use direct or video laryngoscopy for tracheal intubation according to local protocols and rescuer experience.
- Use waveform capnography to confirm tracheal tube position.
- Give the highest feasible inspired oxygen during CPR.
- Give each breath over one second to achieve a visible chest rise.
- Once a tracheal tube or a supraglottic airway (SGA) has been inserted, ventilate the lungs at a rate of 10/min and continue chest compressions without pausing during ventilations. With a SGA, if gas leakage results in inadequate ventilation, pause compressions for ventilation using a compression:ventilation ratio of 30:2.

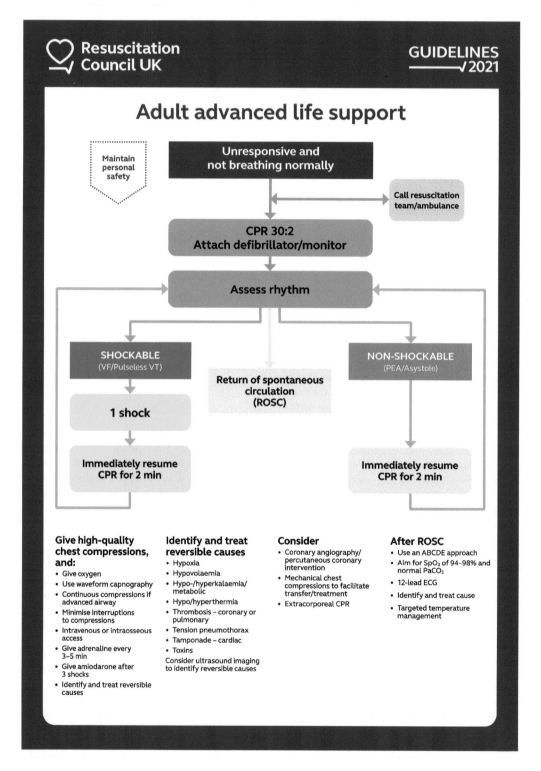

Figure 6.8 Resuscitation UK Adult Advanced Life Support guidelines 2021. Source: With permission of Resuscitation Council (UK)

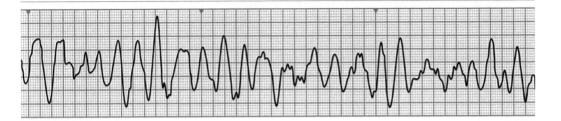

Figure 6.9 Ventricular fibrillation.

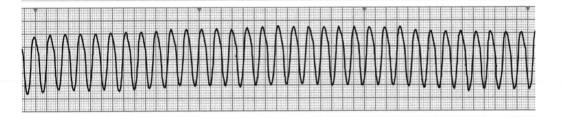

Figure 6.10 Ventricular tachycardia.

If there is a combination of clinical and physiological signs of ROSC such as waking, purposeful movement, arterial waveform or a sharp rise in end-tidal carbon dioxide (ETCO₂), consider stopping chest compressions for rhythm analysis and, if appropriate, a pulse check.

Waveform capnography

Use waveform capnography to confirm correct tracheal tube placement during CPR. Waveform capnography can be used to monitor the quality of CPR. An increase in ETCO$_2$ during CPR may indicate that ROSC has occurred (Figure 6.11). However, chest compression should not be interrupted based on this sign alone. Although high and increasing ETCO$_2$ values are associated with increased rates of ROSC and survival after CPR, do not use a low ETCO$_2$ value alone to decide if a resuscitation attempt should be stopped.

Drugs and fluid use in cardiac arrest

- Attempt IV access first to enable drug delivery in adults at cardiac arrest.
- Consider IO access if attempts at IV access are unsuccessful or IV access is not feasible.

Evidence suggests that the rates of ROSC are the same when either IV or IO access is used, but time to ROSC is longer when only the IO route is used.

Vasopressor drugs

- Give adrenaline 1 mg IV (IO) as soon as possible for adult patients in cardiac arrest with a non-shockable rhythm.
- Give adrenaline 1 mg IV (IO) after the third shock for adult patients in cardiac arrest with a shockable rhythm.
- Repeat adrenaline 1 mg IV (IO) every 3–5 minutes whilst ALS continues.

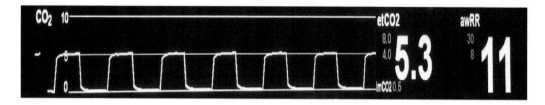

Figure 6.11 A normal capnograph trace such as of a spontaneously breathing patient.

Antiarrhythmic drugs

- Give amiodarone 300 mg IV (IO) for adult patients in cardiac arrest who are in VF/pVT after three shocks have been administered.
- Give a further dose of amiodarone 150 mg IV (IO) for adult patients in cardiac arrest who are in VF/pVT after five shocks have been administered.
- Lidocaine 100 mg IV (IO) may be used if there is a clinical decision not to use amiodarone. An additional bolus of lidocaine 50 mg can also be given after five defibrillation attempts.

Thrombolytics

Consider thrombolytic drug therapy when pulmonary embolus (PE) is the suspected or confirmed cause of cardiac arrest. Consider CPR for 60–90 minutes after administration of thrombolytic drugs. A mechanical CPR device such as a LUCAS chest compression system can help facilitate effective, ongoing CPR for prolonged periods.

Fluids

Give IV (IO) fluids only where the cardiac arrest is caused by hypovolaemia and ensure the resuscitation fluid is appropriate, such as use of crystalloids or blood products.

> Other drugs such as antibiotics (sepsis), calcium chloride and insulin-dextrose (hyperkalaemia) may be required.

CPR in people with obesity

Delivery of effective CPR in obese patients may be challenging due to several factors.

- Vascular access.
- Airway management.
- Quality of chest compressions.

- Efficacy of vasoactive drugs.
- Efficacy of defibrillation.

Provide chest compressions up to a maximum of 6 cm. Change the rescuers performing chest compression more frequently. Consider escalating defibrillation energy to maximum for repeated shocks. Manual ventilation with a bag-mask should be minimised and be performed by experienced staff using a two-person technique – request senior anaesthetic assistance.

Identifying reversible causes

When a patient has an IHCA, it is important to consider the following.

- Medical history: conditions, evidence and degree of organ failure, any specialist care/therapies, documented prognosis/expectations. In any patient over 65, note the Clinical Frailty Score.
- Admission history: why did the patient come in? Any complications? Any incidents such as a medication error/fall? Is the patient expected to leave hospital?
- Any 'Do not attempt cardiopulmonary resuscitation' (DNACPR) decision? If one exists, the resuscitation should be *immediately discontinued*. Treatment/escalation plans? Documented patient and/or family discussions?
- Any identifiable, reversible causes, commonly known as the '4Hs and 4Ts' (Table 6.1).

Many conditions will give rise to a multifactorial cardiac arrest, all of which will need addressing for a successful outcome. An example of this is a patient with septic shock due to pneumonia. The two reversible causes are hypoxia and hypovolaemia, but thrombosis is also possible. In addition, the patient may have acute kidney injury (AKI) with electrolyte and acid–base abnormalities such as hyperkalaemia and/or acidaemia.

Table 6.1 The '4Hs and 4Ts'

4Hs	4Ts
• **H**ypoxia	• **T**hrombosis – coronary or pulmonary
• **H**ypovolaemia	• **T**ension pneumothorax
• **H**ypokalaemia/**H**yperkalaemia	• **T**amponade – cardiac
• **H**ypothermia/**H**yperthermia	• **T**oxins

Intra-arrest point-of-care ultrasound (POCUS) can be used by a skilled operator as long as it does not cause undue delays in resuscitation. POCUS may be useful to diagnose treatable causes of cardiac arrest such as cardiac tamponade and pneumothorax. POCUS may be more valuable peri- and post-arrest.

The four 'Hs'

- *Hypoxia* - minimise by ensuring that the patient's lungs are ventilated adequately with the maximal possible inspired oxygen during CPR. Treat the cause of the asphyxia/hypoxaemia as the highest priority because this is a potentially reversible cause of the cardiac arrest.
- *Hypovolaemia* – PEA arising from hypovolaemia is often caused by severe haemorrhage. This may be precipitated by gastrointestinal bleeding or rupture of an aortic aneurysm. Stop the haemorrhage and restore intravascular volume with fluid and blood products. Sepsis is also an important cause of hypovolaemia and shock. However, only 50% of septic shock cases are fluid responsive.
- *Hypokalaemia*, hyperkalaemia, hypocalcaemia, acidaemia and other metabolic disorders are detected by biochemical tests or suggested by the patient's medical history (e.g. end-stage renal disease, post neck surgery for hypocalcaemia).
- *Hypothermia and hyperthermia* should be suspected based on the clinical context (e.g. hypothermia – cardiac arrest associated with drowning; hyperthermia – drug related), as well as ambient weather conditions.

The four 'Ts'

- *Thrombosis* – coronary thrombosis associated with an acute coronary syndrome (ACS) is the most common cause of sudden cardiac arrest. An ACS is usually diagnosed and treated after ROSC is achieved. If an ACS is suspected, and ROSC has not

been achieved, consider urgent coronary angiography when feasible and, if required, percutaneous coronary intervention (PCI). If venous thromboembolic (VTE) disease associated with massive PE is thought to be the cause of cardiac arrest, consider giving a fibrinolytic drug immediately.
- *Tension pneumothorax* can be the primary cause of PEA and may be associated with trauma or pulmonary causes. The diagnosis is made clinically or by POCUS. Decompress rapidly by thoracostomy or needle thoracocentesis, and then insert a chest drain.
- *Tamponade* – cardiac tamponade diagnosis can be made clinically (e.g. in the setting of penetrating chest trauma) or by POCUS.
- *Toxins* – in the absence of a specific history, the accidental or deliberate ingestion of therapeutic or toxic substances may be revealed only by laboratory investigations. Where available, the appropriate antidotes should be used, but most often treatment is supportive and standard ALS protocols should be followed.

Specific causes

Sepsis during cardiac arrest

Follow standard ALS guidelines, including administering the maximal inspired oxygen concentration via an intubated trachea if this can be done safely. In addition, commence IV crystalloid with further bolus as needed. Give antibiotics early. Do not forget the importance of infection source control (e.g. emergency incision and drainage of collections).

Hypokalaemia and hyperkalaemia

Consider hypokalaemia or hyperkalaemia (especially if known renal disease or AKI) in all patients with an arrhythmia or cardiac arrest. An ECG may be the most readily available diagnostic tool.

Hypokalaemia

Hypokalaemia is defined as a plasma potassium (K) level <3.5 mmol/l.

- Renal K⁺ excretion assessment allows for determination as to whether hypokalaemia is due to renal or extrarenal causes. A spot urine K⁺ <15–20 mmol/l suggests an extrarenal cause of hypokalaemia.
- Consider conditions that cause renal or non-renal K⁺ loss, including diuretic therapy, gastrointestinal loss and chronic alcohol abuse.

Management of hypokalaemia.

- Repeat electrolytes to *verify* the initial result.
- Severity can be assessed by potassium level (e.g. severe generally 2–2.4 mmol/l, critical <2 mmol/l), but other features need to be considered clinically such as chronicity of hypokalaemia and other factors (e.g. co-existing digoxin therapy).
- Associated ECG changes include ST depression, sinus tachycardia, U-waves, abnormal PR interval, high QRS voltage and various atrioventricular and right bundle branch blocks; VT, VF, and cardiac arrest have been reported.
- The goals of treating hypokalaemia are to:
  - prevent life-threatening complications: arrhythmias, paralysis, rhabdomyolysis, diaphragmatic weakness
  - replace potassium deficit (IV initially)
  - correct the underlying cause.

Hyperkalaemia

Hyperkalaemia is defined as a plasma K ≥5.5 mmol/l. Hyperkalaemia is potentially life-threatening and can result in cardiac arrhythmias and sudden death.

Management of hyperkalaemia.

- Severity can be assessed by potassium level (e.g. severe generally 6–7 mmol/l, critical >7 mmol/l).
- Associated ECG changes include peaked T-wave (early), prolonged PR, flattening of P-wave, widening of QRS (increased risk of arrhythmia), absence of P-wave, sine wave (fusion of QRS and T-wave), ventricular arrhythmia and asystole.

A normal ECG does not exclude risk for arrhythmia, as life-threatening arrhythmia can occur without warning.

The UK Renal Association provides guidelines on the management of hyperkalaemia. For a patient in cardiac arrest:

- confirm hyperkalaemia using blood gas analyser if available
- protect the heart: give 10 ml calcium chloride 10% IV by rapid bolus injection. Consider repeating the dose if cardiac arrest is refractory or prolonged
- shift potassium into cells: give 10 units rapid-acting insulin and 25 g glucose IV by rapid injection. Monitor blood glucose. Administer 10% glucose infusion guided by blood glucose to avoid hypoglycaemia
- shift potassium into cells: give 50 mmol sodium bicarbonate (50 ml 8.4% solution) IV by rapid injection.
- Remove potassium from the body: consider dialysis for refractory hyperkalaemic cardiac arrest.

After emergency hyperkalaemia presentation is stabilised, seek and treat the underlying cause(s).

Hypothermia and hyperthermia

Climate change is contributing to disease burdens both directly and indirectly, by intensifying extreme events (e.g. wildfires and floods), enhancing the spread of vector-borne and water-borne diseases, decreasing air quality, increasing food insecurity and displacing populations. Extremes of temperature result in more circumstances leading to hypothermia and hyperthermia.

Hypothermia

Hypothermia is traditionally defined as a core temperature <35 °C.

- Severity – mild 33–35 °C; moderate 28–33 °C; severe <28 °C.
- Hyperkalaemia is an index of asphyxia.
- Management – resuscitate (ABCDE); exclude lethal injury; rewarm.

- Look for secondary causes of hypothermia.
- Consider the old aphorism: 'Not dead until warm and dead'. However, some patients are unfortunately dead when they are cold and dead!

Immediately assess core temperature with a low-reading thermometer (e.g. tympanic in spontaneously breathing, distal oesophageal in patients with an endotracheal tube). Vital signs should be assessed for up to a minute (there may be severe bradycardia). Prehospital insulation, triage, fast transfer to a hospital and rewarming are key interventions.

- Hypothermic patients with risk factors for imminent cardiac arrest (i.e. core temperature <30 °C, ventricular arrhythmia, systolic blood pressure <90 mmHg) and those in cardiac arrest should ideally be transferred directly to an extracorporeal life support (ECLS) centre for rewarming.
- Hypothermic cardiac arrest patients should receive continuous CPR during transfer. Chest compression and ventilation rate should not be different to CPR in normothermic patients.
- If VF persists after three shocks, delay further attempts until the core temperature is >30 °C. Withhold adrenaline if the core temperature is <30 °C. The administration intervals for adrenaline should be increased to 6–10 minutes if the core temperature is 30–34 °C.
- In hypothermic cardiac arrest, rewarming should be performed with an ECLS system.

Hyperthermia

Hyperthermia is traditionally defined as a core temperature >38 °C.
- Due to excessive heat production, failure of heat dissipation or combination of both.
- Severity – severe >40.5 °C with neurological dysfunction.
- Management – resuscitate (ABCDE); close monitoring (e.g. risk of hyperkalaemia and rhabdomyolysis); cooling.

- *Heat syncope* – remove patient to a cool environment, cool passively and provide oral fluids.
- *Heat exhaustion* – remove patient to a cool environment, lie them flat, administer IV isotonic or hypertonic fluids, consider additional electrolyte replacement therapy with isotonic fluids. Replacement of 1–2 l crystalloid at 500 ml/h is often adequate.
- *Heat stroke* – remove patient to a cool environment, lie them flat, immediately actively cool using whole-body (from neck down) water immersion technique (1–26 °C) or other techniques until core temperature is <39 °C. Administer IV isotonic or hypertonic fluids.
- *Malignant hyperthermia, neuroleptic malignant syndrome, serotonin syndrome* – stop triggering agents immediately, follow the ALS algorithm in cardiac arrest and start active cooling. Get expert advice NOW.

Pulmonary embolus

Cardiac arrest following PE commonly presents as PEA. PE may be suggested by clinical context (e.g. known VTE disease, cancer patient, recent prolonged travel), as well as relevant diagnostic findings, including POCUS. Administer thrombolytic drugs for cardiac arrest when PE is the suspected cause of cardiac arrest. When thrombolytic drugs have been administered, consider continuing CPR attempts for at least 60–90 minutes before termination of resuscitation attempts. Use thrombolytic drugs or surgical embolectomy or percutaneous mechanical thrombectomy for cardiac arrest when PE is the known cause of cardiac arrest.

Coronary thrombosis

Acute coronary syndrome (ACS) is a group of conditions that include unstable angina and acute myocardial infarction (AMI). The latter is further classified according to ECG as ST elevation myocardial infarction (STEMI) and non-ST elevation myocardial infarction (NSTEMI). The prerequisite for AMI is troponin release from damaged cardiac myocytes.

Parameters suggesting coronary thrombosis.

- Chest pain prior to arrest.
- Known coronary artery disease.
- Initial rhythm: VF/pVT.
- Post resuscitation: 12-lead ECG showing ST elevation.

Consider performing PCI as part of the resuscitation or administering thrombolysis. In patients with sustained ROSC and a STEMI, arrange primary PCI ≤120 minutes from diagnosis by activating the catheterisation laboratory and transfer patient for immediate PCI. Outside this timeframe, consider thrombolysis and arrange PCI. In the event of a NSTEMI, individualise the decision considering patient characteristics, setting and ECG findings. Consider delayed coronary angiography if there is no suspected ongoing ischaemia and the patient is stable.

Cardiac tamponade

> Cardiac tamponade is accumulation of pericardial fluid under high pressure which compresses cardiac chambers and impairs diastolic filling of *both* ventricles, leading to elevated jugular venous pressure, hypotension and decreased (muffled) heart sounds. Pulsus paradoxus can also be present (>10 mmHg drop in systolic BP during inspiration). Electrical alternans on ECG.

Point-of-care ultrasound echocardiography supports the diagnosis. Decompress the pericardium immediately by resuscitative thoracotomy or POCUS-guided pericardiocentesis.

Tension pneumothorax

> Acute pleuritic pain and breathlessness with diminished breath sounds are the typical features of a pneumothorax. Severe distress with cardiorespiratory compromise suggests a tension pneumothorax. Chest X-ray shows a convex 'pleural line' at the margin of the collapsed lung, with a black gas space containing no lung markings between the collapsed lung and chest wall. A 2 cm rim of air approximately equates to a 50% pneumothorax. POCUS can also be diagnostic.

Diagnosis of tension pneumothorax in a patient with cardiac arrest or haemodynamic instability must be based on clinical examination or POCUS. Decompress the chest immediately by open thoracostomy when a tension pneumothorax is suspected in the presence of cardiac arrest or severe hypotension. Needle chest decompression serves as rapid treatment, and it should be carried out with specific needles (longer, non-kinking). Any attempt at needle decompression under CPR should be followed by an open thoracostomy or a chest tube if the expertise is available.

Chest decompression effectively treats tension pneumothorax and takes priority over other measures.

Toxic agents

Care of the poisoned patient is largely supportive. Manage hypertensive emergencies with benzodiazepines, vasodilators and pure alpha-antagonists. Drug-induced hypotension usually responds to IV fluids (although calcium channel blocker and beta-blocker overdose may cause refractory hypotension and need more nuanced treatment). Use specific treatments where available in addition to the ALS management of arrhythmias. Provide early advanced airway management and administer antidotes, where available, as soon as possible.

Exclude all reversible causes of cardiac arrest, including electrolyte abnormalities which can be indirectly caused by a toxic agent. Measure the patient's temperature because hypo- or hyperthermia may occur during drug overdose. Be wary of injury causing presentation. Be prepared to continue resuscitation for a prolonged period. The toxin concentration may fall as it is metabolised or excreted during extended resuscitation measures. Consult regional or national poison centres for information on treatment of the poisoned patient.

Post resuscitation care

> The immediate management after the ROSC should be considered as a new phase of resuscitation (Figure 6.12).

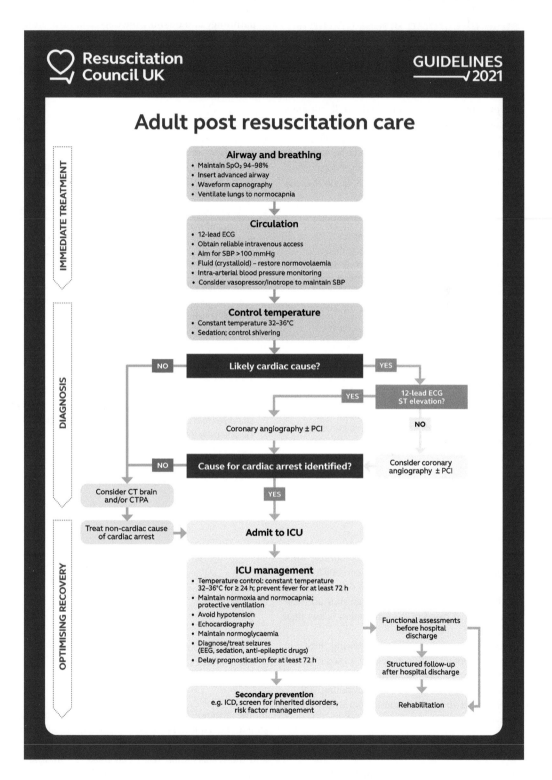

Figure 6.12 Resuscitation UK adult postresuscitation care guidelines 2021. Source: With permission of Resuscitation Council (UK)

Cause of cardiac arrest unknown

- If there is clinical (e.g. haemodynamic instability) or ECG evidence of myocardial ischaemia, undertake coronary angiography first. This is followed by computed tomography (CT) brain and/or CT pulmonary angiography (CTPA) if coronary angiography fails to identify causative lesions.
- If there are signs or symptoms prearrest suggesting a neurological or respiratory cause (e.g. headache, seizures or neurological deficits, shortness of breath or documented hypoxaemia in patients with known respiratory disease), perform a CT brain and/or a CTPA first.

> The transfer of a patient to a scanner or interventional suite can be fraught with risk, including the patient going back into cardiac arrest, so it is essential this is considered in any transfer plans.

Intensive care management

> Postcardiac arrest syndrome is a clinical state that involves global brain injury, myocardial dysfunction, ischaemic reperfusion injury, increased vulnerability to infection and persistent precipitating pathology (i.e. the cause of the arrest).

Airway and ventilation support

Should continue after ROSC is achieved.

- Patients who have had a brief period of cardiac arrest and an immediate return of normal cerebral function and are breathing normally may not require tracheal intubation but should be given oxygen via a facemask if their arterial blood oxygen saturation is less than 94%.
- Patients who remain comatose following ROSC, or who have another clinical indication for sedation and mechanical ventilation, should have their trachea intubated if this has not been done already during CPR.
- Hypoxaemia and hyperoxaemia after ROSC should be avoided.

Circulatory support

- Use arterial line for continuous BP measurements.
- Echocardiography should be performed in all patients to detect any underlying cardiac pathology and quantify the degree of myocardial dysfunction.
- Avoid hypotension.
- Maintain adequate urine output (>0.5 ml/kg/h) and normal or decreasing lactate levels.

Cognitive function

- Monitor electroencephalogram (EEG) – nonconvulsive seizures can occur. If seizures occur post arrest, consider levetiracetam or sodium valproate as first line with/without sedation or general anaesthesia.
- Targeted temperature management (TTM) should be considered for patients unresponsive after ROSC.
  - Maintain a target temperature at a constant value between 32 °C and 36 °C for at least 24 hours.
  - Slows down cerebral metabolism, decreases oxygen consumption and cerebral oedema.

> Brain injury after resuscitation, a common sequela following cardiac arrest, ranges in severity from mild impairment to devastating brain injury and brainstem death. Effective strategies to minimise brain injury after resuscitation include early intervention with CPR and defibrillation, restoration of normal physiology, and TTM. Intensive, tailored rehabilitation after discharge is needed to achieve the best outcomes.

Deciding when to stop CPR

> Clinicians should clearly document reasons for the withholding or termination of CPR.

In the absence of a valid DNACPR, resuscitation should be commenced. The decision whether to continue can be reviewed as information is gathered and the resuscitation team can make an informed decision (Box 6.1). Clinicians should not undertake the deceptive practice of purposely delivering suboptimal CPR (a 'slow code').

Box 6.1 Factors which may inform decision making to terminate the resuscitation attempt

- Safety of the scene and/or personnel cannot be assured.
- Obvious mortal injury or irreversible death.
- The presence of a valid and relevant decision not to proceed with resuscitation.
- Prolonged asystole.
- Initial non-shockable rhythm where the risk of harm outweighs the benefits of ongoing CPR.
- Strong evidence that ongoing CPR would not be consistent with the patient's values and preferences or in their best interests.

Factors that should not, individually, inform decision making to terminate include the following.

- Pupil size.
- CPR duration.
- End-tidal carbon dioxide value.
- Co-morbidity.
- Initial lactate level.
- No heart activity on POCUS.
- Suicide attempt.

What is ReSPECT?

ReSPECT stands for Recommended Summary Plan for Emergency Care and Treatment. The ReSPECT process creates a summary of personalised recommendations for a person's clinical care in a future emergency in which they do not have capacity to make or express choices. Such emergencies may include death or cardiac arrest but are not limited to those events. The process is intended to respect both patient preferences and clinical judgement. The agreed realistic clinical recommendations that are recorded include a recommendation on whether or not CPR should be attempted if the person's heart and breathing stop.

7

Enhanced and critical care Acute Medicine

Glenn Matfin

 KEY POINTS

- Acute medical emergencies are those illnesses that can cause organ failures and death within minutes to hours of their presentation.
- Following initial assessment and delivery of any immediate treatment for a patient presenting with an acute medical emergency, subsequent inpatient care should be on a ward that has facilities appropriate to their clinical condition (i.e. 'right patient – right bed').
- Selecting the appropriate setting for ongoing management should be based on the monitoring and support patients require (i.e. levels of care), rather than the location they are in.
- More recently, the boundaries between the levels of care have become blurred.
- Enhanced care unit (described as level 1+, 1½ or 1a) is an intermediate level of care where a higher level of observation, monitoring and interventions can be provided than on a general ward but not requiring high-dependency care/organ support.
- High-dependency unit (level 2) care is appropriate for patients who require detailed observation or intervention for a single failing organ system.
- Intensive care unit (level 3) care supports failing organ systems when there is potentially reversible disease. It is appropriate for patients requiring advanced respiratory support alone or support of at least two failing organ systems.

Introduction

Critical illness is defined as any life-threatening condition requiring support of vital organ functions to prevent imminent death. This condition can be evoked by a variety of insults such as multiple trauma, complicated surgery and severe medical illnesses. Without modern critical care medicine, critically ill patients would not survive.

Acute medical emergencies are those illnesses that can cause organ failures and death within minutes to hours of their presentation. Acutely ill patients require rapid but careful assessment. Working out how ill the patient is and what needs to happen to them next underpins the effective, safe management of all adult medical emergencies.

Following initial assessment and delivery of any immediate treatment for a patient presenting with an acute medical emergency, subsequent inpatient care should be on a ward that has facilities appropriate to

Acute Medicine: Lecture Notes, First Edition. Edited by Glenn Matfin.
© 2023 John Wiley & Sons Ltd. Published 2023 by John Wiley & Sons Ltd.

their clinical condition (i.e. 'right patient – right bed'). Selecting the appropriate setting for ongoing management should be based on the monitoring and support patients require (i.e. levels of care), rather than the location they are in.

More recently, the boundaries between these levels of care have blurred (Table 7.1). The patient mix and acuity are changing, with a more elderly, frailer population with multiple co-morbidities requiring more complex care. Although the care required in these situations does not fit the criteria for critical care admission to a high-dependency unit (HDU) or intensive care unit (ICU), patients cannot safely be managed in a general ward environment due to the frequency of observations or specialist monitoring required. They would be categorised as requiring level 1+ or level 1½ care. To ensure patient safety and provide a high-quality service, admission to HDU is often required. Consequently, this can lead to disruptions in patient flow: patients in ICU ready to step down cannot be moved if there are insufficient beds, the admission of patients from the emergency department (ED) or wards may be delayed, resulting in capacity issues and care provision in a less than satisfactory environment, and patients requiring critical care admission as part of their perioperative pathway may have their procedure cancelled.

Enhanced care is a pragmatic approach to reducing the risk of patients falling into this service gap: patients who would benefit from higher levels of monitoring or interventions than expected on a routine ward, but who do not require admission to critical care. It can act as a bridge between critical care and normal ward care.

What is enhanced care?

Enhanced care is a relatively new concept. Enhanced care takes place in a ward setting such as the acute medical unit (AMU), by a motivated and upskilled workforce, but provides ready access to the critical care team through established communication links. Enhanced care is an intermediate level of care where a higher level of observation, monitoring and interventions can be provided than on a general ward but not requiring high-dependency care/organ support. It is imperative that such facilities do not exist in isolation from critical care in order to permit the seamless escalation of care, should this be required. Enhanced care needs to become part of the continuum of care from the ward to intensive care.

The National Early Warning Score 2 (NEWS2) and other similar tools should be used to help identify patients who may require enhanced care. Identifying a trigger, where the clinical response includes a senior clinical decision maker, critical care staff or outreach, will be required.

One of the immediate learning points from the COVID-19 pandemic response was the ability to rotate staff into critical care areas to enable rapid learning. Additionally, critical care staff have been 'enablers' to allow the delivery of enhanced care in ward areas. This has been most notably seen in the rapid expansion of medical ward capacity to deal with patients affected by COVID-19 along with additional respiratory support on existing medical wards. This has meant predominantly increased use of continuous positive airway pressure (CPAP) therapy and high-flow nasal oxygen in ward areas.

Table 7.1 Updated levels of care, including enhanced care (level 1+, 1½ or 1a care)

Level	Remarks
Level 0	Patients whose needs can be met through normal ward care in an acute hospital.
Level 1	Patients at risk of their condition deteriorating, or those recently relocated from higher levels of care whose needs can be met on an acute ward with additional advice and support from the critical care team.
Enhanced care	An intermediate level of care where a higher level of observation, monitoring and interventions can be provided than on a general ward but not requiring high-dependency care/organ support.[a] Enhanced advice and support from the critical care team can be accessed.
Level 2	Patients requiring more detailed observation or intervention, including support for a failing organ system or postoperative care, and those stepping down from higher levels of care.
Level 3	Patients requiring advanced respiratory support alone or basic respiratory support together with support of at least two organ systems. This level includes all complex patients requiring support for multiorgan failure.

[a] The level of support should be decided locally and will be dependent on the degree of critical care input.

Admission to critical care

Medical emergencies may present with little warning; however, most in-hospital cardiac arrests and those patients prior to admission to critical care are often predictable and preventable. Although the underlying diagnosis may initially be elusive, the clinical signs that accompany a medical emergency are readily identified (i.e. signs of sympathetic activation; signs of hypoperfusion; signs of organ failure). However, physiological derangement and the need for admission to critical care are not the same thing. It would not be in the best interests of all patients to be admitted to HDU/ICU. Instead, optimising ward care or even palliative care may be required. This decision is based on evidence about prognosis, clinical experience (e.g. recognising when someone is dying), and takes into account any expressed wishes of the patient.

Intensive care unit (level 3) care supports failing organ systems when there is potentially reversible disease. It is appropriate for patients requiring advanced respiratory support alone or support of at least two failing organ systems. HDU (level 2) care is appropriate for patients who require detailed observation or intervention for a single failing organ system. The decision to admit a patient to critical care is informed primarily by clinical factors, such as the potential reversibility of the illness, and the wishes of the patient or their surrogates.

Patient outcomes have significantly improved as a result of the development of critical care services. However, admission to the HDU/ICU does not guarantee a successful outcome. All potential admissions should be assessed by an experienced doctor. Patients who are not admitted to intensive care should have a clear plan and their ward care must be optimised.

Critical care outreach

Generally, acute medical emergencies will be managed in an ED, AMU or equivalent, specialist and general medical wards or acute medical ambulatory care services, as well as more advanced step-up facilities such as enhanced care unit (level 1+, 1½ or 1a care), HDU (level 2 care) or ICU (level 3 care).

Critical care outreach teams offer intensive care skills to patients with, or at risk of, critical illness receiving care in locations outside the HDU/ICU. This can help prevent admission to HDU/ICU or ensure that admission to a critical care bed happens in a timely manner to ensure best outcome. Other potential benefits include enabling discharges from ICU by supporting the continuing recovery of discharged patients on wards.

Enhanced and critical care relevant to Acute Medicine

Effective, early management of acute medical emergencies requires prompt recognition, immediate correction of life-threatening physiological abnormalities, the methodical application of the Control of obvious problem – Airway, Breathing, Circulation, Disability and Exposure (C-ABCDE) approach, and rapid diagnosis and treatment of the underlying condition. The general approach to C-ABCDE management has been outlined in Chapter 5 and Chapter 6.

Occasionally, definitive treatment is not readily apparent or available, or treatments take time to have their full effect. In these cases, adequate organ support to stabilise the patient while the treatment is given becomes the main goal of care.

Respiratory support

Respiratory failure results from inadequate gas exchange in the respiratory system. Hypoxaemia is defined as a lower than normal arterial blood oxygen level, while hypoxia refers to lack of oxygen at a cellular level. Hypoxaemia is a common presentation in critically ill patients, with the potential for severe harm if not addressed early. Determining the nature, cause and severity of hypoxaemia is a key step in enabling effective management. The BLUE protocol (Bedside Lung Ultrasound in Emergency) presents a systematic approach to a patient with respiratory failure to help identify the underlying diagnosis using thoracic and vascular point-of-care ultrasound (see Chapter 11).

Hypoxaemia (arterial partial pressure of oxygen [PaO_2] <8.0 kPa [60 mmHg]) is the most life-threatening facet of respiratory failure. It can occur with (type 2 respiratory failure) or without (type 1 respiratory failure) a high arterial partial pressure of carbon dioxide ($PaCO_2$). It can be due to a failure to ventilate, oxygenate, or both.

The goal of oxygen therapy is to correct alveolar and tissue hypoxia, not breathlessness or acute illness *per se*. Aim for PaO_2 of at least 8.0 kPa (60 mmHg) or oxygen saturations of at least 90% in people who are not at risk of hypercapnic respiratory failure. Aiming for oxygen saturations of 100% is unnecessary (hyperoxia) and can result in harm (e.g. worsened mortality in acute coronary syndromes and stroke). However, certain states may warrant higher oxygen saturations temporarily such as carbon monoxide poisoning, cluster headache and sickle cell crisis.

Apart from oxygen therapy and treatment of the underlying cause, various forms of respiratory support are used in the treatment of respiratory failure. There are two main types of respiratory support – non-invasive and invasive.

- *Non-invasive* respiratory support provides a bridge between simple oxygen delivery devices and invasive ventilation. Non-invasive positive pressure respiratory support consists of bilevel positive airway pressure (BiPAP) or CPAP, usually administered via tight-fitting masks, and high-flow nasal oxygen therapy.
  - CPAP – set positive pressure of air flow to the airways is maintained throughout the respiratory cycle.
  - BiPAP – air flow is delivered at variable pressures that are higher when the person is breathing in (inspiratory pressure) and lower when the person is breathing out (expiratory pressure). BiPAP is a type of non-invasive ventilation (NIV). NIV is the first-line therapy in patients with type 2 respiratory failure secondary to an acute exacerbation of chronic obstructive airways disease (COPD) because it reduces the work of breathing and offloads the diaphragm, allowing it to recover strength.
  - The benefits of non-invasive positive pressure respiratory support include preventing alveolar collapse and lowering cardiac preload (which is helpful in cardiogenic pulmonary oedema). These types of support may prevent the need to intubate patients in respiratory distress.
  - Contraindications to positive pressure respiratory support include that the patient must be able to protect their airway and must have the ability to remove the mask if vomiting (high risk of aspiration). If they have excess secretions (e.g. pneumonia), it may be best to intubate. Associated with aerosol generation, which is a potential risk for nosocomial COVID-19 infection.
- Invasive respiratory support requires tracheal intubation (or alternative) and ventilators which utilise several different ventilator modes depending on the clinical situation.

Respiratory support is indicated when:
- there is a failure to oxygenate or ventilate despite medical therapy:
  - failure to ventilate is treated by manoeuvres designed to increase alveolar ventilation by increasing the depth and rate of breathing (tidal volumes and respiratory rate primarily affect ventilation).
  - failure to oxygenate, however, is treated by increasing fractional inspired oxygen concentration (FiO_2) or by restoring and maintaining lung volumes using alveolar recruitment manoeuvres such as the application of a positive end-expiratory pressure (PEEP) or CPAP
- there is unacceptable respiratory fatigue
- there are non-respiratory indications for tracheal intubation and ventilation (e.g. the need for airway protection such as with decreased conscious level).

Acute respiratory distress syndrome (ARDS)

ARDS is a form of acute respiratory failure caused by permeability pulmonary oedema resulting from endothelial damage due to a cascade of inflammatory events developing in response to an initiating injury or illness.

Acute respiratory distress syndrome develops in response to a variety of injuries or illnesses that affect the lungs, either directly (e.g. aspiration of gastric contents, severe pneumonia) or indirectly (e.g. sepsis, acute pancreatitis). For example, approximately 50% of patients with sepsis develop acute lung injury or ARDS. About 12–48 hours after an initiating event, the patient develops respiratory distress, with increasing dyspnoea and tachypnoea. Arterial blood gases show deteriorating hypoxaemia, which responds poorly to oxygen therapy. Diffuse bilateral infiltrates develop on chest X-ray in the absence of evidence of cardiogenic pulmonary oedema.

Acute respiratory distress syndrome is the most severe end of the spectrum of acute lung injury and is characterised by the following features.

- Acute onset (within one week, although severe COVID-19 infection can present later).
- A history of an initiating injury or illness.

- Hypoxaemia refractory to oxygen therapy.
  - The degree of hypoxaemia may be expressed as the ratio of arterial oxygen tension (PaO_2) to the FiO_2.
  - In ARDS, arterial to inspired oxygen (PaO_2/FiO_2) is <300 mmHg (severe <100 mmHg).
- Bilateral diffuse infiltrates on chest X-ray.
- No evidence of cardiogenic pulmonary oedema (e.g. pulmonary capillary wedge pressure <18 mmHg).

The treatment of ARDS consists of optimal management of the initiating illness or injury, combined with supportive care directed at preserving adequate oxygenation (e.g. target PaO_2 of 55–80 mmHg or pulse oximetry of 88%–95%) and limiting oxygen toxicity (avoiding prolonged FiO_2 >60%), optimizing ventilation with some 'permissive hypercapnia' due to keeping tidal volume low to minimise alveolar barotrauma, maintaining optimal haemodynamic function and compensating for multiorgan failure, which often supervenes.

Other organ support

- *Circulatory* support – treatment of shock requires the restoration of an effective circulating blood volume to reverse decompensation and restore organ perfusion. This process depends on the diagnosis of the underlying condition so that specific therapies can be administered. A useful *aide-mémoire* for the differential diagnosis of shock is to classify this condition into four groups according to the main mechanism of decompensation: 1. Hypovolaemia; 2. Cardiogenic; 3. Obstructive (e.g. pulmonary embolism, cardiac tamponade); and 4. Distributive (e.g. sepsis, anaphylaxis). Whatever the cause and type of intervention (e.g. fluid resuscitation, blood transfusion, vasomotor and inotropic agents, or mechanical support), frequent patient reassessment against relevant clinical endpoints such as peripheral perfusion, pulse, blood pressure (BP) and urine output is essential so that therapy can be titrated, and inadvertent fluid and electrolyte overload can be averted.
- *Renal* support – renal replacement therapy (RRT).
- *Neurological* support – aim of management in acute brain injury is to optimise cerebral oxygen delivery by maintaining normal arterial oxygen content and cerebral perfusion. Secondary insults to the brain, such as hypoxaemia, hyper-/hypoglycaemia and prolonged seizures, must be avoided.

Patient monitoring in enhanced and critical care

Adequate monitoring is a core standard of care for patients receiving enhanced and critical care. When used in addition to vigilance by medical and nursing staff, unfavourable clinical events can be detected quickly and acted upon. Importantly, the use of monitoring in enhanced and critical care does not negate the risk of adverse events but should make them more readily detectable.

General management of the enhanced and critical care patient

The daily assessment is a systems-based approach to assessing a critical care inpatient. This assessment should allow recognition of clinical trends and to inform the short- and long-term management plan. Use standardised patient assessment documentation, which will prompt you to examine all body systems and make it simpler to compare to previous days' assessments.

Before commencing the daily assessment, it is important to familiarise yourself with the patient's clinical history.

- It is useful to note the day of their admission.
- Try to formulate a list of their current clinical issues.
- Is there any relevant past medical history?
- Does the patient have any planned interventions today or outstanding investigations to chase?

Having the above information to hand will make the interpretation of your clinical findings easier. Remember to follow good infection control practices (including wearing the right personal protective equipment) when approaching the patient and to maintain patient privacy.

As part of your daily assessment, it is important to spend a few minutes ensuring that the appropriate elements of routine care are in place for your patient. Routine elements of care can be broadly defined as elements of supportive and preventive care for a critically ill patient which are standardised, regardless of the presenting pathology. This aims to reduce the burden of ICU-acquired complications for patients. The FASTHUGS BID mnemonic serves as a mental checklist to ensure that the bundle of routine care is checked daily for every patient (Table 7.2).

Table 7.2 Routine bundle of daily care of critically ill patient – FASTHUGS BID approach

Component	Consideration for critical care team
Feeding	Can the patient be fed orally, if not enterally? If not, should we start parenteral feeding? Refer to dieticians.
Fluids	Check 24-hour fluid balance and plan for next 24 hours.
Family	Are family, friends, carers up to date? Do we need to plan a meeting with them?
Analgesia	The patient should not suffer pain, but excessive analgesia should be avoided.
Sedation	Delirium is common in the critical care setting. The patient should not experience discomfort but excessive sedation should be avoided; 'calm, comfortable, collaborative' is typically the best.
Thromboembolic prevention	Low molecular weight heparin (LMWH) should be administered to all patients unless there is a contraindication.
Head of the bed elevated	Optimally, 30–45 degrees, which can decrease raised intracranial pressure and risk of aspiration, unless contraindicated (e.g. threatened cerebral perfusion pressure).
Ulcer prophylaxis	Establishing enteral feed is ideal. Proton pump inhibitors are used.
Glucose control	Both hypoglycaemia and hypergycaemia are associated with increased morbidity and mortality. Usual blood glucose goals are between 6 and 10 mmol/l. Remote continuous glucose monitoring (CGM) increasingly used during COVID-19 pandemic. Glucocorticoids are commonly used in critical care patients (e.g. COVID-19) and can be associated with hyperglycaemia even in non-diabetic individuals.
Spontaneous breathing trial	Supplement oxygen. Decrease sedation. Patients who pass a spontaneous breathing trial are assessed for suitability of extubation (endotracheal tube removal).
Bowels	Are they moving? Often enough? Too much? Assess and plan using local protocol.
Indwelling catheter review	Look at all tubes and lines. How long have they been in? Are they still required? Do they need to be changed? Any sign of infection?
Drugs	Medicines reconciliation and de-escalation as needed. Pharmacist critical.

Malnutrition is common in hospitalised patients and is associated with longer length of stay, poorer outcomes and survival, and increased cost of care. The need for nutritional support in malnutrition reflects the following aspects.

- Timing and extent of recent (previous 3–6 months) unintentional weight loss, the degree of depletion of energy stores (in turn dependent on baseline energy stores or body mass index), the presence or absence of clinical markers of stress, and the anticipated time for which the patient will be unable to meet nutritional requirements orally. There is no gold standard for assessing nutrition status.
- In general, any patient who is unable to consume adequate nutrients orally (≥60% nutrition needs) for at least five days in the ICU or 7–14 days in the medical wards should be a candidate for specialised nutrition support. Check with local guidance and get dieticians and speech and language therapy (SALT) teams involved early.

Types of nutritional support.

- Enteral nutrition (EN) – liquid nutritional formulation is given through a tube (i.e. 'tube feeding') into the stomach or small bowel; should ideally be used in patients with a functioning gastrointestinal tract. EN may cause bacterial colonisation of the stomach, high gastric residual volumes with subsequent risk of aspiration pneumonia, and diarrhoea.
- Parenteral nutrition (PN) – which is a solution of IV nutrition compounded to include macronutrients (protein, dextrose, fat), micronutrients (electrolytes, minerals, trace elements, vitamins) and water, should not be given unless anticipated need is for ≥7 days. PN is associated with higher rates of overfeeding, hyperglycaemia and catheter-related infections.
- Both EN and PN have been proven effective in preventing the adverse effects of starvation and malnutrition in hospitalised patients. Whenever possible, EN rather than PN should be used in patients requiring nutrition support.
- Hyperglycaemia is frequently observed in hospitalised patients receiving specialised nutritional support. It is reported that up to 30% of patients receiving EN and more than 50% of patients receiving PN have blood glucose levels above suggested inpatient glycaemic targets. Therapeutic approaches should not only control hyperglycaemia but also have low hypoglycaemia risk.

Refeeding syndrome.
- It is important to monitor for the presence of the refeeding syndrome which is a collection of metabolic derangements that can occur during refeeding in patients who are starved or severely malnourished.
- Metabolic derangements in electrolytes, minerals (especially hypophosphataemia due to intracellular shift in response to calories causing cellular growth) and water-soluble vitamins are common and may be mild or severe.
- Organ compromise can manifest as pulmonary, cardiac, neuromuscular and haematological complications.
- Appropriate monitoring includes daily weight, fluid balance and signs of oedema until stable. Levels of serum potassium, phosphate and magnesium should be measured daily, and any deficiencies replaced. Thiamine should be administered. Overfeeding and excess PN volume and sodium should be avoided.

Ward round and multidisciplinary meeting

Once the daily assessments are complete, a consultant-led ward round takes place. This is an opportunity for multidisciplinary input into the patient's care plan. The overarching aim of the review is to identify the issues that are impeding recovery from critical illness and make alterations to address them. Daily goals should be set and well documented, and clearly communicated to the whole team caring for the patient.

Appropriate handover must occur prior to stepdown from critical care. Discharges from critical care to standard wards should take place within normal working hours to ensure adequate medical and nursing support.

Withdrawal of treatment

In the event of withdrawal of treatment, only interventions that will improve the quality of a patient's remaining life should be offered. If applicable, diagnosis of brain death may be required and consideration should be given to organ donation, termed 'donation after brain death'. All decisions concerning organ donation must follow local legal and ethical requirements. Seek expert help.

Post-ICU considerations

Patients treated in ICU can present with postintensive care syndrome, a spectrum of psychiatric, cognitive and/or physical disability (e.g. muscle weakness, cognitive dysfunction, insomnia, depression, anxiety, posttraumatic stress disorder, delirium, encephalopathy) that affects survivors of critical illness, and persists after the patient has been discharged from the ICU. Appropriate follow-up and rehabilitation are needed.

Long COVID may occur in patients following discharge from enhanced and critical care after being admitted with severe and critical COVID-19 infection. This also requires appropriate specialised management and long-term follow-up.

Example of enhanced and critical care management – sepsis

Early treatment of sepsis with appropriate antimicrobials may improve outcome, but antimicrobial overuse can cause harm and contribute to antimicrobial resistance. The major challenge is identifying patients most likely to benefit from early antimicrobial treatment.

Sepsis is a life-threatening medical emergency with a high mortality. Sepsis is a clinical syndrome which can originate from virtually any infection, resulting in a wide variety of presentations which can sometimes make it difficult to recognise (hence 'think sepsis' campaign). In the UK, it is estimated that there are at least 250 000 cases of sepsis each year, with 52 000 deaths. Sepsis, which can lead to multiple organ failure including septic shock, is thought to cause one in five deaths worldwide each year.

COVID-19 infection – sepsis has been reported in:
- 78% of ICU patients.
- 33% of hospitalised patients.

Definition of sepsis

The definition of sepsis has evolved over the last 30-plus years, with the latest definition aiming to facilitate earlier recognition and timely management of patients (Table 7.3).

Table 7.3 Updated Sepsis-3 definitions

States	Definition
Sepsis	• Life-threatening organ dysfunction caused by a dysregulated host response to infection • For clinical operationalisation, this can be represented by an increase in the sepsis-related organ failure assessment (SOFA) score of 2 or more • In-hospital mortality >10%
Septic shock	• A subset of sepsis in which profound circulatory, cellular and metabolic abnormalities occur • Clinically identified by persisting hypotension requiring vasopressors to maintain a mean arterial pressure of >65 mmHg and a serum lactate of >2 mmol/l in the absence of hypovolaemia • In-hospital mortality >40%

Sepsis is not a specific illness, but rather a constellation of clinical signs and symptoms (i.e. syndrome). It is important to appreciate that sepsis is a multifaceted dysregulated host response leading to life-threatening organ dysfunction, the presentation of which can be modified by pre-existing illness, long-standing co-morbidities, interventions and medication (e.g. immunosuppressants). In sepsis, there are profound immune, cardiovascular, metabolic and coagulation abnormalities that lead to microcirculatory dysfunction and tissue hypoxia, as well as changes in BP and cardiac output. Patients with a normal response to infection (e.g. tachycardia, fever, and high respiratory rate in pneumonia) *do not have sepsis* but they can still be sick and require urgent treatment. On the other hand, patients with sepsis can sometimes look deceptively well, especially to inexperienced clinicians.

Early treatment makes sense if patients risk dying from a dysregulated response to infection, but pre-existing conditions often have a role in sepsis-related deaths. Sepsis diagnosis requires *evidence of infection* and *new organ* damage. However, clinicians often see this combination in people with long-term conditions when a self-limiting or easily treatable infection is exacerbating underlying co-morbidity or frailty rather than causing organ damage through a dysregulated response. In such circumstances, co-morbidities and performance status will be the main determinants of mortality, and early antimicrobial treatment will have limited potential to improve outcome.

Screening tools for sepsis

Guidelines suggest that if a patient has possible sepsis or has a NEWS2 score of 5 or greater, prompt 'immediate review by a senior clinical decision maker to assess the person and think about alternative diagnoses to sepsis is the first step *whenever possible*. 'Is this patient unwell because of an infection?' If the answer is yes and any high-risk (*red flag*) features of sepsis are present (see list below), then the 'Sepsis Six' care bundle should be initiated.

- New altered mental state (i.e. either C, V, P or U on ACVPU assessment).
- BP ≤90 mmHg systolic.
- Heart rate >130/min.
- Respiratory rate ≥25/min.
- Needs oxygen to maintain SpO_2 ≥92% (or ≥88% in known COPD).
- Poor urine output (not passed urine in last 18 h/ urine output <0.5 ml/kg/h).
- Lactate ≥2 mmol/l.
- Recent chemotherapy.
- Non-blanching rash, mottled/ashen/cyanotic appearance.

Another tool – the 'quick SOFA' (qSOFA) score – is designed to rapidly identify patients who are likely to have poor outcomes. The qSOFA score is positive if the patient has two or more of the following.

- Respiratory rate of ≥22/min.
- Altered mentation (GCS <15).
- Systolic BP of ≤100 mmHg.

A positive qSOFA score should prompt clinicians to look for organ dysfunction and initiate or escalate therapy if appropriate. The qSOFA is not a screening tool for sepsis but may be valuable for predicting outcomes in patients *already* diagnosed with sepsis. NEWS2 is preferred to qSOFA (Academy of Medical Royal Colleges, 2022). However, patients often have a raised baseline NEWS2 score, so clinicians need to use their judgement to determine the extent to which abnormal early warning scores reflect serious infection or pre-existing conditions and that early warning scores should *support* and not replace clinical judgement.

Sepsis Six care bundle

The Sepsis Six care bundle refers to six steps in the initial management of patients with suspected sepsis (Table 7.4).

Referral to critical care outreach should occur immediately if after delivering the Sepsis Six bundle, the following apply.

- Systolic BP <90 mmHg.
- Reduced level of consciousness despite resuscitation.
- Respiratory rate over 25 breaths per minute.
- Lactate not reducing.
- If the patient is clearly critically ill at any time.

Management of sepsis and septic shock

Most cases of sepsis require admission to enhanced care or HDU/ICU. They should be referred *early* for advice and escalation of treatment. The Sepsis Six care bundle should be applied. Antibiotic therapy should be tailored at 48 hours depending on results of cultures. The de-escalation of antibiotics should be considered daily as the clinical situation permits.

Patients with shock require urgent resuscitation; a useful mnemonic to describe the important components is the VIP rule.

- Ventilate (oxygen administration).
- Infuse (fluid resuscitation).
- Pump (administration of vasoactive agents).

Sepsis-induced hypotension results from different pathological processes that require different treatments (i.e. at least 50% not fluid responsive). For example, hypovolaemia from intravascular volume loss due to increased vascular permeability requires fluid resuscitation, but vasodilation affecting both venous capacitance and arterial resistance is better treated with vasopressors (i.e. agents that vasoconstrict and increase systemic vascular resistance), and sepsis-related myocardial dysfunction may require inotropes (i.e. increase myocardial contractility).

- Norepinephrine (noradrenaline) is the first-choice vasopressor (Surviving Sepsis campaign, 2021). The target mean arterial pressure is ≥65 mmHg.
- Add vasopressin to norepinephrine and fluids if needed.
- Epinephrine (adrenaline) or dobutamine, which both have inotropic actions, can be used if cardiac dysfunction is contributing to hypotension.

Table 7.4 2021 Sepsis Six care bundle (incorporating Academy of Medical Royal Colleges, 2022 update)

If the patient looks unwell or NEWS2 is 5 or above, ask 'Could this be due to an infection?'.

If there are any high-risk features present (*red flags*), start Sepsis Six.

1 Ensure senior clinician attends: not all patients with *red flags* will need the Sepsis Six urgently. A senior decision maker may seek alternative diagnoses/de-escalate care.

2 Oxygen if required: start if oxygen saturations <92% – aim for saturations of 94–98%. If at risk of hypercapnic respiratory failure, aim for saturations of 88–92%.

3 Obtain intravenous access, take bloods: blood cultures, glucose, lactate, full blood count (FBC), urea and electrolytes, CRP and clotting.

4 Give intravenous antibiotics (do not delay in sick patient and preferably in first hour): maximum-dose broad-spectrum therapy. For possible sepsis and when shock is absent, antimicrobials may be given *within three hours* if concern for infection. Consider: local policy/allergy status/antivirals and antimicrobial stewardship. Source control of infection is important.

Academy of Medical Royal Colleges (2022): Administering antibiotics within one hour may be appropriate for the most severely ill patients with septic shock; however, extending the mandate to *all* patients with presumed sepsis is inappropriate and can cause harm and increased antibiotic resistance. For patients with *possible, probable* or *definite* infection, infection-specific diagnostic tests and administration of antimicrobials should be completed within 6, 3, or 1 hour (outer time limits) of recording a NEWS2 of 1–4, 5–6 or ≥7, respectively.

5 Give intravenous fluids (crystalloids recommended): give fluid bolus of 500 ml (adults). The National Institute for Health and Care Excellence (NICE) recommends using lactate to guide further fluid therapy. Surviving Sepsis campaign also recommends using vasopressors if hypotensive during or after fluid resuscitation to maintain a mean arterial pressure of ≥65 mmHg.

6 Monitor: use NEWS2, measure urine output, which may require a urinary catheter. Repeat lactate at least once per hour if initial lactate elevated (>2 mmol/l) or if clinical condition changes.

- For persistent hypotension, consider re-evaluation of other causes, and point-of-care echocardiogram may indicate whether inotropic support is indicated.
- Glucocorticoids should be used in patients with refractory septic shock.

Example of enhanced and critical care management – COVID-19

COVID-19 disease first emerged as a presentation of severe respiratory infection in Wuhan, China, in late 2019. By January 2020, lower respiratory samples taken from affected patients were sequenced and demonstrated a novel coronavirus (SARS-CoV-2). In March 2020, the World Health Organization (WHO) declared a SARS-CoV-2 pandemic. As with other coronaviruses, SARS-CoV-2 is a ribonucleic acid (RNA) virus which encodes four major structural proteins, including spike proteins which bind to angiotensin-converting enzyme 2 (ACE2) on host cells, and is endocytosed with subsequent release of the viral genome into the cytoplasm.

SARS-CoV-2 is primarily transmitted by person-to-person spread through respiratory aerosols, direct human contact and fomites. Estimates of the basic reproduction number (R) were initially between 2 and 3, although recent estimates for variants (e.g. omicron and subvariants) are even higher. This high transmissibility indicates that stringent control measures, such as active surveillance, physical distancing, mask wearing, early quarantine and contact tracing, are needed in order to control viral spread.

After the initial exposure, patients typically develop symptoms within 5–6 days (incubation period) although about 20% of patients remain asymptomatic throughout infection. Polymerase chain reaction (PCR) tests can detect viral SARS-CoV-2 RNA in the upper respiratory tract for a mean of 17 days, although transmission is maximal in the first week of illness. Symptomatic and pre-symptomatic transmission (1–2 days before symptom onset) is thought to play a greater role in the spread of SARS-CoV-2 than asymptomatic transmission.

In adults, the clinical picture varies widely. A significant proportion of individuals are likely to have mild symptoms and may be asymptomatic at the time of diagnosis. Symptoms are commonly reported as a new onset of cough and fever, but may include headache, loss of smell, nasal obstruction, lethargy, myalgia (aching muscles), rhinorrhoea (runny nose), taste dysfunction, sore throat, diarrhoea, vomiting and confusion; fever may not be reported in all symptomatic individuals. Patients may also be asymptomatic. Progression of disease, multiple organ failure and death will occur in some individuals.

Currently available data suggest that increasing age and male gender are significant risk factors for severe infection. However, there are also groups of patients with underlying co-morbidities (e.g. diabetes, cancer, immunosuppression, poorly controlled asthma) where infection may result in increased risk of serious disease and death. One in five people worldwide are estimated to be at higher risk of adverse COVID-19 outcomes based on the prevalence of chronic conditions. In Europe and the UK, deaths attributed to SARS-CoV-2 have been reported disproportionately from residential care. Other notable risk groups include healthcare workers who may acquire infection both in the hospital or within the community setting.

Health inequalities are unfair and avoidable differences in health among different groups within society. These differences may be segregated by social class, ethnicity, sex, geography and literacy, among other things. The COVID-19 pandemic starkly exposed ethnic health inequality. The disproportionate effect on black and Asian populations, caused by a complex interplay of social and biological factors, resulted in increased exposure, reduced protection and increased severity of illness and a higher risk for death from SARS-CoV-2 infection.

The recognition of the pandemic accelerated the development and testing of several vaccines. Vaccines predominantly focus on immunisation with the spike protein, which is the main target for neutralising antibodies. These vaccines have proven very useful at reducing infections, severity of disease, hospitalisations, the need for ventilation and death. Multiple booster doses have given added and more durable protection (especially in immunocompromised people). Nevertheless, breakthrough infection still occurs.

Many other interventions have also been tested and adopted, including antiviral agents, immunomodulators and antithrombotic agents in response to the multisystem effects of COVID-19 infection.

Management of COVID-19 infection in hospital

Patients who acquire COVID-19 infection after hospitalisation for the management of other conditions may require treatment. The first line treatment is Paxlovid delivered within 5 days of symptom onset. Remdesivir or sotrovimab can also be used.

The field of *covidology* is rapidly evolving and updated local and national guidelines should be used. Considerations for severe COVID-19 infections include the following.

- When a person is admitted to hospital with COVID-19, ensure a holistic assessment is done (such as co-morbidities, clinical frailty assessment and treatment expectations).
- Before escalating respiratory or other organ support, identify agreed treatment goals with the person (if possible), family or carers.
- Use track-and-trigger system (NEWS2) to identify acutely deteriorating patients.
- Basic oxygen therapy (e.g. low-flow oxygen supplementation – oxygen delivered by a simple facemask or nasal canula at a flow rate usually up to 15 l/min) and non-invasive respiratory support should be used where possible, based on the following.
  - How much supplemental oxygen is needed to reach target oxygen saturation?
  - Overall clinical trajectory?
  - Assessment of work of breathing.
  - How well will treatment be tolerated?
  - Treatment preferences after discussion with the person (or family or carers).

- Ensure that pharmacological and non-pharmacological management strategies, including body positioning (e.g. high supported sitting), are optimised before escalating treatment to non-invasive respiratory support.
- Consider offering CPAP to people with COVID-19 when:
  - they have hypoxaemia that is not responding to supplemental oxygen with a FiO_2 of 0.4 (40%) or more, *and*
  - escalation to invasive mechanical ventilation would be an option but it is not immediately needed, *or*
  - it is agreed that respiratory support should not be escalated beyond CPAP.

- Do not routinely offer high-flow nasal oxygen as the main form of respiratory support for people with COVID-19 and respiratory failure in whom escalation to invasive mechanical ventilation would be appropriate.
- Access to critical care providers for advice, review and prompt escalation of treatment if needed (such as when treatment has failed).
- Continue regular assessment and management of other symptoms alongside non-invasive respiratory support.
- Offer dexamethasone, or either hydrocortisone or (methyl)prednisolone when dexamethasone cannot be used (e.g. pregnancy other options preferred) or is unavailable, to people with COVID-19 who:
  - need supplemental oxygen to meet their prescribed oxygen saturation levels
  - continue glucocorticoids for up to 10 days unless there is a clear indication to stop early, which includes discharge from hospital or a hospital-supervised virtual COVID ward.

- Monitor glucose levels.
- Supportive care includes the following.
  - Fluids and electrolytes: use cautious fluid management in adults without tissue hypoperfusion and fluid responsiveness as aggressive fluid resuscitation may worsen oxygenation.
  - Correct any electrolyte or metabolic abnormalities, such as hyperglycaemia or metabolic acidosis, according to local protocols.
  - A hypercoagulable state is one of the hallmarks of disease, particularly in critically ill patients, often manifesting as venous and arterial thromboembolism. Start venous thromboembolism (VTE) prophylaxis in acutely ill hospitalised adults and adolescents, provided there are no contraindications. Monitor patients for signs and symptoms suggestive of thromboembolism and proceed with appropriate diagnostic and management pathways if clinically suspected.

- Consider empirical antibiotics if there is clinical suspicion of secondary bacterial infection (e.g. procalcitonin may be elevated).
- Consider an interleukin-6 (IL-6) inhibitor (e.g. tocilizumab or sarilumab), in combination with a systemic glucocorticoid and initiated at the same time, in patients with severe disease.
- Consider a Janus kinase (JAK) inhibitor (e.g. baricitinib), in combination with a systemic glucocorticoid

and initiated at the same time, in patients with severe disease *and* not on IL-6 inhibitor (except in life-threatening disease).

- Monoclonal antibodies directed at COVID-19 virus may be used in seronegative patients (i.e. no detectable SARS-CoV-2 antibodies), although these agents are generally reserved for early mild–moderate disease.

Critical COVID-19

Admit or transfer patients with critical disease (i.e. presence of ARDS, sepsis, or septic shock) to an ICU.

- Consider interventions as for severe COVID-19 infection noted above.
- Consider endotracheal intubation and mechanical ventilation in patients who are acutely deteriorating despite advanced oxygen/non-invasive ventilatory support measures.
- Mechanically ventilated patients with ARDS should receive a lung-protective, low tidal volume/low inspiratory pressure ventilation strategy.
- Consider prone ventilation (reduces gravity-dependent fluid deposition and atelectasis) in patients with severe ARDS for 12–16 hours per day.
- Consider extracorporeal membrane oxygenation (ECMO) – diverts the patient's circulation through an artificial external membrane to provide oxygen and remove carbon dioxide – according to availability and expertise if the above methods fail.

Multisystem complications of COVID-19

- Cardiovascular complications include arrhythmias, myocardial injury, acute coronary syndrome and heart failure.
- Acute kidney injury is common, particularly in critically ill patients. It can develop at any time before, during or after hospital admission.
- Liver injury may be associated with pre-existing liver disease, viral infection, drug toxicity, systemic inflammation, hypoxia or haemodynamic issues.
- Neurological sequelae are common.
  - Cerebrovascular disease: this includes COVID vaccine-induced thrombosis in association with thrombocytopenia (VITT). Thrombosis in VITT can occur in typical sites of VTE such as pulmonary embolism or DVT in the leg; however, a distinctive feature of the syndrome is thrombosis in unusual sites including the splenic

(splenic, portal, mesenteric) veins and cerebral veins. Arterial thrombosis including ischaemic stroke.
  - Other central or peripheral neurological complications, possibly due to viral invasion of the central nervous system, inflammatory response or immune dysregulation.

- In-hospital cardiac arrest is common in critically ill patients, and is associated with poor survival, particularly among older patients.
- Disseminated intravascular coagulation (DIC) is a manifestation of coagulation failure and related to multiorgan failure. Patients may be at high risk of bleeding or VTE.
- Some patients with severe disease have laboratory evidence of an unregulated inflammatory response similar to cytokine release syndrome ('cytokine storm'), characterised by plasma leakage, increased vascular permeability, DIC and immunodeficiency. These patients have a poor prognosis.

Palliative care

Palliative care interventions should be available for suitable patients with COVID-19.

Example of enhanced and critical care management – hypertensive crises

> Severe hypertension: BP $\geq$180 mmHg or diastolic BP $\geq$110 mmHg.

Hypertensive emergencies are defined by situations of uncontrolled hypertension resulting in acute or looming end-organ damage. Such end-organ involvement includes serious cardiac, vascular, cerebral and renal complications. In the severest forms, a hypertensive emergency can present as or progress to multiorgan failure, cardiovascular collapse and death. Lack of acute life-threatening end-organ damage distinguishes hypertensive emergency, requiring rapid therapeutic intervention, from hypertensive urgency, which may be managed by slower-acting agents and without the necessity for transfer of the patient to an HDU/ICU setting.

Hypertensive encephalopathy is believed to be due to cerebral oedema secondary to failure of the cerebral blood flow autoregulation and rapid elevation of cerebral perfusion. This induces cerebral vasodilation, cerebral oedema and subsequent clinical characteristics of acute lethargy, confusion, headache, visual disturbances and seizures. If untreated, cerebral oedema can progress to cerebral haemorrhage, coma and death

Management of hypertensive emergencies

The key to a successful outcome is the prompt recognition and initiation of treatment. Full medical history and physical examination, including palpation of all peripheral pulses and a fundoscopic examination, are mandatory (Box 7.1). Look for any pointers towards secondary hypertension. Initial investigations should include FBC, electrolytes, urea, creatinine, urine dipstick, chest X-ray and electrocardiogram. Echocardiogram should be performed emergently looking for left ventricular hypertrophy and diastolic dysfunction. These tests should be performed simultaneously with the initiation of antihypertensive therapy.

Box 7.1 First determine the presence or absence of the following

- Neurological symptoms.
  - Generalised: visual disturbance, agitation, delirium, seizures, coma (hypertensive encephalopathy).
  - Focal: stroke (thrombotic, haemorrhagic).
- Fundus: haemorrhage, exudates, papilloedema (malignant hypertension).
- Pain: chest, abdomen, back (aortic dissection, acute coronary syndrome).
- Breathlessness: pulmonary oedema (acute left ventricular failure).
- Nausea and vomiting: increased intracranial pressure (hypertensive encephalopathy).
- Pregnancy: pre-eclampsia, eclampsia.
- Drugs: e.g. cocaine, amphetamine.

Choice of BP lowering agent and BP targets

Hypotensive agents should be administered IV when organ damage is potentially life-threatening. All patients should be admitted to a coronary care unit, HDU or ITU bed, for continuous BP monitoring. The choice of drug will depend on the underlying cause or the organ most compromised.

- In general, for the patient with a hypertensive emergency, quick-acting antihypertensive drugs are required to bring the BP down and prevent the progression of target organ damage. The nature of end-organ involvement dictates the choice of antihypertensive agent and targeted BP falls. For example, aortic dissection carries the highest risk for rapid fatality and requires prompt and aggressive systolic BP lowering to at least 120 mmHg within 20 minutes.
- Specific drug considerations must also take into account the underlying pathology. For example, in the patient with phaeochromocytoma, the serious and potentially lethal cardiovascular complications of these tumours are due to the potent effects of secreted catecholamines. Hence, certain agents, such as beta-adrenergic receptor blockers, are contraindicated.
- Thus, management of the patient presenting with a hypertensive emergency is not only directed at safely lowering BP, but also must be tailored according to affected end-organs and underlying aetiology.

In most cases of hypertensive emergency, the first goal is a *partial reduction* and not necessarily normalisation of BP (e.g. diastolic BP to approximately 100–105 mmHg over 2–6 hours; maximum initial fall not to exceed 25%). However, guidelines also recommend that treatment of hypertensive emergencies should take into consideration the nature of the associated organ damage, with a range in treatment from no or extremely cautious lowering of BP in acute stroke (i.e. *permissive* hypertension) to prompt and aggressive BP reduction in acute pulmonary oedema or aortic dissection.

Rapid lowering of BP is particularly contraindicated in patients with cerebrovascular end-organ involvement, in whom excessive reduction of BP can lead to extension of stroke. Because of this, it has been suggested to consider antihypertensive therapy in patients with ischaemic stroke only when BP exceeds 220/120 mmHg. Even then, BP should be reduced only gradually. Labetalol is most commonly used for this indication. Lower BP thresholds (systolic >180 mmHg) for initiating antihypertensive therapy are, however, called for in patients with cerebral haemorrhage. In contrast, in the patient with aortic dissection, rapid lowering of systolic BP to at least 120 mmHg within 20 minutes has been advocated.

Parenteral antihypertensives are recommended over oral agents in initial treatment of hypertensive emergency, e.g. glyceryl trinitrate (GTN); sodium nitroprusside (caution about cyanide toxicity); labetalol; or calcium channel blocker (such as nicardipine). Choice of agent depends on aetiology and associated target organ damage (and can be combined with oral agents to transition from parenteral route).

Management of hypertensive urgencies

The goal is to reduce BP to <160/100 mmHg over several hours to a day. For known hypertensive patients who are not compliant with their medication, prior therapy should be restarted. For patients taking their medication regularly, therapy should be increased (either by increasing the dose(s) of drugs or adding new drugs). For patients on no treatment, hypertension therapy should be started with oral agents (e.g. monotherapy or combination therapy). Start with nifedipine (extended-release formulations) 10 mg tablets, swallowed whole (DO NOT 'bite and swallow' as per old teaching!). The same dose can be repeated at two hours if required, with maintenance doses of up to 20 mg three times a day. Amlodipine 5–10 mg is a useful alternative. Beta-blockers can be added. Follow-up appointment should be arranged urgently with the hypertension or GP clinic. Monitor renal function frequently initially. Screen for secondary causes of hypertension (including alcohol excess).

8

Acute Medicine in the ambulatory care setting

Glenn Matfin

 KEY POINTS

- Medical emergencies are the most frequent cause of unscheduled hospital admission, and place considerable demands on acute healthcare services.
- Some patients with an acute medical illness can be assessed and treated through ambulatory care pathways without inpatient admission, via same-day emergency care (SDEC).
- Selecting the right patients for SDEC is essential to maintain safety and maximise the impact on emergency flows. Patient selection for SDEC is best provided by a clinical conversation between senior clinicians, often supported by using scoring systems and condition-specific risk stratification tools.

Introduction

Medical emergencies are the most frequent cause of unplanned hospital admission, and place considerable demands on acute healthcare services (including adversely affecting other patient pathways). During times of increased pressure, such as the perennial winter period or waves of the recent COVID-19 pandemic, increased unplanned admissions also negatively affect the delivery of elective services (>7 million waiting in 2022). It is an operational and clinical imperative to maximise capacity within acute care settings, such as by hospital 'front door' (the point of arrival/entry to hospital) reconfiguration measures leading to admission avoidance.

Some patients with an acute medical illness can be assessed and treated through ambulatory care pathways without inpatient admission. Ambulatory emergency care (AEC) provides patients with an acute illness who have been referred to secondary care with the traditional aspects of urgent medical care (i.e. assessment, investigations and management) whilst avoiding overnight inpatient admission. Processes are streamlined, including review by a consultant, timely access to diagnostics and treatments all being delivered within one working day (if needed).

The underlying principle of AEC is to convert traditional inpatient care into *same-day* emergency care. Approximately 80% of SDEC is delivered by the Acute Medicine service in AEC units. This innovative approach to acute medical care at the interface between primary and secondary care has improved both clinical outcomes and patient experience, while reducing costs. Given that SDEC is provided in a clinic-style setting, it can continue to operate during periods of high bed occupancy, alleviating bed pressures and providing timely care for selected patients. Ongoing ambulatory care may be provided either directly through the SDEC unit or by community services, primary care, telemedicine, rapid-access clinics or Hospital at Home.

Acute Medicine: Lecture Notes, First Edition. Edited by Glenn Matfin.
© 2023 John Wiley & Sons Ltd. Published 2023 by John Wiley & Sons Ltd.

SDEC is process-driven, risk-stratified emergency care, seeing the right person in the right place, in a timely fashion, with structured assessment and management using protocolised pathways. SDEC is the process of managing, diagnosing, observing, treating and rehabilitating a proportion of non-elective patients on the same day, without the need for admission to an inpatient hospital bed.

Principles of SDEC services

The structure of SDEC services varies nationally within the UK, and there is no clear evidence regarding the optimum way to design these services. Several models of SDEC are emerging.

The most effective model starts with a clinical conversation between senior clinicians (e.g. doctor or nurse) in the referring area (e.g. emergency department or community care) and SDEC teams to assess clinical severity and suitability for SDEC.

Identification of patients suitable for ambulatory management

Several scoring systems are available to identify SDEC patients from unselected medical admissions (i.e. medical admissions that have not been selected out as belonging to a specific medical specialty), including the Ambulatory Care Score (AMB Score) and the Glasgow Admission Prediction Score (GAPS). The AMB score indicates patients suitable for SDEC based on seven patient characteristics. Both the AMB score and GAPS are designed to be used early in patient pathways before a diagnosis is made. Since 2018, the more nuanced National Early Warning Score (NEWS2), including new-onset confusion and adjusted oxygen saturation ranges in patients with hypercapnic respiratory failure, has been mandated nationally in acute hospitals. The impact of incorporating the NEWS2 score in the AMB score and GAPS (which both use NEWS) has not been evaluated.

The use of scoring systems does not replace clinical judgement or prior experience in ambulatory care. For example, some SDEC units do not use selection scores and take an 'inclusive' approach based on the senior clinical conversation so end up ambulating at higher levels of acuity (but with close senior oversight and up-front diagnostics to support decision making and ambulatory treatment pathways). These scores may inhibit ambulatory care (e.g. being aged >80 years, needing intravenous treatment, having a NEWS of 1 or 2, are all perfectly compatible with an ambulatory care medical model), but they can help units get off the ground if they don't do much SDEC and need to build institutional confidence.

The decision about a patient's suitability for SDEC at the point of referral should be based on the following four questions.

1 **Is the patient clinically stable?** Clear exclusion criteria based on the NEWS2 score used in conjunction with other clinical information should be utilised to maximise effective patient flow to SDEC.

2 **Is the patient functionally capable of being managed in SDEC?** Ability to maintain privacy and dignity in the SDEC unit, including managing toileting needs and nutrition.

3 **Would this patient have been admitted to hospital before SDEC existed?** If no, they should not be referred to SDEC.

4 **Could the patient's clinical needs be better met by another service?**

Organisation of SDEC units

Where possible, the SDEC service should be co-located with the ED and Acute Medical Unit (AMU).

- Staffing (blended medical workforce) and resources should be organised to provide rapid assessment, diagnosis and treatment on the same day. Waiting times for patients in SDEC should be minimised. Patients should have the same access to urgent investigations as inpatients or patients attending the ED. Close interaction with radiology is critical. Point-of-care ultrasound (POCUS) has increasing utility in a range of presentations and clinical management.

- Continued access to senior clinical staff is key for the service to work effectively. A consultant physician should be available on the hospital site throughout the opening times of the SDEC unit to review SDEC patients.

- A key feature of SDEC is the use of ambulatory care pathways, for example the diagnosis and treatment of cellulitis. Clinical pathways can be helpful for high-volume clinical scenarios such as deep vein thrombosis (DVT), chest pain, pulmonary embolism and heart failure, but are less helpful for less

Table 8.1 **Condition-specific risk stratification tools to support patient streaming and early discharge (examples)**

Condition	Risk stratification tool
Acute upper gastrointestinal bleed	Glasgow-Blatchford Bleeding Score
Pulmonary embolism	Pulmonary embolism severity index (PESI), simplified PESI; recommended by the British Thoracic Society
Pneumonia	CURB-65 score; recommended by the British Thoracic Society
Syncope	San Francisco Syncope Rule – 'CHESS' • Congestive heart failure (history of) • Haematocrit <30% • ECG abnormal • Shortness of breath • Systolic blood pressure <90 mmHg If any of the above features are present – patient is NOT IN LOW-RISK group

common presentations or those of diagnostic uncertainty.

- For defined clinical scenarios, there are several validated risk stratification tools (Table 8.1) that can be used to support decision making once the diagnosis is made to facilitate early discharge and therefore suitability for SDEC. Tools are not a replacement for clinical expertise and knowledge but should be a guide to help with objective decision making. They should also be used to assist with auditing of pathways.
- Not all SDEC assessments and treatments need to be delivered within the same day, and patients can return on subsequent days, including for specialist outpatient services. Secondary and primary care services should be geared around patient needs (i.e. patient-centred) and work together to provide ongoing care outside hospital, to avoid a full admission.
- Equity of access. Frail and vulnerable patients, including those with disabilities and mental health problems of all ages, should be managed assertively but holistically with support by a multidisciplinary team (MDT) to cover medical, psychological, social and functional domains and their care transferred back into the community as soon as they are medically fit, to avoid them losing their ability to self-care.
- Comprehensive records must be kept. A same-day discharge summary for a single episode of care should be created at the end of the SDEC episode and sent to the GP and given to the patient. This should include details of investigations undertaken, any new therapies instigated and the follow-up plan required and arranged.
- During the period of care under the ambulatory team, patients should have clear written instructions for actions to take if they feel they are deteriorating

(i.e. safety netting) or if they wish to discuss concerns prior to their next scheduled visit.
- SDEC units should not be bedded overnight to increase inpatient capacity.
- Clear measures must be adopted and monitored to assess impact, quality and efficiency.
- Need to collect patient experience data at regular intervals. Review of SDEC performance should occur using at least the standard metrics as suggested by the Royal College of Physicians of Edinburgh and the Society of Acute Medicine.
- Good communication and staff training are needed across the local healthcare system to ensure that all appropriate patients are directed to the SDEC service.

Benefits of SDEC

The benefits of effective SDEC delivery for teams working to deliver acute care 'at the front door' include the following.

- Reducing unwarranted variation in care pathways.
- Streamlining the patient journey, with most patients completing their care in a single visit.
- Better patient and staff satisfaction.
- Reduction of admissions and improvement of flow in the acute admission pathway. At least 20–30% of 'usual' emergency admissions being converted to SDEC. Decreased 30-day readmission rates compared with standard inpatient care pathways.
- Avoiding the risks associated with inpatient admission.
- Medical trainees get closer consultant supervision (e.g. practical procedures, but also for other competencies like managing uncertainty).

Selection of patients for SDEC

Selecting the right patients for SDEC is essential to maintain safety (risk management) and maximise the impact on emergency flows. However, all patients should be considered for SDEC, with it being the default position until otherwise proven. SDEC should facilitate the right people to be treated in the right place at the right time for that person's condition and is intended to bring about a positive experience and achieve the best outcomes for that patient.

There are several broad categories of patients that can be considered for SDEC.

- Patients to be assessed for diagnostic evaluation (e.g. chest pain, DVT).
- Patients who require treatment provision (e.g. out-patient intravenous antibiotics).
- Patients who require procedural intervention (e.g. pleural effusion management, paracentesis).
- Patients who would benefit from input and intervention from frailty teams (e.g. MDT assessment and interventions for older patients).
- Patients who were discharged early from the AMU or other acute medical care setting (e.g. short-stay ward) who require an earlier review to ensure that they are continuing to improve (e.g. the patient with acute kidney injury who is improving but needs creatinine, urea and electrolytes rechecking).

Selection of clinical diagnoses appropriate for SDEC is evolving and dependent on local circumstances. There should be continued focus on increasing the types of emergency patients and conditions that can be treated on the same day.

9

Acute Medicine in the home

Daniel Lasserson

 KEY POINTS

- Acute Hospital at Home services replace the need for admission (admission avoidance) or enable earlier discharge from hospital (early supported discharge) by delivering hospital-level processes of care in the home or care home.
- Point-of-care testing (blood and ultrasound) supports acute medical decision making in the home.
- Intravenous treatments such as diuretics, antibiotics and fluids as well as oxygen can be delivered in the home, using regimens that are adapted for the home environment.
- Multidisciplinary team working is essential, as most patients are older and live with frailty.

Introduction

Acute Hospital at Home (H@H) was developed to provide an alternative model of care for patients who would otherwise need to be admitted to hospital for acute assessment and treatment. It is most suitable for older patients living with frailty who are at higher risk of complications from treatment in hospital, such as deconditioning and delirium. Patients, their families and carers should make an informed choice over location of care for an acute medical illness, understanding the risks and benefits of both care in-hospital and care at home.

Randomised trials of Acute H@H show that it has an equivalent level of mortality to care in hospital, a reduced incidence of delirium and a reduced probability of needing to move to residential care at six months after acute medical illness. It is also cost-effective and cheaper than inpatient care.

Referral pathways into H@H services

Replacing admission

H@H services that aim to replace admission (named 'admission avoidance') should be referred acutely unwell patients directly from primary care, paramedics or from acute medical call takers who have assessed the potential for a H@H pathway of care. H@H services that replace the need for transfer to hospital require point-of-care (POC) diagnostic tests that can be used in the home and should carry a range of treatments covering the common conditions anticipated from the initial clinical details at the point of referral to the service.

Considerations for H@H service assessment rather than transfer to hospital for assessment should include the following.

- Patient informed choice supported if possible by family member and/or carer.

- Advanced care plan specifying H@H rather than hospital care.
- Suitability of the home environment for healthcare delivery (e.g. absence of safety risks to healthcare staff who may attend the patient alone).
- Acute illness syndrome corresponding to common conditions treated by the local H@H team.

Referrals to H@H for admission avoidance should include key details about presenting symptoms, vital signs, current medications, any available past history and social support. This helps the H@H team plan the initial visit, and whether they need any additional equipment or medication alongside their core drugs.

> Conditions where there is a high risk of deterioration and an advanced care plan includes admission to critical care are *not suitable* for H@H care.

Supporting early discharge

H@H services that support discharge from hospital should be referred patients after an initial hospital-based assessment and treatment, from on-call medical teams, emergency department (ED) teams or ward-based medical teams. Early supported discharge H@H has less requirement for POC testing as patients will have already had extensive diagnostic assessment at the hospital front door. This greater diagnostic certainty at referral means that the referring team can specify an initial medical management plan for the H@H team to deliver.

Referral for early supported discharge H@H should include key information for safe ongoing management in a community setting for an acute medical illness, including diagnosis, results of key investigations, medical management plan, social support, any outstanding investigations and whether the medical responsibility is being passed on to the H@H consultant or retained with the referring consultant.

Presenting syndromes and acute medical conditions treated by H@H

Common presenting acute illness syndromes treated by H@H are related to underlying frailty as well as common medical conditions with localising symptoms.

- Confusion.
- Falls.
- Functional decline.
- New incontinence.
- Breathlessness.
- Fever.

Common underlying conditions diagnosed and treated by H@H include the following.

- Pneumonia.
- COVID-19 pneumonitis (with ceiling of care in advanced care plan).
- Cellulitis.
- Urinary tract infection.
- Bacteraemia with unclear focus (liaison with infectious diseases team required).
- Decompensated acute heart failure.
- Acute kidney injury.
- Dehydration and/or hypernatraemia.
- Atrial fibrillation with fast ventricular response.

Processes of care in the H@H service and acute hospital

Patients treated by H@H should have the same prioritised access to key investigations as patients who are admitted to hospital. This should be a balance between POC tests and, if necessary, single-day attendance at hospital for more advanced tests.

Blood tests

- POC tests in the home: electrolytes, renal function, C-reactive protein (CRP), lactate, gases, glucose and ketones.
- Samples taken at home and sent back to the laboratory: full blood count, liver function tests, blood culture, additional tests as required (e.g. haematinics, thyroid function tests, cortisol).

Imaging

- Point-of-care ultrasound (POCUS) has a major role in H@H care for rapid identification of underlying causes for acute illness syndromes and/or confirming clinical suspicion from physical examination.
- Conditions identified using POCUS include pleural effusion, pneumonia, COVID-19 pneumonitis,

pericardial effusion, reduced left ventricular function, ascites, hydronephrosis, urinary retention, bowel obstruction and deep vein thrombosis.

- POCUS image sharing with specialty teams can support the H@H team in management decisions.
- Transfer to hospital may be needed for plain X-ray (e.g. hip fracture post fall) and computed tomography (CT) scanning (e.g. CT pulmonary angiogram if pulmonary embolus suspected, CT chest/abdomen/pelvis for suspected metastatic malignancy). For the majority of patients transferred for such tests, they can continue at home afterwards under the H@H team, with changes in management determined by imaging results.

Specialist investigations

Other investigations (e.g., gastrointestinal endoscopy) should be performed within the same timeframes as if the patient is in hospital.

Parenteral therapy

- Intravenous (IV) fluid can be given for rehydration, usually 1 Litre boluses of normal saline (0.9% NaCl) or balanced crystalloid over 90 minutes if no risk of circulatory overload and patients are not hypernatraemic.
- For hypernatraemic patients, slow infusions of 'free water' solutions are required, either 5% glucose IV or subcutaneous infusions of 4% glucose/0.18% NaCl.
- IV antibiotics should be approved by the local formulary, adapted to the availability of visiting nurses in the H@H team (e.g. use of once- or twice-daily dosing).
- For antimicrobial stewardship, narrow-spectrum antibiotics should be first line, and if multiple dosing is required, use of 24-hour infusions should be considered (e.g. flucloxacillin 8 g/24 hours).
- Patients with fluid overload requiring high-dose furosemide should have infusions delivered using monitored devices to ensure accurate infusion rates.
- Most patients can be managed with peripheral cannulae, monitored daily for skin reactions and changed when necessary. For prolonged IV treatment, midlines are preferred.

Oxygen

- Short-duration oxygen therapy can be given through H@H. If long-term therapy is subsequently needed, referral should be made to the community respiratory team.
- Portable oxygen concentrators allow flow rates of 4–5 l/min and can be used with Venturi masks for controlled fraction of inspired oxygen (FiO_2) of 24% or 28%.
- Safety assessments must be made about use of oxygen in the home (e.g. smoking).

Multidisciplinary working in H@H

- Older adults with frailty and acute illness managed at home should undergo comprehensive geriatric assessment (CGA) and may require input from physiotherapists, occupational therapists, speech and language therapists, and clinical pharmacists alongside nursing and medical assessment.
- Specialist teams, working in a multidisciplinary team (MDT) format, can support H@H in managing particular patients, including heart failure, respiratory and infectious diseases.

H@H and communication with primary care

- The patient's primary care team should be notified at the point of referral (either admission avoidance or early supported discharge) that they are being managed at home by the H@H team.
- The H@H team should be available on a daily basis to answer queries from primary care about patients they are managing.
- At the point of discharge back to primary care, the H@H team should provide details of diagnosis, progress during treatment and results of key investigations, new medication regimen and changes to existing treatments, further monitoring needed and whether there are changes to the advanced care plan.

10

Effective discharge planning

Glenn Matfin

 KEY POINTS

- It is an operational and clinical imperative to maximise capacity within acute care settings through safe, timely discharge.
- Discharge planning should begin on admission.
- Once the patient is admitted, improving patient flow throughout the hospital should be addressed, such as early senior review of patients in the emergency department; 'pushing' and 'pulling' specialty patients to appropriate specialty wards from the medical assessment and/or internal medicine/outlier wards earlier in the day; and having daily board and/or ward rounds.
- Hospital 'front door' reconfiguration measures can lead to fewer admissions and decrease hospital crowding. Use Alternatives to ED (A-tED) and Admission (A-tA) tools.
- Effective discharge planning by multidisciplinary team interactions with postacute, social and primary care providers can facilitate effective discharge from hospital ('back door') to the most appropriate setting, and hopefully prevent readmission.

Introduction

We are practising medicine at a time of unprecedented demand for medical care, with capacity reaching saturation in primary, secondary, postacute and social care. This has been compounded by the COVID-19 pandemic. It is an operational and clinical imperative to maximise capacity within acute care settings through safe, timely discharge (see Figure 1.1).

The entry point to healthcare is often referred to as the 'front door'. Traditionally, primary care was the starting point for the typical patient journey. However, many patients now begin their patient journey in the beleaguered emergency department (ED) rather than directly through primary care or the main hospital assessment units, such as acute medical unit (AMU). This has several important consequences.

- Pressure on beds in the NHS (and in other countries) results in increased waiting times in ED (so-called 'trolley waits'). This crowding in the ED can lead to ambulances being stuck outside hospitals unable to offload patients, with inevitable

Acute Medicine: Lecture Notes, First Edition. Edited by Glenn Matfin.
© 2023 John Wiley & Sons Ltd. Published 2023 by John Wiley & Sons Ltd.

negative impact on health outcomes (unsafe handover delays and poor patient experience).

- One way to measure crowding in the ED is to use the four-hour ED waiting time target. This operational standard, set in 2010, states that at least 95% of patients attending ED should be admitted, transferred or discharged within four hours. Performance initially remained close to or above the new target. Since the onset of the COVID-19 pandemic, however, the number of EDs reaching this target has fallen dramatically. For example, January 2023 NHS performance data showed only 57% of patients were seen within four hours in major (type 1) EDs, and more than 42 000 patients needing admission waited longer than 12 hours in ED (target is that no patient should wait longer than 12 hours if needing admission).
- Crowding in the ED and other parts of the hospital can lead to patient safety concerns (such as maintaining cleanliness and controlling infections) and is stressful for staff and patients alike (especially as these patients tend to get moved around to accommodate others). In addition, many of these patients are often older, frail high-acuity patients.
- As the various assessment units (e.g. AMU or similar) also become fuller due to increased admissions, cohorting patients to reduce nosocomial COVID-19 infections and an inability to 'push' patients to the most suitable wards (i.e. specialist or internal medicine beds) increase the likelihood that the patient will end up on the 'wrong' ward such as medical outlier wards (i.e. medical patients within the surgical or non-medical bed base).
- The additional burden of staffing these non-medical wards with appropriately skilled medical, nursing and other relevant healthcare professionals (e.g. physiotherapists, occupational therapists) is a major daily challenge.
- All of these (and many other) issues can further delay timely patient access to the right specialty, and discharge-dependent investigative and/or therapeutic procedures.
- In addition, the inability to discharge 'medically fit' older frail patients who have onward community care needs (i.e. postacute care such as rehabilitation, or social care) due to back door 'exit block' is also concerning. More than 13% beds are occupied by patients in this position. This is due to significant issues in postacute and social care delivery and capacity (e.g. chronic underfunding, closure of many facilities and lack of trained staff with more than 165 000 vacancies in social care).

Reducing length of stay

- The number of patients stuck in hospital in the UK because of delays in discharge has increased significantly in recent years. Consequently, the average length of stay in acute medical care in the UK is prolonged compared to many similar countries.
- Reducing length of stay provides patients with a better care experience by ensuring they are discharged from hospital without unnecessary delay.
- Prolonged stays in hospital are bad for patients, especially those who are frail or elderly. Spending a long time in hospital can lead to an increased risk of falling, sleep deprivation, catching infections and sometimes mental and physical deconditioning.
- Reducing the number of long stays (21 days or more) is an important target for the UK NHS. By ensuring patients return to their usual place of residence, or another care setting as soon as it is safe to do so, patient flow will improve right through the system. Beds will be free for those needing quick admission for emergency care, which in turn will have a positive impact on reducing crowding in the hospital.
- The need for a timely discharge, however, should not result in discharges that are unsafe, such as happening overnight, or lead to people not being fully informed as to the next stages of their care.

Avoidance of Acute Medicine admission

It is essential to find innovative ways of avoiding hospital admission (i.e. front door reconfiguration) by best practice streaming. This includes providing early senior advice to GP and ED teams, and helping develop admission avoidance pathways, such as the following.

- Providing patient digital-first access to healthcare service (i.e. digital 'front door').
- NHS 111 was set up as a helpline for urgent medical concerns.
- Improving prehospital care (e.g. paramedic practitioner/urgent care practitioner).
- Improving patient triage from primary care.
- Earlier specialty review and treatment for patients who may otherwise decompensate via telemedicine or rapid-access (hot) clinics.
- Earlier generalist review and treatment in the ED or same-day emergency care (SDEC) unit.

- Improving access to Acute Medicine. Develop services to enable direct access, ensuring clinical conversations are used to direct patients to the most appropriate service/areas to meet their clinical needs.
- Interface Medicine: managing patients with undifferentiated illness who are at an interface between primary and secondary acute care. For example, Hospital at Home is an innovative care model that provides hospital-level care in a patient's home (see Chapter 9). Similarly, 'virtual wards' in the patient's home with monitoring through phone calls or digitally from a team of clinicians, as well as patient monitoring apps, have been useful during and post-COVID-19 pandemic.

Effective discharge planning

Once people no longer need hospital care, being at home or in a community setting (such as a care home) is the best place for them to continue recovery. However, unnecessary delays in being discharged from hospital (exit block) are a problem that too many people experience (flow 'gridlocked').

- Discharge planning should begin on admission and involve as wide a network of health and social care as required to facilitate safe and effective discharge planning.
- All people who no longer meet the clinical criteria to reside for inpatient care in acute hospitals should be discharged as soon as possible on the same day. The Criteria to Reside tool equips clinical teams to have discussions and make decisions on whether a person needs to stay in an acute bed to receive care (Table 10.1).
- Discharge home should be the default pathway. However, people may also be transferred to a non-acute setting as needed.
- Every local health and social care system should have a 'transfer of care' hub (or similar). The hub should link a wide range of health and social care and wider services. It should play a key co-ordinating role to aid discharge and admission avoidance.
- Seven-day care is important too. This can facilitate timely and safe discharge, especially over a weekend and bank holidays.

Table 10.1 Criteria to Reside tool – maintaining good decision making in acute care settings

Every person on every general ward should be reviewed on a twice-daily ward round to determine the following. If the answer to each question is 'no', active consideration for discharge to a less acute setting must be made.

- Requiring critical care?
- Requiring oxygen therapy or non-invasive ventilation?
- Requiring intravenous (IV) fluids?
- NEWS2 score >3?
- Diminished level of consciousness where recovery realistic?
- Acute functional impairment in excess of home/community care provision?
- Last hours of life?
- Requiring IV medication > twice daily (including analgesia)?
- Within 24 hours of an invasive procedure (with attendant risk of acute life-threatening deterioration)?

Clinical exceptions will occur (especially as Hospital at Home services become more widely available) but must be warranted and justified. Recording the rationale will assist meaningful, time-efficient review.

Review and challenge questions for the clinical team

- Is the person medically optimised? Do not use terms 'medically fit' or 'back to baseline'.
- What management can be continued by SDEC or Hospital at Home teams, for example heart failure treatment or IV fluids/antibiotics? Persons with low NEWS2 scores (0–3) – can they be discharged with suitable follow-up?
- Not needing any medical/nursing care after 8 pm.
  - People waiting for results: can they come back or can the results be phoned through or via telemedicine or SDEC?
  - Repeat bloods: can they be done after discharge in an alternative setting?
  - People waiting for investigations: can they go home and come back as outpatients with the same waiting time as inpatients?

Acute Medicine best practice approach to effective discharge planning

> Hospital 'front door' reconfiguration measures can lead to fewer admissions and decrease hospital crowding.

Once the patient is admitted, improving patient flow throughout the hospital, such as early senior review of patients in the ED; 'pushing' and 'pulling' specialty patients to appropriate specialty wards from the assessment or internal medicine/outlier wards earlier in the day; and having daily ward and/or board rounds all help (see Box 1.1).

Effective discharge planning by multidisciplinary team (MDT) interactions with postacute, social and primary care providers can facilitate effective discharge from hospital (back door) to the most appropriate setting, and hopefully will prevent read-mission. Hospital readmissions following discharge are rightly considered an adverse outcome. While a failure of social and other community care may contribute to readmission rates, such events are never-theless regarded as markers of suboptimal healthcare delivery.

Practical arrangements to support safe and timely discharge from acute settings

Follow the five key principles of 'Where best, next?'.

1 Plan for discharge from the start.
2 Involve patients and their families in discharge decisions.
3 Establish systems and processes for frail people.
4 Embed MDT reviews. The MDT needs to manage the interface with community services, including complex discharge planning to clearly describe the support people will require when they are discharged or transferred.
5 Encourage a supported 'Home First' approach.

Other practicalities related to effective discharge.

- Estimate an expected date of discharge at the point of admission.

- A clinical review of all patients seven days a week using the Criteria to Reside tool (see Table 10.1).
- Review 21+ day length of stay patients and work in a co-ordinated way with system partners to ensure people have the support they need to be discharged.
- Implement board-level reporting of length of stay, onward destinations, delays and reasons for delays. Improve and streamline escalation procedures.
- Early planning in relation to transport and take-home medication to enable discharge before 5 pm.
- Create a multidisciplinary triage process at the 'front door' of the transfer of care hub with no sepa-rate routes into or out of the hub. The hub decides the pathway and discharge destination.
- Specialist clinicians should work alongside the ED at peak demand times to own patients from time of arrival at hospital.
- Acute Medicine patients should be appropriately referred to AMU/SDEC.
- Supporting ED colleagues to improve patient flow and reduce crowding.
  - Engaging in flow-enhancing processes such as using SAFER patient flow bundle (Table 10.2), extended hours and seven-day working, and maximising use of ambulatory care can all improve hospital crowding.
  - Contribute to ED capacity/reduce duplication by bringing processes as far forward as possible, such as Acute Medicine medical trainees work-ing in the ED seeing Acute Medicine patients first off.

Table 10.2 Consistent implementation of the SAFER patient flow bundle on all assessment and medical wards

S – Senior Review. All patients will have a senior review before midday by a clinician able to make management and discharge decisions.

A – All patients will have an expected discharge date and clinical criteria for discharge. This is set assuming ideal recovery and assuming no unnecessary waiting.

F – Flow of patients will commence at the earliest opportunity from assessment units to inpatient wards. Wards that routinely receive patients from assessment units will ensure the first patient arrives on the ward by 10 am.

E – Early discharge. 33% of patients will be discharged from base inpatient wards before midday. Effective use of discharge lounge.

R – Review. A systematic MDT review of patients with extended lengths of stay (>7 days – 'stranded patients') with a clear 'Home First' mindset.

- Workforce is aligned to peak hours of demand, and weekend and bank holiday working.
- Ownership of the Acute Medicine take.
- Daily ward rounds on all medical and medical outlier wards to review new and unwell patients and to promote timely discharge (with targeted ward rounds at weekends to support discharge decision making). Start with board rounds (Table 10.3) and consider sick and unstable patients first. The ward round should follow the board round each day. Patients should be seen in a specific order: sick unstable patients first; potential discharges next; and then the remaining patients. A record of the round, with clear management plans, should be written in the patient's notes.
- Ensure twice-daily MDT review (consultant review at least daily) of all people in acute medical beds to agree who no longer meets the clinical Criteria to Reside for inpatient care and therefore should be discharged.
- Specialty teams including cardiac, respiratory, gastrointestinal and frailty teams support patients to be seen in the most appropriate setting, improving delivery of acute care.
- Limited functional assessments should take place in the acute setting. People requiring ongoing support should be discharged to assess.
- Facilitate prompt and accurate information sharing with key stakeholders (e.g. primary and secondary care team) following hospital discharge.

Safety netting

- Conduct patient-initiated follow-up. Give people the direct number of the ward they are discharged from to call back for advice. Do not suggest going back to their GP or going to the ED.
- Request immediate arrangements for discharge with a plan for virtual follow-up where needed. Alternatively, review the patient in the SDEC (or equivalent).
- Manage people virtually or in outpatient clinics under the care of the same team/specialty.
- Request community nursing and/or GP follow-up where appropriate.
- Assess the need for COVID-19 testing prior to discharge (e.g. to a care home).

Always advise patient if the medical condition related to admission (new or existing) impacts on *driving post discharge*. If a patient has a condition that impairs their ability and makes them unsafe to drive, then the doctor has a duty to inform the patient and the patient is legally obliged to inform the Driver and Vehicle Licensing Agency (DVLA). This must be documented in the notes and recorded in the discharge summary.

Criteria-led discharge

Document clear clinical criteria by which the person no longer meets the Criteria to Reside that can be enacted by an appropriate clinician without further consultant review.

Table 10.3 The board round checklist for use on all assessment and medical wards

The board round introduces structure to the day-to-day running of the ward and helps the ward MDT to manage patients safely and effectively.

- Consider sick and unstable patients first – is the patient deteriorating? What actions are required?
- What is the patient treatment plan?
- What are the clinical criteria for discharge?
- What is the expected date of discharge (EDD)? Does it reflect the planned date of discharge (PDD)?
- Will the patient have onward care needs?
- Does the patient agree with their plan and discharge date?
- Are there any patients to be discharged today/tomorrow? What needs to be done to ensure they go before midday?

Self-discharge against medical advice

Make sure you are familiar with the patient's case, so you understand the risks if the patient were to self-discharge. Seek senior support early and security if appropriate. An informed competent patient should be able to refuse admission or leave at will with no prejudice to ongoing care.

- Assess the patient's understanding of their own condition and treatment.
- Ask why they want to leave.
- If the patient is firm that they want to go home, a helpful question can be 'Why would I be worried about you if you were to leave?'. This allows you to assess whether they understand the risks and are willing to take them. If there is a risk of serious harm, then explain and document.
- If a patient has the capacity to self-discharge, is there an alternative that might work, such as Acute Medicine in the ambulatory setting – SDEC or rapid-access clinic? Acute Medicine in the home setting – Hospital at Home, virtual ward, telemedicine?
- All patients who self-discharge should have a discharge letter completed. Ideally, also contact their GP or any relevant specialists directly upon self-discharge (e.g. email). These patients are at high risk of re-presenting and the next team and the GP will need to know what has happened.
- Supply medications if possible.
- Restraint of any kind should be seen as a last resort. Choosing to detain a patient will often escalate the situation. It is important to follow hospital guidelines.
  - o The Mental Capacity Act: allows restraint and restrictions to be used but only if they are in a person's best interests.
  - o Deprivation of Liberty Safeguards (DoLS): extra safeguards are needed if the restrictions and restraint used will deprive a person of their liberty. DoLS ensures people who cannot consent to their care arrangements in hospital are protected if those arrangements deprive them of their liberty.
- If the patient does leave and you have not been able to restrain them, then involve hospital security and police as needed.

11

Point-of-care ultrasound in Acute Medicine

Rasha Buhumaid

 KEY POINTS

- Point-of-care ultrasound (POCUS) is an essential skill for Acute Medicine clinicians.
- The advantages of POCUS are that it is rapid, portable, cost-effective, dynamic, reproducible and with minimal radiation exposure to the patient. It can also be repeated as often as needed. However, its main disadvantage is that image quality and interpretation are dependent on the skills of the operator.
- Thoracic POCUS can aid in the diagnosis (i.e. as part of BLUE protocol) of pneumonia, pleural effusion, interstitial syndrome (e.g. pulmonary oedema), exacerbated chronic obstructive pulmonary disease or asthma, pulmonary embolism and pneumothorax.
- Thoracic combined with focused cardiac POCUS has been especially useful during the management of COVID-19 patients.
- Abdominal and renal POCUS can aid in the diagnosis of intraperitoneal free fluid, hydronephrosis and bladder distension.
- POCUS can be used to diagnose the majority of lower extremity deep vein thrombosis.
- When POCUS is used to guide procedures such as vascular access, thoracocentesis and paracentesis, it improves the success rate and decreases the complication rate.

Introduction

Point-of-care ultrasound is also known as POCUS, bedside ultrasound or clinician-performed ultrasound. POCUS is a form of diagnostic ultrasound examination performed by the clinician at the patient's bedside with real-time application, which aims to answer specific physiological and anatomical questions to establish a clinical diagnosis or guide a procedure.

POCUS is associated with changes in clinical decision making. A recent study showed that POCUS facilitated confirmation of the suspected clinical diagnosis in up to 50% of cases and supported a change in the initial diagnosis in almost a quarter of cases. Clinicians who become proficient in POCUS can also use it to track clinical conditions that may progress rapidly – for example, acute respiratory failure and haemodynamic failure. Specific protocols for POCUS evaluation during cardiopulmonary resuscitation may help to identify potentially reversible

---

Acute Medicine: Lecture Notes, First Edition. Edited by Glenn Matfin.
© 2023 John Wiley & Sons Ltd. Published 2023 by John Wiley & Sons Ltd.

causes (e.g. cardiac tamponade, pulmonary embolism, hypovolaemia, pneumothorax). Absence of cardiac motion on sonography during resuscitation of patients in cardiac arrest is highly predictive of death.

POCUS has many advantages – it is rapid, portable, cost-effective, dynamic, reproducible and with minimal radiation exposure to the patient. The main limitation of POCUS is that image quality and interpretation are dependent on the skills of the operator. Therefore, practising the various POCUS applications that will be discussed in this chapter is essential to achieve proficiency and improve image quality.

POCUS does not replace comprehensive ultrasound examination performed in the radiology department (i.e. *consultative ultrasonography*). Below are some of the main differences between comprehensive ultrasound and POCUS.

- To obtain a comprehensive ultrasound in the radiology department, the physician requests the diagnostic study, the study is performed by the ultrasound technician, the radiologist reports the findings of the exam and then the physician integrates the ultrasound results into the patient's clinical picture. However, when using POCUS, the physician caring for the patient performs the scan at the bedside, interprets the ultrasound findings in real time and immediately integrates the findings into the patient's clinical picture. Performing POCUS saves time, especially in Acute Medicine where establishing a rapid diagnosis is essential and may be life saving.
- During radiology ultrasound examinations, the technician follows a comprehensive protocol that obtains detailed information. However, in POCUS, the physician uses ultrasound to answer very specific dichotomous questions. For example, in a comprehensive renal ultrasound, the report will include detailed information such as the kidney size, location and presence or absence of any pathology. In renal POCUS, the clinician will use ultrasound to answer a specific question such as: 'Does the patient have hydronephrosis?'.

> POCUS is widely used in almost all medical specialties, including Acute Medicine (often termed focused Acute Medicine ultrasound, www.famus.org.uk). It is used across all Acute Medicine care settings, including the patient's home (i.e. Hospital at Home). POCUS is a major required competency in both undergraduate and postgraduate medical training.

Basic ultrasound physics

To be familiar with the language of ultrasonography, it is important to review the basic definitions and physics principles.

Characteristics of sound waves

- *Sound* – is a longitudinal wave that is produced by vibrating objects that travel through a medium.
- *Amplitude (measured in decibels)* – is the peak pressure of the sound wave. It will determine the volume of audible sounds or the strength of returning echoes in diagnostic ultrasound.
  - If the returning echoes have high intensity, the image produced will be brighter/whiter, also known as *hyperechoic*.
  - If the returning echoes have low intensity, the image produced will be grey or black, also known as *hypoechoic* or *anechoic* respectively.
- *Frequency (measured in hertz)* – is the number of wave cycles per second (Figure 11.1). Diagnostic ultrasound frequencies range from 2 to 20 megahertz, which is hundreds of times greater than sounds audible to humans.

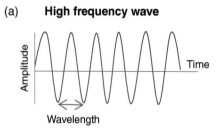

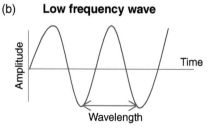

Figure 11.1 Characteristics of sound waves. (a) Characteristics of high-frequency wave. (b) Characteristics of low-frequency wave.

o The higher the frequency of the ultrasound wave, the more wave cycles will be produced, which will consume more energy and travel through shorter distances. This will generate more returning echoes and produce higher resolution images of *shallow* subjects.

o The lower the frequency of the ultrasound wave, the fewer wave cycles will be produced, which will consume less energy and travel through longer distances. This will generate fewer returning echoes and produce lower resolution images of *deeper* structures.

- *Velocity* – is the speed of the wave (velocity = frequency × wavelength). The wave velocity depends on the properties of the medium. Each medium has a constant velocity. Using this principle, the ultrasound machine determines the depth of a structure based on the time it takes for the echoes to return back to the source.

- *Wavelength* – is the distance the wave travels to complete a single cycle. Given that ultrasound velocity is constant in a medium, wavelength is inversely related to frequency. The higher the frequency, the shorter the wavelength and vice versa.

Ultrasound waves behave differently when they travel through different media

Attenuation refers to weakening of the intensity and amplitude of a sound wave as it travels through the medium. The density of the medium is a major determinant of the degree of attenuation.

- In a highly dense medium such as bone, attenuation will be greater than in less dense tissue such as fat or fluid.

- Attenuation of the ultrasound wave can occur in various forms. For example, *reflection* occurs when some of the sound waves are redirected back to the source when they encounter a reflective surface boundary between two media.

o The more echoes returning to the source, the brighter or whiter (hyperechoic) the image produced.

o The fewer echoes returning to the source, the darker (hypoechoic or anechoic) the image produced.

Ultrasound artifacts

To accurately interpret ultrasound images, it is important to understand common artifacts which can be produced in normal and pathological conditions.

- *Acoustic shadowing artifact* – an ultrasound image that displays a hyperechoic structure and posterior to it is an anechoic area. Acoustic shadowing artifact is generated when the ultrasound waves encounter highly attenuating structures, such as bone. Most of the waves are reflected to the source. The ultrasound machine will produce a hyperechoic image of the structure and will perceive the area behind the structure as completely black or anechoic that will appear as a shadow (Figure 11.2).

- *Posterior enhancement artifact* – an ultrasound image that displays an artificially brighter area

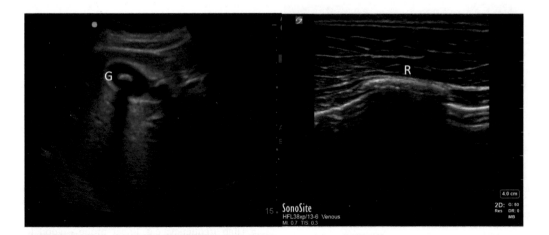

Figure 11.2 Acoustic shadowing artifact caused by a gallstone (G) and a rib (R).

posterior to an anechoic structure. This is generated in conditions when the ultrasound waves travel through low attenuating structures such as a blood vessel or a cyst and therefore don't lose as much energy. The returning echo from the adjacent area will be of higher intensity, therefore appearing artificially hyperechoic (Figure 11.3).

- *Reverberation artifact* – an ultrasound image that artificially displays repeated equally distanced arcs or lines posterior to a structure. This is generated in conditions when the ultrasound waves encounter two highly reflective surfaces and the waves bounce between them. One example is when the ultrasound wave bounces between the skin and the pleura, producing reverberation artifact posterior to the pleura, also known as A-lines (Figure 11.4).

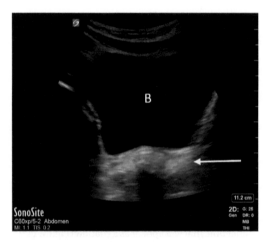

Figure 11.3 Posterior enhancement artifact (arrow) posterior to the bladder (B).

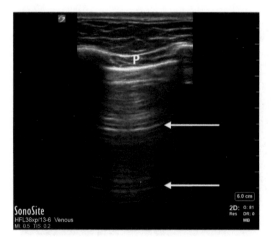

Figure 11.4 Reverberation artifact (arrows) of the pleura (P), also known as A-lines.

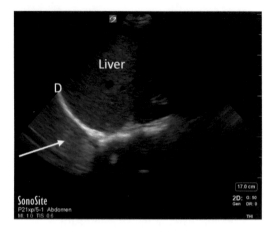

Figure 11.5 Mirror image artifact. Mirror image of the liver (arrow) cephalad to the diaphragm (D).

- *Mirror image artifact* – this is generated in conditions when ultrasound waves encounter highly reflective structures (such as the diaphragm in an aerated lung). Instead of the ultrasound waves returning echoes to the source, they will travel through another structure (the liver). The returning echoes will go back to the diaphragm and then to the probe. The ultrasound machine will falsely perceive the deeper structure to the diaphragm (lung) as the liver and therefore it will appear as a mirror image (Figure 11.5).

Basics of the ultrasound unit and knobology

Place the machine on the patient's right side so you can scan with your right hand and manipulate ultrasound buttons with your left hand. The basic components of an ultrasound unit (Figure 11.6) are as follows.

- Probe (also known as transducer). The ultrasound probe is covered with a thin layer of piezoelectric crystals. Each probe has a characteristic probe marker that corresponds to the screen marker. This will help the sonographer understand the orientation of the image produced (Figure 11.7). Several types of probes are available.
  - Low frequency: e.g. curvilinear and phased array probes – good for imaging deeper structures (e.g. abdomen and thorax).
  - High frequency: e.g. linear probe – good for imaging superficial structures (e.g. blood vessels, nerves).

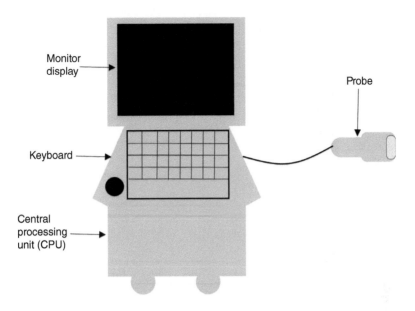

Figure 11.6 Basic components of an ultrasound unit.

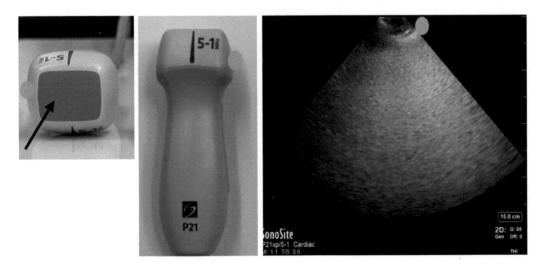

Figure 11.7 Features of an ultrasound probe. It is covered with a thin layer of piezoelectric crystals (arrow) and has a unique probe marker (green dot) that corresponds to the marker on the ultrasound screen (green dot).

- Central processing unit (CPU).
- Monitor display.
- Keyboard and cursor are optional, especially with the new touch-screen devices.

How does the ultrasound machine produce images?

Ultrasound produces images by converting electrical energy to mechanical energy and vice versa (also

known as the piezoelectric effect). This is summarised in six simplified steps (Figure 11.8).

1 The CPU produces electrical energy that travels to the probe.
2 The electrical energy causes vibration of the piezoelectric crystal layer on the probe which generates ultrasound waves.
3 Ultrasound waves travel from the probe through a conducting medium (gel) to the body.
4 The ultrasound waves interact with the body based on the characteristic of the tissue(s) being imaged.

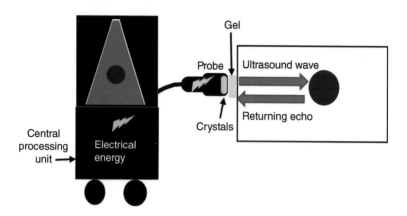

Figure 11.8 How an ultrasound unit produces an image.

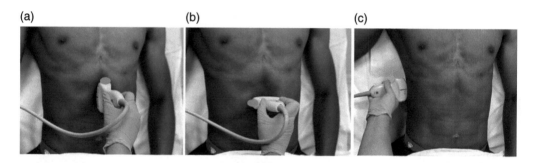

Figure 11.9 Scanning planes. (a) Longitudinal view. (b) Transverse view. (c) Coronal view. The probe marker is highlighted with a green dot.

5 Returning echoes to the probe will lead to vibration of the crystals that generates and transmits electrical energy to the CPU.

6 The CPU processes and translates the electrical energy into a two-dimensional image based on the intensity and time it took the echoes to return.

Scanning planes

Ultrasound produces two-dimensional images of a three-dimensional structure. Scanning in two planes is essential to better evaluate the structure of interest and confirm the findings. There are three main scanning planes used in POCUS.

- *Longitudinal plane* – this view is obtained when the ultrasound probe is placed along the long axis of the body with the probe marker pointing cephalad towards the patient's head (Figure 11.9a). It is also known as sagittal plane.
- *Transverse plane* – this view is obtained when the ultrasound probe is placed along the cross-sectional axis of the body with the probe marker pointing to the patient's right (Figure 11.9b).
- *Coronal plane* – this view is obtained when the probe is placed laterally, with the probe marker pointing cephalad towards the patient's head (Figure 11.9c).

Scanning modes

In POCUS, there are three common scanning modes.

- *Brightness mode (B-mode)* – this is the conventional scanning mode where the ultrasound machine converts the returning echoes into two-dimensional images using the grey-scale converter based on the intensity of the returning echoes (Figure 11.10a).
- *Motion mode (M-mode)* – this is used to analyse a moving structure relative to the probe plane. The ultrasound machine analyses the motion of the returning echoes and produces a waveform image (Figure 11.10b). The motion of the structure being scanned (vertical axis) is plotted over time (horizontal axis).

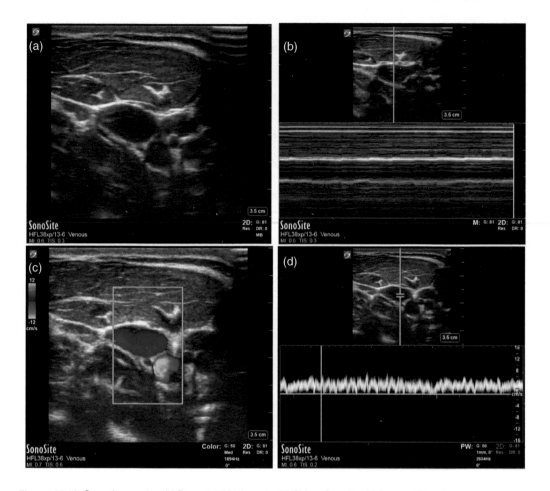

Figure 11.10 Scanning modes. (a) B-mode. (b) M-mode. (c) Colour Doppler. (d) Spectral Doppler.

- *Doppler mode (D-mode)* – this is used to analyse the direction of the moving structure relative to the probe plane. The ultrasound machine analyses the direction of the returning echoes either towards or away from the probe and produces either a colour image (colour Doppler) (Figure 11.10c) or a waveform image (spectral Doppler) (Figure 11.10d). This is commonly used to assess blood flow within vessels or through valves.

Optimising the ultrasound image

It is important to adjust the ultrasound image to obtain the most accurate information from the study. Knobology is a term describing the manipulation of ultrasound knobs and system controls in order to obtain the best image possible from diagnostic ultrasound.

Every machine has programmed presets that adjust the machine setting automatically to obtain the best quality images. For example, when you scan the abdomen, choose the abdominal preset. Novice ultrasound users should learn how to manually adjust at least three basic settings in the ultrasound to obtain the best image.

- *Depth* – the optimal depth is the minimal depth at which the entire structure of interest is included in the image.
- *Gain* – the gain refers to the brightness of the image (Figure 11.11). The optimal gain is achieved when a known anechoic structure appears black on the displayed image.
- *Focal zone* – the focal zone is the area on the screen with the maximum resolution.

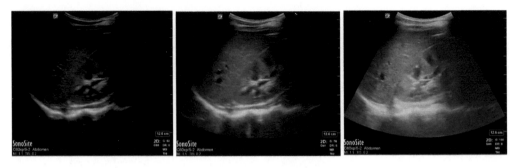

Figure 11.11 Adjusting the overall gain. Increasing gain (brightness) from left to right.

Getting ready to perform POCUS

Prior to starting the ultrasound exam, the most important thing is to make sure you protect yourself and others. The use of personal protective equipment (PPE) and disinfection of ultrasound equipment are especially important during the COVID-19 pandemic. If you are doing a POCUS-guided invasive procedure, make sure you have all the necessary equipment to hand.

Thoracic ultrasound

Thoracic ultrasound is indicated in patients presenting with dyspnoea, chest pain and signs of respiratory distress or respiratory failure.

- Thoracic ultrasound is used for diagnostic purposes and procedural guidance.
- It is used to identify sonographic signs of:
  o pneumothorax
  o pleural effusion
  o interstitial syndrome (e.g. pulmonary oedema)
  o pneumonia (including COVID-19).
- Thoracic POCUS is also used to guide thoracocentesis.

Technique

Probe selection

- High-frequency probes are preferred for the assessment of pneumothorax and pneumonia.

- Low-frequency probes are used to assess for pleural effusion, interstitial syndrome and certain signs of pneumonia.
- Choose the lung preset in the machine to obtain the best image quality.

Probe position

- The hemithorax is divided into three regions: anterior, lateral and posterior (Figure 11.12). Each region is equally divided into superior and inferior zones.
- The views obtained in thoracic ultrasound are longitudinal and coronal views (Figure 11.13).
- To assess for pneumothorax, scan the anterior regions in longitudinal view and the lateral regions in coronal view with the probe marker directed cephalad in both views.
- To assess for interstitial syndrome and pneumonia, scan the anterior and posterior regions in longitudinal view and the lateral region in coronal view with the probe marker directed cephalad in all views.
- To assess for pleural effusion, scan the lateral inferior zone in coronal view with the probe marker directed cephalad.

Normal sonographic anatomy

Longitudinal views using high- and low-frequency probes

The anatomical landmark that must be identified is the pleura between two ribs. A rib appears as a hyperechoic structure with posterior shadowing. The pleura is the hyperechoic line between two consecutive ribs. The two ribs with posterior shadowing ('wings') and pleural line in the middle are referred to as a 'batwing' appearance (Figure 11.14).

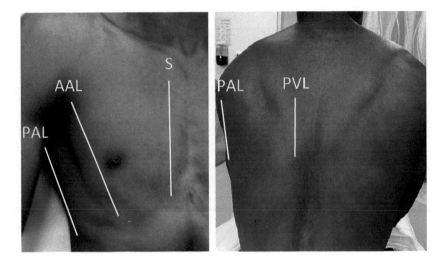

Figure 11.12 The surface anatomical landmarks for thoracic ultrasound. The boundary of the anterior region is the clavicle superiorly, sternum (S) and the anterior axillary line (AAL). The boundary of the lateral region is the AAL and posterior axillary line (PAL). The boundary of the posterior region is the PAL and the paravertebral line (PVL).

(a)   (b)

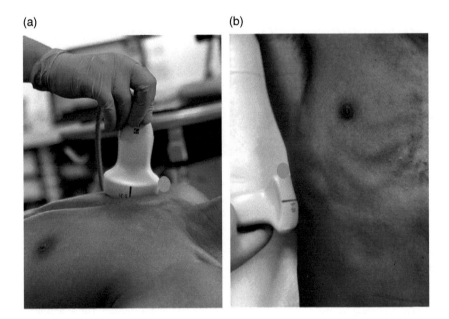

Figure 11.13 Thoracic ultrasound views. (a) Longitudinal view. (b) Coronal view. The probe marker is highlighted with the green dot.

Sonographic findings of a normal aerated lung in longitudinal view

Normal aerated lung shows a 'batwing' appearance, pleural line, lung sliding and A-lines.

- *Lung sliding* – a normal pleura will appear as a thin hyperechoic line that moves with the respiratory cycle. Lung sliding indicates that the visceral and parietal pleura are normal and attached.
- *Seashore sign* – lung sliding can be documented using the M-mode. The subcutaneous tissue and

(a)   (b)

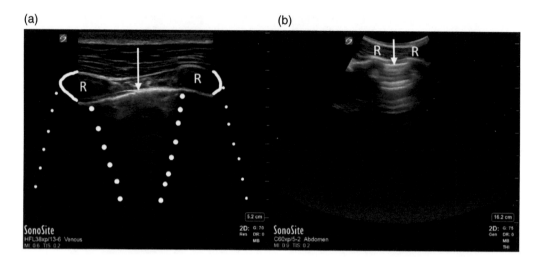

Figure 11.14 Normal longitudinal views of thoracic ultrasound using (a) high-frequency probe (superficial structures) and (b) low frequency probe (deeper structures). The anatomical landmark is the pleural line (arrow) between two ribs (R). The white dotted lines in (a) represents how the 'batwing' may look. In (b) the A-lines are clearly demonstrated below the pleura.

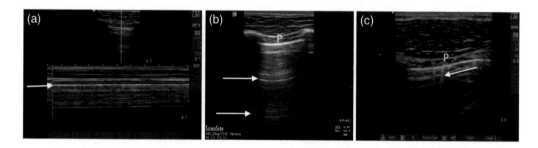

Figure 11.15 Sonographic findings in normal lung. (a) Seashore sign – lung sliding on M-mode appears as coarse lines ('sandy beach') below the pleura (arrow). (b) A-lines are horizontal reverberation artifacts (arrow) of the pleura (P). (c) B-lines or comet tails (arrow) are vertical reverberation artifacts that extend from the pleura (P).

chest wall musculature will produce smooth lines, while the structures deeper to the pleural line will appear as coarse lines due to lung sliding. The interface between the smooth and coarse lines has been described as the 'seashore sign' (Figure 11.15a).

- A-lines – reverberation artifacts that appear as equally distanced hyperechoic horizontal lines that are duplicates of the pleural line (Figures 11.14b and 11.15b).
- B-lines (also known as comet tail) – are also reverberation artifacts generated from the visceral pleura. They appear as hyperechoic 'laser-like' vertical lines that extend from the pleural line to the bottom of the screen (Figure 11.15c). In a normal aerated lung, there should be no more than two B-lines per zone.

Coronal view of the lateral-inferior zone using the low-frequency probe

This is the most dependent part of the lung and is used to look for pleural effusion. The anatomical landmark that must be identified is the diaphragm that appears as a hyperechoic line above the liver (on the right side) or spleen (on the left side). The area above the diaphragm is the pleural space (Figure 11.16a).

Sonographic findings of a normal aerated lung in coronal view

- In a normally aerated lung, the lung will be moving to and fro with respiration. The pleural space will appear as a mirror image artifact of the adjacent abdominal structure (Figure 11.16a).

- The lung parenchyma will be overlapping the abdominal organs during inspiration (also known as the curtain sign) (Figure 11.16b). An aerated lung is like a 'curtain' because as it fills with air, it looks like a curtain sweeping down and over the other organs, momentarily obscuring them from view. The diaphragm, liver or spleen reappear during exhalation.

Sonographic findings of pneumothorax

> POCUS profile of pneumothorax – no lung sliding, M-mode barcode sign, lung point sign (100% specific for ruling in a pneumothorax) and A-lines from intact parietal pleura.

- *Absent lung sliding* – in pneumothorax, the visceral and partial pleurae are separated by air. This will lead to the absence of lung sliding. On M-mode, the absence of lung sliding will appear as a 'barcode' sign with uniform smooth lines (Figure 11.17a). Absent lung sliding is a sensitive sonographic finding for pneumothorax (i.e. if lung sliding is present, you can rule out pneumothorax with 100% sensitivity at that ultrasound point); however, it is not specific. There are many other conditions that can lead to the absence of lung sliding such as large pleural effusion, pneumonia, post pleurodesis or pleurectomy, atelectasis and apnoea.
- *Lung point* – the transition point between the collapsed lung and normal lung, where normal lung sliding is absent and then reappears. In partially collapsed lung, the area of reattachment between

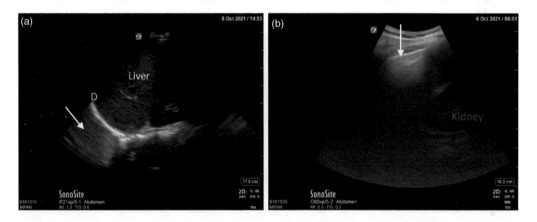

Figure 11.16 Sonographic findings in a normal coronal view of the lung base. (a) The pleural space (arrow) above the diaphragm (D) appears as a mirror image to the liver. (b) Lung parenchyma (arrow) overlapping the spleen during inspiration.

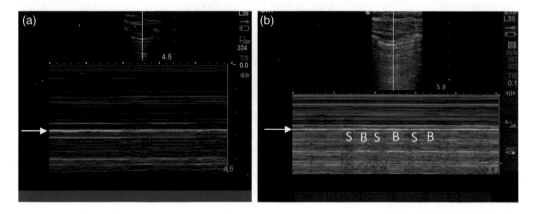

Figure 11.17 Sonographic findings in pneumothorax. (a) Barcode sign: M-mode with absent lung sliding appears as uniform smooth lines below the pleura (arrow). (b) Lung point on M-mode appears as alternating seashore (S) and barcode (B) signs below the pleura (arrow).

the visceral and parietal pleurae will appear as a lung point where part of the pleura will be sliding and the other part will be motionless. The lung point will appear on M-mode as alternating seashore and barcode signs (Figure 11.17b). Though difficult to find, a lung point is 100% specific for ruling in a pneumothorax. The location of a lung point will help quantify the size of the pneumothorax. If it is located in the anterior regions, it indicates that the pneumothorax is small. If it is in the lateral regions, the pneumothorax is large.

Sonographic findings of pleural effusion

- In pleural effusion, fluid will accumulate in the pleural space. In a supine patient, the most dependent areas, the lung bases in the lateral

inferior zone, are the most sensitive location to detect small amount of pleural fluid.
- The appearance of the fluid will depend on the characteristics of the pleural effusion; in a simple effusion, the fluid will be anechoic (Figure 11.18a) and in a complex effusion, the fluid may contain echogenic material (Figure 11.18b).
- *Thoracic spine sign* – in normally aerated lung, the thoracic vertebra will not appear above the hemidiaphragm as air scatters ultrasound waves. However, in pleural effusion, the anechoic fluid collection will transmit the ultrasound waves and therefore the thoracic vertebra will appear as a hyperechoic line that will continue from below to above the diaphragm (Figure 11.18a).
- *Jelly fish sign* – the lung parenchyma may be atelectatic in cases of large pleural effusions. On ultrasound, the atelectatic lung will appear as a homogeneous echogenic structure that is

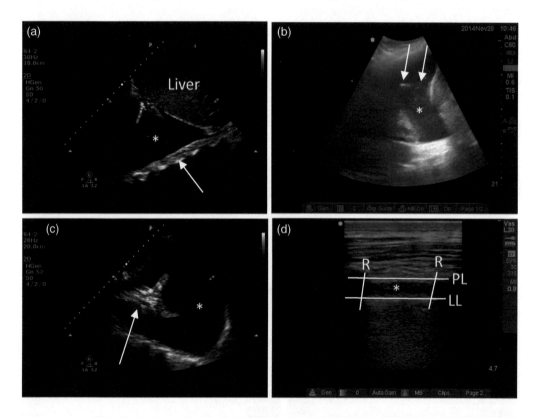

Figure 11.18 Sonographic findings in pleural effusion. (a) Simple pleural effusion on coronal view (*) appears as anechoic fluid. The spine sign (arrow) is when the thoracic spine is visible above the diaphragm. (b) Complex pleural effusion (*) with echogenic material (arrow) in coronal view. (c) Jelly fish sign: atelectatic lung (arrow) within a large pleural effusion (*) in coronal view. (d) Quad sign: in a longitudinal view, fluid collection (*) surrounded by ribs (R), lung line (LL) and pleural line (PL).

floating in a large amount of anechoic fluid (Figure 11.18c).

- *Quad sign* – anechoic fluid collection surrounding by four boundaries: two ribs, the pleural line and the lung line seen in longitudinal view (Figure 11.18d).

Sonographic findings of interstitial syndrome

> Interstitial syndrome is seen in clinical conditions where the alveoli are diffusely filled with fluid rather than air, such as pulmonary oedema and acute respiratory distress syndrome.

- It is important to remember that ultrasound waves are completely scattered and attenuated (absorbed) by the air that fills healthy alveoli. Thus, if the patient has normal lungs, you should not be able to see the texture of the parenchyma (lung tissue) during your scan. However, in certain pathologies such as interstitial lung edema, the accumulated fluid in the interlobular septa results in lung ultrasound artifacts known as 'B-lines'. B-lines form when interlobular septa and lung tissue thicken or fill with fluid. Thus, many clinicians have equated B-lines with 'wet lung' (think: *Kerley B-lines*). Remember, A-lines are horizontal while B-lines are vertical.
- Diffuse bilateral B-lines are seen in interstitial syndrome. There will be three or more B-lines per zone in three or more zones bilaterally. The number of B-lines correlates with the amount of interstitial fluid in the alveoli (Figure 11.19). As more fluid builds ups, it will become increasingly difficult to differentiate between singular B-lines. Thus, as more and more B-lines converge, they can create an appearance of 'confluent' B-lines.

Sonographic findings of pneumonia

> As fluid build-up progresses, sonographic findings will progress from multiple B-lines, confluent B-lines, subpleural consolidation, the shred sign, to a dense consolidation (i.e. completely fluid-filled lung). Once the air is completely gone from the lung and replaced with fluid, this will result in an echogenic structure on ultrasound similar to echogenicity of the liver. This is termed 'hepatisation of the lung'.

- *Subpleural consolidation* – which will appear as irregular, thickened pleural lines with a hypoechoic area (Figure 11.20a).
- *Multiple B-lines* – it is expected to find multiple B-lines (three or more) when scanning areas affected by pneumonia. The distribution of B-lines may be focal or diffuse, depending on the extent of lung parenchymal involvement (Figure 11.20b). B-lines can be unilateral or bilateral (latter more likely viral).

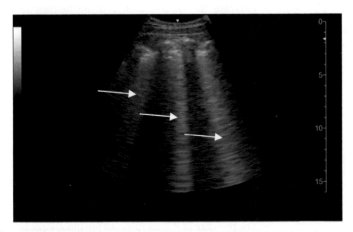

Figure 11.19 Sonographic findings in interstitial syndrome – multiple B-lines (arrows).

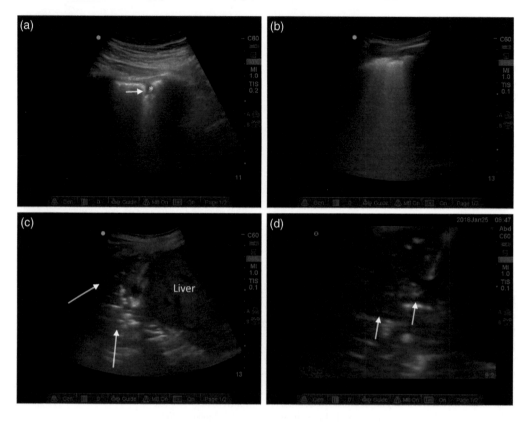

Figure 11.20 Sonographic findings in pneumonia. (a) Subpleural consolidation (*) with shred sign (arrow). (b) Confluent B-lines at the base of the lung. (c) Hepatisation of the lung (arrows). (d) Air bronchogram (arrows).

- *Shred sign* – the irregular line at the margin between normally aerated lung and the subpleural consolidation (Figure 11.20a).
- *Hepatisation* – when the alveoli are filled with purulent fluid, the lung will appear solid with similar echogenicity to the liver (Figure 11.20c).
- *Air bronchogram* – will appear as air within the consolidated area. When the air moves with respiration, this is known as dynamic air bronchogram (Figure 11.20d).

POCUS-guided thoracentesis

POCUS-guided thoracentesis can be static, when ultrasound is used to mark the needle insertion site, or dynamic, when ultrasound is used to visualise the needle entering the pleural space. The dynamic approach is helpful when the effusion size is small.

The advantages of using POCUS to guide thoracentesis are to:

- increase the success rate of the procedure by identifying the area with maximum fluid
- decrease the complication rate by helping to visualise the lung and therefore prevent iatrogenic pneumothorax.

Limitations and pitfalls of thoracic ultrasound

- The lung zones that are scanned by the probe are the only ones assessed for pathology. Therefore, identifying or ruling out pathology will be limited to the scanned zones.
- Absent lung sliding is not specific for pneumothorax. However, the presence of lung sliding rules out pneumothorax at the scanned zones.
- The presence of B-lines rules out pneumothorax at the scanned zone, because B-lines are reverberation

artifacts that require the visceral and parietal pleura to be attached.
- The lung point is the most specific finding that confirms pneumothorax.
- Ultrasound is a sensitive diagnostic tool for pleural effusion. It can detect small effusion (as little as 50 ml) that may be missed on a chest X-ray.
- The ultrasound findings of pneumonia depend on the extent of lung parenchymal involvement with the infection.

Sample clinical protocol for thoracic ultrasound

- The BLUE protocol (Bedside Lung Ultrasound in Emergency or Basic Lung Ultrasound Examination) as described by Lichtenstein presents a systematic approach to a patient with respiratory failure to help identify the underlying diagnosis using thoracic and vascular ultrasound.
- A summary of the BLUE protocol in a patient presenting with dyspnoea is shown in Figure 11.21.

Focused abdominal ultrasound

- Focused abdominal ultrasound is indicated in patients presenting with abdominal pain, abdominal distension or clinical signs of ascites.
- Focused abdominal ultrasound is used for diagnostic purposes and procedural guidance.
- It is used to identify free intraperitoneal fluid and guide paracentesis.

Technique

Probe selection

- Low-frequency probes are used to perform focused abdominal ultrasound.
- Choose the abdominal preset in the machine to obtain the best image quality.

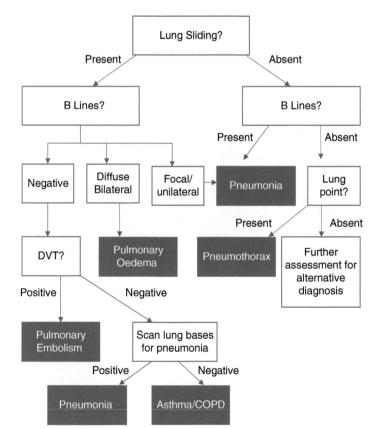

Figure 11.21 Approach to a patient presenting with dyspnoea using the Blue protocol. DVT, deep vein thrombosis; COPD, chronic obstructive airways disease.

Probe position

- Focused abdominal ultrasound involves obtaining three views: right upper quadrant (RUQ), left upper quadrant (LUQ) and pelvic views (Figure 11.22).

- *For the RUQ view* – place the probe in coronal plane at the midaxillary line between the eighth and tenth ribs with the probe marker directed cephalad.

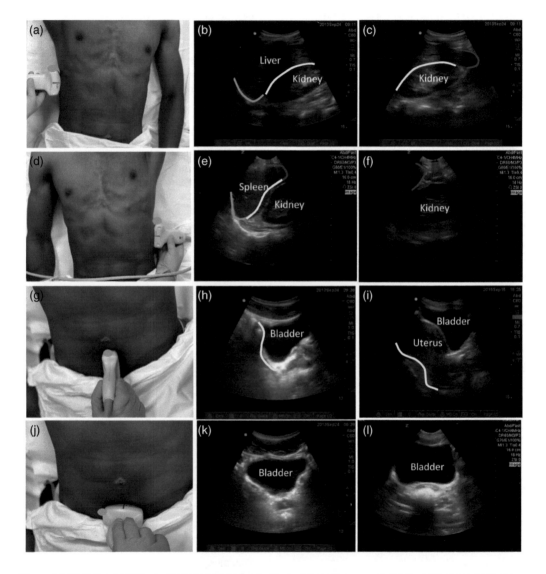

Figure 11.22 Probe positions in abdominal ultrasound with corresponding normal ultrasound findings. (a) Probe position for the RUQ view with the probe marker highlighted by the green dot. (b,c) The three spaces that should be assessed in the RUQ view: hepatorenal space (yellow line), subdiaphragmatic space (green line) and caudal edge of the liver (purple line). (d) Probe position for LUQ view with the probe marker highlighted by the green dot. (e,f) The three spaces that should be assessed in the LUQ view: splenorenal space (yellow line), subdiaphragmatic space (green line) and caudal tip of the spleen (purple line). (g) Probe position for the pelvic longitudinal view with the probe marker highlighted by the green dot. (h) The normal view in a male, highlighting the rectovesical space by the yellow line. (i) The normal view in a female, highlighting the rectouterine space by the yellow line. (j) Probe position for the pelvic transverse view with the probe marker highlighted by the green dot. (k,l) The normal corresponding views in males and female respectively.

- *For the LUQ view* – as the spleen is smaller than the liver, place the probe in coronal plane at the posterior axillary line between the fifth and seventh ribs.
- *The pelvic view* is imaged in two planes – longitudinal and transverse. For the longitudinal pelvic view, place the probe above the pubic symphysis with the probe marker directed cephalad. For the transverse pelvic view, place the probe above the pubic symphysis with the probe marker directed towards the patient's right.

Normal sonographic anatomy

RUQ view

In the RUQ view the following three spaces should be assessed.

- The interface between the liver and the kidney (the hepatorenal space), also known as Morrison's pouch.
- The caudal edge of the liver.
- The subdiaphragmatic space.

Normally there should be no fluid in these spaces (Figure 11.22b, 11.22c).

LUQ view

In the LUQ view the following three spaces should be assessed.

- The interface between the spleen and the kidney (the splenorenal space).
- The subdiaphragmatic space.
- The caudal tip of the spleen.

Normally there should be no fluid in these spaces (Figures 11.22e, 11.22f).

Pelvic view

In the pelvic views the following spaces should be assessed.

- In males, the space posterior to the bladder, also known as the rectovesical pouch (Figures 11.22h, 11.22k).
- In females, the interface between the uterus and rectum, also known as the cul-de-sac, pouch of Douglas or rectouterine pouch (Figures 11.22i, 11.22l).

Normally, there should be no fluid in these spaces. However, in women, a small amount of free fluid in the pouch of Douglas may be due to ruptured ovarian follicles.

Sonographic findings of free fluid in the abdomen

- Free intraperitoneal fluid will accumulate in any of the seven spaces mentioned above.
- Ultrasound is a good tool for detection of free intraperitoneal fluid; it can detect as little as 100 ml.
- Demonstration of free fluid in the RUQ, LUQ and pelvic views (Figure 11.23).
- The appearance of the intraperitoneal fluid will depend on its characteristics; in simple ascites the fluid will be anechoic (Figure 11.24a) and in complex ascites (Figure 11.24b), the fluid may contain echogenic material (fibrin, protein, leucocytes or erythrocytes).

POCUS-guided paracentesis

POCUS-guided paracentesis can be static, when ultrasound is used to mark the needle insertion site, or dynamic, when ultrasound is used to visualise the needle entering the intraperitoneal space. The dynamic approach is helpful when the amount of intraperitoneal fluid is small.

There are numerous advantages for using POCUS to guide paracentesis rather than the blind traditional approach.

- It helps confirm that the abdominal distension is secondary to ascites rather than other pathologies.
- It improves the success rate by identifying the deepest area of intraperitoneal fluid collection.
- It decreases the complication rate by identifying the structures to avoid such as bowel, bladder and vessels (Figure 11.25).

Limitations and pitfalls of focused abdominal ultrasound

- Abdominal POCUS does differentiate between the types of free intraperitoneal fluid (ascites, haemoperitoneum or urine) so correlating the ultrasound finding to the history and clinical picture is important.
- To perform an adequate focused abdominal POCUS, it is important to assess all seven spaces mentioned above to rule out free intraperitoneal fluid. If fluid is identified in one of the spaces, it is enough to confirm the presence of intraperitoneal fluid.

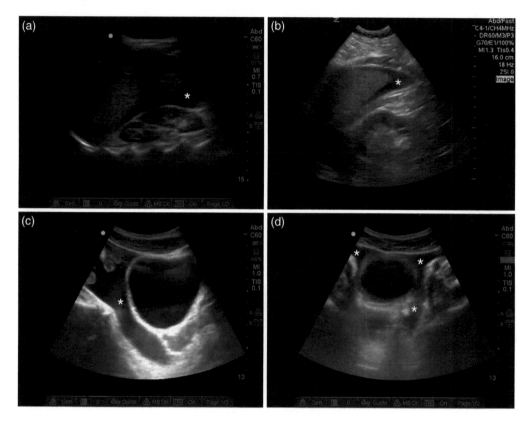

Figure 11.23 Abdominal ultrasound with positive intraperitoneal fluid (*) in the (a) RUQ view, (b) LUQ view, (c) pelvic view longitudinal and (d) pelvic view transverse.

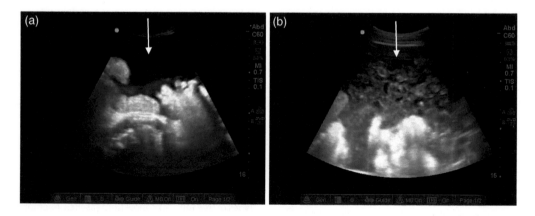

Figure 11.24 Simple ascites will appear as (a) anechoic fluid (arrow) while complex ascites will have (b) echogenic material within the fluid (arrow).

- The RUQ view is the most sensitive for free intraperitoneal fluid.
- Focused abdominal ultrasound has limited utility in detecting retroperitoneal fluid.

- When using the static approach for ultrasound-guided paracentesis, if the patient moves after marking the needle insertion site, this might lead to a dry tap as free fluid shifts with movement.

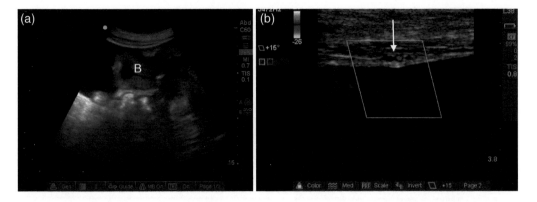

Figure 11.25 Examples of structures that must be avoided during paracentesis. (a) The bowel (B) is very close to the skin, increasing the risk of bowel perforation if paracentesis is performed at this location. (b) The inferior epigastric vessels (arrow) are identified by colour Doppler to avoid injury to the vessels and haematoma formation.

Focused renal ultrasound

- Renal ultrasound is indicated in patients presenting with flank pain, haematuria, urinary retention or anuria.
- Focused renal ultrasound is used to identify hydronephrosis and bladder distension and calculate the bladder volume.

Technique

Probe selection

- The low-frequency probes are used to perform focused renal ultrasound.
- Choose the abdominal preset on the machine to obtain the best image quality.

Probe position

- Focused renal ultrasound involves scanning the kidneys (Figure 11.26) and bladder in two planes (longitudinal and transverse).
- The bladder views (longitudinal and transverse) are similar to the pelvic views discussed in the focused abdominal POCUS section (Figures 11.22j, 11.22g).
- To scan the right kidney, place the probe in longitudinal plane at the midaxillary line below the costal margin with the probe marker directed cephalad, then rotate the probe 90° with the probe marker towards the ceiling to obtain a transverse view.

- The left kidney is more superior and posterior than the right kidney. To scan the left kidney, place the probe in longitudinal plane at the posterior axillary line below the costal margin, then rotate the probe 90° to obtain a transverse view.

Normal sonographic anatomy

- The normal kidney has a characteristic appearance on ultrasound (Figure 11.27).
- It is surrounded by a hyperechoic line which represents the capsule made of complex layers of fascia.
- The renal parenchyma is divided into the renal cortex and medulla. The cortex is homogeneous and appears hypoechoic on ultrasound. The medulla which forms the pyramids are less hypoechoic than the cortex.
- The renal pelvis is a flattened funnel-shaped structure in the centre which appears hyperechoic and bright on ultrasound.

Sonographic findings of hydronephrosis

- In hydronephrosis, urine will accumulate in the renal pelvis and extend proximally because of obstruction to the urine outflow distal to the kidney.
- Hydronephrosis will appear on ultrasound as an anechoic fluid collection in the renal pelvis. Depending on the degree of obstruction, the fluid will move proximally to the renal parenchyma (Figure 11.28).

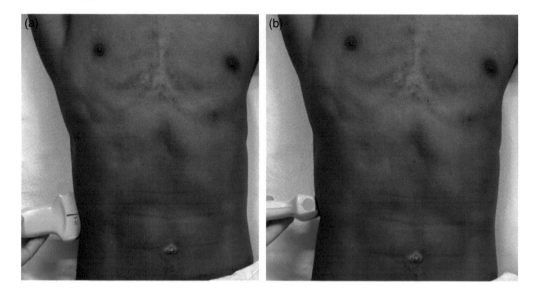

Figure 11.26 Probe position for renal ultrasound. (a) Longitudinal view with the probe marker directed cephalad (green dot). (b) Transverse view with the probe marker directed towards the ceiling (green dot).

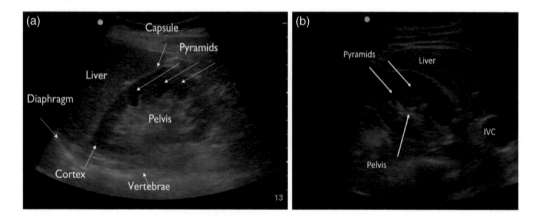

Figure 11.27 Normal renal ultrasound. (a) Longitudinal view and (b) transverse view.

- There are numerous grading systems for hydronephrosis. In POCUS, hydronephrosis is graded by visual assessment into mild, moderate and severe.
  - *Mild* hydronephrosis: the anechoic fluid will be limited to the renal pelvis and calyces without changing its shape.
  - *Moderate* hydronephrosis: the anechoic fluid will extend proximally, leading to the dilation of the pelvis and calyces and flattening of the medullary pyramids.
  - *Severe* hydronephrosis: there is ballooning of the renal pelvis and calyces, with loss of corticomedullary differentiation and thinning of the renal cortex.

Measurement of bladder volume

- POCUS is used to identify a distended bladder. This can be done subjectively by visual assessment of the bladder or objectively by measuring the bladder volume.
- POCUS is one of the tools used to assess postresidual volume.
- Ultrasound estimation of the bladder volume can be achieved using various formulas. The most popular method assumes that the bladder shape is prolate ellipsoid. Based on this assumption, the following formula is used to measure the bladder volume: bladder volume (ml) = height (cm) × width (cm) × length (cm) × 0.52.

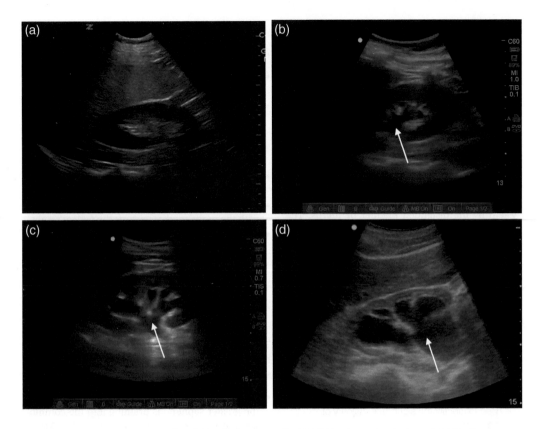

Figure 11.28 Hydronephrosis grading. (a) No hydronephrosis. (b) Mild hydronephrosis (arrow). (c) Moderate hydronephrosis (arrow). (d) Severe hydronephrosis (arrow).

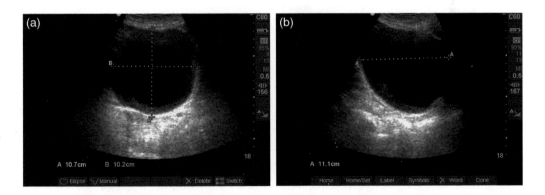

Figure 11.29 Bladder volume measurement. (a) In transverse view, measure the maximum height (A = 10.7 cm) and width (B = 10.2 cm). (b) In longitudinal view, measure the maximum length (A = 11.1 cm). Bladder volume in this case = height × width × length × 0.52 = 630 ml.

- The bladder maximum height and width are measured in transverse view while the maximum length is measured in longitudinal view (Figure 11.29).
- Some machines will calculate the volume automatically once the above measurements are saved.

Limitations and pitfalls of renal ultrasound

- Renal pyramids may be prominent in some individuals. This can be confused with hydronephrosis. In cases of prominent pyramids, the renal pelvis will remain collapsed and hyperechoic, while in hydronephrosis, the renal pelvis will be dilated and filled with anechoic fluid.

- Renal cysts may be confused with hydronephrosis. Renal cysts are usually located in the renal cortex while hydronephrosis starts from the renal pelvis and extends to the cortex in severe obstruction.
- In patients with severe dehydration, hydronephrosis may be missed. The scan should be repeated after hydration.
- Patients with benign prostatic hypertrophy or who are pregnant may have mild hydronephrosis secondary to compression of the renal collecting system by the distended bladder or uterus. The hydronephrosis should resolve once the bladder or uterus has been emptied.

Deep vein thrombosis ultrasound

Deep venous thrombosis (DVT) ultrasound is indicated in patients presenting with lower extremity pain, swelling, erythema or tenderness. It is used to identify the significant majority of lower extremity DVT.

Technique

Probe selection

- The high-frequency probe is used to perform DVT ultrasound.
- Choose the vascular or venous preset on the machine to obtain the best image quality.

Probe position

- Place the patient in a supine position with the knee bent and externally rotated.
- Use a high-frequency probe in transverse plane with the probe marker towards the patient's right.
- The venous anatomy of the lower extremity is scanned at the level of the inguinal ligament and at the level of the popliteal fossa (Figure 11.30).

Scanning protocols

There are various scanning protocols for POCUS DVT. The three-point lower extremity DVT ultrasound helps identify three important locations of the venous system that are high risk for DVT (Figure 11.31).

- *Point 1* – the scan begins proximally at the level of the greater saphenous draining into the common femoral vein, also known as the 'Mickey Mouse sign'.

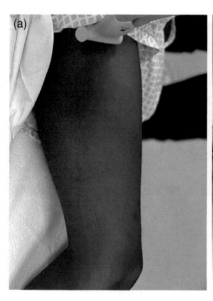
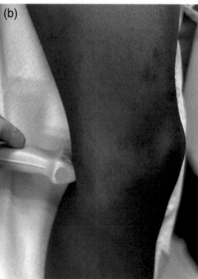

Figure 11.30 Probe positions for DVT ultrasound of the left lower extremity. With the knee bent and externally rotated, (a) scan at the inguinal ligament level with the probe marker directed towards the patient's right (green dot), and then (b) scan at the popliteal fossa level with the probe marker directed towards the patient's right (green dot).

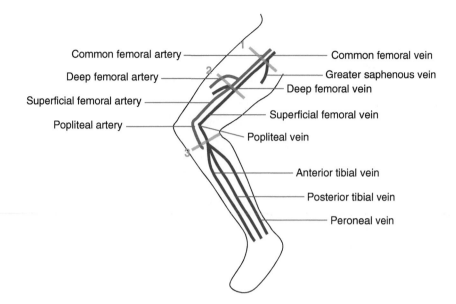

Common femoral artery
Deep femoral artery
Superficial femoral artery
Popliteal artery

Common femoral vein
Greater saphenous vein
Deep femoral vein
Superficial femoral vein
Popliteal vein
Anterior tibial vein
Posterior tibial vein
Peroneal vein

Figure 11.31 The three-point lower extremity DVT scan protocol relevant to the venous anatomy of the lower extremity.

- *Point 2* – the common femoral vein must be traced distally to the junction of the common femoral, superficial femoral and deep femoral veins.
- *Point 3* – at the popliteal fossa, the popliteal vein and artery are identified. The popliteal vein is scanned and traced to its trifurcation into the anterior tibial vein, posterior tibial vein and peroneal vein.

At each point, after identifying the relevant veins by ultrasound, graded compression is applied to the probe to assess vein collapsibility.

Sonographic findings of DVT

A normal vein appears anechoic and should compress completely when applying pressure on the probe. An example of a positive DVT ultrasound scan is shown in Figure 11.32.

- *Direct visualisation of the clot* – the appearance of the clot will depend on its age. Acute thrombus may be anechoic and may be missed on ultrasound. However, when the thrombus ages, it will appear as echogenic material within the lumen of the vein.
- *Non-compressible vein* – when applying sufficient pressure that the artery compresses but the vein does not compress completely, this is probably due to a thrombus in that region.

Limitations and pitfalls of DVT ultrasound

- The three-point DVT ultrasound protocol only assesses for thrombus within the regions that are scanned. Although these are the highest risk areas for DVT, this protocol may miss isolated thrombus in the regions that are not scanned.
- POCUS for DVT is used to 'rule in' the diagnosis, while comprehensive radiology scan is used to 'rule out' the diagnosis.
- The amount of pressure applied to the probe during graded compression must be sufficient to cause the adjacent pulsatile artery to compress a little. Inadequate compression may lead to a false-positive study.
- There are several conditions that may be mistaken for a DVT and lead to a false-positive study, such as superficial thrombophlebitis, inguinal lymph nodes and ruptured Baker cyst. However, they all have unique sonographic features which should allow accurate diagnosis.

Sample clinical protocol for DVT ultrasound

- Due to the limitations of the POCUS DVT scan, it is important to consider the pretest probability of the patient using clinical decision rules such as Wells

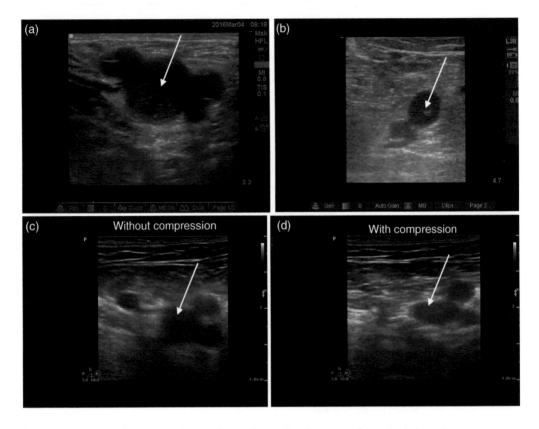

Figure 11.32 Sonographic findings of DVT. (a) Thrombus in the left common femoral vein (arrow) appears as echogenic material in the lumen of the vein. (b) Thrombus in the popliteal vein (arrow). (c) Left common femoral vein without compression (arrow). (d) The left common femoral vein (arrow) is not compressible with graded compression.

criteria for DVT and include other adjunct tests that can help in the clinical assessment of patients with suspected DVT (e.g. D-dimer).

- A representative clinical algorithm for assessment of patients with suspected DVT using a POCUS protocol is outlined in Figure 11.33.

Use of POCUS for guidance in performing procedures

Imaging-guided diagnostic and therapeutic procedures are a mainstay of contemporary clinical practice to reduce morbidity and improve safety, operator effectiveness and immediate symptom relief after thoracentesis, paracentesis, lumbar puncture, central venous access, peripheral venous and arterial access, pericardiocentesis, abscess drainage and joint aspiration.

The availability of portable and hand-held machines permits POCUS to be used for procedural guidance on site by Acute Medicine clinicians across all acute care settings.

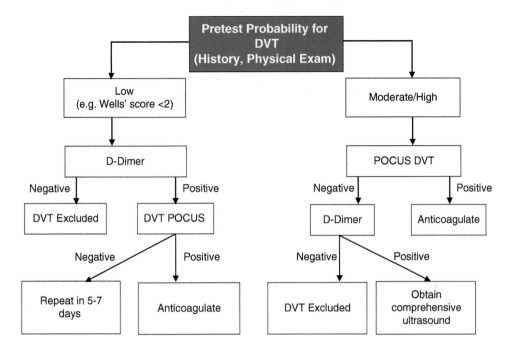

Figure 11.33 Sample clinical protocol for the use of DVT POCUS in patient assessment.

12

Putting it all together – managing the acute medical take

James Piper

 KEY POINTS

- The medical registrar role can be one of the busiest in an acute NHS trust. It is expected that the number of acute medical admissions will continue to rise each year.
- Out of hours, the medical registrar may be the most senior doctor available on a hospital site.
- It is important to focus on the priority roles and responsibilities of the duty medical registrar.
- It is essential to prepare for and manage the acute unselected medical take successfully to maintain patient safety, taking into account patient preferences and the urgency required.
- Maintain close, collaborative relationships with the acute care team and staff in the emergency department – patient care must come first.
- Handovers should be safe, structured and accessible.
- Maintaining your own well-being should be a personal priority.

Introduction

Medical patients make up most of the unscheduled admissions to NHS secondary care hospitals. The number and complexity of these admissions are increasing as the population ages. Acute admissions typically peak between September and February of each year (including the perennial 'winter surge'). The volume of annual emergency department (ED) attendances for a hospital will give an indication of the likely admissions workload. Attendances to UK EDs continue to rise year on year. This situation has been exacerbated by the impact of COVID-19 on health and social care.

Becoming the trainee doctor (i.e. medical registrar) running the acute unselected medical take can feel daunting. The medical registrar is perceived by many to be the busiest role of the hospital, yet the role can seem to lack definition. The expertise of the on-call medical registrar is heavily relied upon by many other hospital and community teams. Developing the capability to perform this role will be essential for those involved in the care of acute medical admissions and ambulatory referrals.

Acute Medicine: Lecture Notes, First Edition. Edited by Glenn Matfin.
© 2023 John Wiley & Sons Ltd. Published 2023 by John Wiley & Sons Ltd.

Managing the acute medical take

Out of hours, the medical registrar may be the most senior decision maker on a hospital site; however, there should always be a consultant physician available for advice. Although the duty registrar may be the most senior medic present, it is important not to allow an overreliance on this by other specialty teams. It is essential to avoid late or poor-quality referrals to the detriment of patients. Good working relationships between acute admission teams and referrers can avoid undue burdens and stress. Hospitals should have standard operating procedures regarding conditions accepted under medical or surgical teams respectively.

Anticipating the need for a medical opinion, and ensuring the request is made in hours, can help relieve the pressure on the medical registrar and prevent crises out of hours. Be mindful of the expertise (and experience) available, especially overnight – routine opinions should be deferred.

Roles and responsibilities of the medical registrar

Roles and responsibilities of the medical registrar (Royal College of Physicians Acute Toolkit) include the following.

Priority

- Leadership and supervision.
  - Leadership of the acute medical take team.
  - Supervision and support of junior medical doctors.
  - Leadership of handover processes.
  - Ensuring appropriate communication and escalation to the medical consultant on call.
  - Communication with senior members of the wider team, including senior nurses and managers.
  - Performing complex clinical procedures.
- Being a senior medical clinical decision maker.
  - Awareness of, and supervision of care for, the most acutely unwell and/or complex patients with medical problems. This can include patients with medical problems across the acute care setting – inpatient and ambulatory.
  - Specialty clinical support and advice to non-medical specialty teams, including GP and staff in the ED.

- Training.
  - Being proactive in seeking training opportunities and ensuring ongoing professional development.
  - Taking an active role in training junior doctors.
  - Supervising junior doctors performing practical clinical procedures.

Non-priority

These are roles that are more appropriately designated to other members of the clinical multidisciplinary team (MDT). This team can include mid-level clinicians (e.g. physician associates).

- Routine clerking of unselected internal medical (or medical specialty) admissions.
- Basic clinical tasks including venepuncture, cannulation, performing electrocardiograms.
- Routine administrative tasks.
- Facilitating routine bed moves.

Preparing for the acute medical take

Acute medical units (AMU) will vary enormously (especially organisationally) so it is important to be aware of how your unit accepts, reviews and manages patients under its care. Prior to or at the beginning of your take shift, try to find out the following.

- What are the referral pathways for your unit – e.g. who takes referrals from GPs? Do *all* referrals come to the medical registrar?
- How is the take list run – e.g. is it a paper book, online spreadsheet or integrated into hospital information technology (IT) systems?
- How do I make referrals to other key specialties such as critical care?
- Are rapid-access services such as for chest pain or diabetes available? And if so, how can I access them?
- Does my unit have ambulatory care pathways? Examples such as deep vein thrombosis (DVT)/pulmonary embolus (PE) and cellulitis are commonplace. If so, is there a designated Acute Medicine same-day emergency care (SDEC) unit for managing these patients?
- Is there a specialist frailty team available?
- Is there an Acute Medicine enhanced care area such as those that deliver non-invasive ventilation? If so, how do you admit a patient to these beds?
- What is the process for accepting patients from another hospital? These transfers are often

complex and should be done at a consultant-to-consultant level.

- Do we have access to procedure packs and point-of-care ultrasound (POCUS) devices?

The acute take shift

The acute take shift can be unpredictable. Here are some points to consider which may help your shift to be as smooth and safe as possible.

- Arrive on time to allow the night team to go home in good time and avoid any other commitments during your shift, especially if there is much to hand over.
- Have a structured handover, introduce each other and identify the skill mix for the shift and allocate tasks accordingly. It is important to be mindful that foundation years (FY) training doctors will need to discuss all their cases with either you or the duty consultant.
- If leading the take, it can be helpful to identify if the trainees have any learning or assessment goals. This will be especially important for rotating trainees such as Acute Care Common Stem (ACCS) who will have specific clinical presentations to see whilst on take.
- Run the take using multiple sources of support: bed managers, senior nurses, critical care, other specialties. Bed or site managers are often a terrific resource for hospital policy or real-time information such as IT systems issues and availability of coronary care unit (CCU)/intensive care unit (ICU) beds.
- Escalate to your consultant on call if you need to; it is a duty of care for them to be available. Avoid apologising or feeling guilty for a situation beyond your control.
- Use colleagues as a 'mirror' to reflect your ideas on (i.e. metacognition – 'making thinking visible' – as part of effective clinical reasoning and decision making). Many registrars on take will be from outside the AMU and will appreciate your expertise and vice versa.
- 'Divide and conquer' strategy: this means reviewing your patient list and allocating them to team members. For example, it may be easier for the registrar or internal medicine training (IMT) doctor to see patients who can go home, since FY1s cannot discharge patients themselves.
- Run through the board/ED patients with the ED nurse in charge and ED registrar, especially if you need to catch up with what's going on. If the ED is busy, there can be many advantages to a single patient clerking rather than double clerking, especially asking an FY1 to see a patient already seen by

a senior doctor. Acting as one big team has many benefits. Avoid seeing ED as the enemy as they will often work with you. Build good relationships.

- Regular team contact such as via WhatsApp or in person. Who can go home? Who can be deferred to AEC/SDEC now or the following day? Who is clinically sick? Prioritise together and share your thought processes. Remember, colleagues can't read minds and junior staff will be looking to you for inspiration and clear communication.
- Try to keep the patients informed and hydrated. ED may keep a patient 'nil by mouth' pending medical review, which is rarely necessary. Patients appreciate a drink, food and up-to-date information. Delivering patient-centred care, including shared decision making, is always critical. An early apology for long delays will be appreciated and make your clerking less stressful.
- If referring to critical care, have an idea of the intervention you're requesting, such as non-invasive positive pressure respiratory/vasopressor support. Critical care rarely appreciates vague referrals. Effective team communication is vital for safe clinical care. The situation, background, assessment, recommendation and readback (SBARR) system of communication should be used.
- Call for specialty input *early* as soon as you think it is necessary. Your colleagues may be in clinic, theatre or at a different hospital. Make a note in the patient records with details and contact information about the encounter.
- Know your local healthcare system: access to tertiary specialties such as trauma, neurosurgery and plastic surgery may be geographically distant from you and each will have its own referral arrangements.
- On a night shift, focus on what's immediately required. If there are multiple patients waiting, patient safety takes precedence. Delegate as need be, but recircle to see all sick patients personally. Five seconds ('five-second rule') critically looking at the patient will tell you more than 10 minutes on the phone.
- Some patients will deteriorate despite what you do – for example, in cardiac arrest the most likely outcome is still unfortunately death.

Sleep and night working

Look after yourself. Working at night is an essential part of providing a comprehensive seven-day, 24-hour service to patients in the NHS. However, night work requires doctors to remain awake and alert when physiologically programmed to be asleep. Working at night, regardless of the shift pattern, can have consequences for both patient and personal safety, as it increases the risk of making poor decisions or even mistakes. Cognitive function is impaired after 16–18 hours awake, leading to a deterioration in the medical worker's ability to interact effectively with patients and colleagues. It is therefore important to learn how to prepare for night shifts and to manage your sleep and general well-being, so that you minimise risk to yourself and your patients. Everyone has different sleeping tactics ahead of and after nightshifts, so find what works best for you. Driving after being awake for 20 hours or more and at the body's circadian low point is as dangerous as driving with blood alcohol levels above the legal limit – please be careful.

Clinical decision making and the acute medical take

There are many factors which can affect our clinical decision making. Either running or being part of the acute medical take is a continuous process of decision making, sometimes under great pressure such as a cardiac arrest or demand for admissions from the ED due to crowding.

The dual-process theory describes two types of decision making:.

- System 1 (type 1) thinking is often rapid and unconscious such as a routine commute to work or phlebotomy. When clerking patients, System 1 thinking is often used as we base our decisions on the types of patients we will have seen before (e.g. a patient presenting with chest pain). System 1 thinking alone, however, can lead to cognitive errors (biases).
- System 2 (type 2) thinking is often much slower, more controlled and involves active, conscious thinking about our decisions.

It is important to understand the possibility of decision-making fatigue and when it may be affecting you. The best calibrated decisions are described as 'rational' – they come from a blend of System 1 and System 2 decisions. Rationality in this context means the best possible decision given the available evidence and the prevailing conditions.

What affects our ability to make rational decisions?

- Lack of time.
- Tiredness.
- Collapse of a team structure.
- Burnout.
- Loss of resilience and short-term coping mechanisms.
- Pressure to provide service.
- Cognitive bias (or 'thinking failures') and previous experiences.

Bias can be conscious or subconscious. We often develop biases (i.e. mental shortcuts like pattern recognition) to enable us to function on the acute take. There are different types of bias, and it is important to be aware of them.

- *Anchoring* – e.g. ignoring the possibility of acute coronary syndrome in a female presenting with gastro-oesophageal reflux disease-like symptoms.
- *Availability* – e.g. assuming everyone has COVID-19 in a COVID-19 outbreak.
- *Diagnostic momentum* – e.g. where the GP, ED and other clinicians diagnose a pneumonia when the patient has an acute abdomen instead. In this case, the bias is accepting that the initial diagnosis was correct. This bias is then transferred between the assessing doctors. In this example, a raised lactate level may be attributed to the pneumonia rather than prompting a detailed reassessment of the patient, and review of imaging and laboratory results.
- *Implicit* – e.g. an initial reaction to a patient such as someone of no fixed abode or a known substance abuser. Implicit biases are unconscious prejudices (microaggressions) individuals might feel about another group or person which can interfere with clinical assessment, decision making and provider–patient relationships such that the health goals that the provider and patient are seeking are compromised. Inclusiveness is important.
- *Overconfidence* – e.g. attributing increasing confusion to a patient's psychiatric diagnosis and not assessing for organic causes. Although rare, not making a timely diagnosis such as encephalitis can have catastrophic results.
- *Confirmation bias* – e.g. inappropriately using a dipstick to diagnose urinary tract infection in an elderly patient.
- *Premature closure* – e.g. seeing an obvious pulmonary apical mass but missing a fractured humerus on a chest X-ray.
- *Framing effect* – in other words, this is 'selling a patient' for example to a radiologist to perform a

computed tomography pulmonary angiogram (CTPA) by emphasising certain points such as female, very high D-dimer result and very short of breath. This also happens in the handover and referral process so objectivity remains crucial for safe care.

- *Hindsight* – e.g. missing a subarachnoid haemorrhage in a previous patient results in all subsequent headache patients having a head CT scan requested even if clinically not indicated (i.e. a change in practice due to one case).

> Reflect on these cognitive biases in your everyday clinical practice and how you can avoid them (i.e. debiasing).

Handover

> Handover, particularly of temporary 'on-call' responsibility, has been identified as a point at which errors are likely to occur. Failure in handover is a major preventable cause of patient harm and is principally due to human factors of poor communication and systemic error. These can lead to inefficiencies, repetitions, delayed decisions, repeated investigations, incorrect diagnoses, incorrect treatment and poor communication with the patient.

A good handover:

- ensures that changes in the clinical teams are not detrimental to the quality of healthcare
- improves communications between all members of the healthcare team, including those with the patient and their family
- identifies unstable and unwell patients, so that their management remains optimal, clear and unambiguous
- improves efficiency of patient management by clear baton passing
- improves patient experience and confidence
- is a teaching and learning opportunity for those in training, who can observe appropriate role models at work.

Features of a standardised clinical handover include the following.

- Embedded in hospital policy and culture (documentation, seminars, discussions, champions).

- Involve training in handover and communication (induction agenda, cross-professional education).
- Tailored to local/unit needs, e.g. different priorities in ED, general ward handovers.
- Recognised as a multiprofessional team activity, reducing repetition within professional silos such as 'Hospital@Night'.
- Command designated time and location within the job plan/shift patterns.
- Determine clear arrangements for ongoing care of patients.
- Define who must be present, including senior (consultant) staff.

The handover process should:

- define leadership responsibility (not necessarily medical staff)
- define who is relinquishing responsibility and who is now responsible for ongoing care (including scope of responsibility and specific tasks)
- standardise an order of proceedings, e.g. proforma to avoid omissions and discourage discussion deviation (e.g. to staff and bed availability)
- standardise the systems of communication, e.g. SBARR, both verbal and documented
- standardise the system of documentation
- define the immediacy of review by incoming team via 'red–amber–green' patient risk assessment, where red is haemodynamic/respiratory instability, unclear diagnosis, sepsis; amber is response to prescribed treatment requires close monitoring; green is stable and discharge planned
- ensure that the handover is communicated effectively to the patient and, where relevant, to family and carers.

The role of debriefing

> If you step back and think about some of the more difficult, upsetting or even anger-inducing events in your training, what did you do afterwards? Did you reflect on what happened? If a team was involved, did the team reflect? Were any learning points reviewed?
>
> Debriefing is often underutilised in medicine but can be a powerful tool for learning as well as identifying ongoing needs of others and any system issues. Debriefing should never be seen as a punitive exercise but an opportunity to share perspectives on a clinical event.

Debriefing helps to explore a clinical event and factors which may have helped or hindered what happened. There should be a particular focus on communication, decision making, situational awareness and/or efficiency. Team members should learn from clinical experiences and agree on actions that would improve patient safety in a positive way, thus also contributing to staff well-being. The power of debriefing as a learning tool is that it can be prearranged or occur spontaneously, for example on exposure to new clinical experiences, good outcomes in a difficult circumstance or after 'near misses' or serious untoward incidents.

Debriefing can be performed in a range of settings but ideally should be held in a private or calm setting. A debriefing can be carried out immediately after a clinical case, at the end of a clinical session or in due course, depending on the circumstances and urgency of the situation.

TALK debriefing

The TALK debriefing was developed in 2014 (www.talkdebrief.org). A TALK debrief has four components.

1 *Target* – the first step is to choose the focus of the discussion, being as specific as possible. Team members share their perspective and agree on what is important to discuss.

- *What shall we discuss to improve patient care?*

2 *Analyse* – team members review the agreed target, in particular how to repeat successful outcomes or identify areas for improvement. As part of this step, team members propose improvement actions.

- *This went very well, how can we do this again?*
- *This was challenging, how can we do things better?*

3 *Learning points* – new insights gained during the clinical experience or the conversation shared by the team members.

- *What can the team learn from this experience?*
- *What have we learned during the conversation?*

4 *Key actions* – team members agree on solutions. They also take responsibility to carry them out and follow them up.

- *What are we going to do?*
- *Who is going to do it?*
- *How will we all know that it has been done?*

Implementing a TALK debrief

- Any team member can initiate a TALK conversation. Don't forget that if the situation to debrief is complex, you can be supported by a debriefing mentor.
- It should take no more than 10 minutes and could be done immediately after a case, at the end of a clinical session or later, depending on the circumstances.
- Prioritising patient care is the most important consideration when having a TALK conversation. Therefore, it is crucial that it is done in a constructive and non-judgemental way.
- Avoid negative comments and behaviours. The aim is that it should be a positive experience for the team, rather than pointing out blame.
- Everybody's input should be valued, no matter what level of experience they have.
- The clinical debriefing should focus on finding solutions to the issues raised. Then the team should decide who within the group will take responsibility for the agreed key actions, and who will ensure they are followed up and completed. This way, we continually improve patient safety, step by step.

Section Two

Acute Medicine in special populations

13

Older persons

Glenn Matfin and Howell Jones

 KEY POINTS

- Demographics have consistently underlined a substantial growing trend in the number of older persons.
- Older people (aged 65+) comprise a relatively small proportion of all patients attending the emergency department but form a substantial proportion (60–70%) of overall hospital inpatients.
- All staff working in Acute Medicine will be familiar with the increasing number of high-acuity, frail older patients with altered physiology, polypharmacy, multimorbidity, cognitive impairment and communication difficulties.
- The acute medical unit and other Acute Medicine care settings (e.g. same-day emergency care) are key areas for initial clinical decision making, and for education and training relevant to older people.
- Different models of care for older people will be suited to different hospitals, but all need to be able to initiate comprehensive geriatric assessment across the various Acute Medicine care settings and to have strong links with community health and social care services.
- Geriatric medicine or frailty liaison teams supporting Acute Medicine services will be able to help identify older people who may be safely managed in the community, improving patient outcomes and reducing hospital bed-days.

Introduction

What is old age? Generally, someone over the age of 65 might be considered an older person. However, it is not easy to apply a strict definition because people can age biologically at different rates so, for example, someone aged 80 may be healthier than someone aged 60. Instead of simply looking at chronological age, we can look at biological age known as 'frailty' which has a bigger impact on the likelihood of the person requiring care and support. From a clinical perspective, frailty may be defined as a person requiring help in activities of daily living.

Advances in healthcare have helped people around the world live longer than ever before. This is good news for all of us but it creates a challenge for the NHS – as we get older, we tend to experience long-term conditions and need more health and social care. Older people (aged 65+) comprise a relatively small proportion (5–10%) of all patients attending the emergency department (ED) but form a substantial proportion (60–70%) of overall hospital inpatients.

In the UK:

- there are now over 13 million people aged 65 or over. The number of the 'oldest old' people is also rising. There are now more than 3 million people aged 80 or over, with more than 600 000 of these aged 90 or over
- around 4 million older people have a limiting long-term illness or disability, and it is estimated that this will rise to over 6 million older people by 2030

- around 850 000 people are living with dementia. One in 14 people over the age of 65 has dementia, and the condition affects 1 in 6 people over 80. Around half of people aged over 70 who are admitted to hospital as an emergency have a cognitive disorder such as dementia and/or delirium.

All staff working in Acute Medicine will be familiar with the increasing number of high-acuity, frail older patients with altered physiology, polypharmacy, multimorbidity, cognitive impairment and communication difficulties. Acute Medicine teams provide a key role in identifying the urgent and important issues which, if addressed accurately and comprehensively, will improve patient outcomes.

One of the most important decisions is where older people requiring acute medical care can be managed most effectively – the patient's home (e.g. 'Hospital at Home' or virtual ward), ambulatory setting (e.g. same-day emergency care, SDEC) or inpatient setting? Accordingly, Acute Medicine clinicians working collaboratively with the multidisciplinary team (MDT), acute geriatric medicine or frailty liaison teams, and community partners need to make a holistic assessment to reduce inappropriate hospitalisations and the need for long-term care in this potentially fragile population.

Evolution of geriatric medicine

In 1965, Bernard Isaacs coined the term 'geriatric giants'. The geriatric giants were commonly known as the '4 Is': immobility, instability, incontinence and intellectual impairment. However, over time a fifth I was added – iatrogenic. These 'giants' have evolved over the past almost 60 years into the geriatric '5 Ms' — a simple construct which defines the core competencies of geriatric medicine in a manner which is memorable for those inside and outside the specialty (Table 13.1).

Careful and thorough clinical assessment can be grouped into five key areas (the geriatric 5 Ms): mind, mobility, medications, multicomplexity and matters most. One of the important components of the geriatric 5Ms is 'matters most', recognising the importance of the patient at the centre of geriatric care delivery. Attention to these areas will assist in timely diagnosis of acute medical problems and development of an appropriate treatment plan.

Frail older people

Frailty is a state of vulnerability to adverse outcomes that helps explain why older people with urgent care needs can experience major functional decline (often after apparently minor stressors). Around one-third of patients in acute medical units (AMUs) are older people living with frailty. Frailty contributes to the oldest patients having the longest lengths of stay, highest readmission rates and highest rate of use of long-term care after discharge. Admission to hospital also adds the specific hazards of more rapid deconditioning, cross-infection, increased risk of falls and associated injury, and worsening of cognitive state due to multifactorial causes. Care at home is often a safer alternative. Thus, if effective medical treatment and care can be provided in the patient's home or ambulatory acute care setting, these additional burdens may be avoided.

What is frailty?

Ageing is characterised by progressive and heterogeneous decline in physiological reserve of all organ systems, albeit at different rates and varying between individuals. There is reduced functional reserve and ability to repair. These changes can be further exacerbated by the presence of multimorbidity. The primary challenge to healthcare systems is not ageing *per se* but the association between ageing and frailty. Not all older people are frail but patients with moderate to severe frailty account for most issues in (e.g. falls, delirium, disability, hospital readmission and care home admission) and use of resources by older people.

Frailty is a multidimensional geriatric syndrome. Common symptoms and signs related to a diagnosis of frailty include the following.

- Shrinking (loss of height or weight).
- Weakness.
- Exhaustion.
- Slowness.
- Low activity.

Multiple age-related hormonal and metabolic changes greatly contribute to the principal age-related chronic diseases and decline in physiological functions. Some of these changes (e.g. low testosterone in men, low 25-hydroxy vitamin D, low insulin-like growth factor-1, elevated cortisol) play a role in the development of sarcopenia (loss of muscle mass) and frailty.

Table 13.1 The geriatric giants (5 Is) versus the geriatric 5 Ms. Both constructs are relevant for the individual older person. However, the increasing recognition of multicomplexity and the primacy of putting the patient first have helped transform older person care

Geriatric giants (5 Is) - circa 1965	Geriatric 5 Ms – current day
Immobility – includes 'Off legs' as well as more chronic mobility issues. 'Off legs' is a frailty syndrome that can represent many diagnoses. As with all the frailty syndromes, there will usually be multiple causes. Potential for becoming house-, chair- or bed-bound with resulting deconditioning and risk of pressure ulcers.	**Mobility** – understanding of baseline mobility/self-care ability and acuity of changes; safety and accessibility of home environment and availability of caregiver support; access to transportation for follow-up care.
Instability – falls and consequences of them such as injury, fragility fractures (osteoporosis) and loss of confidence. Distinguish between syncopal (e.g. cardiac, polypharmacy) or non-syncopal (e.g. strength, balance, vision, proprioception, vestibular and environmental hazards all to be assessed). Note that there is often significant overlap. Most falls are multifactorial.	**Multicomplexity** – medical co-morbidities and geriatric syndromes (frailty, falls, incontinence, skin breakdown); comprehensive physical examination; maintaining a broad differential.
Incontinence – urinary and faecal. This is an unusual acute presentation, but a marker of frailty and a risk factor for adverse outcomes.	**Matters most** – central to all matters related to care is the patient themselves – 'person-centred' care.
Intellectual impairment – cognitive problems such as delirium and/or dementia. These are closely interrelated, but each requires clinically distinct management. Collateral history is key to detecting a recent change in cognition; it is common for delirium to be superimposed on pre-existing dementia. Depression is also common in older people living with frailty.	**Mind** – knowledge of baseline cognitive function is essential in evaluation of acute changes; baseline presence and severity of behavioural symptoms of dementia; presence of substance use and abuse; availability of community and caregiver support and degree of caregiver burden or burnout.
Iatrogenic – polypharmacy with risk of adverse drug events (e.g. medication errors and adverse drug reactions). Adverse drug events lead to increased hospital stay, morbidity and mortality.	**Medications** – review of accurate medication list with focus on psychoactive medications and recent changes, including new or discontinued medications and dose adjustments; medication adherence – is administration supervised and reliable?; be prepared to stop unnecessary or potentially harmful medications (e.g. deprescribing).

Osteoporosis

Sarcopenia is a major predictor of frailty, hip fracture, disability and mortality in older persons. Sarcopenia is defined as age-related loss of muscle mass and function. Prevalence is estimated at 11–50% among people aged >80 years. A diagnosis of sarcopenia is probable when patients are found to have low muscle strength measured by either grip strength or chair stand test together with objective measures of muscle quantity or quality. Sarcopenia specialist groups consider sarcopenia to be the most important cause of frailty in older people.

It is estimated that one in two women and one in five men sustain a fragility fracture after the age of 50. An estimated 500 000 fragility fractures occur in the UK every year. At any one time, hip fractures account for occupation of over 3600 hospital beds across England, Wales and Northern Ireland. Hip fracture is associated with increased risk of death, with only approximately 70% of patients surviving one year after their fracture, and 7% of patients dying within 30 days of admission.

Bone is a dynamic tissue that is under continuous turnover or remodelling, which enables it to repair damage and adjust strength. Osteoclasts and osteoblasts are the two main types of bone cells located on bone surfaces and are responsible for bone resorption and formation, respectively. Bone resorption and bone formation normally are coupled (bone removal equals bone formation) but with excess resorption, a net loss of bone results (i.e. osteoporosis).

Osteoporosis is a generalised skeletal disorder characterised by compromised bone strength, predisposing to an increased risk of fragility fractures. Osteoporotic fractures (fragility fractures, low-trauma fractures) are those occurring from a fall from a standing height or less, without major trauma. Osteoporosis and related fragility fractures represent a major healthcare problem and are a key component of frailty. Fragility fractures are associated not only with the decline in bone and muscle mass, but also frailty syndromes such as delirium and (related) falls. Risk factors for falling and fracture include neurological disorders, impaired vision, impaired hearing, frailty and deconditioning, proximal myopathy, sarcopenia, medications and environmental factors. The impact of fractures may lead to loss of mobility and independence, social isolation and depression.

Initial management of osteoporotic fracture is as follows.

- Refer to fracture liaison services (FLS) when available. FLSs systematically identify people aged 50 and older who have had a 'fragility fracture', with the aim of reducing their risk of further fractures (i.e. secondary prevention). Around 50% of people who experience a hip fracture have had a previous fragility fracture. Identifying people with a previous fracture therefore offers a good opportunity to prevent 'secondary fractures' (25% of which occur within one year of initial fracture).
- Vertebral compression fractures are the most common type of osteoporotic fracture. About two-thirds of vertebral fractures are asymptomatic and are diagnosed as an incidental finding on imaging. In some patients, the presence of vertebral fractures may become apparent because of height loss or kyphosis. Typically, patients present with acute back pain after bending, coughing or lifting. The pain from a vertebral compression fracture may be sharp or dull and often radiates bilaterally into the anterior abdomen in the distribution of contiguous nerve routes. Sitting and movement aggravate the discomfort. Acute episodes of pain usually resolve after 4–6 weeks, but mild pain may persist for up to three months. Vertebral compression fractures should

include pain control, with resumption of activity as quickly as possible, and physical therapy. The evaluation includes assessment for neurological findings.
- Hip fractures are the most devastating osteoporotic fractures and are associated with increased morbidity and mortality. Initial care of the patient with a hip fracture consists primarily of providing adequate analgesia and consulting the perioperative geriatrics service. Because the occurrence of fall and fracture often signals underlying ill health, a comprehensive MDT approach is required from presentation to subsequent follow-up, including the transition from hospital to community.
- A bone mineral density (BMD) scan should be performed on a non-urgent basis if not already done. Initial laboratory testing for osteoporosis should include full blood count (FBC); C-reactive protein (CRP); complete metabolic panel including creatinine, calcium, phosphate, alkaline phosphatase and liver function tests (LFT); 25-hydroxy vitamin D to evaluate for vitamin D deficiency; thyroid-stimulating hormone (TSH); myeloma screen; testosterone in men to test for hypogonadism; 24-hour urine calcium, sodium and creatinine to check for calcium malabsorption or hypercalciuria. This work-up identifies about 90% of occult disorders at a reasonable cost. Patients who have abnormalities on initial laboratory testing or who have suspicious findings on history and physical examination may require additional laboratory tests.
- The diagnosis of osteoporosis can be made by the occurrence of the fragility fracture itself or by a BMD measurement. Osteoporosis is defined as a BMD measurement that is 2.5 standard deviations lower than peak bone mass values (i.e. T-score < -2.5). Osteoporosis treatment may also be offered to patients with osteopenia (i.e. T-score between -1 and -2.5) and increased fracture risk calculated using FRAX country-specific thresholds.
- The therapeutic landscape of osteoporosis continues to evolve with new antiresorptive and osteoanabolic agents (Box 13.1).

Frailty syndromes

The Hospital Frailty Risk Score (HFRS) provides hospitals and health systems with a low-cost, systematic way to screen for frailty and identify a group of patients who are at greater risk of adverse outcomes. Forty percent of non-elective admitted medical patients have a HFRS above 5 and are thus considered frail.

Box 13.1 Management of osteoporosis

- Calcium and vitamin D intake should be optimised.
- Lifestyle – stop smoking, increase weight-bearing exercise and improve nutritional status.
- Reduce falls risk.
- Manage pain and any disability associated with previous fractures.
- Manage underlying disease if secondary osteoporosis.
- The therapeutic landscape of osteoporosis continues to evolve with new antiresorptive and osteoanabolic agents.
  - Bisphosphonates – antiresorptive: various formulations available (e.g. alendronate and zoledronate). Reduce osteoclastic bone resorption by entering the osteoclast, causing loss of resorptive function and accelerating osteoclast apoptosis.
  - Denosumab – antiresorptive: human monoclonal antibody inhibitor of the receptor activator of nuclear factor kappa-B ligand (RANKL). Prevents activation of osteoclasts by RANK/RANKL pathway.
  - Continuous exposure to high levels of parathyroid hormone (PTH) is associated with *catabolic effects* on bone (e.g. as occurs in primary hyperparathyroidism), while intermittent exposure to low doses of PTH has *anabolic effects:* teriparatide – osteoanabolic – recombinant human PTH (1-34); similar findings with PTHrP: abaloparatide – osteoanabolic – analogue of PTH-related peptide (PTHrP).
  - Romosozumab – mixed antiresorptive and osteoanabolic: an antisclerostin agent (sclerostin is a protein involved in the regulation of bone formation).
- A generic oral bisphosphonate will be recommended as the first treatment choice for most people. These treatments are effective at reducing fracture risk at low cost.
- Bone anabolic therapies will benefit osteoporosis patients at very high fracture risk. Anabolic therapy should be followed by antiresorptive therapy (i.e. sequential therapy).

People with frailty may present with acute illness differently from other patients. The presence of frailty syndromes (e.g. falls, immobility, incontinence, multimorbidity and cognitive dysfunction such as delirium or dementia) and the interaction between these and/or associated polypharmacy in the older person presenting to Acute Medicine can make the immediate diagnosis unclear and mask serious underlying pathology. Importantly, these frailty syndromes are usually multifactorial. Both the underlying medical conditions and the presenting frailty syndrome(s) need attention. By identifying all the causes as part of the holistic comprehensive geriatric assessment (CGA) and other evaluations, the management plan will be more effective, thus reducing length of stay – this is good for the patient, the carer and the over-crowded healthcare system.

Multimorbidity

Like frailty, co-morbidities increase with age. By the time people reach their early 80s, only one in seven is free of any diagnosed long-term health condition and, by the age of 85, 80% are living with at least two.

- People with two or more long-term medical conditions are one of the greatest challenges faced by the healthcare service.
- Treating each disease in a patient as if it exists in isolation will lead to less good outcomes and complicate and duplicate interactions with the healthcare system. The resulting polypharmacy can lead to drug adverse events, potentially leading to even more medications to treat the adverse effects. Among Scottish people with two medical conditions, 20.8% were receiving 4–9 medicines and 10.1% were receiving 10 or more medicines.
- Moving from thinking about multimorbidity as a random assortment of individual conditions to recognising it as a series of largely predictable clusters of disease in the same person (i.e. termed *cluster medicine*) will help us to be more systematic in our approach to multimorbidity.
- It is important for each patient to have a personalised assessment and the development of an individualised management plan.

Polypharmacy

Polypharmacy commonly defined as the use of five or more medications daily by an individual. The number definition does not consider the appropriateness of medications, which should be reviewed following medicines reconciliation.

- Patients at highest risk of inappropriate polypharmacy are those with the greatest frailty, on the most medicines and taking high-risk medicines. Polypharmacy can lead to increased 'drug–drug' interactions and problems with treatment adherence and persistence.
- Polypharmacy can be appropriate (e.g. all drugs are indicated) or inappropriate (e.g. when one or more of the drugs is no longer indicated due to prescribing of multiple medicines inappropriately or where the intended benefits from the medicines are not realised).
- The Realistic Medicine 7-Steps approach to polypharmacy is of value in the clinical setting (Figure 13.1).
- Deprescribing, 'the process of withdrawal of an inappropriate medication, supervised by a healthcare professional with the goal of managing polypharmacy and improving outcomes' is important. Stopping potentially inappropriate medications has been shown to result in cognitive improvement, fewer falls and a positive change in a patient's global health, with no evidence of increased mortality. Guides exist to support patients and clinicians; for example, the STOPP/START guidelines or Beers criteria have made progress in aiding clinicians' deprescribing decision making.
- Working within Acute Medicine, close relationships with pharmacy colleagues are vital as they can review patients experiencing polypharmacy for potential inappropriate prescriptions, preferred options and drug–drug interactions.

Falls

> A fall is an *unexpected* event in which the participant comes to rest on the ground, floor or lower level *without known loss of consciousness*. Falls are the most common single reason for older people to present to urgent care.

- Falls account for 17% of all ED presentations in older people.
- Around 40–60% of falls lead to injuries (including 5% fractures).
- Most falls in older people are multifactorial.
- The term *'collapse query cause'* refers to one or more episodes of transient *loss of consciousness* before a thorough evaluation has been made. The major causes of this presentation are acute illness causing syncope and non-syncopal attacks. For example, orthostatic hypotension is common in older people. Defined as a drop of >20 mmHg in systolic blood pressure (BP) or >10 mmHg diastolic BP after standing for three minutes, it is seen in almost a quarter (24%) of ED presentations with syncope. The aim of management is to reduce symptoms and improve standing time, physical function and activity. This takes precedence over optimising standing BP.
- Older people accessing acute care services following a fall, with or without a fragility fracture, should be assessed for reversible causes.
- A multidisciplinary safety assessment before discharge should be routine in patients presenting with an acute fall, or those who have had two or more prior falls in the last 12 months.
- Within Acute Medicine, working closely with physiotherapy and occupational therapy colleagues is essential in delivering patient-centred care. Physiotherapists will focus on mobility and movement whereas occupational therapists will focus on function. They may offer support with regard to interventions to reduce the risk of future falls, such as referral to community falls rehabilitation groups or advice on equipment such as mobility aids.

Figure 13.1 The Realistic Medicine 7-Steps approach to appropriate polypharmacy. The 7-Steps to appropriate polypharmacy demonstrate that the patient review process is not a linear one-off event but cyclical, requiring regular repeat and review. The steps are centred around *what matters to the patient*, as they play a vital part in making informed decisions about their medicines, if they are provided with the right information, tools and resources.

Incontinence

> Incontinence is defined as involuntary loss of urine and is a major concern to older people, their care partners and healthcare systems. Incontinence can cause physical, emotional and social distress. For many older people, incontinence is a stigmatising condition, and they will not volunteer the problem or seek help.

- New incontinence in an older person can be a sign of an underlying condition or the effect of a medication and should not be explained away simply as part of ageing and requires investigation.
- Incontinence can lead to skin breakdown and infection, falls whilst trying to get to a toilet to avoid it and dehydration by limiting fluid intake.
- Most drugs to treat urinary incontinence have a high acetylcholine burden (e.g. oxybutynin) and have been shown to worsen cognitive impairment and dementia, so decisions to initiate pharmacotherapy in older people must take the whole picture into account.
- Patients with ongoing incontinence should be referred to their local community bladder and bowel team for review and ongoing support to advise on interventions to improve symptoms as well as ways to manage it.
- Urinalyses are often obtained when older people present to hospital with non-specific symptoms, leading to erroneous diagnosis of infection, inappropriate antibiotics and increased risk of complications such as *Clostridioides difficile* diarrhoea. Dipstick tests are frequently positive for leucocytes due to the high prevalence of asymptomatic bacteriuria in older adults. Use more objective tests if suspecting urinary tract infection.
- Older people presenting to Acute Medicine should not be routinely catheterised unless there is clear, objective evidence of urinary retention or strict fluid balance measurement is needed.
- Routinely assess older patients on the Acute Medicine service for constipation, request nursing colleagues to keep a record of bowel movements (e.g. Bristol Stool Chart), and prescribe laxatives as required for older people admitted to hospital.

> Urinary tract infections (UTI) are an important cause of morbidity that requires antibiotic use in older adults. There is evidence that hospital admission for UTI is increasing in the UK. In the elderly, recurrent UTIs are associated with frailty.

Dementia

> Dementia is a progressive decline in any of the cognitive domains such as memory, language, perception and executive function.

- Alzheimer's disease (AD) is the most common cause of dementia (50–70% of all dementia cases). Dementia is a progressive disease and patients usually survive for several years; for example, in AD the survival rate is about eight years. Older frail patients, early onset of psychosis and patients with vascular risk factors have a worse prognosis.
  - Key early features include memory loss, language deficits and visuospatial problems.
  - Short-term memory is often most affected, with procedural memory maintained until AD has moderately progressed.
  - Familial forms of AD exist and may present at a younger age. They are autosomal dominantly inherited but account for less than 1% of people living with AD.
  - Treatment includes cholinesterase inhibitors like donepezil or the glutamate antagonist memantine.
- Vascular dementia is common, affecting roughly 4% of people over 65.
  - It may result from either small vessel ischaemia leading to diffuse subcortical white matter changes or multiple recurrent discrete infarcts due to risk factors like hypertension, hypercholesterolaemia and atrial fibrillation.
  - Treatment includes addressing vascular risk factors, as well as antiplatelet or anticoagulant medication where indicated.
- Mixed dementia includes an overlap between AD and vascular dementia, accounting for 20–40% of all cases of dementia.
- Frontotemporal dementia (FTD) accounts for 2–5% of cases.
  - Presents earlier than the previous forms, typically in people in their 50s.
  - Features include personality and conduct change, emotional lability and loss of insight.
  - It also has a familial component, with 40% of people with FTD having an affected first-degree relative.
  - Treatment is focused on managing the associated affective and behavioural symptoms.
- Lewy body dementias (LBDs) include two similar and common subtypes of dementia – dementia with Lewy bodies (DLB) and Parkinson disease dementia (PDD) – accounting for 10–15% of all dementia cases.

- Characterised by visual hallucinations, fluctuating cognitive impairment and parkinsonism.
- LBDs are twice as common in men than women.
- If the motor and cognitive features occur within one year of each other, in either order, it is labelled as PDD.
- In DLB, the cognitive symptoms can predate the motor symptoms by many years.
- Rivastigmine, a cholinesterase inhibitor, is the treatment of choice.

- Alcohol-related dementia is typically a result of prolonged heavy use of alcohol, with alcohol thought to be linked to up to 10% of dementias.
  - The diagnostic criterion is an alcohol intake of more than 35 units a week in men and 28 units a week in women for five or more years.
  - Chronic alcohol use can result in thiamine (B1) deficiency which left untreated can result in Wernicke–Korsakoff syndrome.
  - The Wernicke stage comes first and involves the triad of delirium, ataxia and ophthalmoplegia.
  - The Korsakoff often follows and consist of anterograde and retrograde amnesia and confabulation.
  - Treatment includes abstinence and thiamine replacement, which may result in mild improvements or at least cause symptoms to stabilise.

- Approximately 20% of inpatient beds in a general hospital will be occupied at any one time by people with dementia.
- People with dementia are usually admitted to acute hospitals for management of a new medical condition, acute exacerbation of a chronic disease, adverse drug event (check anticholinergic burden), functional or behavioural crisis, and only rarely, if ever, for diagnosis or management of dementia itself.
- Every effort must be made to provide alternatives to admission (e.g. Hospital at Home), and to expedite discharge as soon as appropriate care can be provided elsewhere.
- Occupational therapists are trained in assessing cognition using validated tools including the Mini-Mental State Examination (MMSE), Montreal Cognitive Assessment (MoCA) and Addenbrooke's Cognitive Examination–Revised (ACE-R), and can be a source of support if you identify patients with undiagnosed memory problems.
- The AMU is not an appropriate place to make a diagnosis of dementia.
  - For most patients presenting with progressive cognitive symptoms, the ideal strategy would be to refer them to local memory services in the community on discharge.

- These teams benefit from the results of routine blood tests (FBC, urea and electrolytes, LFTs), including those for vascular risk factors (lipids, glycosylated haemoglobin [HbA1c]), electrocardiogram (ECG, due to medication affecting the QT interval) and any brain imaging, so communicating these to them directly or on the discharge summary to the GP can hasten this process.
- In some situations, making a formal diagnosis whilst a patient is in hospital is required (e.g. to support an application for care funding), and this should only be done by professionals experienced in diagnosing dementia, typically involving the support of old age psychiatry.

Delirium

> Delirium is a clinical syndrome characterised by a disturbance of perception, consciousness and/or cognitive function, with an acute onset, fluctuating course and severe deterioration arising over hours or days.

- Delirium is usually triggered by a combination of influences including acute illness, surgery, drugs, electrolyte disturbance, metabolic disorders, urinary retention, constipation and environmental factors.
- Typically, delirium is multifactorial.
- Drugs which can cause delirium include opioids, steroids, benzodiazepines, antidepressants, antipsychotics, anticholinergics and Parkinson disease medications.
- It is commonly seen in older people presenting to hospital but can also develop during hospitalisation.
- Predisposing factors include cognitive impairment, frailty and severity of illness.
- For older adults who present with confusion, management and treatment of delirium should be initiated first, rather than labelling the confusion and other symptoms as dementia.
- There are three types of delirium: hypoactive, hyperactive and mixed. Hypoactive delirium, where patients are drowsy or withdrawn, is the most common form, making up 50–70% of delirium cases, but is often missed. Hyperactive delirium is characterised by increased motor activity, agitation and restlessness.
- Delirium is associated with increased morbidity and mortality, prolonged hospital stays, increased likelihood of being discharged to a care home and developing dementia.

- It can take a long time for delirium to resolve and in some cases it never completely resolves.
- Screening for delirium is essential to good care of older people.
  - All patients over 65 years old presenting to hospital should be screened for delirium using the '4AT' tool (Figure 13.2).
  - One parameter of the National Early Warning Score 2 (NEWS2) tool assesses a change in the level of consciousness or the presence of new confusion. The presence of these symptoms would score a '3' and would prompt urgent escalation.
  - To determine if the confusion is new, the 'Single Question to identify Delirium' test should be performed, which is where an able family member, friend or staff member answers 'Is the patient more confused than before?'.
- A history of a patient with delirium should be thorough, exploring the above potential causes of delirium, with focus on a good collateral history usually required.
  - It is important to know the cognitive baseline of the patient and if they have been formally diagnosed with dementia.
  - The onset and course of the confusion are important as well as whether delusions or hallucinations are present.
  - Clarifying if the patient suffers from any sensory deficits, such as hearing, sight and speech deficits, and whether any aids are used.
- In addition to standard examination, consider the following additions to determine the cause of the delirium.
  - Neurological assessment, including level of consciousness and assessing for evidence of head injury.
  - Assessing for evidence of fractures or other bony injuries, in particular hip and pubic rami fracture.
  - Examine for a palpable bladder as a sign of urinary retention and consider a digital rectal examination to look for evidence of faecal impaction.
  - Examine the pressure areas such as sacrum and heels for signs of pressure ulcers.

Investigations for delirium

These investigations are like those for other medically unwell people, such as basic blood tests, including inflammatory markers, glucose and calcium levels, thyroid function and a venous blood gas. An ECG and chest X-ray are often helpful. However, certain other investigations should be considered in specific situations.

- Blood cultures if infection is suspected.
- A coagulation screen if anticoagulated or if there is a history of chronic liver disease or heavy alcohol use.
- Serum vitamin B12 and folate concentrations if not done within the last six months.
- Arterial blood gas only if hypoxia or hypercapnia is suspected and only if the patient is a candidate for respiratory support such as intubation or non-invasive ventilation.
- Urine culture only if signs or symptoms of urinary tract infection as older people are more susceptible to asymptomatic bacteriuria.
- Other microbiological tests such as sputum cultures, faeces culture for bacteria and *Clostridioides difficile*, and respiratory virus nasal swabs, including COVID-19.
- A bladder scan to test for the presence of urinary retention.
- Joint X-rays if there is a concern about fractures.
- If trauma is suspected then a low threshold for whole-body computed tomography (CT) is recommended as older people can experience significant injury from low-impact events such as falling from standing height or from bed.
- Patients with delirium often undergo neurological investigation when it is not warranted, including CT scans of the brain which often do not identify the cause of the delirium or change its management.
  - CT brain scans should not be routinely done for the investigation of delirium unless the patient has focal neurological signs, a reduced level of consciousness, history of a recent fall, evidence of head injury or is anticoagulated.
  - An electroencephalogram (EEG) should only be considered when there is a suspicion of epileptic activity or non-convulsive status epilepticus.
  - A lumbar puncture should not be routinely performed on patients with delirium due to the limited evidence of benefit and the associated risks, unless the history and examination findings suggest an infection of the central nervous system such as headaches, a fever, photophobia or meningism.

Management of delirium

Relatives and carers should be informed early regarding the diagnosis of delirium. AMUs should have written information about delirium to give to families. They should be granted permission to visit their relative at any time to support them whilst in hospital (depending on COVID-19 restrictions, if any).

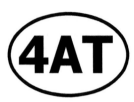

(label)

Patient name:

Date of birth:

Patient number:

**Assessment test
for delirium &
cognitive impairment**

Date: **Time:**

Tester:

CIRCLE

[1] ALERTNESS
*This includes patients who may be markedly drowsy (eg. difficult to rouse and/or obviously sleepy
during assessment) or agitated/hyperactive. Observe the patient. If asleep, attempt to wake with
speech or gentle touch on shoulder. Ask the patient to state their name and address to assist rating.*

Normal (fully alert, but not agitated, throughout assessment)	0
Mild sleepiness for <10 seconds after waking, then normal	0
Clearly abnormal	4

[2] AMT4
Age, date of birth, place (name of the hospital or building), current year.

No mistakes	0
1 mistake	1
2 or more mistakes/untestable	2

[3] ATTENTION
*Ask the patient: "Please tell me the months of the year in backwards order, starting at December."
To assist initial understanding one prompt of "what is the month before December?" is permitted.*

Months of the year backwards	Achieves 7 months or more correctly	0
	Starts but scores <7 months / refuses to start	1
	Untestable (cannot start because unwell, drowsy, inattentive)	2

[4] ACUTE CHANGE OR FLUCTUATING COURSE
*Evidence of significant change or fluctuation in: alertness, cognition, other mental function
(eg. paranoia, hallucinations) arising over the last 2 weeks and still evident in last 24hrs*

No	0
Yes	4

4 or above: possible delirium +/- cognitive impairment
1-3: possible cognitive impairment
0: delirium or severe cognitive impairment unlikely (but
delirium still possible if [4] information incomplete)

4AT SCORE

GUIDANCE NOTES   Version 1.2. Information and download: **www.the4AT.com**
The 4AT is a screening instrument designed for rapid initial assessment of delirium and cognitive impairment. A score of 4 or more
suggests delirium but is not diagnostic: more detailed assessment of mental status may be required to reach a diagnosis. A score of 1-3
suggests cognitive impairment and more detailed cognitive testing and informant history-taking are required. A score of 0 does not
definitively exclude delirium or cognitive impairment: more detailed testing may be required depending on the clinical context. Items 1-3
are rated *solely on observation of the patient at the time of assessment.* Item 4 requires information from one or more source(s), eg. your
own knowledge of the patient, other staff who know the patient (eg. ward nurses), GP letter, case notes, carers. The tester should take
account of communication difficulties (hearing impairment, dysphasia, lack of common language) when carrying out the test and
interpreting the score.
Alertness: Altered level of alertness is very likely to be delirium in general hospital settings. If the patient shows significant altered
alertness during the bedside assessment, score 4 for this item. **AMT4 (Abbreviated Mental Test - 4):** This score can be extracted from
items in the AMT10 if the latter is done immediately before. **Acute Change or Fluctuating Course:** Fluctuation can occur without delirium
in some cases of dementia, but marked fluctuation usually indicates delirium. To help elicit any hallucinations and/or paranoid thoughts
ask the patient questions such as, "Are you concerned about anything going on here?"; "Do you feel frightened by anything or anyone?";
"Have you been seeing or hearing anything unusual?"

Figure 13.2 4AT tool.

- Non-pharmacological preventive measures for delirium should be undertaken for all older people admitted to hospital.
  - These include avoiding non-essential interventions overnight including observations, to aid a normal sleep cycle, optimising medication and co-morbidities, relieving exacerbating symptoms and preventing complications.
  - Restraints should not be used as the associated risks outweigh the benefits substantially.
- Pharmacological agents should not be routinely prescribed to patients who are at risk of delirium.
  - Sedation should only be considered if de-escalation techniques have not worked and the patient is a risk to themselves or others, to conduct essential investigations or to relieve distress in highly agitated patients.
  - Prescriptions should be done on the 'as required' part of the drug chart and be reviewed daily.
  - Local hospital protocol for choice of agent may vary but typically the options include antipsychotics such as haloperidol, which have the benefit of not causing a reduced conscious level.
  - However, antipsychotics are contraindicated in patients with Lewy body dementia, Parkinson disease, arrhythmias, heart failure, seizures and a prolonged QTc interval. In these situations, along with delirium tremens due to alcohol withdrawal, benzodiazepines such as lorazepam are preferable.
  - Patients should have had a recent ECG before treatment with an antipsychotic and if it is not possible to complete one, it is safest to opt for a benzodiazepine.
  - Both options can be given orally or intramuscularly, with oral as the preferred route.
  - It is better to give small doses more frequently than larger doses less frequently.
  - If patients experience an acute dystonic reaction from an antipsychotic, then procyclidine should be given orally or intramuscularly.
  - Patients should not be discharged on a new antipsychotic without a plan for follow-up and review.
  - If sedation is required for more than 24 hours, consider a review by old age psychiatry, to review the diagnosis and consider alternative longer-acting agents such as risperidone, olanzapine or quetiapine.
- Patients with delirium should have formal capacity assessments completed by an appropriate healthcare professional, for example the option to refuse medical treatment, and in England and Wales this will often lead to a 'deprivation of liberty safeguard'

or DoLS being completed. Scotland and Northern Ireland have similar but differing legislation.
- On discharge, patients with delirium should have a follow-up appointment in place with either their GP or an appropriate hospital outpatient appointment to review ongoing symptoms.
- For patients with delirium where there is suspected co-existing undiagnosed dementia, a referral to memory services should be considered.

Assessment of the frail older person

Frail patients should be seen by a senior clinical decision maker as soon as possible to avoid their unnecessary admission, improve care decisions and outcomes, and minimise the time they spend in hospital. Wherever clinically appropriate, care in the older person's home (e.g. 'Hospital at Home' or virtual ward) or in the ambulatory care setting (e.g. SDEC) is preferred.

Atypical presentation of clinical conditions is common in frail older patients. For example, COVID-19 infection in the frail older person can present atypically with delirium, without the well-documented symptoms and signs of cough, breathlessness and fever. Subsequently, clinical assessment of this population is challenging, as they often present non-specifically (for example, with falls, immobility or delirium), which can make the immediate diagnosis obscure. History taking may also be problematic because of sensory impairment, dementia or delirium. Often, additional information and collateral history are needed, which may not be readily accessible in the acute care setting. Time pressures may prevent staff from focusing on anything other than the immediate problem.

The presence of one or more frailty syndromes should prompt early consideration of the need for a fuller assessment by the MDT. The clinical frailty scale (CFS) is a quick and simple tool that identifies degree of frailty based on symptoms and functional status (i.e. patients who score 1 are fit, active and independent; 4–6 are vulnerable; 7 are severely frail and completely dependent; 8 are very severely frail and completely dependent; and 9 are terminally ill with a life expectancy of less than six months). The CFS has value to predict outcome in the short and longer terms, and to prompt an individualised, holistic assessment. However, it has limitations and should not be used as a determinant of frailty in isolation.

Suggested use of CFS scores in clinical care.

- 1–3 are designated as *robust* and patients receive usual care with specialist care referrals as indicated.
- 4–6 are designated as *mild-to-moderate frailty* and it is important to look for frailty syndromes.
- 7–9 are designated as *severe frailty* and frailty syndromes are very prevalent and holistic assessment is required.

Once frailty is likely or has been confirmed, this should prompt the clinician to consider holistic CGA, which considers not only the presenting problems but also the broader factors at play, including prognosis. CGA is a multicomponent intervention where an older person undergoes medical, functional, social and psychological assessment. Frailty and illness severity together are powerful predictors of outcomes, so should be assessed at the first point of contact. The CGA can also generate the information necessary to embark upon an evidence-based management plan with shared decision making. This can lead to better outcomes, including reduced readmissions, reduced long-term care, greater patient satisfaction and lower costs.

> Definition of CGA: 'a multidimensional, interdisciplinary diagnostic process to determine the medical, psychological, and functional capabilities of a frail older person in order to develop a coordinated and integrated plan for treatment and long-term follow-up'.

Acute Medicine best practice approach to older persons

- The first principle is that of what 'matters most' – putting patients first (i.e. person-centred).
- Older people (or designate) should be involved in deciding their own healthcare (i.e. shared decision making).
- Meeting the health needs of older people with respect, dignity and compassion.
- Hospitals should identify patients with frailty soon after their arrival (e.g. using CFS). Once identified, this should prompt the clinician to consider holistic CGA, which considers not only the presenting problems but also the broader factors at play, including prognosis.

- MDT assessment is critical to delivering a holistic overview and arranging ongoing management, either in hospital or in the community (including rehabilitation and post acute care). MDT discussion can occur through various channels, including focused ward and board rounds.
- Collaborate closely with acute geriatric medicine or frailty liaison services, especially during the first 72 hours of care.
- Obtain collateral history.
- Ensure that aids to communication are readily available (e.g. visual aids).
- All older people should be screened for delirium on admission.
- Older patients may benefit from nursing tools such as bowel, food and fluid balance charts as well as Waterlow scores that assess skin to help inform the need for specialist mattresses and how often patients should be turned in bed to prevent the development of pressure ulcers.
- An acute presentation in an older person with frailty should prompt a structured medication review.
- Pain in the older adult population is very common, particularly in acute care settings. Pain can be difficult to assess in older people who have communication barriers – consider using a structured pain scale or empirical analgesic trial. Awareness of renal and gastrointestinal co-morbidities is important in determining choice of therapy. All older people should have as-required analgesia prescribed on admission.
- Intra- and interhospital transfers of older people at night should be minimised. They can increase the risk of delirium.
- The need for Acute Medicine care across the various acute care settings (e.g. home, ambulatory, inpatient) should prompt discussions about advance care planning for the older person.
- Frailty assessment, accompanied by person-centred discussions, can aid decision making with regard to appropriateness for enhanced or critical care escalation.
- Discharge planning. Follow the five key principles of 'Where best, next?'.
  - Plan for discharge from the start.
  - Involve patients and their families in discharge decisions.
  - Establish systems and processes for frail people.
  - Embed MDT reviews. The MDT needs to manage the interface with community services, including complex discharge planning to clearly describe the support people will require when they are discharged or transferred.
  - Encourage a supported 'home first' approach.

- Initiate safeguarding pathways as needed (including elder abuse and neglect).
- It is important to avoid ageist language – 'acopia' and 'social admission' are not diagnoses. This also goes for 'poor historian' (by definition, a historian is someone who records history), which reflects badly on the reviewing clinician.
- Presentation with a frailty syndrome should lower thresholds for COVID-19 testing and early isolation according to local protocols.
- Provide targeted preventive care as needed.
- Refer as needed for common co-morbidities, including referring older people with suspected dementia to memory services.
- Embed older person health and social care education and training for medical students and healthcare professionals working in Acute Medicine.
- Given the prevalence of frailty issues in Acute Medicine, there is justification for a lead Acute Medicine clinician to focus on frailty issues, including education.

14

Perioperative medicine

Robert Grange, Joshua Griffiths and David Shipway

 KEY POINTS

- Physicians in the emerging specialty of perioperative medicine deliver proactive perioperative medical support to surgical teams.
- The aim of perioperative medicine is to deliver the best possible care for patients before, during and after major surgery.
- Frailty is a condition characterised by loss of biological reserve, failure of physiological mechanisms and vulnerability to a range of adverse outcomes, including increased risk of morbidity, mortality and loss of independence in the perioperative period.
- Consultant-led multidisciplinary comprehensive geriatric assessment and optimisation has been shown to reduce mortality, length of hospital stay and postoperative medical complications in older surgical patients.
- When considering a complex or high-risk surgical intervention, it is essential to consider and communicate the potential risks, benefits and burdens of that intervention.

Introduction

Over the next 30 years, epidemiological projections indicate that the population aged ≥80 years old will triple. Ageing is associated with factors increasing surgical risk, such as multimorbidity and frailty. However, indications for surgery, including cancer, degenerative disease and trauma, also increase with age. Societal expectations along with minimally invasive surgical techniques and advances in anaesthesia mean that surgery is increasingly performed in medically complicated, high-risk individuals.

The role of the physician in surgery

> The perioperative period broadly refers to the three phases of the surgical admission: preoperative, intraoperative and postoperative. Subsequently, the aim of perioperative medicine is to deliver the best possible care for patients before, during and after major surgery.

For many physicians, our first involvement in perioperative medicine is when surgical patients develop postoperative medical complications. However, many of these complications are predictable and can be prevented with appropriate medical support.

In the USA, co-management is the shared responsibility, authority and accountability for care of a hospitalised patient. In the case of co-managed surgical patients, the patient's surgeon manages the surgery-related treatments and a hospitalist manages the patient's medical conditions. In the UK, physicians in the emerging specialty of perioperative medicine deliver proactive perioperative medical support to surgical teams. In addition, they support the shared decision-making process before surgery by offering a physician's nuanced view in an enhanced preassessment process.

Acute Medicine: Lecture Notes, First Edition. Edited by Glenn Matfin.
© 2023 John Wiley & Sons Ltd. Published 2023 by John Wiley & Sons Ltd.

The decision to operate – shared decision making

Shared decision making is a process in which healthcare professionals work alongside patients to agree a plan related to their care. Patients often wish to involve their family (or a close friend) in such decisions. For patients who lack mental capacity to make complex decisions, recognising this process should involve patient representatives according to the law of that jurisdiction.

Usually, these decisions are primarily made by the surgeon. But when it is finely balanced or there are many medical issues to consider, the surgeon may ask for a medical opinion.

When considering a complex or high-risk surgical intervention, it is essential to consider and communicate the potential risks, benefits and burdens of that intervention. These issues are particularly challenging in the emergency setting, where more rapid appraisal of the patient's frailty status, values and wishes is required to facilitate true shared decision making.

Risk assessment tools

Specialised risk assessment tools have been developed to quantify risk (although none is perfect) but they should not replace considered clinical judgement.

Commonly used examples include the following.

- American Society of Anesthesiologists (ASA) physical status classification system.
- American College of Surgeons National Surgical Quality Improvement (ACS NSQIP).
- Portsmouth-Physiological and Operative Severity Score for the enumeration of Mortality and morbidity (P-POSSUM).
- National Confidential Enquiry into Patient Outcome and Death (NCEPOD) – Surgical Outcome Risk Tool (SORT).

Those who are living with frailty or who have a predicted hospital mortality of ≥5% should be considered high risk. High-risk patients should receive consultant-delivered care (consultant anaesthetist and consultant surgeon present in theatre), with postoperative care delivered in a critical care setting.

The risk of a surgical procedure must be balanced against the risk of the alternative(s). An example is provided in Table 14.1.

Table 14.1 Example of shared decision-making considerations in a proposed above-knee amputation for a patient with an ischaemic limb

Potential benefits: *What does the patient stand to gain?*	• Resolution of their gangrene? • To relieve their ischaemic pain? • To live longer? What other life-limiting illnesses does the patient have that might influence this?
Potential risks: *What complications may arise from this specific operation occurring on this specific person?*	• Surgical risks: bleeding, infection, pain, delayed wound healing. • Anaesthetic risks. • Medical risks: acute kidney injury, myocardial infarction, stroke, electrolyte disturbance, arrhythmia, delirium, and infection.

Potential burdens:
How might the patient be affected by this operation?
	• It may not produce the benefit intended.
	  ○ Despite a successful operation, they continue to experience pain (e.g. phantom limb pain).
	  ○ They may still succumb to sepsis.
	• Definite outcomes.
	  ○ Loss of limb: may result in a significantly reduced functional state. Will they need carers? Will they be able to return home or will they require nursing home care?

Potential alternatives: *Can we provide the intended benefits by any other means?*	• Analgesia for limb pain. • Antibiotics for gangrene. • Revascularisation. • Palliative approach. • What are the risks/benefits/burdens associated with the alternatives?

It is often beyond the scope of knowledge of a single clinician to provide all necessary detail; an integrated multidisciplinary team (MDT) approach allows the complete picture to be presented to the patient. For example, geriatrician-led MDT comprehensive geriatric assessment (CGA) and optimisation has been shown to reduce mortality, length of hospital stay and postoperative medical complications in older surgical patients.

Improving surgical outcomes

> Preoperative assessment aims to:
> - risk stratify to influence surgical and anaesthetic strategy.
> - predict potential adverse outcomes.
> - formulate perioperative plans to avoid complications.
> - identify and optimise pre-existing disease.

Do not assume that medical conditions are stable and optimally managed. Subjectively assess symptoms, seek objective evidence such as blood pressure (BP) and glycosylated haemoglobin (HbA1c), and ensure chronic co-morbidities are managed as per evidence-based guidelines.

Time will often limit the opportunity to medically optimise a patient for surgery. Planned elective surgery may offer opportunities for prehabilitation and meticulous optimisation of medical co-morbidity.

In contrast, emergency surgery is performed on patients who have an acute condition that threatens life, limb or the integrity of a body structure. Some emergency operations are time-critical and need to be performed immediately (day or night). Emergency surgical care often comprises 40–50% of the workload of some surgical specialties, and can result in additional complications, higher mortality (25%) and increased costs, and is disruptive to elective surgery planning and implementation. The time of occurrence of these emergencies cannot be predicted, and appropriate surgical care must not be unduly delayed. Subsequently, in the context of emergency or urgent surgery (e.g. for cancer), delay for optimisation may worsen overall outcomes.

Of the estimated 300 000 older people living with frailty who undergo surgery each year, frailty is more prevalent in the emergency surgical group than in elective surgical patients. There is an increased incidence of adverse outcomes after emergency surgery compared to elective. This results from acute physiological derangement combined with the limited opportunity to modify patient risk preoperatively. In older people, a large proportion of surgery is non-elective, and optimisation is largely limited to optimising pain, sepsis, renal function, electrolytes, anaemia and medications, managing fluid balance and glucose control.

Each year in the UK, 64 000 adults are admitted with a hip fracture requiring surgery, most of whom are frail. Orthogeriatrics is the largest field of geriatrician input into surgical care and has been associated with improved outcomes, including mortality and length of hospital stay. Even so, the risk of death after hip fracture remains high at around 1 in 20 patients at 30 days and 1 in 5 at one year. Similarly, an estimated quarter of adults undergoing emergency laparotomy and half of patients presenting acutely to vascular services with critical limb-threatening ischaemia are living with frailty. Frailty results in increased rates of postoperative hospital-acquired geriatric syndromes, complications, increased mortality rates and adverse patient-reported outcomes such as quality of life and loss of independence.

Perioperative complications common in those living with frailty (e.g. delirium, falls, hospital-acquired deconditioning, complex discharge issues) may be predicted if frailty is identified early in the surgical pathway (e.g. using the clinical frailty scale, CFS) and mitigated using multidisciplinary CGA and optimisation.

Shared decision making should bring together the clinician's assessment of risk, supported by the CGA, with the patient's priorities for care.

To ensure that emergency surgical patients are directed to the appropriate teams and settings in a timely fashion, a combination of approaches is used. These include national early warning scores (NEWS2), frailty assessment scores, delirium risk assessments (e.g. 4AT) and mortality risk scores. This allows early level 2 and 3 care for the very unwell patient, and proactive involvement from perioperative medicine for patients with geriatric syndromes and multimorbidity.

The following section outlines options for optimising co-morbidities, but they should be considered in the wider context of holistic individualised care.

Specific perioperative issues

Cardiac

Surgery inflicts significant physiological stress on the heart. This may provoke myocardial infarction, arrhythmias or decompensated heart failure. Preoperative cardiac assessment is outlined in Box 14.1.

Box 14.1 Assessment may include the following components

History

- Symptoms: chest pain, dyspnoea, palpitations, orthopnoea, paroxysmal nocturnal dyspnoea, peripheral oedema.
- Background: ischaemic heart disease, heart failure, hypertension, diabetes, stroke, peripheral vascular disease, atrial fibrillation, obesity, smoking, alcohol.
- Exercise tolerance and functional ability: consider assigning metabolic equivalents (METS) based on a patient's activity estimate or using tools such as the Duke Activity Status Index (DASI) to objectively quantify function.

Examination

Pulse rate and rhythm, BP, murmurs, assess fluid status: jugular venous pressure, auscultation for crepitations/wheeze, peripheral oedema.

Investigations

- ECG: ischaemic changes, arrhythmias.
- Chest X-ray: cardiomegaly, pulmonary oedema.
- NT-proBNP: may be used to screen for heart failure (e.g. <125 pg/ml has a high negative predictive value); abnormal results should prompt echocardiogram.
- Echocardiogram: cardiac function and valvular pathology.
- Stress testing: e.g. dobutamine stress echocardiography.
- Cardiopulmonary exercise test.

Ischaemic heart disease

Poorly controlled ischaemic heart disease may manifest as angina, dyspnoea or fatigue.

- Medical optimisation should include the following.
  - Beta-blockers.
  - Angiotensin-converting enzyme (ACE) inhibitors/angiotensin receptor blockers (ARB).
  - Statins.
  - Antiplatelets.
- Asymptomatic/stable coronary artery disease (CAD).
  - The benefits of aspirin monotherapy usually exceed the risks of surgical bleeding. Aspirin therefore should be continued (except in neurosurgery, prostate, ophthalmic or other surgery associated with very high risks of bleeding).
  - Prophylactic revascularisation for stable disease (such as coronary artery bypass grafting, percutaneous coronary intervention or balloon angioplasty) does not improve perioperative outcomes, so is not typically recommended preoperatively.
  - In high-risk surgery, where asymptomatic proximal stenoses have incidentally been diagnosed (e.g. left main stem artery) affecting a large myocardial territory, there may be a role for prophylactic revascularisation. Such situations are complex and require case-by-case discussion with cardiology to balance the benefits of revascularisation with the risk of delaying surgery.
- Unstable CAD/recent non-ST-elevation myocardial infarction (NSTEMI).
  - Discussion with cardiology is essential.
  - Recent NSTEMI or unstable cardiac chest pain is an important risk factor for perioperative cardiac complications. NSTEMI or unstable angina should be treated appropriately preoperatively. This may require coronary intervention and/or dual antiplatelet therapy (DAPT).
  - Surgery should be deferred, except where immediate, emergency surgery is needed to save life or limb.
  - Stopping DAPT prematurely is associated with high risks of in-stent thrombosis and perioperative MI. This risk is highest in the first month after stent deployment, after which the risks associated with modern drug-eluting stents dissipate.
  - Wherever possible, surgery should be delayed until indication for DAPT has elapsed (usually six months).
  - Where surgery is urgent (e.g. cancer), after a minimum of one month of DAPT following treatment for acute coronary syndrome, the DAPT can be temporarily replaced by a single antiplatelet agent (aspirin) to facilitate urgent surgery (clopidogrel stopped five days before surgery, ticagrelor three days, prasugrel seven

days). The patient must be counselled that cardiac risks are elevated (stent thrombosis). Rapid access to coronary revascularisation services should be available if needed.

- o DAPT should be resumed for the remainder of the indicated duration postoperatively once haemostasis has been achieved 24 hours after surgery.
- o For emergency surgery, consult with haematology and cardiology.

> *Clinical pearl*: if a patient is identified as taking DAPT, always confirm the indication and duration of treatment. It is not uncommon for patients to remain on DAPT for longer than initially intended.

Valvular heart disease

The presence of valvular heart disease is a risk factor for perioperative cardiac complications. Risk is dependent on severity and type of valvular disease. Patients with established or suspected valvular disease should undergo echocardiogram evaluation prior to surgery to evaluate the severity, inform risk and influence anaesthetic practice.

- Severe aortic stenosis.
  - o Aortic valve replacement, transcatheter aortic valve implantation (TAVI) or balloon valvuloplasty should be considered in all patients prior to high-risk elective surgery.
  - o Low-to-intermediate risk surgery may be performed so long as the patient is asymptomatic; exercise testing may be required for functional evaluation.
  - o If surgery is required for urgent, life-threatening conditions, it may be necessary to proceed with surgery prior to treatment of the aortic stenosis. This will require invasive intraoperative haemodynamic monitoring and BP control by an experienced anaesthetist.
- Mitral valve stenosis.
  - o Patients undergoing intermediate or high-risk surgery may benefit from mitral valve commissurotomy or open repair if they have severe mitral valve stenosis with symptoms or raised pulmonary artery pressures (>50 mmHg).
  - o Meticulous fluid balance management and avoidance of tachyarrhythmias are required due to the high risk of developing pulmonary oedema.
- Aortic and mitral regurgitation.
  - o In the absence of symptoms or heart failure, surgery may be performed safely.

- o If heart failure is present, the patient should be medically optimised preoperatively (see below).

Heart failure

Patients with known heart failure are at risk of decompensation in the perioperative period. Preoperative NT-proBNP levels correlate strongly with postoperative mortality and can also be used to screen patients in whom heart failure is suspected. Echocardiogram should be considered in patients undergoing high risk surgery.

Medical optimisation includes:

- beta-blocker
- ACE inhibitor/ARB
- mineralocorticoid antagonists
- diuretics aiming for preoperative euvolaemia
- sodium-glucose co-transporter-2 (SGLT2) inhibitors.

Where a new diagnosis of heart failure is made, elective surgery should, where possible, be delayed by three months to allow appropriate titration of the above medication(s).

Meticulous fluid balance management is required during intraoperative and postoperative periods, aiming to maintain euvolemia. Planned critical care admission may be advised.

Arrhythmias

Patients with a history of structural heart disease or previous arrhythmia are at increased risk of developing intraoperative or postoperative arrhythmias.

Electrolytes such as potassium, magnesium and calcium must be maintained within their reference ranges and antiarrhythmic drugs should continue and be given on the day of surgery (*even if nil by mouth*).

Where new arrhythmias are identified, management will depend on the type of rhythm and haemodynamic stability of the patient.

Hypertension

The long-term cardiovascular benefits of hypertension control are well established. However, it remains unclear what effect, if any, hypertension has on perioperative mortality. Guidelines suggest BP should be maintained below 160/100 mmHg in the preoperative period; elective operations should be allowed to proceed with BP up to 180/110 mmHg.

Antihypertensives (except for ACE inhibitors/ARB) should be continued perioperatively. Failure to do so risks rebound hypertension.

Pacemakers

Diathermy may interfere with permanent pacemakers (PPM) or implantable cardiac defibrillators (ICD). Surgery may be safely performed with the following precautions.

- Ensure PPM/ICD battery check is performed within three months of planned surgery.
- Avoid monopolar diathermy where possible (use bipolar).
- Liaise with local pacing department to arrange PPM reprogramming/ICD deactivation.
- In an emergency setting, a magnet may be placed over the device to deactivate the ICD and switch the PPM to asynchronous setting.
- Ensure an external defibrillator is available whilst ICD is deactivated.
- Ensure ICD is reactivated/PPM reprogrammed (or magnet removed) prior to the patient leaving theatre.

Respiratory

Perioperative respiratory complications are common and a significant cause of mortality. Atelectasis may ensue during general anaesthesia, increasing the risk of pneumonia and respiratory compromise. Pulmonary preoperative assessment is outlined in Box 14.2.

Box 14.2 Assessment may include the following components

History
- Symptoms: dyspnoea, wheeze, recurrent chest infections, daytime somnolence, recurrent respiratory infections.
- Background: known respiratory conditions, smoking, industrial exposure, obesity.
- Exercise tolerance and functional ability.

Examination

Clubbing, asterixis, cyanosis, accessory muscle use, wheeze, crepitations, chest wall deformity, features of right heart failure, pulse oximetry, body mass index.

Investigations
- ECG – right bundle branch block, right ventricular hypertrophy.
- Chest X-ray – consolidation, hyperexpansion.
- Spirometry.
- Echocardiogram – features of pulmonary hypertension.
- Cardiopulmonary exercise test.

Chronic obstructive pulmonary disease (COPD) and asthma

The risk of complications is related to disease severity. Spirometry and history determine disease severity (exercise tolerance, home oxygen/nebulisers, frequency of respiratory exacerbations, infections/hospitalisations/oral steroid use, previous non-invasive or invasive ventilation).

Management may include the following.

- Smoking cessation.
- Inhaler therapy (bronchodilators/corticosteroids) as per the British Thoracic Society guidelines.
- Pulmonary (p)rehabilitation.
- Early postoperative mobilisation.
- Controlled oxygen therapy (aiming for oxygen saturations 88–92% in patients at risk of carbon dioxide retention).
- Consider risk of endogenous adrenal suppression secondary to recurrent steroid use.

Obstructive sleep apnoea (OSA) and obesity hypoventilation syndrome (OHS)

Obstructive sleep apnoea and OHS should be considered in all obese patients (body mass index [BMI] >30). The STOP-BANG tool can be used to predict risk of OSA. Ask about daytime somnolence, witnessed apnoeic episodes and snoring. Patients with OHS have daytime hypercapnia, i.e. partial pressure of arterial carbon dioxide ($PaCO_2$) >6 kPA (45 mmHg), whereas those with OSA do not.

- For non-urgent elective surgery, patients who are high risk of OSA should be referred for sleep studies.
- Patients with established OSA/OHS should bring their continuous positive airway pressure (CPAP) machine with them to hospital.
- Ensure the anaesthetist is aware of OSA/OHS; this may alter anaesthetic technique.
- Patients may require extended theatre recovery or postanaesthetic CPAP due to the risk of developing type 2 respiratory failure (hypoxia with CO_2 retention).

Pulmonary hypertension

The risk of perioperative complications and mortality is high. Patients undergoing elective surgery should:

- be discussed in an MDT meeting, with specific consideration given to non-operative solutions and local/regional anaesthetic techniques

- where possible, be managed in a centre with access to specialist pulmonary hypertension support, including those with expertise in pulmonary hypertension anaesthetic techniques and postoperative intensive care
- optimise vasodilator therapy where appropriate.

Gastrointestinal

Gastrointestinal conditions may negatively impact surgical outcomes via a variety of mechanisms. History and examination should target the underlying disease.

Chronic liver disease

Risk is determined by Child–Pugh status. Complications of chronic liver disease can be predicted by considering the consequences of impairment of the many functions of the liver.

- Bile production – impairment in absorption of fat-soluble vitamins such as vitamin K leading to coagulopathy and poor nutritional state.
- Drug metabolism – anaesthetic and analgesic challenges.
- Glycogen storage – perioperative hypoglycaemia.
- Inactivation of toxins – encephalopathy/delirium.
- Synthetic function – hypoalbuminaemia resulting in challenging fluid management, thrombocytopenia secondary to diminished thrombopoietin levels.
- Other issues – oesophageal varices, electrolyte disturbance (especially hyponatraemia).

Liver disease preoperative assessment is outlined in Box 14.3.

Management should include the following.

- Early involvement of a hepatologist.
- Preoperative anaesthetic review – avoid neuromuscular blocking agents and inhalation agents that are primarily metabolised by the liver.
- Correction of coagulopathy – intravenous (IV) vitamin K (blood products may be necessary in emergency surgery).
- Correction of thrombocytopenia – see thrombocytopenia section.
- Laxatives – aim for bowels to open at least twice daily to avoid encephalopathy.
- Maintain euvolaemia and consider treating hypovolaemia with 20% human albumin solution. Monitor renal function carefully – risk of hepatorenal syndrome.
- Patients with chronic liver disease have increased risk of infection and sepsis.
- Dietician support; early nasogastric tube feeding may be required.

Box 14.3 Assessment may include the following components

History
- Symptoms: haematemesis/melaena, weight loss, ascites.
- Background: alcohol history, aetiology of liver disease (e.g. alcohol, metabolic, autoimmune), previous decompensation, ensure under surveillance for hepatocellular carcinoma if indicated.

Examination
- Suspected diagnosis: assess for features of chronic liver disease (jaundice, spider naevi, gynaecomastia, leuconychia, anaemia, raised jugular venous pressure, caput medusae, hepatosplenomegaly).
- Established disease: assess for features of decompensation (asterixis, ascites).

Investigation
- Liver function tests, albumin, clotting screen.
- Ultrasound liver/fibroscan in suspected disease.

Risk assessment
- A Child–Pugh status should be assigned based on the patient's bilirubin, albumin, international normalised ratio (INR), prothrombin time and presence of encephalopathy. This can then be used to predict perioperative mortality rates: Child–Pugh A 10%; Child–Pugh B 30%; Child–Pugh C 76–82%.

Clinical pearl: patients with cirrhosis and an elevated INR are not 'auto-anticoagulated'. They are still at risk of thrombotic events – seek haematological advice regarding venous thromboembolic prophylaxis.

Alcohol misuse

Alcohol misuse is common. It may precipitate trauma via intoxication, ataxia or peripheral neuropathy and complicate admission due to withdrawal and alcohol-related co-morbidities such as liver disease, peptic ulcers and dementia.

Identification of problematic alcohol consumption can be screened for using tools such as the Alcohol Use Disorders Identification Test-Concise (AUDIT-C) or CAGE alcohol questionnaire.

Management includes:

- reducing alcohol preoperatively; aim for abstinence

- referral to alcohol services
- monitoring for signs of withdrawal using tools such as the Clinical Institute Withdrawal Assessment for Alcohol (CIWA) and managing with benzodiazepines (chlordiazepoxide/lorazepam).
- IV vitamin B substances (Pabrinex®).

Nutrition

Patients may be malnourished due to reduced intake (dementia, dysphagia), impaired absorption (inflammatory bowel disease, coeliac disease, previous bariatric surgery) or increased metabolic activity (neoplastic disease).

Poor nutritional state impairs wound healing and is an independent risk factor for postoperative mortality and morbidity.

Patients should be screened for malnutrition using the Malnutrition Universal Screening Tool (MUST). High-risk patients should receive dietician assessment; where possible, surgery should be delayed until nutritional optimisation is achieved.

Endocrine

Surgery initiates the 'stress response', a collection of neuroendocrine, metabolic and inflammatory changes that seek to maintain homeostasis under physiological challenge. This is achieved through volume expansion, liberation of metabolic substrate (such as glucose) and diversion of metabolic pathways away from anabolism towards tissue repair.

Diabetes mellitus

Diabetes mellitus is a collection of diseases characterised by absolute or relative endogenous insulin insufficiency and resultant hyperglycaemia. Poor diabetic control risks perioperative infection, poor wound healing and longer length of admission. The following recommendations and tables are adapted from the Centre for Perioperative Care 2021 Guideline 'Perioperative Care of People with Diabetes Mellitus Undergoing Elective and Emergency Surgery'.

General principles of perioperative diabetes management – *before surgery.*

- HbA1c should have been checked within the last three months.
- Elective surgery with acceptable glycaemic control would be the preferred option for people with diabetes requiring surgery.
  - HbA1c <69 mmol/mol (<8.5%).
  - Ambient glycaemic levels within ranges defined by local guidelines.
  - No evidence of diabetes-related acute decompensation such as hypoglycaemia, diabetic ketoacidosis (DKA), hyperosmolar hyperglycemic state (HHS) or electrolyte disturbance.
- Patients with HbA1c >69 mmol/mol (8.5%) and those with insulin pumps should be referred to diabetes specialists for optimisation.
- Ensure early referral to preoperative assessment for perioperative planning.
- Minimise periods of fasting (e.g. first on the operative list).
- The management goal is to optimise metabolic control through close monitoring, adequate fluid and caloric repletion, and judicious use of insulin (usually IV in this setting but the subcutaneous route, including insulin pumps, is also used).
- Avoiding pressure damage to the feet during surgery and recovery is also critical.
- Capillary blood glucose (CBG) monitoring is usually performed before meals and at bedtime.
- Pre-prescribe treatment for hypoglycaemia (e.g. CBG <4 mmol/L) and hyperglycaemia (CBG >12 mmol/L).
- If the patient was taking long- or ultra-long-acting basal insulin (human or analogue) prior to admission, then this should generally be continued.
- Consider variable rate insulin infusion (VRII).
  - If the fasting patient is going to miss more than one meal.
  - Suboptimal diabetes control, e.g. HbA1c >69 mmol/mol (>8.5%).
  - Requiring emergency surgery.
  - Persistent hyperglycaemia in the perioperative period in the context of acute decompensation.
- Medication adjustments as per Table 14.2.

General principles of perioperative diabetes management – *during surgery.*

- CBG should be at least hourly during the procedure and in the immediate postoperative period.
- Aim for CBG 6–10 mmol/l.
  - Target 4–10 mmol/l may be acceptable if patient is not taking glucose-lowering therapy known to cause hypoglycaemia.
- Capillary ketones should be checked.
  - If CBG is >13 mmol/l on two consecutive readings.
  - Patient becomes unwell.
  - Daily in patients taking SGLT2 inhibitors due to risk of euglycaemic ketoacidosis.
- Medication changes as per Table 14.2.

General principles of perioperative diabetes management – *after surgery*.

- CBG should continue to remain in the target range of 6–12 mmol/l.
- The aim is to restore usual diet and normal diabetes medication as soon as clinically safe to do so. This can be achieved through early 'DREAMing' (DRinking, EAting and Mobilising), which is the cornerstone of postoperative care.
- Do not stop VRII in a person with type 1 diabetes unless ALL the following criteria are met.

  - Basal subcutaneous insulin has been given (at least two hours before; six hours is preferred for U300 insulin glargine and 2–4 hours for U100/U200 insulin degludec).
  - CBG <10 mmol/l.
  - Ketones <0.6 mmol/l.

- Prior to hospital discharge, the patient should be made aware that the metabolic and endocrine effects of surgery may last for several days because of ongoing changes in the amount that they eat, their activity levels and the levels of stress hormones.

Table 14.2 Suggested diabetic medication adjustments during the perioperative period

Intermediate and (ultra)long-acting insulins

e.g. Abasaglar®, Humulin I®, Insulatard®, Lantus®, Levemir®, Toujeo®, Tresiba®, Insuman basal®

Insulin regime	Day prior to admission	Day of surgery
Once daily (morning)	No adjustment necessary	Give 80% of dose and blood glucose to be checked on admission
Once daily (lunchtime)	Give 80% dose	Restart insulin at normal dose when eating and drinking start.
Once daily (evening)	Give 80% dose[a]	No dose adjustment necessary.
Twice daily	Morning dose stays the same, evening dose 80%	Morning dose will need to be 80% and blood glucose to be checked on admission. The evening dose will remain unchanged.

Premixed insulin prepared by manufacturer

e.g. Humulin M3®, Humalog Mix®, Hypurin Porcine 30/70 Mix®, Insuman Comb®, Novomix 30®

Insulin regime	Day prior to admission	Day of surgery
Twice daily	No adjustment necessary	Halve usual morning dose. Blood glucose to be checked on admission. Resume usual insulin with evening meal if eating a normal meal. If eating a half/small meal, give half usual dose. If not eating, give basal only component of the usual mixed insulin.
Three times daily	No adjustment necessary	Halve usual morning dose. Blood glucose to be checked on admission. Omit lunchtime dose. Resume normal insulin with evening meal if eating a normal meal. If eating a half/small meal, give half usual dose. If not eating, give basal only component of the usual mixed insulin.

Self-mixed insulin prepared by patient/carer

e.g. **Short-acting:** Actrapid®, Humalog®, Humulin S®, Porcine Neutral®, Lyumjev®, NovoRapid® **AND intermediate-acting:** Humulin I®, Hypurin®, Porcine Isophane®, Insulatard®

Insulin regime	Day prior to admission	Day of surgery
Twice daily	No adjustment necessary	Calculate the total dose of both morning insulins and give half of this total dose as intermediate-acting insulin only, in the morning. Blood glucose to be checked on admission. Resume usual insulin with evening meal if eating a normal meal. If eating a half/small meal, give half usual dose. If not eating, give basal only component of the usual mixed insulin.

Table 14.2 (Continued)

Short-acting or (ultra)rapid-acting insulin

e.g. Actrapid®, Humalog®, Humulin S®, Porcine Neutral®, Insuman Rapid®, Lyumjev®, NovoRapid®

Insulin regime	Day prior to admission	Day of surgery	
		AM surgery	**PM surgery**
Short-acting insulin with meals (1–4 doses a day), e.g. as part of basal-plus or basal-bolus regime	No adjustment necessary[a]	Omit morning dose if no breakfast is eaten.[a] Blood glucose to be checked on admission. Omit lunchtime dose if not eating and drinking normally. Resume normal insulin with evening meal if eating a normal meal. If eating a half/small meal, give half usual dose. If not eating, give basal only component of the usual regimen.	Take usual morning insulin dose with breakfast.

Non-insulin glucose-lowering therapy

Medication	Day prior to admission	Day of surgery	
		AM surgery	**PM surgery**
Acarbose	Take as normal	Omit morning dose if not eating.	Give morning dose if eating.
Meglitinide (repaglinide or nateglinide)	Take as normal	Omit morning dose if not eating.	Give morning dose if eating.
Metformin (AND eGFR >60 ml/min/1.73m² OR procedure not requiring use of contrast media)	Take as normal	If taken once or twice a day, take as normal. If taken three times per day, omit lunchtime dose.	
Sulfonylurea (e.g. gliclazide, glipizide)	Take as normal	Omit on morning of surgery. If taken twice daily, take evening dose if eating.	Do not take on day of surgery.
Pioglitazone	Take as normal	Take as normal	Take as normal
DPP4 inhibitor (e.g. sitagliptin, vildagliptin, linagliptin)	Take as normal	Take as normal	Take as normal
GLP-1 receptor agonist (e.g. liraglutide, dulaglutide, semaglutide) Subcutaneous daily/weekly administration Oral semaglutide is available	Take as normal	Take as normal	Take as normal
Dual GIP/GLP-1 receptor agonist (e.g. tirzepatide) Subcutaneous weekly administration	Take as normal	Take as normal	Take as normal
SGLT-2 inhibitors (e.g. empagliflozin, dapagliflozin, canagliflozin)	Omit	Omit	Omit

[a] **Worked example:** Patient is awaiting a morning operation. They will only miss breakfast on the day of surgery. They usually take 40 units of long-acting insulin in the evening with 8 units of short-acting insulin three times a day with meals. The day before their surgery, they should take 32 units (80% of usual dose) of long-acting insulin and 8 units (usual dose) of short-acting insulin with their evening meal. Omit morning short-acting insulin and restart when eating normally.
eGFR, estimated glomerular filtration rate.

About 100000 emergency surgical procedures are performed per annum in the UK on people with diabetes. Unfortunately, many patients who require emergency surgery will have suboptimal glycaemic control. However, this is not necessarily a contraindication to the timely performance of potentially life-saving surgery.

- An IV access should be secured and immediate blood specimens should be sent for glucose, electrolyte and acid–base assessment.
- Gross derangements of volume and electrolytes (e.g. hypokalaemia, hypernatraemia) should be corrected.
- Surgery should be delayed (must discuss with the surgeon planned timing of surgery), whenever feasible, in patients with DKA, so that the underlying acid–base disorder can be corrected or, at least, ameliorated. Patients with HHS are markedly dehydrated and should be restored to good volume and improved metabolic status before surgery.

hypothalamic-pituitary-adrenal axis. Failure to produce adequate levels of cortisol (adrenal insufficiency) may lead to an Addisonian crisis. Features include hypotension, hypoglycaemia, hyperkalaemia, hyponatraemia, fever and impaired consciousness. It can also present with abdominal symptoms and signs that mimic a surgical abdomen but resolve with glucocorticoid therapy. This is a medical emergency which can rapidly result in death if not correctly identified and managed.

Patients with known adrenal insufficiency or taking ≥5 mg prednisolone (or equivalent) for ≥4 weeks should:

- receive 100 mg IV hydrocortisone at induction, followed by a 200 mg/24-hour infusion (or 50–100 mg 6 hourly IV or intramuscularly)
- once able to take medications orally, be prescribed glucocorticoid at double the presurgical dose for 48 hours (if recovery is uncomplicated) or up to a week otherwise.

Neurological

Parkinson disease

Parkinson disease (PD) is a common, progressive, multisystem neurological disorder which is often associated with increased perioperative mortality. As well as this, patients are often at increased risk of postoperative delirium, aspiration pneumonia and a prolonged length of stay.

In order to minimise the risk in patients with PD, recommendations include the following.

- Early PD specialist involvement.
- Avoid missed doses of medication. If absolutely necessary, consider converting oral medication using the OPTIMAL calculator to transdermal rotigotine. Seek expert advice.
- Operate early in the day (ideally first) to reduce the risk of missed medications.
- Remain aware of aspiration risk; if appropriate, refer to the speech and language therapy (SLT) team.
- Avoid potential medications that may worsen PD symptoms, such as metoclopramide and haloperidol.
- Early involvement of therapy teams to reduce risk of functional decompensation. Sitting out of bed will also aid in respiratory rehabilitation.
- Recognition and treatment of potential causes of delirium (as below).

Thyroid disease

Patients with known thyroid disease should have their thyroid-stimulating hormone (TSH) level checked within six months of surgery (routine testing of asymptomatic patients without known thyroid disease is not required). If euthyroid, no further measures are necessary.

- Management of hyper/hypothyroidism will depend on the severity of thyroid disease and urgency of operation.
- Urgent and elective surgery may proceed in subclinical hypothyroidism and subclinical hyperthyroidism. The latter may require perioperative beta-blockade (e.g. atenolol 25–50 mg) in patients at the extremes of ages but this should be weaned postoperatively.
- In more severe disease, elective surgery should be delayed until euthyroid state is achieved.
- If surgery cannot be delayed, endocrinology opinion should be sought. Treatment aims to avoid rare complications associated with severe hypothyroidism and hyperthyroidism such as myxoedema coma and thyroid storm respectively.

Adrenal suppression

A key component of the stress response is the release of cortisol through stimulation of the

Stroke

Mortality secondary to stroke in the perioperative period can be as high as 26%. It is therefore crucial that the risk of stroke is minimised as much as possible. Risk factors include previous stroke/transient ischaemic episode (TIA), advanced age, ischaemic heart disease and atrial fibrillation (AF).

For patients who have previously had a stroke, the main considerations include the following.

- Timing of surgery in relation to stroke. Higher perioperative mortality is associated with surgery within nine months of a stroke. Where surgery is not urgent, it should be deferred depending on urgency between 3–9 months.
- Perioperative medication management.
  - Cessation of anticoagulants and antiplatelets before surgery increases the risk of recurrent perioperative stroke but must be balanced with perioperative bleeding risk.
  - Antiplatelets: stop clopidogrel seven days before surgery, replace with aspirin (except in neurosurgery, prostate, ophthalmic or other surgery associated with very high risks of bleeding).
  - Anticoagulation: patients may require bridging therapy if they have had a recent stroke (within three months) or have AF and are at high risk of stroke (see anticoagulation section).

Dementia

Population projections indicate that within the next two years, there will be ≥1 million people living with dementia in the UK. These patients are at high risk of developing perioperative complications including delirium, pneumonia, acute kidney injury (AKI) and stroke. They are also at higher risk of a prolonged length of stay, nutritional, cognitive and functional decline. Consent must be carefully sought, with a test of mental capacity adhering to the legislation of the local jurisdiction. Where capacity is found to be absent, the decision to operate must be carefully considered and judged to be in best interests.

Delirium

Delirium is characterised as an acute (typically fluctuant) confusional state with evidence of clouded consciousness, disorientation, cognitive impairment, emotional lability and disordered thinking. This can also present with a hypo- or hyperactive psychomotor response and may be the first or only sign of acute medical illness in older people. Early identification of

> **Box 14.4 PINCH ME mnemonic for causes of delirium**
>
> **P**ain
>
> **I**nfection
>
> **N**utrition
>
> **C**onstipation
>
> **H**ydration
>
> **M**edication
>
> **E**nvironment

delirium (e.g. using the 4AT delirium assessment tool) is essential because a protracted course is associated with an increased risk of death, functional decline and institutionalisation. Since the medical causes are usually reversible, early investigation and treatment are essential to promote rapid resolution.

Once delirium has been identified, understanding the cause/predisposing factors is essential to guide management. **PINCH ME** is a very useful mnemonic (Box 14.4).

Non-pharmacological management of delirium is a priority. This typically involves identification of the causes, which are usually multiple. Additionally, environmental nursing measures have been shown to be effective; these include reorienting the patient, providing usual sensory support (such as hearing aids or glasses), encouraging mobility and engaging family or friends in the management and care for the patient.

In some cases, agitated behaviour can become a threat to self or others; in this instance, temporary pharmacological management may be required, and should be discussed with either geriatric or psychiatry specialists. Since sedation with even low-dose lorazepam (0.5 mg) or haloperidol (0.5 mg) is associated with increased risk of falls and increased mortality, sedation should be considered a treatment of last resort and not an alternative to quality nursing care.

Epilepsy

Patients with epilepsy are at an increased risk of seizures during the perioperative period. Anticonvulsant medication should be continued throughout the perioperative period. Where the gastrointestinal route is lost, a parenteral route will be required. Early discussion and dose conversion with pharmacy and/or neurology are advised.

Haematological

Anaemia

Anaemia is associated with significantly increased perioperative risk. Intra- or postoperative transfusions are effective, but do not come without risk.

Preoperative optimisation.

- Early haemoglobin check (at least four weeks prior to surgery) will allow time to correct causes of vitamin or iron deficiency anaemia.
- Check urea and electrolytes, ferritin, iron studies, B12, folate, thyroid function tests, LFT and a blood film.
- If evidence of iron deficiency, consider IV or oral iron replacement. IV iron is often the preferred treatment method in patients expected to have poor compliance or reduced absorption of oral preparations.
- If there is evidence of significant renal failure (anaemia of kidney disease), discuss with nephrology for consideration of erythropoietin.
- If cause of iron deficiency is unknown, consider coeliac screening and ensure postoperative plan for investigation.

Intraoperative measures.

- Consider cell salvage, acute normovolaemic haemodilution and meticulous surgical control of haemostasis to minimise blood loss.

Postoperatively.

- Patients should have a set restrictive red blood cell transfusion threshold of usually 70 or 80 g/l with posttransfusion targets of 70–90 g/l or 80–100 g/l respectively.
- Patients may require transfusion at higher haemoglobin levels if they are symptomatic of anaemia.

Some patients may decline the use of blood products (e.g. Jehovah's Witnesses).

- ensure they are appropriately informed of the potential risks
- discuss which interventions they may accept (e.g. cell salvage, autologous blood transfusion).

Thrombocytopenia

Thrombocytopenia may occur due to decreased platelet production (e.g. bone marrow suppression, infection, liver disease), increased destruction (e.g. immune thrombocytopenia, heparin-induced thrombocytopenia, sepsis) or platelet sequestration or dilution (IV fluids, splenomegaly).

Where possible, the aetiology should be sought as this will guide management. Patients with platelets $<100\times10^9$ should be discussed with haematology. Management includes platelet transfusion and in some cases of immune thrombocytopenia, steroid or immunoglobulin therapy may be indicated.

Most surgery can be performed with platelets $>50\times10^9$. However, in operations where even a small quantity of blood loss may have catastrophic consequences (e.g. spinal, ocular or neurosurgical procedures), platelet transfusion should be given to maintain a level $>100\times10^9$. Spinal anaesthesia requires a level $>80\times10^9$.

Anticoagulation

> Perioperative anticoagulation management must balance the surgical bleeding risk with the potential consequences of thromboembolism.

Most surgical procedures carry a high bleeding risk and will therefore necessitate interruption of the patient's anticoagulation. This should be executed carefully.

Warfarin

- For elective surgery, the last warfarin dose should be given six days before surgery.
- If bridging is required (Box 14.5), this should be started three days before surgery. Administer either of the following.
  - Treatment dose low molecular weight heparin (LMWH), at 0800 am daily until 24 hours before surgery (final dose may be half treatment dose if surgery carries very high bleeding risk) *or*
  - Unfractionated heparin infusion (UFH) until six hours before surgery. This necessitates admission to hospital for three days before surgery.
- INR should be checked the day before surgery to allow for oral vitamin K to be given if INR $\geq$1.5. If given, recheck INR on the day of surgery.
- Warfarin can be restarted on the evening of surgery or the day after surgery if the surgeon is satisfied that adequate haemostasis has been achieved.
- Where bridging is not necessary, administer prophylactic dose LMWH on the evening of surgery or day after surgery if indicated (for venous thromboembolism prophylaxis) and continue until INR $\geq$2.0.
- If bridging is required, administer treatment dose LMWH (or start UFH) no sooner than 48 hours after surgery and continue until INR $\geq$2.0.

Direct oral anticoagulants (DOACs)

- For elective surgery, patients with normal renal function should take their last dose of anticoagulation either 24 hours (low surgical bleeding risk) or 48 hours (high surgical bleeding risk) before surgery.
- Patients with renal impairment will need to discontinue their anticoagulation at varying times depending on renal function, type of anticoagulant and surgical bleeding risk (Table 14.3).
- Prophylactic LMWH should be given if indicated on either the evening of surgery or the day after surgery before being replaced by treatment dose DOAC at 48 hours.

Reversal of anticoagulation

If urgent surgery is required for patients taking anticoagulation, reversal of the anticoagulant is likely to be required. Discuss with haematology. This will involve the use of reversal agents such as:

- vitamin K (warfarin): time to effect for oral and IV administration is 24 hours and eight hours respectively. Fresh frozen plasma (contains all coagulation factors) and 4-factor prothrombin complex concentrate (contains factor 2, 7, 9, and 10) can also be used.
- idarucizumab (dabigatran)
- andexanet alfa (apixaban/rivaroxaban).

The last two significantly reduce anticoagulation effect within 2–5 mins.

Venous thromboembolism prophylaxis

All patients being admitted to hospital should be risk assessed for VTE and bleeding risk. Pharmacological agents (such as LMWH, UFH and in some cases DOACs) along with early mobilisation are the mainstay of VTE prophylaxis.

Devices such as graduated compression stockings and intermittent pneumatic compression devices may be used as adjuncts alongside pharmacological agents in high-risk patients. Alternatively, they may serve as monotherapy in patients who have a contraindication to pharmacological agents (e.g. those undergoing neurosurgery and some patients with major trauma).

Patients undergoing major abdominal, pelvic or orthopaedic surgery may require extended VTE prophylaxis for 28–35 days postoperatively.

Renal

Acute kidney injury (AKI)

The kidneys face many potential assaults during the perioperative period (Table 14.4). Chronic kidney disease is a risk factor for the development of AKI. This risk can be mitigated through appropriate cessation

Table 14.3 Time to withhold direct oral anticoagulation (DOAC) before surgery in hours

DOAC	Renal function (creatinine clearance, ml/min)	Time to discontinue DOAC before surgery (hours)	
		Low surgical bleeding risk	High surgical bleeding risk
Dabigatran	≥80	24	48
	50–79	24–48	48–72
	30–49	48–72	96
Rivaroxaban/apixaban/edoxaban	≥30	24	48
	<30	48	72

Table 14.4 Diagnostic schema for potential causes of acute kidney injury

Pre-renal	Renal	Postrenal
Hypovolaemia (haemorrhage, third spacing, insensible losses, overdiuresis)	**Drugs** (antibiotics, furosemide, non-steroidal anti-inflammatory drugs)	**Related to reason for surgery** (tumour, prostatic enlargement, calculi)
Hypotension (low systemic vascular resistance secondary to anaesthesia)	**Inflammation**	**Surgical damage**
Sepsis	**Endogenous nephrotoxins** (haemoglobin, myoglobin)	**Urinary retention** (constipation)
Decreased cardiac output (cardiac failure, cirrhosis, anaesthesia, increased intra-abdominal pressure)	**Radiocontrast agents** (disputed)	
	Acidosis	
	Anaemia	
Drugs (antihypertensives)	**Fluid solutions** (chloride-rich solutions)	

of nephrotoxic agents, intraoperative BP management and meticulous fluid balance management, aiming for euvolaemia.

Endstage renal disease

- Ensure early nephrology involvement.
- Correct anaemia (using IV iron infusion or erythropoietin).
- Optimise cardiovascular risk factors.
- Preoperative anaesthetic review.
- Aim for haemodialysis to be performed the day before surgery and for patient to be at their dry weight.
- Exercise extreme caution in the use of IV fluids in anuric patients.

Renal transplant

- Ensure early nephrology involvement.
- Continue immunosuppressive medication throughout perioperative period.
- Be vigilant for signs of typical and atypical infection.
- Be mindful of drug–drug interactions between immunosuppressive agents and commonly encountered surgical drugs such as antimicrobials.
- Uptitrate corticosteroids – see section on adrenal suppression.

Immunosuppression

Immunosuppression and immunomodulatory medication may be encountered in patients with solid organ transplants and inflammatory disorders such as rheumatoid arthritis or inflammatory bowel disease (Table 14.5).

Steroid use

The risk of adrenal suppression has been discussed in the adrenal suppression section. Perioperative steroid use is associated with poor wound healing, hyperglycaemia, hypervolaemia, gastric ulcers, local and systemic infections.

Analgesia

Effective surgical analgesia is essential for prompt recovery. Not only is it humane, but it supports early mobilisation and avoidance of respiratory complications, VTE and physical deconditioning which can lead to delayed discharge.

Analgesia may be titrated in line with the World Health Organization analgesic ladder.

- Step one (mild pain) – non-opiate analgesia, e.g. paracetamol, non-steroidal anti-inflammatory drugs (NSAIDS).
- Step two (moderate pain) – step one + weak opiate, e.g. codeine, tramadol.
- Step three (severe pain) – step one + strong opiate, e.g. morphine, oxycodone.

Considerations

- Some medications may not be appropriate for your patient.
  - NSAIDs should be avoided in the elderly, except in exceptional circumstances.
  - Opiates should be used with caution in renal and liver impairment.

Table 14.5 Immunosuppression and immunomodulatory medication in perioperative period

	Example medication	Recommendations
Conventional synthetic agents	Methotrexate Leflunomide Hydroxychloroquine Azathioprine	Continue throughout perioperative period; risk of inflammatory disease flare outweighs risk of postoperative infection. Medication can be held for a short period in serious infection.
Biologic agents	Adalimumab Infliximab Etanercept Abatacept Rituximab Tocilizumab	Risks of postoperative infection must be balanced against the risk of postoperative flare of inflammatory disease. For most biologics, consider performing surgery after one dosing interval has elapsed (except rituximab and tocilizumab which should be held 3–6 months and 2–4 weeks respectively). Restart after surgery when: • surgical wound has healed • sutures/staples have been removed • there is no evidence of infection.
Transplant medication	Tacrolimus Sirolimus	Do not stop antirejection medication; early involvement of transplant team is essential.

- Consider co-prescribing laxatives and antiemetics with opiates.
- Many surgical or trauma patients will suffer from severe pain from the outset. In this instance, proceed directly to step 3. It is reasonable to bypass weak opiates, which are often constipating, deliriogenic and have limited pain efficacy.
- In this instance, low-dose strong opiates (e.g. 2.5 mg oral morphine four times per day) are more effective and allow rapid titration with a single agent.
- In severe pain, consider alternative methods of analgesia including patient-controlled analgesia or regional/local anaesthesia.

15

The obstetric woman in the acute setting

Siara Teelucksingh, Emma Page and Anita Banerjee

KEY POINTS

- All women of childbearing potential presenting with acute medical conditions should have a pregnancy test.
- The leading causes of maternal mortality are indirect maternal deaths including cardiovascular disease, neurological disease and venous thromboembolic diseases.
- Multimorbidity, mental health disorders and a constellation of social vulnerabilities predispose pregnant women to increased risk and often, inequitable care.
- There are a few nuances to be aware of when reviewing a pregnant woman, including a National Maternity Early Warning Score (MEWS) and some pregnancy-specific afflictions.
- The acute care of pregnant women should not be compromised due to uncertainty and clinical inertia in the assessment and management.

Introduction

> Maternal mortality is estimated to be one death every two minutes worldwide. Two-thirds of maternal deaths are attributable to an indirect (medical or psychiatric) cause.

Pregnant women are at least equally susceptible to all common acute medical conditions compared with the non-pregnant population. Pregnant women can present to any acute hospital service at any time during their pregnancy or the postpartum period, which is up to 12 months post delivery. Women may present with acute medical problems that may need to be managed differently because of pregnancy. In addition, there are a host of obstetric syndromes that can necessitate acute admission to hospital. Timely and appropriate assessment is key to successful outcomes for these women, e.g. Acute Medicine in the ambulatory setting such as same-day emergency care (SDEC) or inpatient setting such as an acute medical unit (AMU).

High-risk pregnancies are also becoming more common as the pregnant population is reflective of:

- advancing maternal age
- increase in assisted conception

Acute Medicine: Lecture Notes, First Edition. Edited by Glenn Matfin.
© 2023 John Wiley & Sons Ltd. Published 2023 by John Wiley & Sons Ltd.

- increasing prevalence of chronic disease. Obesity is the most common health problem in women of reproductive age
- a constellation of vulnerabilities including:

  o lower socioeconomic class
  o black, Asian, ethnic minority groups
  o mental health conditions
  o substance misuse disorders
  o women born outside the UK.

Physiological changes in pregnancy

During pregnancy, a woman undergoes significant anatomical and physiological changes in order to nurture and accommodate the developing fetus. These changes occur in response to many factors: hormonal changes, increase in oxygen demand, increase in the total blood volume and increase in fetal size.

It is important to differentiate between normal physiological changes and disease pathology to identify and treat acute presentations (Table 15.1).

National Maternity Early Warning Score (MEWS) tool in obstetrics

Pregnant women are known to compensate substantially until they can no longer do so and can rapidly deteriorate. The window of opportunity to treat may therefore be narrow. Recognising an acutely unwell deteriorating pregnant woman may be challenging. A modified early warning score in maternity is therefore used to identify women at risk of deterioration. Importantly, this should not be used in isolation but rather attention must also be paid to the woman's entire clinical picture.

Physiological track and trigger monitoring of women who are pregnant and require acute assessment should use the National Maternity Early Warning Score (MEWS) tool. MEWS is a scoring system specifically for pregnant women, similar to the National Early Warning Score (NEWS2).

Radiological investigations in pregnancy

- The first-line radiological investigation of a woman with breathlessness or chest pain is a chest X-ray (CXR).
- Radiation from a CXR is equivalent to a week's exposure to background radiation in London and is therefore safe throughout pregnancy.
- Ultrasound, computed tomography (CT) scans of head and chest, and magnetic resonance imaging (MRI) are safe throughout pregnancy.
- Gadolinium contrast should be avoided.

Table 15.1 **Physiological changes and normal findings in pregnancy**

Parameter	Normal physiological change in pregnancy
Heart rate	An increase of 10–20 beats per minute, particularly in third trimester.
Blood pressure	Can decrease by 10–15 mmHg by 20 weeks but returns to pre-pregnancy levels by term.
Respiratory rate (RR)	• Unaltered in pregnancy. • If RR >20 breaths per minute, consider a pathological cause. • Mild, fully compensated respiratory alkalosis is normal during pregnancy.
Oxygen saturations	Unchanged throughout pregnancy.
Electrocardiogram	• Sinus tachycardia. • 15 degree left axis deviation due to diaphragmatic elevation. • T-wave changes – commonly T-wave inversion in leads III and aVF. • Non-specific ST segment changes (e.g. ST segment depression).
Chest X-ray	• Prominent vascular markings. • Raised diaphragm due to gravid uterus.

- For women with suspected pulmonary embolism (PE) and a normal CXR, a ventilation/perfusion (V/Q) lung scan should be requested in preference to CT pulmonary angiography (CTPA), because the radiation dose to maternal lung and breast tissue is lower.

Safety of commonly used imaging investigations in pregnancy

Fetal and maternal radiation exposure from common imaging procedures is as follows (Table 15.2).

- Threshold for fetal damage is 50 mGy. 1 mGy increases the risk of fatal childhood cancer up to the age of 15 years by 0.006%.
- Radiation to mother's breasts. 10 mGy increases the lifetime risk of developing breast cancer by 13.6%.

Table 15.2 Fetal and maternal radiation dose from common imaging procedures

Imaging modality	Fetal radiation dose	Radiation to mother's breasts
Chest X-ray	0.0005–0.01 mGy	0.04 mGy
CTPA	0.1 mGy	3 mGy
V/Q scan	0.32–0.74 mGy	0.22–0.28 mGy

Breathlessness in pregnancy

> Breathlessness occurs in more than 75% of pregnant women, and in most cases is physiological.

All pregnant women presenting with shortness of breath to acute care should have:

- emergency department (ED) and/or Acute Medicine (SDEC or AMU) assessment
- MEWS
- electrocardiogram (ECG)
- CXR
- arterial blood gas (ABG) if hypoxic.

> **Breathlessness: alarm signs and symptoms**
> - Stridor.
> - Raised respiratory rate >20/minute.
> - Oxygen saturation <94% on room air or falls to <94% on exertion.
> - Orthopnoea.
> - Sudden-onset breathlessness.
> - Chest pain or syncope.
> - Associated tachycardia.

Upper airway obstruction

- If any upper airway obstruction (e.g. anaphylaxis/upper airway oedema):
  - treat as peri-arrest scenario and obstetric and neonatal emergency; requires senior obstetric anaesthetist
  - follow Resuscitation Council UK Anaphylaxis algorithm as per non-pregnant population (see Figures 6.3 and 6.4).
- Airway compromise (e.g. angioedema, compressive neck mass): immediate obstetric anaesthetist assessment.

Exacerbation of asthma

- Aim for target saturation >94% (unless known carbon dioxide retainer).
- Consider ABG if hypoxic.
- Pharmacological management.
  - Salbutamol nebulisers.
  - Steroids (dose as per non-pregnancy).
  - Magnesium sulfate ($MgSO_4$) 2 g in 0.9% sodium chloride.
  - Consider antibiotics (consult local guidelines).
- Peak flow monitoring (unaffected by pregnancy).
- Consider cause of exacerbation.
- Admit: respiratory nurse review for fractional exhaled nitric oxide (FeNO) test if new diagnosis (indication of eosinophilic inflammation in the lungs used to support the diagnosis of asthma), and check inhaler technique and adherence.

Pulmonary oedema

- Important not to miss.
- Always ask about orthopnoea.
- Careful assessment of fluid status including intake and output charting.
- Avoid injudicious use of intravenous (IV) fluids.

- Mainstays of management.
  - Oxygen.
  - Stop IV fluids.
  - Nitrates.
  - Consider diuretics.
  - Beware of assuming that wheeze equates with airways disease.
- Urgent investigations.
  - CXR.
  - Brain natriuretic peptide (BNP).
  - Echocardiogram.
- Aetiology.
  - Cardiogenic causes: ischaemia, valvular, congenital, cardiomyopathy (including peripartum).
  - Non-cardiogenic: drugs (e.g. tocolytics), iatrogenic (fluid overload).
  - Adult respiratory distress syndrome (ARDS): pre-eclampsia, sepsis, haemorrhage, amniotic fluid embolism, COVID-19 pneumonitis (Box 15.1).

Box 15.1 Pregnant women with COVID-19 infection

- Pregnant women with COVID-19 infection are at greater risk of severe disease than their non-pregnant peers. Minority ethnicity has consistently been identified as being associated with a higher risk of being admitted to hospital with COVID-19 in pregnancy.
- The basic principles of diagnosing and managing COVID-19 are the same as for non-pregnant patients, (see Chapter 7) and a multidisciplinary, expert team approach is essential to ensure optimal care.
- During pregnancy, treatment with corticosteroids should be modified to use non-fluorinated glucocorticoids (e.g. prednisolone, methylprednisolone or hydrocortisone). Fluorinated glucocorticoids such as dexamethasone readily cross the placenta, and repeated doses in pregnancy have been associated with neurocognitive and neurosensory disorders in childhood.
- Interleukin-6 inhibitors and monoclonal antibodies, together with specific antiviral therapies, may also be considered.
- Prophylaxis against venous thromboembolism is important.
- Women may require respiratory support with oxygen, non-invasive ventilation, ventilation in a prone position (either awake or during invasive ventilation), intubation and ventilation, and extracorporeal membrane oxygenation (ECMO).

- Decisions regarding timing, place and mode of delivery should be taken with a multidisciplinary team experienced in the care of COVID-19 in pregnancy.

Pulmonary embolism

See the section on venous thromboembolism (VTE).

Common systemic causes of breathlessness in pregnancy

- Physiological breathlessness of pregnancy (affecting up to 75% of women).
  - Diagnosis of exclusion.
  - Normal oxygen saturation.
  - Worse at rest/talking, relieved by mild exertion.
- Anaemia.
- Infection (typical/atypical/aspiration).
- Thyrotoxicosis.

Chest pain

All patients presenting to acute care with chest pain during pregnancy should have:

- ED, AMU or SDEC assessment
- MEWS
- ECG
- CXR.

Chest pain: alarm signs and symptoms
- Pain requiring opioids.
- Pain radiating to arm, shoulder, back or jaw.
- Sudden-onset, tearing or exertional chest pain.
- Associated with haemoptysis, breathlessness, syncope or abnormal neurology.
- Abnormal observations.
- Cardiac risk factors.
- Multiple attendances.

Further investigations/management are suggested according to differential diagnosis (Table 15.3). Any patient who is discharged must have safety-netting advice and appropriate follow-up in place.

Table 15.3 Differential diagnosis and management of chest pain in pregnancy and postpartum period

Diagnosis	Risk by trimester	Critical investigation	Urgent action
Acute coronary syndromes (ACS): • Unstable angina (UA) • Non-ST-elevation myocardial infarction (NSTEMI) • ST-elevation myocardial infarction (STEMI)	Greater risk in T3/PP	Troponin (is NOT elevated in normal pregnancy)	STEMI: • Activate Primary Angioplasty in Myocardial Infarction (PAMI) pathway • Follow ACS algorithm NSTEMI or UA: • Treat as ACS
Aortic dissection	Greater risk in T3/PP	CT-aorta	Type A: prep for theatre Type B: control blood pressure
Pulmonary embolism (PE)	T1/T2/T3/PP	V/Q scan or CTPA	Massive PE: • 2222 peri-arrest call, resuscitate • Consider systemic thrombolysis Sub-massive PE: • Admit plus consider catheter-directed thrombolysis Non-massive PE: • Suspected or confirmed, admit
Epigastric pain	T1/T2/T3/PP	Troponin, amylase/lipase, glucose Ultrasound scan abdomen	Consider ACS, PUD, gallbladder disease, pancreatitis, GORD (most common in 3rd trimester – treat symptomatically, e.g. lifestyle advice, antacids, PPI, antiemetics)
Musculoskeletal	T1/T2/T3/PP	Reassuring MEWS plus CXR plus ECG	Clinical assessment suggestive plus no red flag alarm features, discharge

CTPA, CT pulmonary angiography; GORD, gastro-oesophageal reflux disease; PP, postpartum period; PPI, proton pump inhibitor; PUD, peptic ulcer disease; T1, 1st trimester; T2, 2nd trimester; T3, 3rd trimester.

Aetiology of acute coronary syndrome in pregnancy
- Atherosclerosis.
- Spontaneous coronary artery dissection.
- Coronary artery vasospasm.
- Thrombophilia.
- *In situ* thrombosis.
- Paradoxical embolism.

Alternative causes of raised troponin in pregnancy
- Pre-eclampsia.
- Pulmonary embolism.
- Arrhythmias.
- Myocarditis.
- Sepsis.
- Heart failure.
- Renal failure.

Causes of pleuritic chest pain in pregnancy
- Pleural disease.
  - Pneumothorax and pneumomediastinum: can occur in pregnancy due to hyperemesis gravidarum and following spontaneous vaginal delivery.
  - Pleural effusion.
- Pulmonary embolism.
- Pneumonia.
- Musculoskeletal.

Palpitations

Palpitations are a common symptom during pregnancy.

History and examination

- Frequency and duration? Pattern of onset/resolution, time of day.
- Triggers for symptoms? For example, exertion, caffeine, alcohol, stress.
- Associated symptoms? For example, shortness of breath, chest pain.
- Current heart rate and rhythm?
- Audible murmur suggesting underlying structural heart disease?

Palpitations: alarm features
- Presyncope or syncope.
- Chest pain.
- Pre-existing heart disease – ischaemic, congenital, structural, valvular, heart failure, arrhythmia, previous cardiac surgery.
- Family history of sudden cardiac death <40 years.
- Exertional symptoms.
- Abnormal resting ECG (left bundle branch block, left ventricular hypertrophy, Q-waves).
- Persistent, severe tachycardia.

Obtain symptom-ECG correlation

- While not always possible for patients who report very infrequent or short-lived episodes of palpitations, ECG recording during palpitations, or 'symptom-ECG correlation', forms the mainstay of diagnosis.
- Choosing the method and duration of ambulatory monitoring with the greatest likelihood of capturing an individual patient's symptoms is important in efficiently making the diagnosis.
- Consider the frequency of symptoms and the individual patient's ability to activate a recording device to guide which type and duration of ambulatory cardiac monitoring is most appropriate.

Initial assessment

All pregnant women presenting with palpitations must have the following.

- ED, AMU or SDEC assessment.
- MEWS.
- Twelve-lead ECG.
- CXR.
- Full blood count (FBC), C-reactive protein (CRP), urea and electrolytes (U&E), bone profile, magnesium, thyroid function tests (TFT) and venous blood gas (VBG).

Palpitations: systemic causes
- Physiological.
- Hypovolaemic states.
- Anaemia.
- Thyrotoxicosis.
- Sepsis.
- Phaeochromocytoma.
- Pulmonary embolism.

Common arrhythmias in pregnancy

Treatment of tachyarrhythmias in pregnancy differs very little from a non-pregnant adult, and treatment of unstable arrhythmias should follow Resuscitation Council UK guidelines (Table 15.4 and Figure 6.1). Pregnant women with pathological arrhythmias need to be cared for by a multidisciplinary team, including obstetricians, obstetric anaesthetists, specialist midwives, cardiologists and obstetric physicians.

Common tachyarrhythmias in pregnancy include the following.

- Tachycardia: e.g. supraventricular tachycardia (SVT), atrial flutter, atrial tachycardia, ventricular tachycardia.
- Atrial fibrillation (AF): consider anticoagulation, rate control (first-line beta-blocker).

Nausea and vomiting in pregnancy and hyperemesis gravidarum

Nausea and vomiting are common in early pregnancy, affecting almost 80% of pregnant women.

- When nausea and vomiting in pregnancy are severe or prolonged, it is called *hyperemesis gravidarum*.

Table 15.4 Tachyarrhythmias in pregnancy – management

If tachyarrhythmia **Narrow QRS (<120 ms)** *plus* **NO** haemodynamic compromise:
- Vagal manoeuvres.
- Adenosine (6/12/12 mg to be given in large-bore antecubital cannula, followed by a 10 ml rapid flush with ECG strip recorded during administration).
- If atrial flutter/atrial fibrillation/atrial tachycardia and no response, rate control.
  - Beta-blocker (e.g. metoprolol) or calcium channel blocker (e.g. verapamil).

If tachyarrhythmia **Wide QRS (≥120 ms)** *plus* **NO** haemodynamic compromise.
- Discuss with cardiology.

If tachyarrhythmia *plus* haemodynamic compromise, need **synchronised direct current cardioversion (DCCV)** – think **6 As**.

1 **Access**
- Multiple adequate gauge cannulae.
- Blood group and cross-match.

2 **Anatomy**
- Left lateral tilt to maximise venous return.
- Pads position (avoid gravid uterus and lower lateral pad; consider AP placement).
- Levocardia or dextrocardia?
- Adjust around existing cardiac devices.

3 **Anticoagulation**
- Already established?
- Adherence?
- Duration of arrhythmia?
- Thrombogenic anatomy?
- Transoesophageal echocardiogram needed?

4 **Anaesthetist**
- General anaesthetic needed?
- Obstetric anaesthetist plus cardiac anaesthetist.

5 **Ability to pace**
- Risk of bradyarrhythmia requiring pacing?
- Use defibrillator with pacing capability.

6 **Appropriate area**
- Theatres, hospital birth centre/delivery suite.
- Level 2/3 bed often required.
- Facilities for fetal monitoring and emergency caesarean section must be available.

- Hyperemesis gravidarum is a clinical diagnosis after the exclusion of other causes.
- Incidence is 0.3–1%.
- Symptoms usually begin at 6–8 weeks, peak at 12 weeks and usually resolve by 20 weeks gestation.
- New symptoms appearing after 12 weeks should not be attributed to hyperemesis and other diagnoses should be considered.

Clinical features of hyperemesis gravidarum

Typical symptoms and signs suggestive of hyperemesis gravidarum are shown in Table 15.5.

Table 15.5 Symptoms and signs suggestive of hyperemesis gravidarum

Symptoms	Signs
- Nausea - Vomiting - Ptyalism (inability to swallow saliva) - Food and fluid intolerance - Lethargy	- Ketonuria (2+ ketones on urine dip) - Weight loss >5% and muscle wasting - Tachycardia - Postural hypotension - Signs of dehydration

Differential diagnosis of nausea and vomiting in pregnancy

- Urinary tract infection (UTI) and pyelonephritis.
- Gastroenteritis.
- GORD, peptic ulcer disease and gastroparesis.
- Pancreatitis.
- Hepatitis.
- Diabetic ketoacidosis (DKA).
- Addison disease (primary adrenal failure).
- Hyperthyroidism – Graves' disease (may predate the pregnancy).
- Hypercalcaemia.
- Acute fatty liver of pregnancy.

Initial assessment

- ED, AMU or SDEC assessment.
- MEWS.
- Weight (>5% weight loss from pre-pregnancy or booking weight is significant).

- Hydration status – mucous membranes, skin turgor.
- Urinalysis – confirms ketonuria and need to rule out significant glycosuria (e.g. exclude DKA).
  - Send midstream urine (MSU) if urinary symptoms or positive for nitrites or leucocytes.

PUQE score

- The Pregnancy-Unique Quantification of Emesis (PUQE) index should be used to assess severity of symptoms in the last 24 hours.
- The total score is the sum of replies to each of the three questions.
- The PUQE-24 score breakdown.
  - Mild ≤6
  - Moderate 7–12
  - Severe 13–15
- If the PUQE score is >12, then rehydration with IV fluid is recommended.

Investigations

- FBC.
- U&E.
- Transvaginal ultrasound scan (TV USS) to rule out multiple/molar pregnancy.
- Liver function tests (LFT).
- Bone profile (corrected calcium and phosphate).
- Magnesium.
- Glucose (capillary or venous, especially if glycosuria).
- TFT.
- Amylase/lipase (if associated abdominal pain).
- VBG – only required in refractory vomiting.

Management of nausea and vomiting in pregnancy

Suggested multimodality management and escalation are outlined in Table 15.6.

> **Hyperemesis gravidarum: alarm features and criteria for inpatient admission**
> - Continued nausea and vomiting and inability to keep down oral antiemetics; Associated with ketonuria and/or weight loss (>5% of body weight), despite oral antiemetics; Confirmed or suspected co-morbidity (e.g. diabetes).

Table 15.6 Management of nausea and vomiting in pregnancy

Treatment	Details
Intravenous fluids	• Sodium chloride 0.9% or Hartmann solution should be used for initial rapid rehydration (1 l over 1–4 hours). • Sodium chloride 0.9% with potassium chloride 20–40 mmol/l should then be infused (1 l over 4–12 hours) depending on fluid status and serum electrolytes. • If potassium is low (i.e. <3.5 mmol/l), use sodium chloride 0.9% with potassium chloride 40 mmol/l at no greater than 250 ml/hour (1 l over 4 hours).
Antiemetics	*First line* • Cyclizine or prochlorperazine with metoclopramide or ondansetron prescribed when required (PRN). • Cyclizine 50 mg three times daily (oral/IM/IV) or prochlorperazine 5–10 mg three times daily (oral) or 12.5 mg three times daily (IM). *Second line* • Add further regular antiemetic if symptoms do not improve. • Ondansetron 4 mg three times daily or PRN (oral/IV) or metoclopramide 10 mg three times daily or PRN (oral/IM/IV). • There is a risk of acute dystonic reactions such as oculogyric crisis with prochlorperazine and metoclopramide. If it occurs, treat with procyclidine 5 mg IV or IM (usually effective in 5–10 minutes but may need 30 minutes for full relief). • Metoclopramide is not suitable for teenagers (<18 years old). *Third line* • Xonvea® (doxylamine succinate/pyridoxine hydrochloride) 10 mg/10 mg 2 tablets oral at night to be uptitrated carefully if needed to 1 tablet in the morning, 1 tablet in the mid-afternoon and 2 tablets at bedtime. • Not always readily available. *Fourth line* • Hydrocortisone (IV) 100 mg twice daily and once clinical improvement occurs, convert to prednisolone (oral) 30–40 mg once daily (reducing dose by 5 mg weekly).
Vitamins	To prevent Wernicke encephalopathy and neural tube defects: • Thiamine 50 mg three times daily (oral) for duration of hyperemesis. • If unable to tolerate tablets, give IV Pabrinex® (B vitamins and ascorbic acid). One pair of Pabrinex ampoules IV three times a day, diluted in 100 ml 0.9% NaCl and given over 30 minutes.
Antacids	• Peptac 10 ml PRN. • Histamine 2 receptor antagonists. • PPI (e.g. omeprazole 20 mg once daily).

Thromboprophylaxis	• Thromboprophylaxis if patient is being admitted to ward.
	  ○ Antiembolic (TED) stockings for all women.
	  ○ Low molecular weight heparin. Adjust dose in renal impairment.
	• Continue thromboprophylaxis on discharge if ongoing dehydration or immobility or if additional risk factors for VTE are present.

Other	• Folic acid 5 mg once daily (oral) for duration of hyperemesis. • Consider stopping or reducing iron-containing preparations (e.g. ferrous sulfate/fumarate) as can exacerbate nausea and vomiting.

Headache

Headaches are common in pregnancy. The challenge lies in distinguishing between primary headaches and potentially life-threatening causes.

1 History: time, character, cause, response and health between attacks (for each headache type).
2 Examination/investigations.
   - Full neurological examination.
   - Bloods: VBG including carboxyhaemoglobin, FBC, U&E, LFT.
   - Urine dip (exclude proteinuria).
3 Are there any alarm features present (Table 15.7)?

Treatment of headaches in pregnancy

- If no alarm features, probably primary headache: treat with simple analgesia: paracetamol, non-steroidal anti-inflammatory drugs (NSAIDs) (up to 32/40 weeks gestation) and triptans (check local formulary).

Table 15.7 Alarm features for headaches in pregnancy

History	Physical examination
- Sudden onset/ thunderclap or worst headache ever.	- Blood pressure >140/90 mmHg at >20/40 weeks gestation.
- Headache persisting >48 hours/longer than usual to resolve.	- Fever.
	- Nuchal rigidity.
	- Papilloedema.
	- Neurological deficit.
- Vomiting.	- Seizure/altered mental status.
- Associated fever, seizures, focal neurology, photophobia, diplopia.	
- Excessive use of opioids.	

- If alarm features present, seek involvement of senior decision makers and imaging according to primary differential (Table 15.8).

Table 15.8 Differential diagnosis of headaches presenting during pregnancy

Primary headaches: migraine, tension, cluster	- Most common in first trimester; treat with simple analgesia.
Meningitis	- Can occur at any point during pregnancy plus postpartum. - Do not delay antibiotics – ensure cover for *Streptococcus pneumoniae* and *Listeria monocytogenes* as more common during pregnancy.
Idiopathic intracranial hypertension (IIH)	- Can occur throughout pregnancy and can worsen as weight increases. - Acetazolamide is safe in pregnancy.
Pre-eclampsia	- Consider if gestational age >20/40, most common 27–40/40. Defined as BP >140/90 mmHg + urinary protein:creatinine ratio >50 (+ve urine dip adequate). - Maintain BP 140–155/90–105 mmHg (labetalol/hydralazine); give IV magnesium to minimise risk of eclamptic seizure. - Refer to obstetric team.
Posterior reversible encephalopathy syndrome (PRES)	- Occurs in the presence of pre-eclampsia. - Associated with headaches, seizures and cortical blindness caused by vasogenic brain oedema. - Treat hypertension, give IV magnesium.
Subarachnoid haemorrhage (SAH)	- Can occur throughout pregnancy/postpartum; most common in third trimester.
Cerebral venous sinus thrombosis	- Can occur throughout pregnancy/postpartum; most common in third trimester.
Stroke	- Can occur throughout pregnancy; most common in third trimester plus postpartum. - No contraindication to thrombolysis, thrombectomy or stenting during pregnancy for ischaemic stroke. Refer as per local stroke pathway.

(continued)

Table 15.8 (Continued)

Reversible cerebral vasoconstriction syndrome (RCVS)	• Self-limiting condition. Treat with nimodipine; resolves within 1–3 months of onset. • Associated with severe hypertension and recurrent thunderclap headaches. • Multifocal segmental cerebral artery vasoconstriction on cerebral angiography.
Postdural puncture headache	• Can occur <5 days after dural breach (i.e. from regional anaesthetic procedure – spinal/epidural). • Contact obstetric anaesthetist.

Collapse

All pregnant women presenting with collapse should have:

- ED, SDEC or AMU assessment
- MEWS.
- lying and standing BP
- ECG
- blood glucose.

Major differential of collapse in pregnancy

- Syncope.
  - Vasovagal.
  - Orthostatic: dehydration, antepartum haemorrhage (APH) and postpartum haemorrhage (PPH), postural orthostatic tachycardia syndrome (POTS).
  - Cardiogenic: arrhythmia; structural heart disease; peripartum cardiomyopathy.
  - Amniotic fluid embolism.
- Seizures.
  - Infection.
  - Acute vascular events (stroke): intracranial bleeds, dissection, venous sinus thrombosis.
  - Raised intracranial pressure.
  - Epilepsy and non-epileptic seizure disorders.
  - Hypoglycaemia.
  - Eclampsia: emergency – seek multidisciplinary expert help now (Box 15.2).

Management of collapse in pregnancy

- All women should be admitted for a period of observation to ensure:
  - Neurology observations *plus* symptom control *plus* specialist input *plus* robust follow-up and safety netting.

Box 15.2 Eclampsia emergency management

- Seek expert help.
- Admit.
- Secure airway.
- IV magnesium: initially 4 g (over 5–15 mins) then IV infusion 1 g/hour for 24 hours.
- If seizure recurs – additional 2–4 g IV over 5–15 mins.
- Treat BP: IV labetalol, IV hydralazine.

Common seizure precipitants in pregnancy

- Non-adherence with medications.
- Subtherapeutic drug levels (antiepileptic drugs tend to be increased in pregnancy to achieve therapeutic drug levels).
- Illicit drug use.
- Alcohol.
- Nausea and vomiting in pregnancy, inability to keep medications down.
- Electrolyte imbalance.
- Intracranial event (stroke/dissection/thrombosis).
- Intercurrent infection (including COVID-19).
- Sepsis/intracranial infection.
- Space-occupying lesion.

- *All patients should receive a written advice leaflet.*
  - Do not drive, inform the Driver and Vehicle Licensing Agency (DVLA), avoid swimming/watersports, take showers rather than baths, avoid locking the bathroom door.
- If actively seizing:
  - secure airway
  - oxygen
  - IV access
  - bloods (FBC, U&E, LFT, CRP, bone profile, magnesium, antiepileptic drug levels)

o MEWS
o urine toxicology screen
o ECG, CXR, urine dip, blood glucose
o consider need for imaging
o pharmacological management: first line – benzo-diazepines (e.g. lorazepam, diazepam, clobazam, clonazepam); second line – levetiracetam commonly used (*avoid sodium valproate*)
o discuss with Neurology/Obstetric Medicine
o ensure obstetric on-call and maternity unit aware.

Risk factors for sudden unexpected death in epilepsy (SUDEP)

Epilepsy-related risk factors
• Uncontrolled seizures.
• Tonic clonic seizures.
• Nocturnal seizures.

Treatment risk factors
• Infrequent epilepsy reviews and engagement with an epilepsy clinician.
• Ineffective antiepileptic drug (AED) treatment.
• Frequent medication changes.
• Subtherapeutic doses of AEDs.

Individual risk factors
• Living alone or sleeping alone.
• Not taking medication as prescribed.
• Sleep deprivation.
• Stress.
• Alcohol or substance misuse.
• Learning disability.

Sepsis

• The empirical 'Sepsis Six' is considered in women presenting with infective symptoms and signs at any gestation.
• Peripartum sepsis considerations.
  o Chorioamnionitis.
  o Full sepsis screen is recommended including blood cultures and high vaginal swab.
  o Note whether woman has had a history of Group B Strep.
• Fluid resuscitation.
  o Up to 1.5l fluid resuscitation is usually safe, but there are large amounts of fluid shifts to the extravascular space.
  o Low threshold for referral to intensive care unit (ICU) for inotropes/pressors.

o Careful fluid balance monitoring is needed as these high degrees of fluid shifts can lead to pulmonary oedema.
• Early anti-infective agents and source control.
  o Antibiotics (*plus* medical/radiological/surgical intervention as indicated).
  o UTI should be appropriately investigated and managed.
  o Intrauterine death.
  o Midtrimester chorioamnionitis.
  o COVID-19.
• Preterm prelabour rupture of membranes (PPROM) as a cause.
  o Appropriate rapid intervention.
  o Erythromycin is used for membrane stabilisation, not for treatment of chorioamnionitis.
  o Further antibiotics should be prescribed for chorioamnionitis according to local guidelines.

Cardiac disease

Cardiac disease remains the leading cause of maternal mortality in the developed world.

Physiologic cardiovascular changes:

• Bounding or collapsing pulse.
• An ejection systolic murmur, present in over 90% of pregnant women.
• Third heart sound.
• Peripheral oedema due to hyperdynamic state; note sudden onset more concerning for pre-eclampsia.
• Heart rate - an increase of 10–20 beats per minute, particularly in third trimester.
• BP - can decrease by 10–15 mmHg by 20 weeks but returns to pre-pregnancy levels.

Normal Findings on ECG in pregnancy
• Sinus tachycardia.
• Atrial and ventricular ectopic beats.
• Q wave (small) and inverted T wave in lead III.
• ST-segment depression and T-wave inversion in the inferior and lateral leads.
• Left-axis shift of QRS.

Cardiac conditions affecting pregnancy

The rise in maternal mortality due to cardiac disease has been attributed to increasing numbers of women undertaking pregnancy at advanced maternal age, co-morbid pre-existing conditions such as diabetes mellitus and hypertension, and the growing number of women with congenital heart disease surviving to childbearing age. Early and specialised multidisciplinary care in the antepartum, peripartum and postpartum periods is essential to improve cardiovascular outcomes and reduce maternal mortality up to the first year post partum.

- Structural heart disease.
  - Adult congenital heart disease.
  - Cardiomyopathies: dilated cardiomyopathy (DCM), hypertrophic obstructive cardiomyopathy (HOCM), arrhythmogenic right ventricular cardiomyopathy (AVRC).
- Hypertensive heart disease.
- Ischaemic heart disease.
- Valvular heart disease.
- Myocarditis/endocarditis.
- Aortopathy.
  - Aneurysms.
  - Connective tissue disease: Marfan syndrome, Ehlers–Danlos syndrome (EDS) IV (vascular).
  - Dissection.
- Acute coronary syndromes.
  - Spontaneous coronary artery dissection.
  - Coronary artery disease.
  - Myocardial infarction with non-obstructive coronary arteries (MINOCA) – spasm, *in situ* thrombosis, paradoxical embolism.
  - Other aetiologies (e.g. antiphospholipid syndrome).
- Heart failure.
  - Pulmonary oedema: cardiogenic vs non-cardiogenic (e.g. sepsis, ARDS, pre-eclampsia).
- Peripartum cardiomyopathy.
  - Occurs late in pregnancy.
  - Left ventricular dysfunction confirmed on echo with ejection fraction (EF) <45%.
  - Diagnosis of exclusion.
  - Management: nitrates, beta-blockers, diuretics. If *in extremis*, bromocriptine. Avoid angiotensin-converting enzyme (ACE) inhibitors/angiotensin receptor blockers (ARB) in pregnancy but can start enalapril once the woman has delivered.

Hypertension, pre-eclampsia and eclampsia

Hypertensive disease is one of the major contributors to maternal mortality worldwide. Morbidity and mortality are preventable and usually due to:

- stroke
- eclampsia
- pulmonary oedema
- renal/hepatic impairment.

Pre-existing/chronic/essential hypertension in pregnancy

- Hypertension that occurs before conception or within the first half of pregnancy.
- Consider secondary causes: 5–10% of hypertension in pregnant women is secondary to conditions of the kidneys (majority of cases), endocrine system, heart and arteries.

Background

- BP falls in healthy pregnancy.
- This occurs as early as the first trimester, sometimes one week following conception.
- Some women with chronic hypertension have dose reduction in medications within the first two trimesters of pregnancy.

Antihypertensive treatment

- Stop ACE inhibitors or ARBs within two working days of notification of pregnancy and offer alternatives.
- Start aspirin 75–150 mg once daily from 12 weeks.
- Offer antihypertensive treatment to women with sustained BP of ≥140/90 mmHg.
- Use labetalol, nifedipine or methyldopa. Base the choice on any pre-existing treatment, side-effect profiles, risks (including fetal effects) and the woman's preference.
  - Labetolol, first line: 100 mg twice daily to 500 mg four times daily (caution: asthma).
  - Nifedipine modified release (MR), second line: 10–40 mg twice daily MR preparation.
  - Alpha-blockers (doxazosin), third line: 1 mg once daily to 8 mg twice daily.

○ Hydralazine, third line: 25 mg three times daily to 75 mg four times daily.
- Aim for target BP ≤135/85 mmHg.

Assessment of proteinuria

- Interpret proteinuria measurements in context of full clinical review and other investigations for pre-eclampsia.
- If dipstick screening is positive (1+ or more), use protein:creatinine ratio to quantify proteinuria.
- If using protein:creatinine ratio, use 30 mg/mmol as a threshold for significant proteinuria.

Pre-eclampsia

Pre-eclampsia affects up to 6% pregnancies, with severe pre-eclampsia developing in around 1–2% of UK pregnancies.

- Pre-eclampsia is a disease of the vascular endothelium associated with placental stress.
- Many other conditions are associated with abnormal maternal vascular endothelium dysfunction (e.g. COVID-19).

Diagnosis

Defining pre-eclampsia is difficult because it is a syndrome characterised by a group of clinical features that, when they occur together, lead to diagnosis and treatment.

- Hypertension *plus:*
  ○ evidence of endothelial disease, e.g. proteinuria, evidence of biochemical (elevated liver enzymes) or haematological (thrombocytopenia, disseminated intravascular coagulation) abnormalities
  ○ symptoms/signs of target organ damage (e.g. acute kidney injury)
  ○ fetal growth restriction
  ○ angiogenic biomarkers: offer placental growth factor (PLGF)-based testing if pre-eclampsia is suspected between 20 and 35+6 weeks of pregnancy (NICE approved).

General principles of management

- Careful surveillance.
- Maintain safe BP.
- Early identification of multisystem disease.
- Assess fetal well-being.
- Prevent/treat seizures.
- Avoid pulmonary oedema.
  ○ Avoid aggressive fluid resuscitation/fluid challenges.

○ Oliguria is a part of pre-eclampsia and fluid challenges can be more harmful.

Pre-eclampsia: alarm signs and symptoms
- Sustained systolic BP ≥160 mmHg.
- Any maternal haematological or biochemical investigations.
  ○ Fall in platelet count (<150 000 × 10^9/l).
  ○ Rise in creatinine (≥90 μmol/l or more, ≥1 mg/dl).
  ○ Rise in alanine transaminase (>70 IU/l, or twice upper limit of normal range).
- Signs of impending eclampsia.
  ○ Headache.
  ○ Blurred vision.
  ○ Right upper quadrant pain.
- Pulmonary oedema.
- Fetal compromise.

Eclampsia

- Seizures, altered mental state, hyperreflexia, clonus.
- $MgSO_4$ 4 g IV.
- Treat BP.

Venous thromboembolism in pregnancy

- VTE is the leading direct cause of maternal death in the UK, with rates of 1.48/100 000 maternities being reported in the 2016–2018 triennium.
- For every woman who dies of PE in pregnancy, a further 50 suffer non-fatal PEs and deep vein thrombosis (DVT) which may be associated with long-term morbidity.
- These rates reflect women of increasing maternal age entering pregnancy with increased numbers of risk factors for VTE.
- There is also demonstrable scope for improved prevention and treatment of VTE in pregnancy.
- Of all VTE in pregnancy, 10.1% occur in the first trimester, 10.4% in the second, 28.4% in the third and 49.3% in the first six weeks post partum.
- However, of those who die of VTE in pregnancy, 16% die in the first trimester.
- It is therefore essential to ensure that women who need to commence prophylaxis as soon as

they become pregnant have clear pathways to access prescriptions and support to enhance compliance.

Management of acute thrombosis in pregnancy

- Risk assessment should be performed on all pregnant patients (Royal College of Obstetricians and Gynaecologists green top guideline).
- D-dimer levels increase in most women in pregnancy and should therefore not be used in pregnancy.
- Clinical decision tools, e.g. Wells score, Pulmonary Embolism Severity Index (PESI) score, are not validated in pregnancy.

Deep vein thrombosis

- Clinical features are particularly unreliable in pregnancy.
- Ninety percent of DVTs in pregnancy are on the left and 70% are iliofemoral (which are more prone to lead to PE and postthrombotic syndrome).
- Compression duplex ultrasound *plus* treatment dose low molecular weight heparin (LMWH) should be administered until the diagnosis is excluded by objective testing.
- If ultrasound is negative and there is a low level of clinical suspicion, anticoagulant treatment can be discontinued.
- If ultrasound is negative and a high level of clinical suspicion exists, anticoagulant treatment should be discontinued but the ultrasound should be repeated on days 3 and 7.
- When iliac vein thrombosis is suspected (groin pain and swelling of the entire limb), magnetic resonance direct thrombus imaging may be considered.

Pulmonary embolus

- ECG and CXR should be performed. In women with suspected PE who also have symptoms and signs of DVT, compression duplex ultrasound should be performed.
- If compression ultrasonography confirms the presence of thrombus, no further investigation is necessary, e.g. a CTPA or V/Q single-photon emission CT (SPECT) is not required because it will not change the need for anticoagulation and treatment for VTE should continue.

- In women with suspected PE without symptoms and signs of DVT, a V/Q SPECT or CTPA should be performed.
- When the CXR is abnormal and there is clinical suspicion of PE, the case should be discussed with a nuclear medicine consultant to consider whether a CTPA may be required in preference to a V/Q SPECT (V/Q SPECT may still be possible if there are minor CXR abnormalities).

High-risk PE (previously called massive PE)

- Massive PE occurs when a patient is haemodynamically compromised by PE.
- Collapsed, shocked patients need to be assessed by a team of experienced clinicians, including the obstetric team, who should decide on an individual basis the management plan, including systemic thrombolysis or catheter-directed lysis or thoracotomy and surgical embolectomy dependent upon local expertise.
- An urgent portable echocardiogram or CTPA within one hour of presentation should be arranged.
- If massive PE is confirmed or, in extreme circumstances, prior to confirmation, immediate thrombolysis should be considered.

Postnatal management with a new VTE

- After delivery, the non-pregnant dose of LMWH can be used.
- Treatment should be continued until at least 3–6 months of treatment has been given in total.
- Women should be advised that in a future pregnancy, they will require LMWH throughout their pregnancy from a positive pregnancy test to six weeks post partum.

Treatment of VTE post partum (as with non-pregnant)

- Women should be offered a choice of LMWH or oral anticoagulation with warfarin for postnatal therapy (for those not breastfeeding, a direct oral anticoagulant [DOAC] can be considered) after discussion about the need for regular blood tests for monitoring of warfarin, particularly during the first 10 days of warfarin treatment.

- Women should be advised that LMWH and warfarin are not contraindicated in breast feeding.
- DOACs are contraindicated if women are breast feeding.

Abnormal liver function tests in pregnancy

Consider the patient's medical history, previous pregnancy history and gestation of pregnancy when interpreting abnormal liver function tests in pregnancy. Clinical pointers include the following.

- Hypertension and proteinuria – consider pre-eclampsia/HELLP (haemolysis, elevated liver enzymes and low platelet count).
- Pruritus – consider intrahepatic cholestasis of pregnancy.
- Nausea and vomiting in first trimester – consider hyperemesis gravidarum.
- New medication – think of drug-induced liver injury (DILI).
- Obstetric haemorrhage – think of ischaemic hepatitis.

Metabolic emergencies

- Diabetes mellitus is the most common endocrine disorder in pregnant women. Urgent acute medical challenges include the following.
  - DKA in pregnant women can occur rapidly and at lower blood glucose concentrations than in non-pregnant individuals.
  - Hypoglycaemia is more common in women with pre-existing diabetes when pregnant and is treated as in the non-pregnant population.
- Starvation ketoacidosis can occur in the third trimester in association with a short duration of vomiting or reduced oral intake. Treatment is with IV glucose.
- Serum sodium levels fall by 4–5 mmol/l in pregnancy, for a variety of reasons. Hyponatraemia is common in labour, often related to excessive fluid intake in combination with the antidiuretic hormone-like effects of high oxytocin levels. Hypertonic sodium chloride is reserved for symptomatic cases of severe hyponatraemia and should be administered in a high-dependency unit setting with expert specialist input.

Mental health crises in pregnancy and postpartum

- The UK Mothers and Babies: Reducing Risk through Audits and Confidential Enquiries (MBRRACE) reports reveal that mortality is increasingly caused by:
  - suicide
  - depression
  - domestic violence.
  - homicide.
- Take the opportunity to enquire after a woman's mental well-being when she presents to acute medical services during pregnancy and the postpartum period.
- Those with a history of mental health disease such as postpartum psychosis and bipolar affective disorder are more likely to develop new symptoms during pregnancy and the postpartum period, even if they have been well for a number of years.
- Anxiety and depression are also common.
- Specialist perinatal psychiatric services have expertise in this area for women who experience symptoms during this time.

> **Psychiatric disorders: alarm signs and symptoms**
> - Recent significant change in mental state or emergence of new symptoms.
> - New thoughts or acts of violent self-harm.
> - New and persistent expressions of incompetence as a mother or estrangement from the baby.

Drugs commonly prescribed in pregnancy

Always check the relevant section in the British National Formulary or seek expert advice.

- Prenatal and first trimester.
  - Preconception and pregnancy multivitamins.
  - Folic acid 400 μg or 5 mg in high-risk patients.
  - Vitamin D supplementation in high-risk patients.

- Analgesia.
  - Paracetamol and dihydrocodeine are safe.
  - NSAIDs can safely be used up to 30 weeks gestation.
  - Opiates: generally safe but risk of withdrawal in the baby. Rarely, breastfed babies have developed sedation, respiratory depression and bradycardia – advise the mother of this; use dihydrocodeine.
- Antibiotics.
  - Avoid trimethoprim and tetracyclines.
  - All others safe.
- Antiemetics: all safe in pregnancy.
- Antiplatelets.
  - Aspirin in those at risk of pre-eclampsia; prescribed after 12/40 weeks gestation to reduce the risk of preterm pre-eclampsia.
  - Clopidogrel and dipyridamole are safe.
- Antihypertensive agents.
  - Avoid ACE inhibitors and ARBs throughout pregnancy.
  - Enalapril has been shown to be safe post partum if breast feeding.
  - Evidence is lacking for other ACE inhibitors in breast feeding.
- Antiarrhythmic agents: adenosine, beta-blockers, flecainide and verapamil are all safe.
- Anticoagulants.
  - Twice-daily dosing of LMWH for VTE treatment in pregnancy, once daily post partum.
  - Warfarin is teratogenic, and only used in exceptional circumstances under expert supervision. It is safe in breast feeding.
  - DOACS: there is insufficient evidence to support the use of DOACS in pregnancy and breast feeding.
- Antiepileptic agents.
  - Sodium valproate contraindicated.
  - For status epilepticus, IV benzodiazepines or levetiracetam safe.
- Bronchodilators: all safe.
- Steroids.

- Prednisolone or hydrocortisone are the preferred steroids for a maternal indication in pregnancy as they are metabolised and do not cross the placenta in significant amounts.
- Dexamethasone and betamethasone do cross the placenta and thus are used as IM doses to aid fetal lung maturation.
- Risk of gestational diabetes mellitus, pregnancy-induced hypertension and infections.
- If >7.5 mg per day prednisolone equivalent >3 weeks needs intrapartum stress dose steroid cover.

Maternal resuscitation

Maternal resuscitation should follow the Resuscitation Council UK guidelines using the standard Airway (A), Breathing (B), Circulation (C) approach with some modifications to consider during pregnancy (Figure 15.1). The obstetric team and neonatology team (>22 weeks gestation) should be called at the time of the arrest call.

The same defibrillation energy should be used as in a non-pregnant woman. There should not be any alteration to the algorithm of drugs or doses administered. Reversible causes should be considered throughout resuscitation and therapy directed to correcting cause.

For pregnant women >20 weeks, two further important actions are added to the standard algorithm.

1 *Manual displacement of the gravid uterus* – to decrease the effect of aortocaval compression on venous return.
2 *Perimortem caesarean section* – if there is no response to correctly performed cardiopulmonary resuscitation (CPR) *after the first cycle*, delivery should be performed to assist maternal resuscitation, by reducing oxygen consumption, improving venous return and making compressions and ventilation easier, thus improving chances of maternal survival.

Obstetric Cardiac Arrest

Resuscitation Council UK — MBRRACE-UK

Alterations in maternal physiology and exacerbations of pregnancy related pathologies must be considered. Priorities include calling the appropriate team members, relieving aortocaval compression, effective cardiopulmonary resuscitation (CPR), consideration of causes and performing a timely emergency hysterotomy (perimortem caesarean section) when ≥ 20 weeks.

START

1 Confirm cardiac arrest and call for help. Declare 'Obstetric cardiac arrest'
- Team for mother and team for neonate if > 20 weeks

2 Lie flat, apply manual uterine displacement to the left
- Or left lateral tilt (from head to toe at an angle of 15–30° on a firm surface)

3 Commence CPR and request cardiac arrest trolley
- Standard CPR ratios and hand position apply
- **Evaluate potential causes (Box A)**

4 Identify team leader, allocate roles including scribe
- Note time

5 Apply defibrillation pads and check cardiac rhythm (defibrillation is safe in pregnancy and no changes to standard shock energies are required))
- If VF / pulseless VT → defibrillation and first adrenaline and amiodarone after 3rd shock
- If PEA / asystole → resume CPR and give first adrenaline immediately
- Check rhythm and pulse every 2 minutes
- Repeat adrenaline every 3-5 minutes

6 Maintain airway and ventilation
- Give 100% oxygen using bag-valve-mask device
- Insert supraglottic airway with drain port –or– tracheal tube if trained to do so (intubation may be difficult, and airway pressures may be higher)
- Apply waveform capnography monitoring to airway
- If expired CO₂ is absent, presume oesophageal intubation until absolutely excluded

7 Circulation
- I.V. access above the diaphragm, if fails or impossible use upper limb intraosseous (IO)
- See **Box B** for reminders about drugs
- Consider extracorporeal CPR (ECPR) if available

8 Emergency hysterotomy (perimortem caesarean section)
- Perform if ≥ 20 weeks gestation, to improve maternal outcome
- Perform immediately if maternal fatal injuries or prolonged pre-hospital arrest
- Perform by 5 minutes if no return of spontaneous circulation

9 Post resuscitation from haemorrhage – activate Massive Haemorrhage Protocol
- Consider uterotonic drugs, fibrinogen and tranexamic acid
- Uterine tamponage / sutures, aortic compression, hysterectomy

Version 1.1

Box A: POTENTIAL CAUSES *4H's and 4T's* (specific to obstetrics)

Hypoxia	Respiratory – Pulmonary embolus (PE), Failed intubation, aspiration Heart failure Anaphylaxis Eclampsia / PET – pulmonary oedema, seizure
Hypovolaemia	Haemorrhage – obstetric (remember concealed), abnormal placentation, uterine rupture, atony, splenic artery/hepatic rupture, aneurysm rupture Cardiac – arrhythmia, myocardial infarction (MI) Distributive – sepsis, high regional block, anaphylaxis
Hypo/hyperkalaemia	Also consider blood sugar, sodium, calcium and magnesium levels
Hypothermia	
Tamponade	Aortic dissection, peripartum cardiomyopathy, trauma
Thrombosis	Amniotic fluid embolus, PE, MI, air embolism
Toxins	Local anaesthetic, magnesium, illicit drugs
Tension pneumothorax	Entonox in pre-existing pneumothorax, trauma

Box B: IV DRUGS FOR USE DURING CARDIAC ARREST

Fluids	**500 mL IV** crystalloid bolus
Adrenaline	**1 mg IV** every 3-5 minutes in non-shockable or after 3rd shock
Amiodarone	**300 mg IV** after 3rd shock
Atropine	**0.5-1 mg IV** up to 3 mg if vagal tone likely cause
Calcium chloride	**10% 10 mL IV** for Mg overdose, low calcium or hyperkalaemia
Magnesium	**2 g IV** for polymorphic VT / hypomagnesaemia, **4 g IV** for eclampsia
Thrombolysis/PCI	For suspected massive pulmonary embolus / MI
Tranexamic acid	**1 g** if haemorrhage
Intralipid	**1.5 mL kg⁻¹ IV** bolus and **15 mL kg⁻¹ hr⁻¹ IV** infusion

Obstetric Anaesthetists' Association
Promoting the highest standards of anaesthetic practice in the care of mother and baby

GUIDELINES ✓ 2021

Figure 15.1 Obstetric cardiac arrest. Source: With permission of Resuscitation Council (UK)

16

Adolescents and young adults

Glenn Matfin

 KEY POINTS

- Healthcare needs in adolescents and young adults (AYAs) aged 16–24 years old span prevention to treatment of acute, emerging and long-term conditions.
- The transition of care for adolescents and young adults from a pediatric, family-centred model to an adult, patient-centred model can be challenging.
- AYAs are increasingly accessing acute care in adult settings, including Acute Medicine.
- Caring for adolescents and young adults presents unique challenges in the Acute Medicine care setting, due to their distinct biological and psychological profiles.
- Acute Medicine staff have a key role in identifying the urgent and important issues which, if addressed accurately and comprehensively, should improve health outcomes for AYAs.

Introduction

Healthcare needs in adolescents and young adults (AYAs) aged 16–24 years old span prevention to treatment of acute, emerging and long-term conditions. AYAs are potentially vulnerable, with increased morbidity and mortality compared with adults. Current provision is also often suboptimal, with many AYAs feeling left out of decision making and not being treated with respect and dignity.

The transition of care for AYAs from a pediatric, family-centred model to an adult, patient-centred model marks an important milestone in the lives of patients with chronic disorders managed from a young age. The transition should be a 'purposeful, planned movement'. The timing and tempo of transition require special consideration of the physical, psychological and social changes occurring in AYAs. No current single approach is effective for all patients (although the 'Ready Steady Go' programme enables the delivery of all the over-arching principles outlined by National Institute for Health and Care Excellence) and can be challenging alongside other life transitions for AYAs (e.g. leaving education, leaving home, parenthood).

In addition to chronic care, AYAs are increasingly accessing acute care in adult settings, including acute medical units (AMU). For some AYAs, the AMU may be their first adult experience of healthcare, and thus there is a need to ensure that the environment of the AMU and the training of staff are appropriate. Acute Medicine staff have a key role in identifying the urgent and important issues which, if addressed accurately and comprehensively, should improve health outcomes for AYAs.

Acute Medicine: Lecture Notes, First Edition. Edited by Glenn Matfin.
© 2023 John Wiley & Sons Ltd. Published 2023 by John Wiley & Sons Ltd.

How do AYAs present to Acute Medicine?

Certain patterns have been recognised.

- New presentations of acute disease – particularly gastrointestinal, renal and respiratory illnesses (including COVID-19).
- New presentations of chronic disease – for example:
  - endocrine (e.g. type 1 diabetes)
  - neurological (e.g. epilepsy)
  - gastrointestinal (e.g. inflammatory bowel disease)
  - oncology (e.g. 25% of cancer diagnoses in AYAs now occur in the acute care setting)
  - mental health problems are common.
- As a result of risk-taking behaviour – such as alcohol, drug and substance abuse. Traumatic injuries are also common.
- Less frequent presentations of patients with chronic, complex disease, experiencing either exacerbations of disease or other intercurrent illnesses (e.g. cystic fibrosis, sickle cell disease).
- Less frequent presentations of patients with newly diagnosed or chronic inherited metabolic disorders (IMDs).
- Patients with severe and complex disabilities.
- Patients receiving end-of-life and palliative care.
- Patients with medically unexplained physical symptoms.

Challenges of managing AYAs in Acute Medicine

Caring for AYAs presents unique challenges in the Acute Medicine care setting, due to their distinct biological and psychological profiles.

- AYAs are often 'invisible' on the AMU, being perceived as independent and self-caring, or cared for by their parent or carer. This contrasts with other patients who may demand higher levels of input from acute medical staff such as acutely unwell, confused, frail elderly patients.
- Clinical assessment of AYAs may be challenging. Building a rapport with an AYA may take additional time and communication skills from talking to older adults. In addition, time and space constraints may make it difficult to see the AYA alone, and staff must sensitively balance the involvement of parents and carers.
- AYAs may have a different disease management approach compared with other adults. For example, treatment of diabetic ketoacidosis or severe hyponatraemia differs in AYAs compared with adults due to increased risk of cerebral oedema in the younger patient.
- AYAs may have traditionally childhood conditions, for example IMDs, for which the optimal management may be unfamiliar to the acute medical staff.
- AYAs may have different social needs. Peer support is very important for AYAs, and the ability to see or contact their friends is vital. Restricted access to mobile phones and the internet may also be a problem.
- AYAs often have different sleep patterns from adults, which can make the routine of the ward challenging. AMUs also often have problems providing overnight accommodation for parents and carers for AYAs with chronic/complex needs, which can be a source of frustration.
- AYAs with complex needs are a particular challenge on the AMU, where unfamiliar equipment, protocols or regimens can lead to potential difficulties.
- Safeguarding and child protection concerns. Acute medical staff may be unfamiliar with the transition between children's and adult legal frameworks and service provision for AYAs with safeguarding and child protection concerns. Recognising new AYA maltreatment and how to raise concerns may also be challenging for predominantly adult-focused healthcare professionals within Acute Medicine care.

Acute Medicine best practice approach to AYAs

- A joined-up experience of care is critical, whether AYAs are accessing acute episodic care or transitioning from paediatric to adult services in the management of long-term conditions.
- Ensure that, in any setting, AYAs with urgent or emergency care needs receive the earliest possible review by an appropriately experienced senior clinical decision maker.
- Identify designated leads from among medical and nursing staff within acute medical care for service delivery and training in AYA care, with a similar lead in paediatrics to co-ordinate care.

- Involve AYAs and parents or carers in the planning of care and ask what is important to them, such as assessing individual patients' readiness and preparedness for adult care, including acute medical care.
- If AYAs are managed in the AMU in an integrated approach with other adults, AYAs should be cared for in single rooms when possible or with other AYAs and in a separate area from both older patients with confusion and patients in the last stages of life.
- It is important that acute medical staff are aware of the support services available for AYAs. This should include pathways of referral to Child and Adolescent Mental Health Services (CAMHS).
- Most AMU staff have not been trained in the care of AYAs, yet AMU staff often see AYAs when they are at their most vulnerable. Education and training should provide staff with the knowledge, skills and attitudes necessary to provide developmentally appropriate care for AYAs, including basic training on communicating with younger patients. Training on safeguarding and child protection is also critical.

17

People with learning disabilities

Glenn Matfin

 KEY POINTS

- People with learning disability have a lower intellectual ability and impaired social and adaptive functioning, with onset in childhood. This affects someone for their whole life.
- There are varying degrees of learning disability (mild, moderate, severe, profound), and consequently the intensity of support needs differs widely.
- People with learning disabilities frequently suffer from multiple health issues.
- Safeguarding patients with learning disabilities is critical. Remember that children and adults with a learning disability can be especially vulnerable in hospital.

Introduction

There are three core criteria which must be met for the term 'learning disability' to apply.

- Significant impairment of intellectual function, usually with IQ <70 (learning new information and skills, remembering and recalling dates, issues, events that would be expected for their age and culture).
- Significant impairment of adaptive and/or social functioning (ability to cope on a day-to-day basis with the demands of their environment and the expectations of age and culture).
- Age of onset before adulthood.

A learning disability is a permanent condition. There are more than 1 million people with learning disability in England alone or 2% of the adult population. The aetiology includes genetic and chromosomal conditions, antenatal and perinatal problems, and incidents in the early years of life, such as meningitis or trauma.

There are varying degrees of learning disability (mild, moderate, severe, profound), and consequently the intensity of support needs differs widely.

A person with a learning disability might also have mental health problems or learning difficulty but these are separate issues. Learning difficulties affect the way someone learns and processes information. They are not related to intelligence, although they can have a significant impact on education and learning. Examples of learning difficulties include dyslexia and attention deficit hyperactivity disorder (ADHD).

How does a learning disability affect everyday life?

The person affected may:

- be less able to understand and retain information
- require the use of simple language
- need unfamiliar things to be explained
- have swallowing difficulties.

Acute Medicine: Lecture Notes, First Edition. Edited by Glenn Matfin.
© 2023 John Wiley & Sons Ltd. Published 2023 by John Wiley & Sons Ltd.

- be less able to communicate pain or discomfort
- rely on others to meet some, or all, of their basic needs or to maintain their safety.

What are the indicators of a possible learning disability?

These may include:

- difficulties following instructions
- difficulties understanding abstract concepts, like time and directions.
- difficulties with phrases in conversation, repetition and/or expanding on content
- confusion about appointments.
- challenges when doing more than one task at a time.

What are the health needs of people with a learning disability?

> People with learning disabilities frequently suffer from multiple health issues. They are more likely to have mental illness, epilepsy, dementia and physical and sensory disabilities (vision and hearing, gait and postural problems, and difficulties with communication). In addition, many people with learning disabilities are not getting their annual health check, and may face increased risk factors for a number of diseases as a result.

People with learning disability may experience the following.

- Die around 20-plus years younger than their peers. It is 10–20 years younger still in people from minority ethnic groups.
- Greater risk of death from amenable causes; 40% of deaths in people with a learning disability are due to pneumonia. This also includes a higher risk from COVID-19-related admission and mortality compared with the general population. Problems with dysphagia and choking are common; 70% of hospitalised patients with a learning disability have some form of dysphagia which can lead to aspiration pneumonia. A dietician or speech therapist should provide guidance as to the consistency and type of food that the patient can and cannot safely swallow.
- Are more likely to fall.
- Have low take-up for national cancer screening programmes and immunisations. For example, may be unaware of lumps in their testicles or breasts, significant change in bowel habit (constipation is common), rectal bleeding, haematuria.
- Polypharmacy is common. Medications should be reviewed during the acute hospital admission, paying particular attention to drugs that worsen cognition, increase the risk of falls or cause constipation. Tend to be overmedicated with psychotropic medicines. STOMP stands for Stopping Over Medication of People with a learning disability, autism or both with psychotropic medicines. It is estimated that every day about 30 000–35 000 adults in England with a learning disability are taking psychotropic medicines when they do not have the health conditions the medicines are prescribed for.
- Some adults with a learning disability are more vulnerable to forms of abuse and might require safeguarding.
- Some causes of intellectual disability can have specific associations; for example, a patient with Down syndrome is at increased risk of hypothyroidism, cardiovascular disease, leukaemia, premature dementia, etc.

What is the role of a carer in an acute hospital?

Carers play an important part in supporting people with learning disabilities whilst in an acute hospital. They can:

- facilitate effective communication, including supporting the person to comprehend information
- provide emotional support, especially during clinical investigations or treatment
- support the patient to make decisions and/or give consent.

Acute Medicine best practice approach to patients with learning disabilities

- The first principle is that of putting patients first (i.e. patient-centred).

- People with learning disabilities (and their carers) should be involved in deciding their healthcare when appropriate (i.e. shared decision making).
- There is a risk of implicit bias, and practitioners need to take active steps to reduce this.
- Use primary care records/hospital alert system to help identify, on admission, all patients with a learning disability.
- Ask if the patient has a hospital passport. This provides important information about a patient with a learning disability, including personal details, the type of medication they are taking, and any pre-existing health conditions.
- Fifty percent to 90% of people with a learning disability have communication difficulties. The hospital passport includes information about how a person communicates and their likes and dislikes, which can be very important when they are first admitted to hospital. This can include any communication aids and how they can be used so health staff can communicate clearly. They can also show how the person expresses things such as happiness, sadness, pain and discomfort. Enhance communication with people with learning disability by the following methods.
  - Use straightforward and clear language.
  - Use pictures and drawings to help explain.
  - Use family or carers to support the person.
  - Look people in the face; make eye contact, so they can read your expressions.
  - Listen to the person and observe their body language.
  - Use gestures and objects or sign language to help explain.
  - If the patient is wearing hearing aids or glasses, make sure they are on before communicating with them.
  - Be respectful and polite; do not shout or patronise.
  - Give the family and patient time to ask questions.
  - Check for understanding.
- Distressed or 'challenging' behaviour is often experienced as physical or verbal aggression, self-harming or socially unacceptable behaviours that have a negative impact on the person or those around them. These behaviours can be a means of patients communicating physical illness.
- Making reasonable adjustments is a legal requirement and a way to ensure that every individual has equal access to health services. An adjustment is any action that reduces or alleviates a disadvantage. Tailoring your practice aims to remove barriers that prevent disabled people from receiving an equal health service. Healthcare professionals are required to make reasonable adjustments to any of their provisions, criteria or practices that place a disabled person at a particular disadvantage compared to non-disabled persons. Hospital passports allow health staff to understand the needs of the individual and help them make the necessary reasonable adjustments to the care and treatment they provide. Simple adjustments can make a difference. To consider reasonable adjustments for your patients, you can use the TEACH acronym to help you think this through.
  - **T**ime: allow more time for consultations. This includes extra time and support when consenting to a procedure or investigations.
  - **E**nvironment: move to a quieter area if possible.
  - **A**ttitude: consider more open visiting or sharing caring duties in hospital. Consider less frequent monitoring of vital signs or laboratory tests when the patient is stable. Demonstrate a physical exam on yourself or a carer.
  - **C**ommunication: make information accessible and try to provide it in advance.
  - **H**elp: refer to the Acute Liaison Nurse Service for Learning Disabilities for additional help and support.
- Interact with the patient's named lead practitioner. This may be a named contact such as a social worker or community learning disability team, or community learning disability nurse, who gets to know the person and co-ordinates support with other members of the multidisciplinary team to meet their long-term needs.
- Support their carers. You can do this by:
  - using straightforward and clear language
  - ensuring they are aware that they have certain rights, including the right to a carer's assessment
  - allowing them to make choices about their caring role
  - identifying and supporting people with carers responsibility
  - keeping carers informed of the person's condition.
- Capacity to consent must be assumed unless assessed otherwise. It is essential to remember that each decision is time, location and decision specific. The capacity to make decisions about one's own medical care is fundamental to the ethical principle of autonomy. The criteria for decision-making capacity may be remembered with the 3 C's: Comprehension (of medical condition and proposed treatments); Consequences (of accepting or refusing proposed treatments); and Choice. If the capacity of an individual over the age of 18 is in question, health professionals need to carry out a

four-point capacity test, in accordance with the Mental Capacity Act (2005). It should be established if the person is able to:

o understand the information relevant to the decision

o retain the information long enough to make the decision

o use or weigh up the information

o communicate their decision.

- If your patient lacks capacity, you must act in the patient's best interests, using the least restrictive alternative to achieve this. Any decision about resuscitation must also be made in their best interests. When making best interest decisions, encourage the person to participate in decision making. Ideally, this involves consulting the patient's relatives, carers and advocate. Consider referring to an independent mental capacity advocate (IMCA) if no family/carer is available. The decision to act in the patient's best interests and what those interests are should always involve a discussion with your senior. Any decisions made in 'best interests' must be carefully documented.

- Safeguard patients with learning disabilities. Remember that people with a learning disability can be especially vulnerable and experience poorer patient safety outcomes in hospital. Make sure a Datix is completed when reporting an incident or near miss involving a person with a learning disability.

- Patients with a learning disability do not have a higher pain threshold. Be proactive, prescribe pain relief or sedation as you would for other patients. The hospital passport may reveal how the person expresses pain and discomfort. Consider pain tools, for example the Abbey pain scale.

- Be aware of diagnostic overshadowing: in the context of learning disabilities, this means that 'symptoms of physical ill health are mistakenly attributed to either a mental health/behavioural problem or as being inherent in the person's learning disabilities'.

- Adults with a learning disability typically experience age-related difficulties at different ages, and at a younger age than the general population.

- Prompt access to COVID-19 testing and healthcare is warranted for this group, and prioritisation for COVID-19 vaccination and other targeted preventive measures should be considered.

- Discharge planning – include other members of the health and social care MDT for effective and safe discharge planning. Is the patient safe to discharge? Do you need to clarify aspects of the history? Have you given the patient the essential information in the form they are most likely to understand? Update and share care plans in a way that is understood by the person, family and their main carers and share with the GP.

- Embed learning disabilities education and training for medical students and healthcare professionals working in Acute Medicine.

18

Inclusion health

Glenn Matfin

KEY POINTS

- Inclusion health focuses on people who are socially excluded, and are in extremely poor health due to poverty, marginalisation and multimorbidity.
- Inclusion health includes people who experience homelessness, drug and alcohol dependence, Gypsies and Travellers, sex workers, people in contact with the criminal justice system and migration-related concerns.
- Inclusion health involves integrated care that considers patients' physical, psychological and social care needs, with complexity managed by individual care co-ordination supported by a multidisciplinary team to address related clinical problems and signpost into care within and beyond admission.
- Recognise that all clinicians must be involved in helping patients to improve their health, not just by medical treatment but through advocacy, interprofessional working and engagement with public health.

Introduction

- *Health equity* – means that everybody should have the opportunity to lead the healthiest life possible. This requires removing obstacles to health such as poverty, discrimination and their consequences, including powerlessness and lack of access to good jobs with fair pay, quality education and housing, safe environments and healthcare.
- *Social justice* – is fairness as it manifests in society. That includes fairness in healthcare, employment, housing and more. The four interrelated principles of social justice are equity, access, participation and rights. Physicians should work actively to eliminate discrimination, whether based on ethnicity, gender, socioeconomic status, religion or any other social category.

Inclusion health is a research, service and policy agenda that aims to prevent and redress health and social inequities among people in extremely poor health due to poverty, marginalisation and multimorbidity (i.e. two or more diseases or disorders occurring in the same person).

Acute Medicine: Lecture Notes, First Edition. Edited by Glenn Matfin.

Healthcare alone cannot transform health inequalities. It requires societal change, reducing poverty and inequality to tackle the root causes of homelessness and multiple disadvantages.

Inclusion health

Inclusion health is a 'catch-all' term used to describe people who are socially excluded, typically experience multiple overlapping risk factors for poor health (such as poverty, violence and substance abuse), experience stigma and discrimination, and are not consistently accounted for in electronic databases (including healthcare records). Inclusion health is a universal concept but responds to local needs.

- Inclusion health includes any population group that is socially excluded. This can include people who experience homelessness, drug and alcohol dependence, Gypsies and Travellers, sex workers, people in contact with the criminal justice system and migration-related concerns.
- These experiences frequently lead to barriers in access to healthcare.
- People belonging to inclusion health groups frequently suffer from multiple health issues.
- This leads to extremely poor health outcomes, often much worse than the general population, a lower average age of death, and it contributes considerably to increasing health inequalities.
- A key challenge within inclusion health is providing integrated health and social care to socially complex patients who have high levels of physical and mental health multimorbidity complicated by chaotic lifestyles and frequent use of emergency services.
- Inclusion health aims to prevent harms of extreme inequity and address the health needs of the most vulnerable through innovative, clinically focused service models, research, teaching and advocacy.
- Frontline NHS and care professionals can do a lot to improve access and appropriate use of services by people who are socially excluded. Small actions can lead to considerable improvements in health outcomes, reduced inequalities and reductions in cost for services.

Homelessness

The scale of homelessness is a notoriously difficult thing to quantify.
- Homelessness is a global phenomenon. An estimated 100 million people are homeless worldwide, and this number is rising.
- In the UK, almost 300 000 households are homeless or at risk of becoming homeless. This is a staggering 1 in 200 people.
- In the USA, around half a million people live in a state of homelessness.
- More than 70% of homeless people are young adults (<50 years of age).

The legal definition of homelessness is that a household has no home available and reasonable to occupy. Homelessness does not just refer to people who are sleeping rough and is not just a problem found in high-value housing markets (e.g. London, San Francisco).

Examples of homelessness are shown in Box 18.1.

The causes of homelessness are typically described as either structural or individual and can be interrelated and reinforced by one another. However, it is ultimately the result of the convergence of individual vulnerabilities and structural factors leading to a broken social support network and relative poverty (Table 18.1). Causes and their relationship vary across the life course.

Box 18.1 Types of homelessness

- Rooflessness (without a shelter of any kind, rough sleeping such as on the streets, or in doorways, parks or bus shelters).
- Houselessness (with a place to sleep but temporary, in bed and breakfast, hostels or a shelter).
- Living in insecure housing (threatened with severe exclusion due to insecure tenancies, eviction, domestic violence or staying with family and friends, known as 'sofa surfing').
- Living in inadequate housing (in caravans on illegal campsites, in unfit housing) or other places not designed for habitation (such as barns, sheds, car parks, cars).

Table 18.1 Causes of homelessness

Structural factors include:	Individual factors include:
• Poverty • Inequality including structural racism • Housing supply and affordability • Unemployment or insecure employment	• Disability – in the USA, almost 40% of homeless are disabled • Poor physical health • Mental health problems • Experience of violence, abuse, neglect, harassment or hate crime • Drug and alcohol problems • Bereavement • Relationship breakdown • Experience of care or prison • Refugees

Health consequences of homelessness

The health and well-being of people who experience homelessness are poorer than those of the general population. They often experience the most significant health inequalities. The longer a person experiences homelessness, particularly from young adulthood, the more likely their health and well-being will be at risk. Death rates can be up to eight times higher than in the general population. Recent UK statistics show that the mean age of death of homeless people is almost 40 years lower than the general population, at 45 years, and even lower for homeless women, at just 43 years. One in three deaths of people who are homeless are preventable. Homeless patients are also overrepresented amongst frequent attenders in Acute Medicine and emergency departments.

Homelessness and tri-morbidity

Chronic homelessness is an associated marker for tri-morbidity, complex health needs and premature death. Tri-morbidity is the combination of physical ill health with mental ill health and drug or alcohol misuse. This complexity is often associated with advanced illness at presentation, in the context of a person lacking social support who often feels ambivalent about both accessing care and their own self-worth.

Homelessness is associated with increased incidence of serious chronic conditions such as hepatitis C, heart disease, asthma, chronic obstructive pulmonary disease, epilepsy, human immunodeficiency virus (HIV) infection and tuberculosis (TB). There is also a lack of screening and testing, with 65% having not had a sexual health check in the past 12 months and most having not been tested for HIV, hepatitis C or TB. Furthermore, a majority have not had their hepatitis A or B vaccinations. Women, young people and gender-diverse people living on the street also experience an increased incidence of violence, including sexual violence and forced or coerced sexual activity.

Mental health problems in people who are homeless are twice as high as the general population, with 86% of people who are homeless reporting a mental health condition yet only 44% having a formal diagnosis. People who are homeless are also nine times more likely to take their own lives than the general population, making it the second most common cause of death.

The third part of the tri-morbidity is problematic alcohol or drug use, which is reported in 27% of the population of people who are homeless generally, increasing to over 40% in those specifically that sleep rough.

Direct impact of lack of housing on health

Frontline health and care professionals already witness firsthand the detrimental impact that lack of housing has on our unhoused patients, whose health is routinely compromised by:

- restricted access to resources
- crowded and unsafe living conditions
- exposure to serious environmental and situational hazards.

Tragically, these factors have only intensified during the COVID-19 pandemic (Box 18.2).

Acute Medicine approach to homelessness

Simply housing people who have been long-term homeless (although an essential first step) does not, of itself, resolve the underlying problems. When homeless people die, they do not commonly die because of exposure or other direct effects of homelessness; they die of treatable medical problems, HIV-related disease, liver and other gastrointestinal

> **Box 18.2 Homelessness and COVID-19**
>
> Shelters are often crowded, poorly ventilated indoor spaces with high numbers of people passing through each day and sleeping on cots just a few feet apart. Not surprisingly, shelters were identified as hotspots for COVID-19 transmission early in the pandemic. People living in homelessness shelters are at higher risk of being hospitalised with COVID-19, because of the presence of co-morbidities and systemic barriers that prevent equitable access to healthcare. When hospitalised, homeless people face substantial obstacles to safe discharge and recovery, particularly amidst this pandemic. This can lead to excess length of hospital stays, morbidity and costs, and limiting acute care access within some communities.

disease, respiratory disease or acute and chronic consequences of drug and alcohol dependence.

Health and care professionals play an important role, working alongside other members of the multidisciplinary team (MDT), to:

- identify the risk of homelessness among people who have poor health and prevent this
- minimise the impact on health from homelessness among people who are already experiencing it
- enable improved health outcomes for people experiencing homelessness so that their poor health is not a barrier to moving on to a home of their own.

Frontline health and care professionals can have an impact on an individual level by:

- enquiring about the household's housing circumstances and ensuring this is recorded
- fulfilling the requirements of the new public sector duty to refer where a person or household is homeless or threatened with homelessness
- using the Homeless Assessment Tool, an instrument recently developed by Gloucestershire Hospitals NHS Foundation Trust to help standardise and more comprehensively evaluate the needs of this vulnerable group. As the model of care in the UK moves to integrated care systems, this provides opportunities to treat these patients in a more holistic fashion (Figure 18.1).

Services for homeless people should include the provision of 'respite care' – community-based residential medical facilities for homeless people with significant and complex healthcare problems. Pathway has published standards for medical respite in England.

Migration-related concerns

> A migrant is a person who moves away from his or her place of usual residence, whether within a country or across an international border, temporarily or permanently, and for a variety of reasons. Migrants number more than 300 million worldwide. People migrate for diverse reasons, which makes them a heterogeneous group.

The term 'vulnerable' is used to describe those who have been adversely affected by circumstances leading to or resulting from migration and refers to their circumstances rather than being an attribute of a person themselves. Vulnerable migrants include the following.

- Asylum seekers (i.e. protection by a state on its territory to individuals outside their country of nationality or habitual residence, who are fleeing persecution or serious harm or for other reasons) and failed asylum seekers.
- Refugees (i.e. any person who is outside the country of their nationality and is unable or unwilling to return to that country due to persecution and violence).
- Internally displaced people who have sought refuge within the borders of their nation state.
- People who are undocumented.
- People who are trafficked.

New migrants frequently face adversity before, during and after arrival in the host country, resulting in complex service needs. Perceptions of migrants are increasingly influenced by racism and xenophobia. This contributes to increasingly restrictive policies for all forms of migration. Establishing more inclusive migrant healthcare is critical to supporting health as a human right regardless of migratory status.

> Trafficking is the movement of people by means such as force, fraud, coercion or deception with the aim of exploiting them. It is a form of Modern Slavery. People can be trafficked for many different forms of exploitation such as forced prostitution, forced labour, forced begging, forced criminality, forced marriage, domestic servitude and forced organ removal.

HOMELESS ASSESSMENT TOOL

This is an adjunct to the clerking proforma, designed as an opportunistic prompt to ensure we are delivering the best care for our homeless patients.

Please note this is to be used as a **resource only**. It is an example of best practice. It is not an official trust document. It therefore **cannot be used** in the as documentation in trust medical notes.

Homeless Team:	DART:	Homeless Cupboard GRH Code:
Mental Health Liaison:	Alcohol Liaison:	Safeguarding:
Housing Officer:	P3 Hospital In-Reach Navigator:	
Emergency Duty Team OOH:	P3 Housing Support:	

ADMISSION CHECKLIST

HISTORY	☑/☒	COMMENTS
Place of sleep / Safe place	☐	
Partner / Children / NOK / Pets	☐	
Contacts / Organisations / Case Workers / Support involved	☐	CGL ☐ Housing ☐ George Whitfield Centre (Homeless Health Centre) ☐ Domestic Abuse ☐ Dental ☐ Other ☐
Alcohol, drugs & replacement	☐	
Sexual health	☐	
MMSE / Capacity / Cognition assessed	☐	
Mental health	☐	
Past suicide attempt or overdose	☐	
Safeguarding: neglect, risk from others	☐	
Trafficking / Slavery	☐	
If patient wants to self-discharge: explore needs, reasons & risk	☐	
Follow-up required if self-discharges	☐	

EXAMINATION	☑/☒	COMMENTS
Neurology, head injuries & gait	☐	
Mouth & dentition	☐	
Head, neck & lymph nodes	☐	
Skin, feet & injection sites	☐	
Peripheral vascular exam	☐	
Nutritional status	☐	

TESTS & TREATMENT	☑/☒	COMMENTS
Frequent attender / Management plan	☐	
BBV (HIV, hep B&C)	☐	
Sexual health screen & β-hCG	☐	
CXR & TB	☐	
Pain, nicotine, drug replacement & withdrawal (CIWAS, COWS)	☐	
Vaccinations (Covid, flu, hep A/B)	☐	
Supplements & risk of refeeding	☐	

REFERRALS TO MAKE	☑/☒	COMMENTS
Homeless Team / Housing Officer	☐	
Mental Health Liaison	☐	
Drug & Alcohol In-Reach Team / ALT	☐	
Safeguarding Team / Social Work	☐	
Dietitian	☐	
Tissue Viability	☐	
Vascular	☐	
Dentist / Max Fax	☐	
Chronic Pain Team	☐	
Already known to a specialty	☐	

Figure 18.1 Homeless Assessment Tool developed and used by Gloucestershire Hospitals NHS Foundation Trust.

How does migration affect health?

Migrants individually and collectively are affected by a range of factors that affect health and their access to, and experiences of, healthcare.

- Life in the host country before migration: migrants bring a 'health footprint' with them, including ethnic and family susceptibility, different disease patterns, as well as varying quality of previous healthcare.
- The migration process: migration is a difficult process, regardless of the motivations behind it, and it has a variety of potential physical and psychological health impacts.
- Establishment in the host country after arrival: a range of health problems may occur after migration, associated with changes in living and working environments, social stress and changes in personal behaviours. In addition, migrants are often simultaneously struggling with poor access to healthcare and limited social services.

Health problems of vulnerable migrants are frequently related to destitution and lack of access to services, rather than to complex or long-standing ill health.

Which areas of health are affected by migration?

Vulnerable migrants are often described as facing a 'triple burden' of infectious diseases, non-communicable diseases, and mental health issues.

- Infectious diseases: there is a significant burden of active and latent TB, HIV, hepatitis B and C, parasitic infections (e.g. strongyloidiasis in people from Afghanistan) and vaccine-preventable diseases in migrant populations. Special concerns arise about infectious diseases in dynamic populations. As population mobility increases, diseases spread wider and more quickly.
  - NICE recommends that new entrants aged under 65 from high-incidence countries, such as Afghanistan, are screened for latent TB using interferon-gamma release assay via a single blood test; this is most suitable for underserved groups (including refugees and asylum seekers).
  - Patients who are febrile or unwell: consider a wide range of differentials, including the infections mentioned above, as well as malaria and typhoid.
- Non-communicable diseases may be undiagnosed or poorly controlled: certain disorders are more prevalent in migrants when moving to host countries (e.g. premature diabetes and cardiovascular disease are especially common in Asian and Hispanic migrants when moving to middle- and high-income countries due to genetic/epigenetic predisposition, chronic stress, poor food adaptation and drastic lifestyle changes).
- Mental health problems: depression, anxiety, substance abuse and other mental health problems are common.

Other issues related to migrants

- Healthcare access.
  - The 'Overseas Visitors NHS Cost Recovery Programme' is now a legal obligation on NHS trusts. Although immediately necessary and urgent treatment should always be provided, concerns remain that vulnerable migrants may be dissuaded from accessing care because they fear charges or coming to the attention of immigration authorities.
  - Language and cultural barriers also can present obstacles to appropriate care. Migrants will often not be able to speak, read or understand English fluently. This can cause problems with consent and explaining the options available to them, obtaining an adequate and relevant medical history, and ascertaining payment status or explaining payment options.
- Occupational illnesses and injuries: many migrants work in industries with increased risks, including agriculture, construction, transportation and domestic services.
- Consider nutritional deficiency (e.g. anaemia, vitamin D deficiency), oral health, reproductive health (e.g. female genital mutilation, cervical screening, gender-based violence), pregnancy and contraception.
- Survivors of human trafficking.
  - High levels of physical and sexual violence, and workplace injury.
  - High rates of depression, anxiety and posttraumatic stress disorder (PTSD), attempted suicide.
  - Chronic threats, excessive work hours, poor living conditions and severe curtailment of freedoms.

Immigration detainees have been found to have high levels of PTSD that are very closely associated with their detention, and which frequently lead to anxiety, depression, self-harm, suicidal ideation and suicide attempts. Survivors of torture and trafficking have often experienced extreme circumstances in which they have been exposed to uncontrollable and unpredictable events, which can result in severe and longer-term PTSD. Migrants' high risk of homelessness and destitution creates circumstances that further exacerbate their already fragile mental health.

workers meet the criteria for PTSD – this is in the same range as victims of torture and combat veterans undergoing treatment.

Despite street sex workers having significantly higher rates of health service use compared with the general population, a comparatively low percentage of female sex workers have had routine health checks such as cervical screening or attend antenatal checks when pregnant. Psychological and institutional barriers to accessing healthcare include fear of criminalisation, institutional factors (e.g. opening hours, location), stigmatisation and discrimination.

Contact with criminal justice system

In 2022, the UK has approximately 80 000 prisoners at any one time. In comparison, almost 2 million US adults and youth are incarcerated – more than any other nation. Prisoners have high all-cause mortality and mortality from injuries, self-harm and suicide, COVID-19 and poisonings. Part of the reason will not be prison itself but the multiple problems that prisoners have, including the risk of substance use disorder, mental illness and violent behaviour, all of which increase an individual's risk of imprisonment.

Criminal justice services can provide an excellent opportunity for engagement with healthcare if there is an appropriate non-judgemental attitude. When criminal justice services offer healthcare, this can be a positive starting point at which to assess general health status, stabilise conditions and begin treatment(s).

Sex workers

This includes commercial 'street-based' and 'parlour-based' sex workers. Sex workers are likely to experience poor health because of the risks associated with their work. Female sex workers in London have a mortality rate that is 12 times the national average. Up to 95% of female sex workers are problematic drug users and 68% of female sex

Gypsies and other Travellers

'Gypsies and Travellers' is a commonly used 'catch-all' term that includes people from a variety of groups, all of whom were – or are – nomadic. In total, around 63 000 people in the UK identified themselves as members of these groups, of which 58 000 were living in England and Wales. These include:
- Romany (English/Welsh) Gypsies (the majority group in England and Wales)
- Scottish Gypsies/Travellers
- Travellers of Irish heritage (Irish Travellers)
- Roma (Romany people from European countries)
- miscellaneous, including fairground and show people, circus people, and watercraft/canal boat Travellers.

Today, although nomadism ('travelling') is an important part of Gypsy and Traveller people's culture and history, the word 'Gypsy' or 'Traveller' is more accurately a description of ethnic identity and distinct culture(s) – social organisation, value system, shared history, language, traditions, etc. – rather than a description of actual daily activities or an identifier of nationality. An estimated two-thirds of Gypsies and Travellers in the UK today live among the 'settled community' in permanent housing, with a further significant portion living on permanent sites, either privately or publicly provided.

All Gypsies and Travellers have the same rights as other UK residents to access NHS and social care services, whether they are nomadic or living in permanent settlements. Despite this, Gypsies and Travellers have significantly poorer health outcomes compared with the general population of England and with other English-speaking ethnic minorities. This is due to several reasons.

- They are frequently subject to structural racism and discrimination.
- There is a serious underprovision of official trailer sites for Gypsies and Travellers across the country and so community members may find themselves living in irregular locations, for instance under motorways or next to sewage works. Consequently, they face health hazards uncommon in the general population, such as lack of sewage disposal and limited access to water.
- Gypsies and Travellers may not be literate, so information concerning treatment and appointments may need to be explained.
- Gypsies and Travellers have high rates of mental health issues including suicide, substance misuse issues and diabetes, as well as high rates of heart disease and premature morbidity and mortality.
- Travellers are less likely to receive effective, continuous healthcare.

Acute Medicine best practice approach to inclusion health patients

- The first principle is that of putting patients first (i.e. patient-centred).
- They should be involved in decisions on their condition (i.e. shared decision making), including taking into account social and cultural norms especially for multiethnic populations (i.e. cultural distinction).
- Meeting the health needs of excluded groups with respect, dignity and compassion. Show kindness and empathy during all encounters.
- Use non-discriminatory language. This includes words and phrases that treat all people equitably and fairly. It does not discriminate against people.

- Signpost patients to services and voluntary support.
- Offer translator and appropriate translated health information (e.g. educational, consent forms) as needed.
- Ensuring prompt access to emergency care for all.
- Address cost recovery only *after* the patient receives urgent treatment.
- Integrated care that considers patients' physical, psychological and social care needs, with complexity managed by individual care co-ordination supported by an MDT to address related clinical problems and signpost into care within and beyond admission.
- Initiate safeguarding pathways as needed (including physical violence, exploitation and Modern Slavery).
- Offer GP registration to all who need healthcare.
- Provide targeted preventive care as needed.
- Supporting individuals to attend appointments and engage in treatment.
- Inclusion health services should work closely with public health departments, particularly in relation to serious communicable diseases (e.g. TB, COVID-19, monkeypox or blood-borne virus transmission). Catch-up immunisation and COVID-19 vaccination should be offered.
- Refer as needed for common co-morbidities (e.g. oral health, eye and skin problems, sexually transmitted infections).
- Discharge planning should begin on admission and involve as wide a network of health and social care as required.
- Ensure that all clinicians involved in the care of complex patients receive adequate communication to ensure safe and effective discharge – including liaison with named lead clinician in adult and/or older persons mental health services.
- All admitted patients should be asked 'Do you have somewhere safe to stay when you leave hospital?' and staff should be trained and supported to help people who say 'No'.
- Embed inclusion health in the education and training of medical students and healthcare professionals working in Acute Medicine.

19

Lesbian, gay, bisexual, transgender, queer or questioning, and others (LGBTQ+)

Howell Jones and Glenn Matfin

 KEY POINTS

- All physicians, regardless of specialty, should be trained in the fundamentals of lesbian, gay, bisexual, transgender, queer or questioning, and others (LGBTQ+) health.
- Approximately 3.6 million people in the United Kingdom identify as LGBTQ+.
- LGBTQ+ people may experience social exclusion, stigma and discrimination.
- They may experience challenges when seeking medical support, including difficulty accessing care and discrimination from healthcare professionals, resulting in health inequalities.
- People belonging to the LGBTQ+ community frequently suffer from multiple health issues. They have poorer health outcomes and lower average age of death compared to their heteronormative counterparts.
- Promote good practice in using non-discriminatory language in an inclusive way, which shows respect for, and sensitivity towards, all members of the LGBTQ+ community.
- Consider exploring and recording of sexual orientation, gender identity, preferred name and pronouns as part of routine Acute Medicine consultations if relevant and the patient feels comfortable to do so.

Acute Medicine: Lecture Notes, First Edition. Edited by Glenn Matfin.
© 2023 John Wiley & Sons Ltd. Published 2023 by John Wiley & Sons Ltd.

Introduction

> There are approximately 3.6 million people in the UK who identify as lesbian, gay, bisexual, transgender, queer or questioning, and others (LGBTQ+) and are considered to be in sexual and gender minority groups.

Despite the strides we have made towards LGBTQ+ equality in recent years, many LGBTQ+ people still face significant barriers within both healthcare and wider society. They often experience social exclusion, stigma and discrimination.

Homosexuality was made illegal in England in 1533 and was not decriminalised until 1967 in England and Wales, 1980 in Scotland and 1982 in Northern Ireland. The Civil Partnership Act was passed in the UK in 2004, with same-sex marriage finally legalised in 2014 in England, Wales and Scotland. It took until 2020 for Northern Ireland and all the Channel Islands to do so.

The results of these and other laws have had the impact of increasing awareness of LGBTQ+ rights, with the first Pride rally held in London in 1972. The first case of acquired immunodeficiency syndrome (AIDS) was recorded in the UK in 1981. The human immunodeficiency virus (HIV) epidemic led to the passing of Section 28 of the Local Government Act, meaning the local authority could not 'promote homosexuality' or 'promote the teaching in any maintained school of the acceptability of homosexuality as a pretended family relationship'. The impact of this legislation is still discernible today, directly affecting LGBTQ+ people's health and how they interact with healthcare services. To combat this, groups like Stonewall UK were created to campaign for LGBTQ+ rights. The most recent change was in 2021, as gay men in closed (monogamous) relationships can now donate blood without a deferral period, in line with heterosexual counterparts.

LGBTQ+ people face challenges when seeking medical support, including difficulty accessing care and discrimination from healthcare personnel. In a 2018 UK survey, one in eight LGBTQ+ people experienced some form of unequal treatment from healthcare staff because they were LGBTQ+, and almost one in four LGBTQ+ people witnessed discriminatory or negative remarks against LGBTQ+ people by healthcare staff. In addition, many healthcare professionals are also not knowledgeable or experienced in caring for the specific needs of LGBTQ+ people. Overall, this results in increasing health inequalities for LGBTQ+ people.

Acute Medicine professionals can improve LGBTQ+ patient care experience by developing an awareness of the challenges that this group often face in acute care settings, knowing and using appropriate terminology, and providing best practices in care. It must be acknowledged that LGBTQ+ patients are not a homogeneous group, and a person-centred approach is required.

Definitions

In healthcare, the following definitions are used.

- *Sex* – refers to the biological distinctions that exist between male, female and intersex people with respect to reproductive anatomy, sex chromosomes and/or specific genes. Based on these biological distinctions, most infants are assigned a sex at birth according to the binary framework of male or female.
- *Gender* – refers to a socially constructed set of ways in which people understand and express themselves along the continuum of masculinity, femininity, both or neither.
- *Gender identity* – refers to an individual's internal sense of self as female, male, neither, both or some other gender. Gender identity may or may not reflect the biological sex assigned at birth.
- *Gender expression* – refers to the way a person expresses their gender identity, typically through their name, pronouns, appearance, dress and behaviour.

Terms used to describe an individual's gender, gender identity and gender expression

The most common of these are defined below.

- *Cisgender* – someone whose current gender identity aligns with the sex they were assigned at birth. In other words, someone who is not agender or transgender.
- *Transgender* – someone whose current gender identity does not align with the sex they were assigned at birth.
  - A transgender woman (or transwoman) was assigned male sex at birth but identifies as a woman.

○ A transgender man (or transman) was assigned female sex at birth but identifies as a man.

○ Some individuals have a gender identity that is not the traditional binary of male and female, encompasses both or may change over time; these individuals may identify as gender fluid or genderqueer.

- *Non-binary* – someone who identifies their gender outside the binary of *man* and *woman*, because they identify as both masculine and feminine, because they identify as neither masculine nor feminine, or because they identify in a way that does not conform with the normative views of sex and gender in their culture and historical period.

- *Agender* – someone who does not identify themselves as having a particular gender; someone who is neither cisgender nor transgender.

- *Transitioning* – refers to the process of shifting gender expression to more closely align with gender identity, which can include social transition (such as new names, pronouns and clothing) and/or medical transition (such as hormone therapy or surgery).

One important expression of gender is through the use of personal pronouns. Pronouns are words that can be used by a person to describe themselves and it is validating when people show care and understanding of them. These may include he/him for those who identify as a man, she/her for those who identify as a woman whilst they/them may be used for those who identify as non-binary. Some people may feel comfortable with combinations of pronouns, or other pronouns known as neo-pronouns, which can take the form of many different words such as ze/zir and xe/xir. Disregarding a person's pronouns is disrespectful and discriminatory. For further information visit www.MyPronouns.org.

Terms used to describe an individual's sexual orientation

Sexual orientation is how a person describes the gender or genders of people they are attracted to. Common terms used to describe sexual orientation include the following.

- Straight or heterosexual – a person who is mostly or exclusively attracted to partners of the opposite binary gender.

- Bisexual – a person who is attracted to people of two or more genders.

- Gay or homosexual – a person attracted mostly or exclusively to someone of their same gender. This word is used more often by gay men to describe their sexuality than gay women (many of whom identify as lesbian).

- Lesbian – a woman attracted mostly or exclusively to other women.

- Pansexual or 'pan'– people who are attracted to people regardless of gender.

- Queer – a reclaimed, positive and affirming term used to describe people who are neither cisgender nor heterosexual as a unifying umbrella term inclusive of everyone in the LGBTQ+ community. In some cases, the term *queer* is used to describe multiple people (e.g. 'the queer community'); in other cases, individuals use it as their term of choice in describing their sexual orientation and/or gender identity (e.g. 'she is a queer woman'; 'they are queer'). This is a term with a long history and not accepted by all LGBTQ+ people and should therefore only be used with people who feel comfortable using it.

- Asexual or 'ace' – a person who experiences little or no sexual attraction, of which there are several subtypes.

None of the terms above are mutually exclusive – often, people will identify with multiple labels, and the ways in which these terms are used are often fluid and context dependent. It is best practice to ask patients how they refer to themselves and to mirror their language.

What are the health needs of the LGBTQ+ community?

People belonging to the LGBTQ+ community frequently suffer from multiple health issues. They have poor health outcomes, often much worse than the general population, a lower average age of death, and it contributes considerably to increasing health inequalities. These experiences can also lead to barriers in access to healthcare. Intersecting minority statuses (such as poverty and unemployment) have a synergistic effect on the health and health-seeking behaviours of LGBTQ+ patients.

Mental health problems

LGBTQ+ people are at higher risk than the general population of experiencing common mental health problems such as depression, anxiety, suicidal thoughts or attempts. These are highest amongst trans people, with 29% attempting suicide in their lifetime, 22 times higher than the national average. This can be related to experiences of discrimination, harassment and bullying in day-to-day life, rejection from one's family and community and being subjected to hate crimes including physical and sexual violence.

Eating disorders are also more common amongst LGBTQ+ people, often to provide a sense of control. They are especially common amongst trans people as a way to try and conform to societal stereotypes of body type and to reduce dysphoria. Anorexia nervosa has the highest mortality rate of any psychiatric condition, with 20% of people experiencing it going on to develop a lifelong chronic form of the disease. LGBTQ+ people are also more likely to be neurodiverse and have a diagnosis of autistic spectrum disorder (ASD) or show traits of ASD. This again is more common amongst trans people, with a study showing that 23.8% of trans people had a diagnosis of autism, compared to 6.9% of cisgender men and 4.4% of cisgender women.

LGBTQ+ people are also more likely to experience intimate partner violence.

> It is important to address the unique needs of LGBTQ+ patients in acute psychiatric settings, including inclusive and affirming communication and culturally competent history taking, risk assessment, treatment environments and discharge considerations.

Substance use

Substance use is common amongst LGBTQ+ people, with higher rates of tobacco and alcohol dependence. The use of recreational drugs is more common particularly amongst gay and bisexual men, particularly during sex, commonly known as 'chemsex'. The three main drugs people take as part of chemsex are methamphetamine, mephedrone and GHB/GBL (gamma hydroxybutyric acid/gamma butyrolactone). These drugs can have both direct and indirect effects as well as acute and long-term impacts on people's health and are common reasons for acute medical presentation.

Gay and bisexual men may also use image- and performance-enhancing drugs (IPEDs) such as anabolic steroids and testosterone to change their appearance or weight. Due to long waiting times for gender identity clinics (GIC), many trans people self-source hormone treatments.

> Working within Acute Medicine requires an understanding of common drugs used, terminology and ways of taking to recognise the signs of use as well as feeling confident talking to people about them (see Chapter 22).

Medical transition

Transgender and gender diverse people often seek medical therapies to better align their bodies with their gender identity. These are overseen by GICs but prescribed and monitored by GPs.

The average time from referral to a GIC to receiving hormone replacement therapy (HRT) is currently 5.5 years. GPs have guidelines with regard to bridging hormones whilst waiting but many trans people still face barriers to receiving this care.

Gender-affirming treatments include HRT and hormone blockers. These hormonal interventions aim to reduce endogenous hormone production and induce secondary sex and physical characteristics congruent with gender identity. Sex hormone therapy for transgender women (if used) primarily involves exogenous oestrogen agents, with some also using testosterone blockers. The latter are only required for people with testes. Sex hormone therapy for transgender men consists of exogenous testosterone, which suppresses oestrogen's effects leading to body changes associated with masculinity.

All trans people are subject to unique adverse effects of hormone therapy and require routine monitoring for hormone levels and the presence of side-effects (including cardiovascular disease and venous thromboembolic complications). Monitoring is similar to other HRT indications, with regular checks of hormone levels, renal and liver function and blood pressure. For those with uteruses taking testosterone therapy, it is advised that they have an ultrasound scan of the uterus every two years due to the increased risk of endometrial cancer. In a recent observational study of transgender women and transgender men receiving gender-affirming hormone therapy, the mortality risk was twice as high as in cisgender people and has not decreased in the past five decades. Higher observed deaths than expected deaths overall and for categories of cardiovascular disease, lung cancer, HIV and suicide in transgender women and increased overall deaths in transgender men are seen compared with the general population.

> One of the biggest barriers to trans-inclusive healthcare relevant to Acute Medicine is 'trans broken arm syndrome'. This is when healthcare providers assume that all medical issues are a result of a person being trans and the medication they may choose to use. Trans people should be treated the same as cisgendered patients, with all potential differential diagnoses considered prior to attributing symptoms to solely being trans.

Cancer

LGBTQ+ patients continue to experience inequalities throughout the cancer pathway, from routine cancer screening (e.g. breast, cervix, prostate) through to late effects and end-of-life care. The invitation letters to attend screening are generated according to the patient's gender marker on their NHS record. Changing your gender marker in the NHS results in a new NHS number. Invitations to screening are based on this record, meaning that often trans people are left to advocate for themselves to receive screening.

Transwomen should undergo breast screening if they develop breast tissue on gender-affirming hormonal treatment, whilst transmen should also undergo screening if they retain breast tissue. Transmen should also be offered cervical screening where relevant. Both groups should undergo screening for bowel cancer and abdominal aortic aneurysms.

Some LGBTQ+ patient groups have higher cancer risk factors, for example obesity, alcohol and tobacco consumption, and can have complex competing co-morbidities, such as anxiety and depression, which affect their engagement with healthcare services.

LGBTQ+ people have a much higher rate of human papilloma virus (HPV)-related cancer. These include head and neck, penile, cervical, vulval, vaginal and anal cancer. The cervical cancer screening programme aims to identify HPV-related changes called cervical intraepithelial neoplasia (CIN). Currently, there is no anal intraepithelial neoplasia (AIN) for gay and bisexual men, as well as trans and non-binary people who have sex with men. Gay and bisexual men as well as trans and non-binary people who have sex

with men are eligible for vaccination against HPV up until age 45 to reduce the risk.

Finally, the common screening test for prostate cancer is prostate-specific antigen (PSA) which can be elevated in people with prostates if they are the receptive partner in anal sex, so patients should be advised to not have sex for one week before having a PSA test when possible. Prostate Cancer UK has good resources for gay, bisexual, non-binary and trans people.

Infection

Increased prevalence of sexually transmitted infections, COVID-19 infection, Monkeypox, HIV, hepatitis A, B and C, and syphilis is also more common within the LGBTQ+ community. Gay and bisexual men as well as trans and non-binary people who have sex with men should be vaccinated against hepatitis A and B. They are also eligible for pre-exposure prophylaxis (PrEP) medication which can be taken to reduce the risk of HIV acquisition.

Acute Medicine best practice approach to LGTBQ+ people

- The first principle is that of putting patients first (i.e. patient-centred).
- LGBTQ+ patients should be involved in deciding their own healthcare (i.e. shared decision making).
- Meet the health needs of excluded groups with respect, dignity and compassion.
- Promote good practice in using non-discriminatory language in an inclusive way, which shows respect for, and sensitivity towards, all members of the LGBTQ+ community.
  - Correctly using LGBTQ+ health vocabulary makes an important contribution to the celebration of diversity.
  - As well as avoiding offence, it is about treating each other with dignity and as equal members of an integrated community.
  - Language is both fluid and deeply personal; not all LGBTQ+ patients refer to themselves with similar terms, and the ways in which these terms are used may change over time.
  - Gender-neutral language avoids stereotyping people according to their sex.

- When addressing any patient for the first time, respectfully ask your patient how they prefer to be addressed. Ask people what pronouns they use. Apologise if you make a mistake of terminology or otherwise.
- Encourage the recording of preferred name and pronouns as part of routine Acute Medicine consultations as well as sexual orientation and gender identity, where relevant.
- Create inclusive clinical environments that are affirming to LGBTQ+ patients, staff and students.
- Initiate safeguarding pathways as needed (including physical and sexual violence, exploitation).
- Provide targeted preventive care as needed (including COVID-19 vaccination).
- Refer as needed for co-morbidities (e.g. sexually transmitted infections, mental health issues).
- Encourage local training in equality and diversity with feedback from LGBTQ+ patients as this has been shown to be most effective in improving patient experience.
- Embed LGBTQ+ education and training for medical students and healthcare professionals working in Acute Medicine.
  - There remains a massive knowledge gap among most practising physicians when it comes to LGBTQ+ health, and a lack of people competent to teach what needs to be taught.
  - LGBTQ+ vocabulary, social and behavioural determinants of LGBTQ+ health, creation of welcoming and inclusive healthcare spaces, legal issues for unmarried partners, strategies to prevent HIV transmission and care of transgender patients.
  - All physicians, regardless of specialty, should be trained in these fundamentals of LGBTQ+ health.

20

People living with HIV

Nadia Ahmed and Robert Miller

 KEY POINTS

- Human immunodeficiency virus (HIV) infection and acquired immune deficiency syndrome (AIDS) are a spectrum of conditions caused predominantly by infection with HIV-1.
- People living with HIV are still often stigmatised and discriminated against.
- The widespread use of combined antiretroviral therapy (ART) has dramatically improved the life expectancy of people living with HIV.
- People living with HIV can present to Acute Medicine services because of: (a) non-HIV-related acute medical issues; (b) acute seroconversion illness; (c) opportunistic infections and malignancy associated with untreated HIV infection or disease progression; (d) immune reconstitution occurring after ART initiation (early or late); (e) complications of ART (i.e. adverse drug reactions); (f) non-AIDS-related long-term cardiometabolic complications and malignancies; and (g) predisposition to more severe COVID-19 infection as a result of immunosuppression and/or co-morbidities.
- Acute Medicine clinicians caring for people with HIV must seek expert advice with any queries related to ART. Care must be taken to avoid 'drug–drug' interactions in this patient group. Needlestick injuries and 'splash' contamination involving people living with HIV need prompt systematic management, including consideration of HIV postexposure prophylaxis.

Introduction

Human immunodeficiency virus (HIV) infection and acquired immune deficiency syndrome (AIDS) form a spectrum of conditions caused predominantly by infection with HIV-1. The HIV epidemic has seen significant advancements since the first case was described in 1981. Largely propelled by the advent of combined antiretroviral therapy (ART), HIV has been transformed from a death sentence to a manageable condition with a near normal life expectancy. AIDS is no longer the dominant health issue in HIV infection, in countries where ART is available and accessible. However, disparities in ART access exist internationally, particularly in resource-limited settings.

Globally, there are 37.7 million people living with HIV, with adults accounting for 95% of infections. Gender disparities are seen, disadvantaging women and girls

---

Acute Medicine: Lecture Notes, First Edition. Edited by Glenn Matfin.

by just over half of all cases, and are more evident in sub-Saharan African countries that also see the highest rates of HIV. In 2020, an estimated 106 890 people were living with HIV in the UK. Of these, an estimated 5150 were unaware of their infection. The COVID-19 pandemic has changed patterns of sexual behaviour, HIV testing and access to sexual health and HIV services in the UK.

HIV transmission

HIV can only be transmitted through sexual fluids (pre-cum, semen, vaginal fluids, anal mucus), blood and blood products, and from mother to child during vaginal or caesarean section delivery or via breast feeding.

The risk of transmission depends on the type of exposure, that is, the risk behaviour, membrane involved and if the person living with HIV is on ART with an undetectable HIV viral load. Our understanding of HIV transmission, in the context of HIV viral loads, has transformed the way in which HIV is considered, with implications not only for living with HIV but preventing it. For transmission of HIV to occur:

- firstly, HIV must come in contact with a mucous membrane inside the mouth, vagina, penis or rectum, or damaged tissue, or be directly injected into the bloodstream from a needle or similar
- secondly, there needs to be a detectable HIV viral load. If the HIV viral load is controlled on ART, transmission will not occur.

This forms the basis of the HIV treatment paradigm: Undetectable = Untransmissible, or U = U.

Course of infection

Once HIV has gained entry into the body, it infects and destroys cells of the immune system. It specifically infects CD4+ T helper lymphocytes, but also monocytes, macrophages and microglial cells. It uses these cells to replicate, which in turn infect other cells, continuing and maintaining the cycle of life of HIV in the body. The CD4 cell dies two days after it

Box 20.1 Stages of HIV infection (without ART)

1 *Seroconversion* – this occurs in the first few weeks, usually 2–8 weeks after acquisition of HIV. Symptoms include a flu-like illness, fever, lymphadenopathy, aches and tiredness, and can be so mild that they go unnoticed or so severe that hospital admission is necessary. This stage also sees very high levels of HIV, significantly increasing the risk of onward transmission of HIV.

2 *Asymptomatic HIV* – if left untreated after the first stage of seroconversion, asymptomatic HIV infection follows. During this stage persistent generalised lymphadenopathy may also be present.

3 *Symptomatic HIV* – as the immune system continues to weaken, patients can experience recurrence of infections and conditions not necessarily specific to HIV, such as recurrent ear infections, flares/worsening of eczema, diarrhoea, etc., as well as starting to develop opportunistic infections. Constitutional symptoms such as night sweats, weight loss and fatigue may also be experienced.

4 *AIDS* – also known as advanced HIV infection, this stage is when the CD4 count is less than 200 cells/mm^3, giving rise to an increased risk of opportunistic infections and cancers. Definitions do vary; for example, in the USA, AIDS is defined as being diagnosed with HIV and a CD4 count less than 200 cells/mm^3, or an AIDS 'indicator' disease, while in the UK, AIDS is defined as a diagnosis of HIV and having an AIDS indicator disease, irrespective of CD4 count.

has been infected by HIV. The immune system therefore slowly becomes depleted, increasing the risk of infections, as well as cancers.

The course of HIV infection (without ART) has four key stages (Box 20.1).

Anyone at any stage of HIV is considered as having chronic HIV infection when they start ART and continue to take it on an ongoing daily basis.

Opportunistic infections

Opportunistic infections are seen more commonly when the CD4 count is less than 200 cells/mm^3. Many of the causative organisms are the same as those commonly acquired by people with normal immune systems, with asymptomatic or mild primary infections that then lie dormant. Reactivation occurs in the presence of a weakened immune system, as seen in stage 4

HIV infection, albeit with severe presentations. Other organisms that occur in normal immune systems may have a more atypical or severe presentation when seen in people living with HIV (e.g. herpes simplex virus, shingles).

Certain infections are seen below certain CD4 counts. Some of the key opportunistic infections are outlined in Table 20.1. Investigations mentioned are those that are key for diagnosis and tailored according to resources. The management options shown in the table only include an example of typical first-line recommendations. Local and national guidelines should be referred to and specialist physicians consulted.

Management of people living with HIV

Improved access to ART is what has really enabled continued efforts in ensuring that HIV remains a chronic condition that can be successfully managed long term, while also reducing the risk of new infections. The care of people living with treated HIV now focuses primarily on suppression of replication of HIV, restoration of the immune system, and management of the chronic health issues that can be associated with treated HIV infection. While we are seeing a reduction in AIDS-related mortality, deaths due to non-AIDS-related illnesses are on the rise, with a significant number of people living with HIV dying from cardiovascular disease, non-AIDS malignancies and liver disease.

With the introduction of ART to treat HIV infection, there has been a paradigm shift from infections and malignancies to complications associated with ART and immune reconstitution inflammatory syndrome (IRIS). IRIS is a hyperinflammatory reaction to organisms/antigens as the immune system starts to recover after starting ART in a person living with HIV. Toxicities related to ART can vary substantially between different antiretroviral medications, medication classes and individual patient susceptibility.

The aims of ART

The primary aim of ART is the prevention of HIV-associated mortality and morbidity with a low level of drug toxicity (British HIV Association guidelines 2022).

The aims of ART are to:

- reduce the plasma viral load to suppression, namely undetectable (e.g. <50 copies/ml). Viral loads should generally be undetectable by six months
- restore the immune system (CD4 count >500 cells/mm^3). CD4 counts take longer to improve than reductions in plasma HIV viral load, with some never recovering to normal range
- reduce morbidity and mortality from both HIV-related and non-HIV-related conditions
- reduce the risk of transmission to others.

Nowadays, the recommendation is for anyone to start ART regardless of their CD4, viral load and/or stage of infection. Many countries follow the 'test and treat' strategy, whereby ART is initiated for a patient on the same day that HIV infection is identified. Generally, the lower the CD4 count, the quicker ART should be commenced (usually recommended within two weeks of diagnosis) but this needs to be done with caution in the presence of opportunistic infections where there is a risk of IRIS. Two types of IRIS are seen when ART is started (Box 20.2).

Generally, ART is recommended after two weeks of treating opportunistic infections, and after four weeks in those with infections of the central nervous system. Local and national guidelines should be referred to and specialist physicians consulted.

Triple therapy is the norm, with two nucleoside reverse transcriptase inhibitors (NRTIs) and a third agent from another class. Dual therapy is increasingly being used. Local guidelines should be consulted for specific ART regimens.

Adverse effects of currently available ART are not as notorious as they use to be, with experiences naturally

Box 20.2 Types of IRIS

- 'Unmasking' – is when an underlying, undiagnosed infection presents itself.
- 'Paradoxical' – where there is a worsening of a previously treated infection.

Table 20.1 Summary of key opportunistic infections

CD4 count (cells/mm³)	Opportunistic infection	Symptoms and signs	Key investigations	Management
<200	Pneumocystis jirovecii pneumonia	Progressive shortness of breath, dry cough, desaturation on exercise	Chest X-ray, CT thorax, beta D glucan, induced sputum or bronchoscopy	Co-trimoxazole + adjunctive steroids if have low oxygen saturations
	Cryptosporidium	Profuse watery diarrhoea	Stool for MCS, OCP and PCR	Supportive management as well as opiates, octreotide, paromomycin
	Candida	Oral white lesions that can be scraped		Fluconazole
<100	Toxoplasmosis	Headaches, visual symptoms, seizure, low GCS +/- focal neurology	CT or MRI head	Sulfadiazine and pyrimethamine with folinic acid
	Candida oesophagitis	Odynophagia, dysphagia	Endoscopy +/- biopsy	Fluconazole
<50	Cytomegalovirus (CMV) infections	Visual symptoms, encephalitis, pneumonitis, oesophagitis, enteritis	Detectable CMV plasma viral load with evidence of end-organ disease	Valaciclovir/ganciclovir
	Cryptococcal meningitis	Headaches, visual symptoms, seizure, low GCS +/- focal neurology	Serum/CSF cryptococcal antigen, lumbar puncture: India ink/mucicarmine	Liposomal amphotericin B and flucytosine, serial lumbar punctures
	Mycobacterium avium intracellulare	Night sweats, weight loss, malaise, lymphadenopathy, organomegaly, diarrhoea	Blood cultures, tissue biopsy culture	Seek expert input based on local antibiotic sensitivities

CT, computed tomography; GCS, Glasgow Coma Scale; MRI, magnetic resonance imaging; MCS, microscopy, culture and sensitivity; OCP, ova, cysts and parasites; PCR, polymerase chain reaction.

varying from person to person, and given the availability of so many options, ART can be switched to something else if not tolerated.

Adherence with ART is crucial and cannot be stressed enough. Adherence of less than 95% risks:

- viral non-suppression leading to ART resistance with the potential for needing more complex/costly regimens. ART resistance occurs due to HIV having the highest mutation rate seen for any biological entity
- viral non-suppression leading to the risk of HIV transmission
- immunosuppression leading to the risk of opportunistic infections and death.

> ART should never be started, switched or stopped without input from a specialist. Drug interactions should always be checked (www.hiv-druginteractions.org/), including prescribed, over the counter (OTC), supplements, herbal and recreational drugs, and managed with specialist input.

Acute Medicine best practice approach to people with HIV

- The first principle is that of putting patients first (i.e. patient-centred).
- People living with HIV should be involved in deciding their own healthcare (i.e. shared decision making).
- Meeting the health needs of stigmatised and discriminated groups with respect, dignity and compassion.
- Perform thorough history and physical exam in all patients known to be living with HIV.
- Consult HIV and other specialists as needed.
- People living with HIV can present to Acute Medicine services because of the following.
  - Non-HIV-related acute medical issues.
  - Acute seroconversion illness – HIV testing.
    - Many tests are now available for HIV testing, differing not only in how the test is taken but the marker of infection tested (antibody and/or antigen), the speed of the result and accuracy according to 'window periods'.
    - The 'window period' can be defined as the time from the initial HIV infection to when a test can accurately detect the infection. It differs according to the marker of infection used, that is, an antigen or antibody. If someone is tested during the window period for that particular test, they may have a negative test result, but still have HIV, and at a very infectious stage of the course of the infection such as during seroconversion. It is important when testing someone to explain the 'window period' according to the test used, and whether they would therefore have a follow-up test.
    - Regardless of the test used, a HIV-positive result should always be confirmed using a different platform of testing.
  - Opportunistic infections and malignancy associated with untreated HIV infection or disease progression.
  - IRIS occurring after ART initiation (early or late).
  - Complications of ART (i.e. adverse drug reactions).
  - Non-AIDS-related long-term cardiometabolic complications and malignancies.
  - Predisposition to more severe COVID-19 infection as a result of co-morbidities such as obesity, diabetes, cardiovascular disease, a current AIDS-defining illness or a CD4 count less than 200 cells/mm^3.
- Acute Medicine clinicians caring for people with HIV must seek expert advice with any queries related to ART, when patients are critically ill and are admitted to the intensive care unit (ICU).
- Care must be taken to avoid 'drug–drug' interactions in this patient group. Take a comprehensive drug history covering OTC, supplements, herbal and recreational drugs.
- Provide targeted preventive care as needed (including COVID-19 vaccination).
- Refer as needed for common co-morbidities (e.g. sexually transmitted infections including monkeypox, mental health issues).
- Occupational needlestick (percutaneous) injuries and 'splash' contamination (skin, eye, mouth) involving people with HIV (Box 20.3).

Box 20.3 Dealing with needlestick and 'splash' contamination

- First aid.
  - Wash with soapy water.
  - Squeeze to make bleed (don't suck).
  - Irrigate eye.
  - Cover.
- Incident form.
- Current UK law does not permit testing the infection status (i.e. HIV, hepatitis B or C) of an incapacitated patient solely for the benefit of a healthcare worker involved in the patient's care.
- Estimated risk of transmission from HIV infected person following:
  - needlestick injury ~0.3%
  - mucous membrane 'splash' exposure ~0.6%.
- Needlestick – greatest risk of HIV transmission.
  - Hollow needle.
  - Visible blood on needle.
  - Deep penetration of tissue.
  - Patient has high HIV viral load (e.g. acute seroconversion or advanced disease).
- Postexposure prophylaxis (PEP).
  - PEP consists of a combination of three drug ART given after a potential risk (similar to emergency contraception) and according to risk, within 72 hours for 28 days, and has been found to be up to 80% effective.
  - When should it be started? Ideally <1 hour after exposure; in practice, usually 4–6 hours after exposure; sometimes 24 hours after exposure.
  - 5 Day 'starter' packs. Keep packs in readily accessible sites such as intensive care unit, labour ward, emergency department, HIV/infectious disease (ID) ward.
  - Example PEP regimen: tenofovir 245 mg + emtricitabine 200 mg and raltegravir 1200 mg once daily for 4 weeks duration.
  - Follow-up: occupational health; HIV or ID physician – experienced in use of ART; advice regarding contraception; emotional/psychological support; and advice regarding returning to work.
  - Labs performed at baseline (including pregnancy test) and repeated after PEP treatment.
  - Important to retrain regarding safe practice (e.g. handling sharps).

If the person with HIV has an undetectable viral load, PEP may not be recommended.

21

The poisoned patient

Glenn Matfin

KEY POINTS

- Toxicological presentations are broad and heterogeneous and the mainstay of management is supportive.

- Toxidrome thinking may enable early decontamination, antidote administration, enhanced elimination and improved supportive care.

- A proportion of patients, particularly those with low conscious level and refractory shock, will require critical care support, for which there are emerging supportive treatment options.

- Acute Medicine physicians deliver frontline care to toxicology patients and must remain vigilant to changing threats (e.g. novel psychoactive substances, nerve agents) and therapeutic options and protocols (e.g. SNAP 12-hour N-acetylcysteine regimen for treatment of paracetamol overdose).

In the United States, drug overdose is the leading cause of accidental death. More than 100 000 people per year die of drug overdose. Psychoactive drugs, painkillers, cardiovascular (CV) drugs and alcohol are the major agents causing death. However, nearly 7 out of 10 of these overdose deaths are due to *opioids*. The misuse of and abuse (i.e. addiction) of opioids – including prescription pain relievers, heroin and synthetic opioids such as fentanyl – is a serious international crisis. A recent UK study found that 14.6% of people given opioids for the first time became long-term opioid users within a year.

Poisoning is an important public health issue in the UK, with approximately 160 000 presentations occurring annually as a result of poisoning, which may include self-harm, accidental exposures, medication errors and drug misuse. Many more patients are managed in the community. Although the management is largely supportive, a knowledge of the constellation of signs and symptoms that constitute specific poisonings, referred to as *toxidromes*, may enable early empirical decontamination, antidote administration, enhanced elimination and supportive care, and may also predict the clinical course.

Most frontline medical staff would have used Toxbase, the online poisons information database provided by the National Poisons Information Service (NPIS), or contacted a clinical toxicologist through the 24-hour telephone advice service.

Introduction

Accidental and intentional poisoning from over-the-counter, prescribed, illicit and recreational organic substances remains a major cause of morbidity and mortality worldwide.

Clinical toxicology

Clinical toxicology is a rapidly evolving field with new information emerging daily – be it novel psychoactive substances, needle injecting date-rape drugs in

Acute Medicine: Lecture Notes, First Edition. Edited by Glenn Matfin.
© 2023 John Wiley & Sons Ltd. Published 2023 by John Wiley & Sons Ltd.

nightclubs, household chemicals, poisonous plants or bioterrorism agents. For example, paediatric melatonin ingestions reported to US poison control centers increased 530% from 2012 to 2021.

The NPIS therefore invests heavily in maintaining Toxbase as a source of up-to-date, evidence-based information. In addition, a registry of the effects of drug and chemical exposures in pregnancy is provided by the UK Teratology Information Service.

> The branch of medicine that deals with the detection and treatment of poisons is known as Toxicology. Clinical toxicologists specialise in the prevention, evaluation, treatment and monitoring of injury and illness from exposure to drugs and chemicals, as well as biological and radiological agents.

General toxicological definitions

Toxicity

- A toxic agent is anything that can produce an adverse biological effect.
- A toxic substance (i.e. toxicant) is simply a material that has toxic properties.
  - *Toxin*: peptides or proteins produced by living cells or organisms (e.g. plant, microbes, animals). A venom is a toxin injected into another living organism.
  - *Poison*: substance that through its chemical properties usually kills, injures or impairs an organism.
  - Toxins are poisons, but not all poisons are toxins (i.e. not all produced by living cells).
- Toxicity is the degree to which a substance (toxicant) can harm humans.

> Botulinum neurotoxin is the most potent known toxin – it causes botulism.

Time course of toxicity

- *Acute* toxicity – involves harmful effects in an organism through a single or short-term exposure (e.g. radiation, bioterrorism agent, drug misuse (abuse) including overdose).
- *Chronic* toxicity – involves more long-term exposure (includes environmental).

Poisoning

Poisoning occurs when a poison interferes with normal body functions after it is swallowed, inhaled, injected or absorbed.

> 'Toxidrome' is the pattern of symptoms and/or signs (i.e. syndrome) that suggest a specific class of drugs or chemicals causing poisoning. For example, the opioid toxidrome includes the triad of pinpoint pupils, respiratory depression and decreased conscious level.
>
> Other toxidromes include cholinergic, anticholinergic, serotonergic, hallucinogenic and sedative/hypnotic.

Acute poisoning is common and accounts for ~10–15% of hospital attendances in UK. Most admissions are drug or substance (e.g. alcohol)-related poisoning (Box 21.1).

> **Box 21.1 Drug and substance poisoning**
>
> - Drug or substance misuse (use of a drug/substance for a purpose not consistent with legal or medical guidelines, i.e. to alter a person's mood or cognition).
> - Drug or substance abuse (chronic misuse begins impairing specific aspects of life, such as health complications, physical dependence, withdrawal symptoms and 'cravings').
> - Intentional drug overdose (e.g. suicide or parasuicide attempt). Mixed overdoses (+/- alcohol) are common.
> - Non-intentional (or accidental) drug and/or substance overdose.

Poisons *not meant* for human ingestion or other exposure

Include car anti-freeze, battery products or household cleaning products.

Carbon monoxide (CO)

Carbon monoxide is termed a 'silent killer' because it is odourless and colourless.

- Poisoning can occur with incomplete combustion, house fires and vehicular exhaust fumes (intentional or accidental).

- Pathophysiology.
  - CO binds avidly to haemoglobin with >240 times greater affinity than oxygen; high levels lead to tissue hypoxia.
  - Arterial blood gas sampling required; oximetry may appear falsely normal and fail to reveal hypoxia.
  - Measured carboxyhaemoglobin (HbCO) levels >10% abnormal. Levels correlate poorly with severity of exposure, although levels in excess of 30% are generally considered severe.
- Clinical features.
  - Most common symptoms of CO poisoning are headache, dizziness, weakness, upset stomach, vomiting, chest pain and confusion. CO symptoms are often described as 'flu-like'. Pink rosy skin discoloration can occur.
  - Late features can develop over 2–40 days and include delayed neurological symptoms, which often last for a year or longer with symptoms including loss of memory, disorders of movement, low mood, dementia and psychosis.
- Treatment.
  - 100% oxygen. Hyperbaric oxygen may be considered if there are markers of severity, such as HbCO levels greater than 30%, electrocardiogram (ECG) evidence of myocardial infarction or persistent acidosis.
  - Supportive care. Managing patients who have been exposed to fire may be complex and often requires a dedicated multidiscplinary team and a structured ABCDE approach to management. Patients with a hoarse voice, soot in the mouth, facial burns or stridor usually require immediate tracheal intubation as laryngeal oedema tends to progress over the first 24 hours. Peripheral burns may require input from plastic surgery teams.
- Prevention – CO monitors, keep rooms ventilated, service boilers, etc.

Cyanide

Related to medication, occupational exposure/accident (e.g. Bhopal, India) or smoke inhalation during fires (Box 21.2).

Poisons *meant* for humans to ingest or other exposure

- Foods (e.g. poisonous mushrooms, Japanese puffer fish tetrodotoxin is more toxic than cyanide).
- Medicines (e.g. drug overdose).
  - A drug overdose (i.e. when you take more than the normal or recommended drug amount) may

---

Box 21.2 Cyanide exposure

The most common cause of death in *fires* is the inhalation of noxious gases rather than thermal injury. Each fire generates its own particular composition of chemicals depending on the combusting materials.

- It is estimated that 50–75% of fire-related injuries have a component of CO poisoning.
- Co-existent cyanide poisoning is also common. Cyanide poisoning causes tissue hypoxia through inhibition of mitochondrial function. The cardinal feature is the presence of lactic acidosis not explained by any other features of the patient's presentation. Cyanide antidotes all have a significant side-effect profile and data on their efficacy is limited, which may restrict their use to patients most severely affected. Hydroxycobalamin is the safest therapy.

---

result in serious, harmful complications or death.
  - Drugs can either be *prescribed* or *non-prescribed* (e.g. OTC or drug misuse/abuse).
  - If an overdose is taken *on purpose*, it is called an intentional or deliberate overdose; some are associated with suicidal intent or self-harm.
  - If an overdose is taken *accidentally*, it is called an unintentional or accidental overdose.

What are the most common substances implicated in poison exposures?

Poisoning affects *all* age groups, from infants to seniors. For adult poison exposures:
- pain medications lead the list of the most common substances implicated
- sedatives and sleeping medications, antidepressants and CV medications follow
- these exposures are often *intentional*.

General principles of poisoning management

General management

- Check for your own safety. It may be necessary to decontaminate the area or the skin of toxins

---

Box 21.3 Approaches to poisoning

ABCDEFGH *approach*

- **A**irway.
- **B**reathing.
- **C**irculation – cardiac monitoring critical and serial ECGs with particular emphasis on arrhythmias, PR, QRS and QT intervals. Treat prolonged: QRS - IV sodium bicarbonate; QT - IV magnesium.
- **D**isability (conscious level) – Glasgow Coma Scale (GCS) or ACVPU (*A*lert, *C*onfusion, *V*oice, *P*ain, *U*nresponsive); **D**econtamination (if applicable).
- **E**xposure – **E**xamination and **E**valuation; **E**mergency antidote.
- **DEFGH** – '**D**on't **E**ver **F**orget **G**lucose and **H**eroin (opioids)' if comatose.

RRSIDEAD *approach*

- **R**esuscitate – *A*irway, *B*reathing, *C*irculation, *D*etect and correct (seizures, hypoglycaemia, hyper/hypothermia) and *E*mergency antidote.
- **R**isk assessment – agent(s), dose, time since ingestion, clinical features, patient factors. Always consider the *worst-case scenario* when conducting the risk assessment.
- **S**upportive care.
- **I**nvestigations – ECG, paracetamol levels and glucose.
  - ECG: acute coronary syndrome (e.g. cocaine); QT prolongation (e.g. antipsychotic drugs) – risk of torsades de pointes is better described by the absolute rather than corrected QT; QRS prolongation (e.g. sodium channel blockade with phenytoin); bradycardia (e.g. beta-blockers, calcium channel blockers) and tachyarrhythmias.
  - Paracetamol level: required at least four hours after any ingestion, a salicylate level is only advocated if they have taken aspirin, have an unexplained respiratory alkalosis (direct action on the central nervous system) or metabolic acidosis.
  - A pregnancy test is indicated in certain individuals, and a creatine kinase level in those patients with hyperthermia (Hyperthermic toxidromes have worst prognosis) or risk of rhabdomyolysis.
- **D**econtamination.
- **E**nhanced elimination.
- **A**ntidotes.
- **D**isposition.

(e.g. fentanyl), and use appropriate personal protective equipment in the acute phase. Protect yourself and others from needlestick injuries.
- Supportive care – includes eye and mouth care if decreased conscious level, and urinary catheterisation as indicated.
- General approach to poisoning (Box 21.3).

Consider 'Coma Cocktail' if low GCS (<8) or unresponsive on ACVPU scale.

- Dextrose (hypoglycaemia).
- Thiamine (Wernicke encephalopathy).
- Naloxone (opioid antagonist).
- Oxygen (hypoxia including CO poisoning).
- Poisoning is a common cause of coma, especially in younger people, but it is important to exclude other potential causes (e.g. head injuries, trauma or acute neurological events/infections), unless the aetiology is certain.

Identify poison or toxidrome

Identify poison or toxidrome if possible.

- You can consider calling dedicated toxicologists such as the NPIS, to discuss unexplained toxidromes, polypharmacy overdoses or poisoning with uncommon toxins, as well as subsequent possible management strategies.
- Single toxin overdose may be managed with online resources such as Toxbase for which most hospitals have a dedicated login, with in-depth advice. There is also guidance in online resources including the Royal College of Emergency Medicine and the British National Formulary (BNF).

Decontamination

Decontamination is carried out along with diagnosis and supportive therapy.

- Skin – clean with soap and water.
- Gastrointestinal – depending on the nature of the toxicant (Box 21.4).

Elimination

Elimination helps to minimise injury and enhance excretion of presumed toxicant.

- Haemodialysis to enhance elimination of compounds that are already in the circulation (e.g. salicylates). It may also be necessary to use renal replacement therapies due to refractory metabolic disturbances or acute kidney injury.
- ECMO (extracorporeal membrane oxygenation) may also have a role in improving survival in severe states such as refractory hypotension.
- Urine pH manipulation – acidic compounds better excreted in alkaline urine (e.g. salicylates).

Lipid rescue therapy – IV fat emulsion (intralipid) used in life-threatening arrhythmias/cardiac arrest caused by lipid-soluble drugs (especially local anaesthetics).

Antidotes and symptomatic treatment

- Counteract with specific antidotes if available or clinically indicated or toxicant known (Table 21.1).
- Symptomatic treatment as needed (e.g. for hypotension, seizures, arrhythmias).

Refractory hypotension – many medications in overdose are associated with cardiovascular toxicity although severe refractory hypotension is most associated with calcium channel blockers (CCB), beta-blockers and TCAs. Patients may appear surprisingly well until the moment they become unstable, by which point they are often refractory to conventional treatment. This is particularly true for CCB overdose and there should be a low threshold for alerting critical care early. Fluid challenge and calcium is the first-line treatment for CCB toxicity. However, the physiological basis for use of high-dose insulin euglycaemic therapy (HIET) in CCB toxicity is compelling.

- HIET doses of insulin of up to 5–10 units/kg/h (plus dextrose) improve glucose uptake by cardiac myocytes, promoting sarcoplasmic reticulum-associated calcium ATPase activity and enhanced calcium uptake by mitochondria, which serves to improve excitation–contraction coupling and contractility without increasing oxygen demand. Close monitoring, particularly for hypoglycaemia and hypokalaemia, is critical. Aim for systolic blood pressure (SBP) >90mmHg.
- Glucagon is mainstay of treatment for significant beta-blocker overdose (and can be used in CCB).
- Lipid rescue therapy – antidote of last resort in cardiotoxic overdoses of lipophilic agents, which include CCBs, beta-blockers and TCAs.

Psychiatry review

Identifying patients at risk of further attempts at suicide/self-harm. All patients need psychiatry review. Special focus on those with:

- suicidal ideation
- evidence of psychiatric disease
- evidence of addiction (e.g. illicit drugs, alcohol).

Taking a history in poisoning: what, when, how much and why?

- What poison(s) have been taken and how much?
- What time were they taken and by what route?
- Has alcohol or any drug of misuse been taken as well?
- Obtain details from witnesses of the circumstances of the overdose (e.g. family, friends, paramedics), including any trauma, suicide note, pill bottles, needles or other drug use paraphernalia (e.g. syringes and pipes/bongs, or residual evidence of drugs or toxins including empty packets).

Table 21.1 Antidotes or management strategy for common toxicants (see Table 22.2 also)

Toxin	Antidote or management strategy	Mechanism	Notes
Anticoagulants: vitamin K antagonists warfarin	Vitamin K	Reversal of vitamin K antagonist, may take time.	Look at indication for anticoagulation and bleeding to determine treatment
	Prothrombin complex concentrate (PCC)	PCC should correct INR within an hour	
	Fresh frozen plasma		
Direct-acting oral anticoagulants (DOACs): dabigatran rivaroxaban apixaban	Specific DOAC antibodies available		
Beta-blockers	Beta-agonists Glucagon HIET		
Calcium channel blockers	Calcium HIET		
Carboxyhaemoglobin	High-flow oxygen Hyperbaric oxygen		Available on most blood gas results Consider if from older houses/camping/fires
Cyanide	Sodium thiosulfate Hydroxocobalamin Dicobalt edetate		Consider in house fires
Digoxin	Digoxin specific antibody fragments	Antibody binds poisons	May cause yellow vision (Xanthopsia), confusion and arrhythmias
Ethylene glycol/Methanol	Ethanol Fomepizole	Competitive inhibition	High anion gap
Insulin	Dextrose Glucagon		If intramuscular, may consider excision (e.g. myomectomy)
Iron	Desferrioxamine	Chelates iron	May cause GI strictures
Paracetamol	N-acetylcysteine (NAC) Oral glutathione	Deactivation of active metabolite	Levels should be taken at 4 hours or more after ingestion. SNAP 12-hour NAC regimen now preferred (see text)
Tricyclic antidepressants	Sodium bicarbonate	Stabilisation of myocardium and increased excretion	Monitor potassium levels closely and replace

GI, gastrointestinal; HIET, high-dose insulin euglycaemic therapy; INR, international normalised ratio.

- Assess mental capacity to make decisions about accepting or refusing treatment.
- Ask the general practitioner for background and details of prescribed medication and pertinent history (e.g. drug abuse, depression and virus-borne illnesses).
- Establish past medical history, drug history and allergies, social and family history.
- Assess suicide risk (full psychiatric evaluation mandatory when patient has physically recovered).

Identifying toxidrome

The most commonly encountered toxidromes are anticholinergic, cholinergic, opioid, sedative-hypnotic and sympathomimetic (also known as adrenergic or stimulant).

Cholinergic toxidrome

'Wet and weak' or 'wet opioid' (Box 21.5).
   Examples include the following.

- Organophosphate poisoning – insecticide inhalation, skin contact, ingestion; common cause of self-harm.
- Bioterrorism/warfare – nerve agents, e.g. Novichok (UK 2018; Russia 2020 and more contemporary).

Mechanism of action of organophosphate poisoning.

- Acetylcholinesterase inhibitors – prevent breakdown of acetylcholine. High probability of death without treatment.

Management includes the following aspects.

- Decontamination.
- Supportive care.
  - Diazepam for seizures, etc.
  - Atropine: first-line treatment (good for excess secretions). Blocks muscarinic receptors.
  - Pralidoxime: cholinesterase reactivator.

Box 21.5 Cholinergic toxidrome

DUMPSS

Diarrhoea; **U**rination; **M**iosis; **P**aralysis; **S**eizure; **S**ecretion(s).

SLUDGE (muscarinic symptoms)

Salivation; **S**weating; **L**acrimation; **U**rination; **D**iarrhoea; **G**atrointestinal distress/cramping; **E**mesis.

Other toxidromes

- Anticholinergic.
  - Dry mouth, mydriasis, urinary retention, reduced bowel sounds.
  - Examples: TCA, antihistamines.

- Sedative/hypnotic.
  - Depressed conscious level, ataxia, dysarthria.
  - Examples: alcohol, benzodiazepines, GHB (gamma hydroxybutyrate – 'date rape' drug)/ GHL (gamma butyrolactone).
- Sympathomimetic/stimulant.
  - Tachycardia, sweating, anxiety, seizures.
  - Examples: amphetamines, cocaine, legal highs.

Paracetamol overdose

Approximately 100 000 people attend UK emergency departments every year for paracetamol (acetaminophen) overdose, with half (50 000) admitted.

- Approximately 10% have liver transaminase elevation, whilst ~1:1000 develop acute liver failure (ALF).
- Risk factors for ALF include late presentation (antidote should be started within eight hours ideally), malnourishment, chronic alcoholic abuse, enzyme-inducing drugs.

Paracetamol basic facts.

- Therapeutic plasma level ~15 mg/l.
- Toxic plasma level >100 mg/l after four hours if immediate-release formulation; repeat levels at 8–10 hours if extended-release (XR) formulation taken.
- Maximum adult dose: 4 g in 24 hours (although lower doses preferred with chronic alcoholism, enzyme-inducing drugs and severe liver disease).
- Major toxicity: hepatotoxicity at higher doses.
- Overdose common: ~160 000 Toxbase views in the UK/year.

Mechanisms of hepatotoxicity with paracetamol overdose

- Around 95% of paracetamol (acetaminophen) is normally metabolised by sulfonation and glucuronidation to non-toxic metabolites (Figure 21.1).
- Around 5% of paracetamol (acetaminophen) is converted to a toxic metabolite – N-acetyl-p-benzoquinone imine (NAPQI) – by cytochrome P450 enzymes (e.g. CYP2E1, 1A2, 2A6, 3A4).
- NAPQI is usually conjugated and detoxified by endogenous glutathione.
- Glutathione is depleted at higher doses of paracetamol (acetaminophen).
- Excess NAPQI binds covalently to macromolecules in liver cells, resulting in oxidative damage, mitochondrial dysfunction, inflammatory response that propagates hepatocellular injury, and eventually liver necrosis.

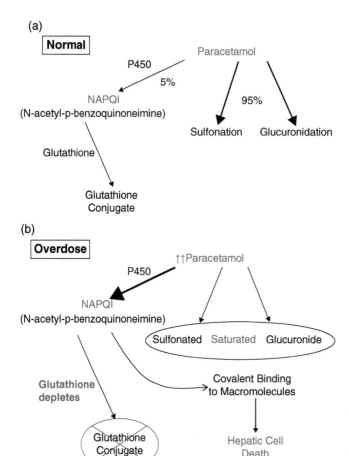

Figure 21.1 (a) Metabolism of paracetamol (acetaminophen) under normal circumstances. (b) Mechanism of action of paracetamol (acetaminophen) overdose damage of the liver.

Clinical features of paracetamol poisoning

Phase I (0–24 hours): nausea and vomiting, but most asymptomatic.

Phase II – Latent stage (~24–48 hours): subclinical increase in transaminases, bilirubin, international normalised ratio (INR) and other biomarkers.

Phase III – Hepatic stage (~3–4 days): liver failure, right upper quadrant pain/discomfort, vomiting, jaundice, coagulopathy, hypoglycaemia, renal failure and metabolic acidosis.

Phase IV – Recovery stage or death (~4 days–3 weeks): resolution of hepatic and multisystem dysfunction or posttransplantation or death.

Management of paracetamol poisoning

It is important to start treatment prior to levels coming back from the lab. Serious paracetamol toxicity is usually associated with ingestion of more than 150 mg/kg in any 24-hour period, although rarely toxicity can occur with ingestions between 75 and 150 mg/kg within any 24-hour period.

Activated charcoal can adsorb paracetamol and is useful as a decontaminant if given within one hour of ingestion. N-acetylcysteine (NAC) is the specific antidote, given IV in the UK typically over 12–21 hours; it can be extended if there is significant liver damage. NAC is a glutathione precursor and repletes glutathione levels, resulting in increased conjugated NAPQI, and prevents cellular damage if given within eight hours of paracetamol overdose.

Bloods should be sent for paracetamol level, blood gas analysis, transaminases, bilirubin, prothrombin

> **Box 21.6 Paracetamol overdose – criteria for specialist liver team referral**
>
> **TAPSHOE:**
>
> **T**hrombocytopenia
>
> **A**cidosis pH <7.3
>
> **P**rolonged prothrombin time – INR >4.5 or >3.0 at 48 hours
>
> **S**ystolic BP <80 mmHg
>
> **H**ypoglycaemia
>
> **O**liguria or creatinine >200 µmol/l
>
> **E**ncephalopathy

time/INR and urea and electrolytes. There is a nomogram available to decide who to treat (only valid for acute overdoses – paracetamol must all be taken within one hour). All patients are now treated as if they are high risk.

Staggered overdoses are when paracetamol is taken multiple times during a timeframe greater than one hour. Historically, it was common practice to treat all staggered overdoses for at least 21 hours pending blood results. It is now agreed that if it is four or more hours since the last paracetamol was ingested, their paracetamol level is <10 mg/l, ALT and renal function are normal, INR less than 1.3, and no clinical features of liver disease (e.g. encepthalopathy), patients can have their NAC discontinued and can be potentially discharged.

If the patient does not satisfy all these criteria (and all other patients with acute, non-staggered overdose) then Toxbase previously recommended treatment with total NAC dose 300 mg/kg given over 21 hours before further risk stratification for liver damage with blood testing for INR, plasma creatinine, venous pH or plasma bicarbonate and ALT. Features suggesting referral to dedicated liver services are shown in Box 21.6.

What's new in paracetamol overdose?

Biomarkers for liver injury

Identifying patients at risk of subsequent liver injury (i.e. risk stratification) at first presentation to hospital is challenging, especially with staggered overdoses (nomogram invalid), late presentations or unknown details (e.g. timing, dose, other drugs).

- Acute liver injury biomarkers – miR-122, HMGB1 and K18 (measured at four hours or later

presentation) have superior sensitivity compared with the current gold standard marker (e.g. ALT >50–100 U/l or doubling at end of initial NAC treatment).

ADRs decreased with modified SNAP regimen

> Adverse drug reactions (ADRs) with 21-hour NAC infusion are common, such as nausea and vomiting (e.g. managed with pretreatment ondansetron) and anaphylactoid reactions (i.e. non-immune-mediated mast cell degranulation – leads to allergic-type reactions – occurs in one-third of patients). Dose dependent to some degree as high doses are given initially then slower infusion.

SNAP regimen.

- Still give same total dose (300 mg/kg NAC) as old regimen but now over 12 hours. IV NAC 100 mg/kg over two hours, then 200 mg/kg over 10 hours. Fewer side-effects and ADRs.
- If adverse effects occur, temporarily stop NAC and can restart at lower dose, consider antiemetic and/or antihistamine. Allows shorter length of stay for most patients based on labs at 10 hours.
- If labs are similar to those noted above for staggered paracetamol overdose and no clinical features of ALF, patients can be considered for discharge (psychiatry review needed).
- If any of the labs are abnormal or suspicious clinical features, a third NAC bag (200 mg/kg) is administered over 10 hours and repeat bloods.
- Can discontinue treatment after third bag (22 hours after commencing NAC) if:
  - INR is 1.3 or less *AND*
  - ALT is less than two times the upper limit of normal *AND*
  - ALT is not more than double the admission measurement.
- If ALL these criteria are not met:
  - continue infusion at same dose and rate
  - discuss with NPIS
  - discuss with liver unit if not already involved.

> SNAP now appears on Toxbase and is the default NAC regimen. It is increasingly being used across the UK and overseas.

22

Alcohol, drugs and substance abuse

Nick Murch

 KEY POINTS

- Alcohol use disorders including intoxication, withdrawal and chronic misuse, are common factors in presentations to healthcare and have huge financial and clinical implications for healthcare providers.
- Drugs of misuse may be bought legally, 'over the counter', prescribed, shared or obtained illegally.
- Newer psychoactive substances may be missold to users as household chemicals. Subtle differences in their structure and potency make them difficult to detect and their effect may therefore be difficult to assess accurately.
- There is an overlap between recreational and toxic effects depending on therapeutic windows and user characteristics. Some effects may be apparent acutely; others may manifest after chronic use.
- Accurate recognition of acute and chronic toxidromes may help healthcare professionals identify how to manage toxic effects. However, the use of multiple drugs is common so they may not be absolute.

Introduction

Acute Medicine is the specialty concerned with the initial assessment, diagnosis and management of adult patients with urgent medical needs, and it would be unlikely to have a full clinical session without at least one patient presenting with the effects of alcohol (by this is meant ethanol unless otherwise indicated) or drug use or toxicity from both prescribed and non-prescribed substances. Use of over-the-counter (OTC), prescribed, illicit or recreational substances remains a major cause of morbidity and mortality worldwide. A knowledge of the constellation of signs and symptoms that constitute specific intoxications, withdrawals and potential overdoses (referred to as *toxidromes*) may enable early correct diagnosis, supportive care, decontamination where appropriate, antidote use, withdrawal regimen and enhanced elimination where indicated.

Paracelsus, a Swiss physician, stated that 'Solely the dose determines that a thing is not a poison'. Therefore, many useful medications are poisonous if they either chronically or acutely accumulate within the body. Reduced excretion of drugs may happen if someone develops worsening renal or hepatic function, or if they have lost weight and are malnourished. Some drugs have a narrow therapeutic window, so it is not difficult for someone to develop problems if pharmacokinetics (i.e. what the body does to the drug) change. It is therefore important to have a certain index of suspicion if a patient has access to these medications.

Drug, alcohol and toxin consumption

Drug, alcohol and toxin consumption, whether acute, chronic or historic, encompasses a broad and heterogeneous group of presentations that may pose several challenges for the treating clinician. There may be cultural influences or social taboos associated with their use. Patients may be unable or unwilling to reveal what they use, and may not consider that, for example, marijuana is a drug. Often patients, friends or relatives can reveal exactly what they have taken, including the regularity, timing, dosage, compound, preparation (such as modified release for prescribed medication), and combination with other drugs such as alcoholic beverage ingestion.

The use of alcohol, drugs or illicit drugs has an intimate connection with mental health and will often have a profound two-way relationship with psychological and psychiatric disorders and well-being. Safeguarding, child safety and protection issues may all be affected by the use of these substances with obvious effect. Alcohol, drug and substance use may lead to criminality, directly, indirectly or by association due to the nature of the chemicals themselves, the cost implications and overall effects on society. The use of drugs and alcohol and the pharmacodynamic effects on the body (sedation, seizures, slowed reflexes, high levels of risk-taking behaviour, etc.) mean that they are a major factor in accidents, especially road traffic accidents.

Alcohol

In the UK, more than one million hospital admissions per year are related to alcohol-related disorders.

Alcohol misuse has gone up in recent years, with a culture shift from drinking in formal establishments such as pubs, bars and nightclubs to increased evidence of drinking at home. This change has happened for a number of reasons, including price discrepancies, increased availability and ease of home delivery, and social isolation associated with the rules and self-perceived risks of the recent pandemic. It is well recognised that self-poured drinks have more generous quantities, so this may often be an underestimate.

Chronic alcohol use may be a complicating factor in those presenting with other medical and surgical problems, with acute withdrawal often precipitated by hospitalisation for other illnesses. A failure to recognise this condition may result in severe disability or even death.

As such, it is important that an accurate alcohol history is taken in all acute assessments. This should include the type and strength, as well as frequency and volume of the alcoholic beverage contained – particular beer types, for example, may commonly range from 3% to 8% alcohol by volume (ABV). The self-reported or documented evidence of issues such as fatty liver, peptic ulcers and other gastro-oesophageal disease, or cirrhosis with or without varices, can help to correctly delineate the clinical picture of the effects on the patient's body (Box 22.1).

Acute alcohol intoxication

Top tip: Ethanol is a clear odourless liquid, therefore patients can only be described as smelling of 'alcoholic beverage'.

It is common for patients to present to the emergency department (ED) with acute alcohol intoxication. It is very important not to discount other conditions, as alcohol can mask clinical pictures and introduce cognitive bias to the minds of the treating healthcare professionals. Trauma, including head injuries, and hypothermia, as well as other drugs and metabolic disorders must be considered amongst other causes if there is a a reduced level of consciousness. Blood ethanol levels can be useful clinically, but the medicolegal implications need to be carefully considered. If there is a reduced level of consciousness, it is important to ensure that the airway and cardiovascular systems are supported appropriately. Hypothermia and rhabdomyolysis can also manifest in these patients and often need to be closely monitored and corrected.

Box 22.1 Potential clinical manifestations of alcohol overuse

Direct toxic effects
- Cardiovascular: dilated cardiomyopathy, hyperlipidaemia (LDL), hypertension
- Gastrointestinal: dyspepsia, gastro-oesophageal reflux disease, peptic ulcer disease
- Haematology: anaemia, thrombocytopenia
- Hepatology: alcoholic liver disease (hepatitis, steatosis, cirrhosis), pancreatitis
- Immunology: immunocompromise
- Malignancy: including breast, head and neck cancers, oesophagus and rectum
- Musculoskeletal: osteoporosis, proximal myopathy
- Neurological: cerebellar syndromes, peripheral neuropathy
- Obstetric: fetal alcohol spectrum disorders, low birthweight, miscarriage, prematurity

Signs of chronic misuse (in order of examination)
- Dermatology: caput medusa, palmar erythema, gynaecomastia, hyperpigmentation, jaundice, spider telangiectasias/naevi, striae from pseudocushing picture and weight gain
- Hands: liver flap, nail changes including clubbing (rare), tremor
- Mouth: gingival inflammation, parotid swelling, stomatitis
- Eyes: jaundice, nystagmus (as part of cerebellar disorder), ophthalmoplegia (perhaps as part of Wernicke–Korsakoff syndrome)
- Abdominal: ascites, liver enlargement/shrunken liver, splenomegaly
- Neurocognitive: encephalopathy
- Neuropsychiatric effects:
  - Absenteeism
  - Anxiety disorders
  - Cognitive impairment
  - Depression/low mood
  - Insomnia/frequent waking
  - Paranoia/psychosis (perhaps as part of Wernicke–Korsakoff syndrome)
  - Relationship and behavioural difficulties

Classic laboratory markers that might provide clues to alcohol use
- Hypomagnesaemia (and other markers including hypocalcaemia, hypokalaemia and hypophosphataemia)
- Raised mean corpuscular volume (MCV) (often 100–110 fl, normal range 80–100 fl)
- Raised gamma-GT and AST/ALT (with ratio often >1 in alcoholic liver disease) – these may be low in advanced cirrhosis when liver is largely non-viable (when synthetic function, such as prothrombin time and albumin, may become deranged)
- Thrombocytopenia

Once the acute episode has been managed, it may be useful to assess for dependence and conduct a brief intervention with screening tools as below. If problematic drinking habits are identified, then an offer of advice may be indicated in the ED (alcohol brief intervention), including:

- highlighting alcohol unit calculations
- government guidance for safe drinking levels – currently 14 units per week for both sexes, spread over three or more days. A unit of alcohol is defined as 10 ml or 8 g of pure alcohol, which equates roughly to the amount of alcohol the average adult can metabolise in an hour.

Follow-up plans should ideally be offered both as an outpatient and in the community to try to ensure either abstinence or reduced problematic drinking habits in the future, with associated health benefits and lower risk levels.

Acute alcohol withdrawal

> In the central nervous system, alcohol promotes the inhibitory gamma-aminobutyric acid (GABA) pathways and reduces the excitatory N-methyl D-aspartic acid (NMDA) system, resulting in the relative relaxing, sedative effects of intoxication.

The regular use of alcohol-containing beverages can, through affecting these pathways, lead to tolerance. The period of time taken to attain this tolerance may depend on factors such as the individual's alcohol and other substance intake, genetic predilection and prior history of dependence. The period of time required, especially in those who have had dependence before, may be as little as 10–14 days.

Risk factors and approximate levels of consumption suggesting relative risk of alcohol dependence/withdrawal are as follows.

- Daily alcohol use or high weekly use.
- Male sex.
- Single marital status.
- Co-dependency or use of other substances.
- Co-existing psychiatric disorders.

If a person with this physical tolerance has an acute reduction in their alcohol consumption, this imbalance in the competing systems from reduced GABA system activity and upregulation of the NMDA system can lead to anxiety and insomnia, and neuronal excitation and reduced seizure threshold respectively. In addition, noradrenaline released during the acute withdrawal period can cause sympathetic overactivity, and dopamine-related neural pathways may be the reason for visual, auditory or tactile hallucinations (often called 'insects under the skin') during this time (Table 22.1).

Delirium tremens (DTs)

Delirium tremens is the most severe form of alcohol withdrawal, manifested by altered mental status (global confusion) and sympathetic overdrive (autonomic hyperactivity), which can progress to cardiovascular collapse.

- DTs occurs in about 5% of patients during withdrawal, usually 2–5 days after alcohol cessation or reduced alcohol intake.
- DTs is fatal in 15–20% of inappropriately managed patients, whilst prophylactic and proactive sedation reduces mortality to 1–5%.
- Symptoms and signs include agitation, fever, hallucinations, confusion and seizures (see Table 22.1).

Wernicke encephalopathy

Wernicke encephalopathy refers to the presence of neurological symptoms caused by biochemical lesions of the central nervous system, after exhaustion of B vitamin reserves, in particular thiamine. It classically presents with the triad of confusion, ataxia and ophthalmoplegia, but only 10% of patients present with all three features. It may develop rapidly or over a number of days. Inappropriately managed, it is the primary (or a contributory) cause of death in up to 20% of patients and results in permanent brain damage (Korsakoff psychosis) in 85% of survivors.

Management of acute alcohol withdrawal

In order to manage the features of acute alcohol withdrawal, a planned, graded withdrawal regimen may be required. This may take the form of a tapering regime of either alcohol itself or medications that can control the physical and cognitive/perceptual features, with the aim of preventing potentially life-threatening episodes such as seizures or DTs.

Table 22.1 Some common features of acute alcohol withdrawal

Autonomic hyperactivity	Cognitive/perceptual	Gastrointestinal
Fevers (usually low-grade)	Anxiety	Alcoholic ketoacidosis
Hypertension	Delirium (may be part of delirium tremens [DTs])	Anorexia
Insomnia	Delusions	Dyspepsia
Seizures	Hallucinations	Nausea
Sweating	Vivid dreams	Vomiting
Tachycardias		
Tremor (may be part of DTs)		

Patients with known alcohol dependence should be warned of the risks of unsupported acute abstinence in the community. Community-based detoxification with medications can be difficult due to the possible presence of alcohol in the home setting, so an organised residential placement is often preferable. An added benefit of these units is that they are often better at addressing the psychosocial and emotional elements of alcohol withdrawal, which are often key to the success with ongoing abstinence. Arranging these residential detoxes can be difficult, as they have long waiting lists, so many patients attend the acute hospital instead. All hospitals should have a dedicated practitioner for drugs and alcohol who can signpost support networks in the community; often these networks and groups are supported by the charity sector.

Not all those admitted with 'withdrawal' require support with specific medications. Those who do usually exhibit the signs and symptoms noted above within 24 hours, with a peak around 30 hours, although DTs can develop later than this. It is key to have a high clinical suspicion of withdrawal.

Medical detoxification regimes aim to reduce the signs and symptoms of withdrawal (Table 22.1), often by masking the effects with drugs active on the GABA pathway. Benzodiazepines are often used for this effect, with common ones used including oxazepam, chlordiazepoxide, diazepam and lorazepam. These drugs may accumulate, causing drowsiness, reduced Glasgow Coma Scale (GCS) or paradoxical agitation. It is important to monitor patients' vital signs, including conscious level and respiratory rate. Concomitant use of other sedatives, including alcohol, is precluded. Benzodiazepine-sparing strategies that are sometimes advocated include clomethiazole (a sedative hypnotic), carbamazepine (an anticonvulsant) and gabapentin (an anticonvulsant used for neuropathic pain), amongst others. Clonidine, an alpha-2-adrenergic agonist, may be helpful as an adjunct to benzodiazepines, to reduce the effects of sympathetic overactivity.

Historically, it was more common to see a fixed reducing dose regime applied to all those with alcohol withdrawal. More recently, self-reported symptom-triggered dose reduction regimes, based on, for example, pharmaceutical requirements for withdrawal in the first 24 hours, can help to decide which reducing regime to follow. Scoring systems used include the Clinical Institute Withdrawal Assessment for Alcohol revised (CIWA-Ar). Symptom-triggered regimes tend to use lower cumulative doses of pharmaceuticals, but can be resource intensive for trained staff in the initial symptom-triggered stage.

Withdrawal seizures can be managed with intravenous (IV) benzodiazepines (such as lorazepam). Phenytoin should be avoided. DTs can be managed with oral or IV benzodiazepines. All patients, especially those who are malnourished, should have IV thiamine considered (such as Pabrinex®, a high-potency vitamin B/C infusion, two pairs three times daily for 3–5 days) with ongoing oral thiamine prescribed.

During the admission, those with established liver disease should have a consultation with local hepatology (or gastroenterology) services. An alcohol liaison nurse should ideally be available to counsel patients and signpost community support.

Alcohol co-dependency

There are a number of tools for review of whether a patient has alcohol-related co-dependency. A common example is CAGE (Box 22.2).

Not all patients with an alcohol misuse disorder will have dependency. Binge drinking affecting normal social and professional participation, regularly losing consciousness or committing socially unacceptable or criminal activity may also be signs of an alcohol-related disorder.

Other recreational drugs (excluding tobacco)

In addition to established recreational drugs, there are a growing number of novel psychoactive substances derived from parent compounds whose chemical structure is manipulated to cause a range of pharmacological effects. They are potent addictive

---

Box 22.2 CAGE questionnaire screening test

Two or more of the following may suggest a need for further tests/tools.

- **C**onsidered cutting down?
- **A**ngry when drinking discussed?
- **G**uilty about amount drunk?
- **E**yeopener required (drink needed first thing in morning)?

Table 22.2 Management strategy for common toxins

Toxin	Potential antidote or management strategy	Notes
Benzodiazepines (e.g. alprazolam, diazepam, lorazepam, temazepam)	Flumazenil	Consider avoiding antidote use in polypharmacy overdose as may uncover seizures
Alkyl nitrates ('poppers') or other drugs causing acute acquired methaemoglobinaemia	Methylene blue High-flow oxygen	Methaemoglobin level available on many blood gas results Consider if has risk factors/taken drugs, e.g. 'poppers' Blood gas often out of keeping with saturations
Nitrous oxide	Vitamin B12	Measured B12 level may be normal due to functional deficiency
Opiates (e.g. buprenorphine, codeine, fentanyl, morphine [heroin], oxycodone, tramadol)	Naloxone	Effect of antidote may be much shorter than toxin so repeats/infusion often needed Caution needed in chronic opiate users (may induce acute pain)

drugs that evade detection by conventional hospital methods. Management of common toxins is outlined in Table 22.2.

Cannabis/marijuana

Cannabis/marijuana is also known as green, hash, herb, Mary Jane, skunk (often more potent) or weed; all these terms may depend on local slang and on preparation/potency.

- Psychoactive drug from a plant native to Central and South Asia. Often not viewed as a drug so need to ask specific question regarding usage.
- Main active agent is THC (tetrahydrocannabinol) but there are many others, including cannabidiol (CHB).
- Often smoked with tobacco (and associated effects) or via a high-temperature water pipe ('bong'), vapourised or ingested.
- May cause relaxation, euphoria, altered states of mind and increased appetite.
- High doses may precipitate anxiety, delusions, hallucinations and paranoia.
- Physical side-effects of long-term use include bullous lung disease, emphysema and risk of pneumothorax.
- May be used medicinally for nausea and analgesia. However, regular smoking can paradoxically cause cannabinoid hyperemesis ('dancing man') syndrome where the patient is agitated, unable to stay still and has chronic bouts of abdominal pain and vomiting, often with multiple admissions/scans. Cessation is advised to prevent recurrence.

Synthetic/novel highs

GBL/GHB

Gamma-butyrolactone (GBL)/gamma-hydroxybutyrate (GHB) – also known as GBH, Geebs and liquid ecstasy.

- Closely related drugs with similar sedative and anaesthetic effects; GBL is converted to GHB in the body after ingestion.
- GHB is synthetic, colourless and odourless so may be used to 'spike' drinks. Has been implicated in criminal activity ('Date rape'). GBL has a strong taste.
- May be sold as paint stripper or odour remover. GHB may be used medically for narcolepsy.
- Usually ingested.
- Narrow therapeutic window so easy to overdose.
- May cause relaxation, euphoria, altered states of mind and increased sexual appetite. May also cause grinding of teeth.
- May cause features of increased sympathomimetic function (hyperpyrexia, hypertension, tachycardias).
- Nose bleeds may be caused by snorting.
- Side-effects of long-term use not understood yet.

Mephedrone

Also known as drone, M-Cat, meow-meow and white magic.

- Synthetic stimulant of amphetamine and cathinone (like khat plant) classes, so effects are similar to those of amphetamines/cocaine/3,4-methylenedioxymethamphetamine (MDMA).

- May be sold as 'bath salts' or 'plant food' as a powder, capsules or tablets. Often taken orally but can be snorted, smoked, taken rectally or injected.
- May cause euphoria, elevated mood and increased sexual appetite.
- May cause confusion and disorientation.
- Mixing with other sedatives may heighten effects and make them more unpredictable.
- Side-effects of long-term use not yet understood.

Spice

Also known as black mamba, fake weed, incense, K2, pot pourri and synthetic cannabis.

- SCRA (synthetic cannabinoid receptor agonist) that is relatively cheap, without odour (so easily hidden), and sometimes perceived as natural.
- Can be difficult to test for, meaning relatively high use in homeless, prison inmates, those on probation, in the military or in sport.
- Often smoked after coating in a herbal mix, but can be vaped, ingested, sprayed and used topically; high affinity binding means it is much more potent than THC in cannabis.
- Effects include agitation, psychosis, anxiety, palpitations, tachyarrhythmias, bradycardias, hyper- or hypotension, seizures, acute kidney injury (related to acute tubular necrosis and interstitial nephritis) and cannabinoid hyperemesis.

Nitrous oxide

Also known as balloons, chargers, hippie crack, laughing gas, nox and whippits.

- Makes user relaxed and giggly but risk of anxiety and paranoia. Can cause headaches, fainting or even loss of consciousness in overdose.
- Widely legally available medically, or in small silver metal whipped cream or beer canisters often seen discarded by the side of the road (Figure 22.1). Often inhaled via balloons.
- Prolonged use may cause a functional B12 deficiency (measured levels may be normal) with associated sensorimotor peripheral neuropathy with demyelination features or subacute combined degeneration of the cord. Diagnosis can be made with history and raised levels of homocysteine and/or methylmalonic acid. Treatment is with intramuscular (IM) vitamin B12 (see Table 22.2).

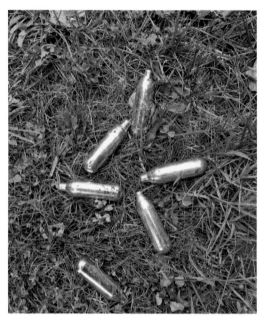

Figure 22.1 'Whippits' discovered by the side of a road.

Chemsex

Chemsex is a term for often intentional, prolonged, sex under the influence of drugs such as crystal methamphetamine, GBL/GHB or mephedrone, among others. Most often, but not exclusively, voluntarily involving more than two male participants, these drugs can lead to diminished inhibitions (including sharing needles, not using condoms or allowing filming) and increased pleasure. However, it may also lead to lack of control and having multiple sexual partners at once, with overdose sometimes causing loss of consciousness. Sensitive history taking may be required; sexual health screens and support should be offered to those individuals who disclose participation, especially if presenting after overdose during chemsex. Sometimes, they cannot recollect all the prior events.

Alkyl nitrates

Also known as amyl, liquid gold, poppers, rock hard, thrust and TNT.

- Inhalation usually for short-term euphoria or during sexual intercourse (can vasodilate, giving a 'high' as well as relaxing the anus and vagina). Sometimes it is more problematic if ingested.

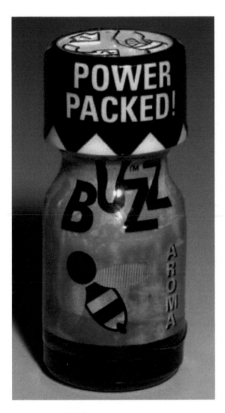

Figure 22.2 Amyl nitrates may come in brightly coloured packaging and be advertised alternatively so it may not be immediately obvious to healthcare providers which chemicals are active.

- May be sold legally for other uses such as deodorisers, leather cleaners or room aromas (Figure 22.2).
- Originally prescribed for angina-type pain, they are called 'poppers' as there was a 'pop' when the original glass vials opened.
- Usage may cause an acute acquired methaemoglobinaemia. This diagnosis can be made with history of use but needs a high clinical suspicion and review of the blood gas. The measured partial pressure of oxygen in arterial blood (PaO_2) is often out of keeping with the peripheral measured oxygen saturations on pulse oximetry (which are low despite high PaO_2). The patient may have a blue-grey cyanotic discolouration, with chocolate brown blood on sampling. Treatment is usually with high-flow oxygen, methylene blue (see Table 22.2).

Stimulants

Stimulants are drugs that result in increased activity in the body so may informally be known as 'uppers'.

Caffeine is a commonly used legal stimulant, but there are many other legal and illegal stimulants available.

> With all these drugs, a concern is hyperthermia, which is a medical emergency. Passive and/or active cooling is indicated, supportive care and benzodiazepines, and in severe cases, discussion with anaesthetics for consideration of paralysis.

Amphetamines

Amphetamines – also known as base, Billy, speed, whizz; and methamphetamine – also known as crank, crystal meth, glass, ice, meth, Tina and Christine.

- Amphetamine-derived drugs are often used to treat conditions such as narcolepsy or attention deficit hyperactivity disorder (ADHD) but are also drugs of misuse.
- Can be used to abate the need for sleep and suppress appetite and are usually snorted.
- Methamphetamine is a highly addictive derivative that is often found in crystal form and is smoked or injected. If injected, there are all the risks associated with IV drug use (IVDU). Its initial euphoric rush is rapidly followed by a crash, such that concomitant use of other drugs may be found.
- Chronic misuse can cause dependence but also physical effects such as severe pruritus, broken teeth ('meth mouth') and cognitive impairment.

MDMA

Also known as E, ecstasy, mandy, MD, mitsubishis, pills, X and XTC.

- MDMA is a psychoactive drug that can cause altered sensations, increased energy, empathy and pleasure.
- Comes as a powder or in pills that often have designs such as emoticons.
- Acute water intoxication and excessive dancing/sweating can cause hyponatraemia and cerebral oedema.
- Can cause hepatic and renal dysfunction.
- Long-term use may cause memory problems, depression or anxiety.

Cocaine

Also known as blow, C, Charlie, ching, coke, crack, freebase, pebbles, rocks, sniff, snow, stones and white.

- A highly addictive derivative of the South American coca plant.
- Usually snorted as a white powder or smoked in the crystallised rock form known as 'crack'.
- May cause increased speed of talking and overt risk taking.
- Signs of cocaine use include excitability, dilated pupils, running nose and nose bleeds or even nasal septal defects, as well as weight loss.
- Cocaine misuse has increased markedly.
- Medical issues that can be encountered with cocaine are outlined in Box 22.3.

Sedatives

Sedatives or depressants are drugs that result in decreased activity in the body, so may be informally known as 'downers'. They generally make individuals feel sleepy, relaxed and calm.

Benzodiazepines

Also known as alprazolam, benzos, blues, diaze, rohypnol, roofies, temazes, Valium®, vallies and Xanax®.

- May be legally prescribed, often for many years, or bought illegally.
- Occasionally, users may have paradoxical agitation which needs to be monitored.

Box 22.3 Medical consequences related to cocaine

Acute medical issues

- Agitation and tachycardias, severe hypertension with evidence of end-organ dysfunction including coronary spasm, acute myocardial infarction, arterial dissection or subarachnoid haemorrhage.
- Acute management can include non-pharmaceutical measures such as placing the patient in a quiet, reassuring environment with additional use of benzodiazepines.
- Evidence of severe end-organ dysfunction or systolic hypertension over 200mmHg may require the use of IV nitrates and avoidance of beta-blockers.

Chronic use

- May cause accelerated cardiovascular disease with premature atherosclerosis as well as depression and low mood.
- Smoking crack may cause chronic lung disease, known as 'crack lung'.

Purity?

For illicit drugs, there may often be purity issues, with drugs supplied illegally being either too pure or adulterated with other ingredients such as talc or levamisole (an antihelminthic drug that is often found alongside cocaine and can cause an antineutrophil cytoplasmic antibody-positive vasculitis, sometimes with involvement of the nasal septum, but often peripheral necrotic-looking black lesions on nose, ears, limbs, etc.). Anticoagulants have been discovered with synthetic cannabinoids. Other contaminants commonly include caffeine, paracetamol, sugars such as glucose and even laxatives. There have been reports of heroin contaminated with anthrax spores from being transported in the hides of infected camels.

Herbal stimulants

Some drugs may be used culturally amongst certain groups. Knowledge of their use can be invaluable when assessing these patients. Betel nut, khat and to a lesser extent coca leaves (used culturally in South America with effects related to cocaine) are relatively common drugs used in more cosmopolitan, urban areas in the UK.

Betel nut is the fruit of the areca palm. It is a stimulant drug which may be chewed with tobacco or other natural materials, and is commonly culturally used in South-East Asia. It is used as an 'energy boost' and can cause dependence. Short-term effects can include anxiety and tachycardias. Longer term effects can include tooth discolouration (orange), gum disease, oral cancer and cardiovascular disease, including hypertension.

Khat is a flowering plant native to East Africa that is chewed to release the alkaloid cathinone, which can cause excitement, suppression of appetite and euphoria. It can have side-effects of constipation and dilated pupils. Short-term effects include tachycardia and hypertension; longer term use can precipitate greenish tooth discolouration, oral ulceration, insomnia and anorexia. Occasional hypomanic episodes have been reported.

- When prescribed for sleep disturbances, they may reduce time to get to sleep but do not generally improve the quality of sleep.

- Ingestion with alcohol has the risk of central nervous system depression.
- Withdrawal may cause reflex agitation and even seizures similar to those of alcohol withdrawal (where benzodiazepines are often the treatment of choice due to their effect on the GABA system receptors). Benzodiazepines are often the mainstay for withdrawal from most other drugs in a healthcare setting. Withdrawal for benzodiazepine users may require prolonged reducing/tapering regimes with extremely high doses compared to those for alcohol.
- They are used in healthcare settings for managing seizures, anxiety, for sedation and mild amnesic effect usual with some procedures.
- Reversal is possible with flumazenil in this setting, but use of the reversal agent in mixed purposeful overdose needs careful consideration as it may be the only thing stopping the patient from having seizures (see Table 22.2).

Z drugs (zolpidem, zopiclone)

- These so-called 'Z' drugs may be used for similar effects on the GABA receptors to those of the benzodiazepines.
- The reversal effect of flumazenil has been reported.
- Management is usually supportive.

Opioids

> **Top tip**: Opiates are generally 'natural' versions derived from the opium poppy, such as heroin, morphine and codeine. Opioids are synthetic and semi-synthetic versions, including oxycodone and methadone. Most opioids are 'controlled drugs'; however, codeine is available over the counter in co-codamol.

- Opioids can be either prescribed or illicit, and if not used for analgesic effect, can be highly addictive.
- They are potent pain relievers and as such are used extensively in healthcare. There is also the opportunity for their use to be abused. These pharmaceutical-grade drugs are also sold illegally alongside those from less formalised and perhaps less rigorously tested manufacturers.
- Morphine may be taken orally, usually as a fast-acting liquid (such as Oramorph®) or slower release (MST, morphine sulfate tablets). Codeine is converted to morphine in the body of those who can metabolise it (approximately 90% of individuals). Heroin (also known as brown, gear, H, horse, skag,

smack) is diamorphine and is often smoked, injected or snorted.
- Methadone is a synthetic opioid agonist that is often used to replace other opioids and in withdrawal, but also occasionally for pain relief. It is usually taken orally (and often under direct observation by the pharmacist) or given in small amounts to last a short duration. It is available to buy illegally, so it is important to determine if the patient is taking other drugs or medications alongside any prescribed.
- Opioids may be in the form of synthetic tablets such as oxycodone or OxyNorm®, which can be highly addictive, or as patches including buprenorphine. Fentanyl is a potent opioid that can also be misused, and is often a contaminant in other drug preparations.
- If a patient who is on opioids presents with reduced GCS, confusion or reduced respiratory rate (including type 2 respiratory failure) then a trial of naloxone may be indicated (see Table 22.2). In sepsis, or other causes of peripheral vasodilation, it is possible to increase the absorption from opioid patches, so it is important to consider a dose reduction or removal of patches (often many may be discovered). The excretion may be reduced in those with liver or kidney dysfunction, so again, this should be reviewed.

> Naloxone is the antidote of choice for all opioids, but has a short half-life so may need to be administered repeatedly, or an infusion considered. If the patient is a long-term user for pain, lower doses of naloxone should be considered to reduce the risk of rebound pain.

Opioid withdrawal

When a patient attends acute healthcare services, they may have the risk of withdrawal from either illicit or prescribed (e.g. methadone) opioids. It is important to try to accurately clarify prescribed doses, as well as the total current use including type, administration, amount, frequency, duration, time of last use and withdrawal symptoms previously. It is important to enquire about other drug and alcohol use as well as blood-borne virus status and immunisation records. Testing for urinary opioids will allow healthcare practitioners to assess if these drugs are in the system.

> Methadone or buprenorphine can be prescribed acutely for opioid withdrawal, in the lowest dose possible, whilst monitoring for toxic effects.

Risks of IV drug misuse

- Drug related.
  - Dependency (with potential risk to relationships, housing and social support networks, as well as necessitating involvement with criminals).
  - Overdose potential.
  - Risk of contaminants causing problems.
- Local trauma related (site dependent).
  - Damage to local structures, e.g. arteries (potential for pseudoaneurysms or obliteration or embolisation peripherally), nerves, skin and muscles.
  - Deep vein thrombosis (with associated risk of infection and embolisation).
  - Local sclerosis secondary to trauma and noxious chemicals (leading to 'poor veins' for future healthcare interactions).
  - Thrombophlebitis.
- Infection related (have a low threshold for imaging with CT angiography, thoracic CT, and echocardiography in people who inject drugs presenting with acute infections).
  - Abscesses.
  - Bacterial endocarditis (often, but not always, right heart valves).
  - Blood-borne viruses and infections including hepatitis B and C viruses, and human immunodeficiency virus (HIV).
  - Cellulitis.
  - Disseminated infections including septic emboli and discitis with bacteraemia.
  - Fungal infections, especially *Candida*.
  - Mycotic aneurysms.
  - Septic thrombophlebitis.

Other drugs of misuse

- LSD (lysergic acid diethylamide) – also known as acid, Lucy, rainbows and trips. Usually sold as a liquid on blotter paper or as a liquid or pellet. It causes the user to feel energised and excited with strange sensations and feelings towards colours, sounds and objects. Users have been known to self-harm due to these effects. Tolerance is commonly reported, with the need for higher doses.
- Ketamine – also known as donkey dust, green, K, ket, special K and vitamin K. A powder that is usually snorted and similar in appearance to cocaine that leads to feelings of detachment and being chilled out. Ketamine occasionally comes as a liquid and is sometimes injected IM. It has an anaesthetic effect, meaning it is possible to harm oneself whilst under the influence of the drug, and also the reason why it is sometimes used by healthcare staff in medical emergencies. Chronic use may cause bladder problems, including haemorrhagic cystitis, abdominal pain and liver dysfunction.
- Magic mushrooms – also known as liberties, liberty caps, magics, mushies and shrooms. Ingested either fresh or dried. It is well reported that poisonous mushrooms can be ingested by accident, and a high level of clinical concern is needed. Magic mushrooms cause the user to feel relaxed and chatty, but can also cause anxiety and nausea. They augment the current emotional state. Tolerance can become an issue, so higher numbers are needed.
- Intravenous cyclizine can cause a short-term buzz so be careful if patients actively request this or have self-reported 'allergies' to all other antiemetics without proper evidence.
- There are multiple other drugs that are misused, for which it is not possible to create an exhaustive list. Almost any medication can be misused, including thyroxine for weight loss, gabapentin and derivatives for relaxation or euphoria, or to enhance the effects of other drugs. It is not uncommon for patients to admit to taking medications purchased off the internet or social media, especially for weight loss. These may have unknown contents, potency, effects and legality.

Special circumstances

Body packers

Body packers are individuals who either voluntarily or under coercion swallow or insert drug-filled packages in order to transport them across secured borders in a covert fashion. Common drugs implicated include cocaine and heroin. Body packers may attend healthcare services in custody if detained, or voluntarily if they have medical complications such as intestinal obstruction or suspected leakage. The latter will often cause a fatal overdose. Careful history taking and examination as well as imaging may be useful to ensure their well-being (Figure 22.3). Active interventions including laxatives, manual evacuation, retrieval or surgical intervention need to be carefully considered as rupture may be lethal.

(a) (b)

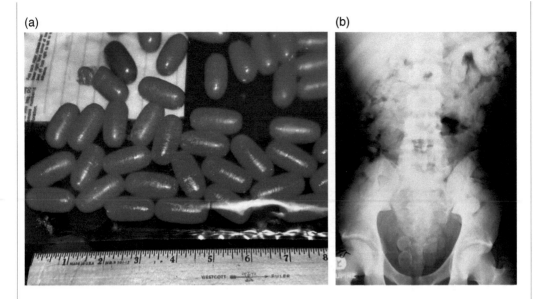

Figure 22.3 A 31-year-old man was admitted with a one-day history of dull intermittent abdominal pain. Most body packers or 'mules' are asymptomatic and management is focused on the passage of drug-filled packages. (a) In this case, each latex packet contained 10 grams of cocaine. (b) Plain abdominal X-ray showed multiple spherical latex packages.

Gym drugs/weight loss including diuretics

Drug use and misuse are increasingly common in sports teams and gyms. It is important to ask about use of drugs including anabolic steroids, growth hormone, insulin, appetite suppressants and fat strippers (such as ephedrine or high-dose caffeine), and diuretics, particularly prior to body-building competitions ('stripping', which can cause dehydration and acute kidney injury).

Generic management of patient where toxins suspected but unproven

Examination of patients with drug misuse

- *General*: evidence of drug paraphernalia including needles, syringes and pipes/bongs, or residual evidence of drugs or toxins including empty packaging. If the patient has purposely ingested drugs for trafficking, they may exhibit signs of undue stress or even leakage. This needs careful evaluation. Check the patient's skin for noxious substances, injection sites/blebs and any patches that may need removal. Hyperthermia ominous sign.
- *Hands*: there may be traces of drugs themselves or tar scarring, or the stigmata of liver disease. It is also important to note if there is evidence of Dupuytren contracture. There may be evidence of stigmata of infective endocarditis in IVDU. Cyanosis despite oxygen therapy may suggest methaemoglobinaemia (with precipitants such as alkyl nitrates).
- *Ophthalmic*: check conjunctivae for jaundice, Roth spots for endocarditis and pupillary response (see toxidrome chart, Table 22.3).
- *Respiratory*: measure respiratory rate (see Table 22.3). There may be evidence of emphysema from tobacco or marijuana use, vaping or shisha damaged lungs, crack lung or other pathology.
- *Cardiovascular*: pulse and blood pressure: (see Table 22.3). Listen carefully for murmurs. Inspect groins and other potential injection sites for possible areas of infection, track marks, sinuses or possibly infected pseudoaneurysms. Patients with history of IVDU may be very possessive of their vasculature and often know which veins are best for taking bloods.

Table 22.3 Potential common toxidromes

Toxidrome and example causative agents	Signs and symptoms of toxicity				Possible antidotes available
	Neuro	Observations	Pupils	Other features	
Sympathomimetic *Amphetamines, caffeine, cocaine, MDMA (ecstasy), mephedrone, theophylline*	Agitation Paranoia Seizures	Increased temp Increased HR Increased BP	Large	Piloerection Sweating Hyperactive bowel sounds	Alpha then beta blockage
Serotonin syndrome *SSRIs, synthetic cannabinoids, Tricyclic antidepressants*	Hunter's criteria including: clonus, agitation, diaphoresis, tremor, hyperreflexia, hypertonia	Increased temp Increased HR Increased BP	Large	Fast onset (<24 hours) Loose stool	Cyproheptadine (Serotonin antagonist)
Anticholinergics *Antihistamines, Parkinson medications*	Agitation Paranoia Seizures	Increased temp Increased HR Increased BP	Large	Dry skin Reduced bowel sounds Urinary retention	Physostigmine
Psychedelic/dissociative *Ketamine, LSD*	Hallucinations Synaesthesia	Increased HR Increased BP	Large		None
Cannabinoid *Cannabis, synthetic cannabinoids*	Agitation Paranoia Seizures	Increased HR	Varies	Red eyes Dystonia Coagulopathy	None
Sedative-hypnotic *Benzodiazepines, GHB/GBL*	Sedation Ataxia Confusion	Reduced RR Reduced HR Reduced BP	Varies	Dry skin	Flumazenil Naloxone may have some effect on GHB/GBL
Opioid *Buprenorphine, codeine, fentanyl, morphine (heroin), oxycodone, tramadol*	Depressed conscious level	Reduced RR Reduced HR Reduced BP Reduced temp	Small	Constipation Pulmonary oedema (rare)	Naloxone (may need repeat doses/infusion). Caution in chronic use
Cholinergic *Mushrooms*	Confusion Weakness Fasciculations Seizures	Variable BP	Small	Salivation Lacrimation Urination Diarrhoea GI discomfort Emesis	Atropine Pralidoxime

BP, blood pressure; HR, heart rate; GI, gastrointestinal; RR, respiratory rate; SSRI, selective serotonin reuptake inhibitor.

- *Neurological*: examination including GCS may identify potential causes (see Table 22.3). Monitor for seizures, postictal states, subacute combined demyelination of the spinal cord, neuropathies, neuropsychiatric disorders including Wernicke–Korsakoff syndrome as well as acute withdrawal or intoxication.

Laboratory tests

Drug screening and drug levels are often not rapidly available and are often unhelpful in the acute situation. This means that clinical acumen and the recognition of toxidromes are key (see Table 22.3). There is currently a lack of readily available or reliable assays for many drugs, especially the newer synthetic compounds. In the Emergency and Acute Medicine departments, there will often be a carboxyhaemoglobin and methaemoglobin level (percentage) generated on the blood gas machine results. Urinalysis toxin screens or serum levels of some drugs such as benzodiazepines or opioids may be available, but often not until after the initial acute phase.

Liaison with local or national toxicology experts (such as the NPIS) can help to target acute management and appropriate investigation.

Generic care of those with drug use

- Monitoring ABCDE – closely for a defined period of time, often designated by Toxbase, with serial blood gases, cardiac monitoring and serial electrocardiograms (ECGs) with emphasis on arrhythmias and ECG morphology.
- Gastric lavage/activated charcoal – via nasogastric tube if indicated.
- Eye and mouth care if unconscious.
- Intubation and ventilation for patients for a period of time whilst effects of an (un)identified toxin wear off.
- Urinary catheterisation – if the patient has reduced GCS or urinary retention.
- It may be appropriate to consider psychosocial aspects and offer psychiatric assessment once medically optimised.
- Further investigations may include the following: a capillary blood glucose and urea and electrolytes; a pregnancy test is indicated in those of childbearing age, and a creatine kinase level in those patients with hyperthermia or risk of rhabdomyolysis.

Malnutrition in those with drug or alcohol misuse

It is not uncommon for alcohol and drug users to either forget to eat or replace their meals with the 'empty calories' associated with alcoholic beverages. Money may be spent on alcohol or drugs rather than nutritious meals. Social dynamics and withdrawal from family and community networks mean that malnutrition is relatively common even in those with a normal, or raised, body mass index (BMI). The combination of chronic disease, including pancreatitis, gastro-oesophageal disease and poor diet means a high index of suspicion, monitoring and prophylaxis may be required.

B vitamins

- Thiamine (vitamin B1) deficiency may manifest as an acute decompensation in the form of Wernicke syndrome, a triad of ophthalmoplegia, ataxia and confusion. It is usually a clinical diagnosis, but blood for either thiamine level or red cell ketolase may be useful. Chronic deficiencies may present rarely as beri-beri (the 'wet' form causing cardiac failure, the 'dry' form presenting with confusion and a painful peripheral neuropathy). Treatment (and also prophylaxis) is with IV thiamine (usually in the form of Pabrinex, a high-potency vitamin infusion – ascorbic acid, pyridoxine, nicotinamide, thiamine, riboflavin and glucose; two pairs three times a day for 3–5 days) with ongoing dietary advice, oral thiamine and consideration of a multivitamin.
- Vitamin B12 may need assessment and replacement IM if there is evidence of neuropathy, including subacute combined degeneration of the spinal cord or a megaloblastic anaemia (MCV usually >110 fl; normal range 80–100). Measured blood levels may be low, or at the lower end of normal in functional deficiency.
- Other oral vitamin B supplements, such as vitamin B co-strong, are not routinely indicated.

Vitamin C

- Scurvy, or deficiency of vitamin C, may manifest with lethargy, oedema, spontaneous bleeding especially from the gums, corkscrew hairs and painful limbs.

- It is usually a clinical diagnosis, but blood levels (often delayed) may be useful.
- Treatment is with intravenous vitamin C (often in the form of Pabrinex) with subsequent dietary advice and oral supplementation.

Folate

- Folate levels may need assessment and replacement orally if there is a megaloblastic anaemia (MCV usually >110 fl; normal range 80–100). If required, ensure B12 is replaced, before replacement with folic acid if needed, as this can precipitate subacute degeneration of the cord.
- Measured blood levels may be low or at the lower end of normal in functional deficiency.

Iron

- Poor oral intake, reduced uptake due to chronic inflammation or upregulation of hepcidin (which can block intestinal absorption and macrophage recycling of iron) as well as increased blood loss may cause iron deficiency.
- If there is evidence of high hepcidin, and evidence that oral iron may not be absorbed adequately, then IV iron may be indicated (note risk of persistent hypophosphataemia). Need to exclude B12/folate

deficiency first. Oral iron may be tolerated and effective in some cases.

- Investigation of potentially co-existing conditions such as coeliac disease and gastrointestinal bleeding may need addressing.

Other trace elements/vitamins

- *Calcium* – may be low and drop lower in refeeding syndrome. Consider checking calcium, vitamin D and magnesium levels and replacing if appropriate.
- *Copper* – can present with neurological disorders, such as myelopathy, optic neuropathy or peripheral neuropathy, as well as anaemia. Measuring serum levels and replacement may be indicated.
- *Magnesium* – may be low and drop lower in refeeding syndrome. Low levels can cause refractory hypocalcaemia.
- *Phosphate* – hypophosphataemia is common in those with alcohol withdrawal and can be exacerbated by refeeding syndrome, so checking levels and replacement may be indicated.
- *Vitamin D* – excessive alcohol intake is often associated with deficiency, even in those with normal liver function. This may be partially due to reduced dietary and environmental (sunlight) exposure. Vitamins A, D, E and K are fat soluble, therefore uptake may be reduced in those with pancreatic exocrine dysfunction.

23

People with diabetes and other hormonal disorders

Glenn Matfin

 KEY POINTS

- Diabetes and stress hyperglycaemia are common in the inpatient setting and are associated with increased risk of complications and mortality.
- Most people with diabetes are admitted for a reason other than diabetes. Less than 10% require admission for a diabetes-specific cause.
- The most common reasons for diabetes-specific admissions are foot ulceration, hypoglycaemia, hyperglycaemia, diabetic ketoacidosis and hyperosmolar hyperglycaemic state. Other reasons for admissions to hospital in the diabetes population include newly diagnosed diabetes (especially during the COVID-19 pandemic), cardiovascular disease including acute coronary syndromes and stroke, and end-of-life care (e.g. endstage renal disease).
- For a variety of reasons, achieving good glycaemic control during hospitalisation presents a significant challenge. Effective education of Acute Medicine healthcare providers is key.
- Patients rarely present to Acute Medicine with endocrine and metabolic disease in isolation. Rather, hormonal disorders occur in combination with other conditions such as critical illness, frailty or cancer, which directly or through their treatments precipitate endocrine disease or elicit physiological responses that alter hormonal pathways.
- Hospitalised patients are also increasingly complex, with high-acuity presentations. This setting is rife with stress-related hormonal responses and is rarely appropriate for the methodical evaluation of endocrine and metabolic conditions.
- Consequently, in the acute care setting, the emphasis has shifted to acute management of endocrine and metabolic emergencies such as hypoglycaemia and hyperglycaemia, hyponatraemia, hypocalcaemia and hypercalcaemia, adrenal insufficiency and thyroid storm.

Acute Medicine: Lecture Notes, First Edition. Edited by Glenn Matfin.
© 2023 John Wiley & Sons Ltd. Published 2023 by John Wiley & Sons Ltd.

Introduction

> Endocrine and metabolic conditions such as obesity, diabetes mellitus and thyroid disorders are everyday medical problems managed in the Acute Medicine setting.

The number of inpatients with diabetes in the UK continues to grow. Hyperglycaemia in this setting is associated with increased risk of complications and mortality.

The most recent UK National Diabetes Inpatient Audit (NaDIA) revealed the following.

- Almost one-fifth of hospital beds were occupied by people with diabetes; in many hospitals it already exceeds 30%.
- In addition, other patients may develop transient hyperglycaemia detected during admission that normalises after discharge, so-called 'stress hyperglycaemia'.
- Taken together, the number of people in hospital with either diabetes or transient hyperglycaemia is large, with a prevalence of 32–38% on general wards and 28–80% of patients with critical illness or undergoing cardiac surgery.

For a variety of reasons, achieving good glycaemic control during hospitalisation presents a significant challenge. Reasons include changes in the patient's daily routine, the size and timing of their meals, reduction in carbohydrate intake from emesis or interruption of enteral feeding, periods of fasting for procedures, the effect of stress associated with illness and/or surgery, and alteration in insulin sensitivity due to use of new medications such as steroids. Since over 90% of patients with diabetes are admitted for reasons unrelated to diabetes (e.g. pneumonia or heart failure), they will be cared for by non-diabetes specialist staff who may not be familiar with insulin dose adjustment or proper prescribing, the need to tailor diabetes medications during illness (e.g. reviewing the risk of continuing metformin with worsening renal function or during contrast procedures), and the effective management of hypoglycaemia and hyperglycaemia.

Added to this, new classes of diabetes medications, new combinations of existing medications and biosimilar and concentrated insulins with new names have made diabetes management more complex, presenting a significant challenge for specialist and non-specialist alike (e.g. almost 40% of drug charts in NaDIA for insulin-treated inpatients had one or more insulin medication errors).

However, patients rarely present to Acute Medicine with endocrine and metabolic disease in isolation. Rather, hormonal disorders occur in combination with other conditions such as critical illness, frailty or cancer, which directly or through their treatments precipitate endocrine disease or elicit physiological responses that alter hormonal pathways. This setting is rife with stress-related hormonal responses and is rarely appropriate for the methodical evaluation of endocrine and metabolic conditions. Consequently, in the hospital setting, the emphasis has shifted to acute management of endocrine and metabolic emergencies such as hypoglycaemia and hyperglycaemia, hyponatraemia, hypocalcaemia and hypercalcaemia, adrenal insufficiency and thyroid storm.

Effective education of Acute Medicine healthcare providers is key. For example, many patients presenting to the acute care setting with severely abnormal values, such as very high levels of glucose, low sodium, low plasma osmolality and high blood pressure, are corrected back to 'normal' as quickly as possible. This practice can lead to increased morbidity and mortality depending on whether adaptive changes have occurred, such as the complication of osmotic demyelination syndrome (ODS) occurring with overrapid correction of chronic hyponatraemia. Preventing overrapid and overcorrection can lead to improvements in patient outcomes.

Basic clinical endocrinology

Disturbances of endocrine function usually can be divided into two categories – *hypofunction* and *hyperfunction*. Endocrine disorders in general can be divided into *primary* and *secondary*.

- *Primary defects* of endocrine function – originate in the target gland responsible for producing the hormone. For example, total thyroidectomy produces a *primary* deficiency of thyroid hormones.
- *Secondary disorders* of endocrine function – the target gland is essentially normal, but its function is altered by deficient or excessive levels of stimulating hormones or releasing factors from the hypothalamic-pituitary system. For example, removal or destruction of the pituitary gland eliminates adrenocorticotropic hormone (ACTH) stimulation of the adrenal cortex and brings about a *secondary* deficiency in cortisol (major glucocorticoid – also known as corticosteroid or 'steroid').

Basic endocrine evaluation

Endocrine function can be assessed:

- *directly* by measuring specific hormone levels
- *indirectly* by assessing the effects that a hormone has on the body; for example, assessment of insulin function through measuring blood glucose (BG) levels.

Endocrine dynamic stimulation and suppression tests are widely used in the ambulatory setting but have a limited role in the inpatient setting (Box 23.1).

Laboratory considerations

The clinical laboratory has an integral role in the management of patients with acute and critical illness. This group of patients has diverse presentations, multiorgan dysfunction is frequent and some of the life-threatening pathophysiological disruptions may be occult. The laboratory is necessary to detect many of these conditions and is essential for both monitoring responses to treatment and detecting or avoiding deleterious consequences of therapy, such as hypoglycaemia and hypokalaemia due to insulin treatment for diabetic ketoacidosis (DKA).

Many factors combine to increase the complexity of endocrine and metabolic testing in the acute and critically ill patient, not only in terms of laboratory service provision but particularly in the interpretation of results. Critically ill patients are prone to metabolic derangements and alterations to endocrine systems that are unique. Several factors contribute to these changes.

- The stress of acute illness may augment (e.g. HPA) or attenuate (e.g. hypothalamic-pituitary-gonadal) the activity of hormone axes.
- In addition to changes in hormone secretion, hormone metabolism and clearance can be altered by reduced circulation and renal function, hypoxia or other insults.
- The normal diurnal variation that occurs with a number of hormones is also disrupted.
- Acute and critically ill patients usually receive numerous therapeutic agents, some of which may alter endocrine homeostasis.
- During acute and critical illness, the amount of hormonal binding protein(s) may change considerably, and the direction of the change (increase or decrease) is dependent on the underlying condition(s). In addition, the amount of binding of hormone to carrier protein (e.g. thyroid hormones or cortisol) can be affected by numerous factors.
- The sensitivity of target tissues to hormones may be modified by changes in the binding capacity and the affinity of cellular hormone receptors. For these reasons, measured hormone concentrations that are obtained during illness may not correlate well with cellular hormone activity.
- The use of reference intervals derived from healthy populations is often inappropriate for interpreting hormone results during illness.
- Dynamic function tests in the critically ill patient may be contraindicated and in practice, other than the short ACTH stimulation test, are rarely performed in this setting.

Point-of-care testing

Measuring patient samples at the bedside, termed point-of-care (POC) testing, is usually performed using blood or urine samples and is of value in certain circumstances, such as BG and serum ketone measurements for diagnosing and monitoring response to DKA management. POC testing provides rapid results and can be used in the Acute Medicine inpatient, ambulatory and home settings (i.e. Hospital at Home), but the compromise is often considerably reduced accuracy.

Hypothalamic-pituitary disorders

> Common symptoms and signs to consider in a patient with suspected pituitary disease include those related to pituitary hormone excess, hormone deficiency and/or local complications (e.g. headaches, visual field defects and diplopia, acute pituitary infarction/enlargement due to pituitary apoplexy).

Because of its complex control mechanisms over vital hormonal functions, and its strategic location at the base of the brain, endocrine and metabolic emergencies related to the pituitary are important clinical problems, and are regularly encountered. The pituitary gland can be affected by tumours (primary and metastatic); trauma to the head; haemorrhage, vasospasm and vascular insufficiency; infection; inflammatory and autoimmune processes; the influence of drugs, and surgical and radiation therapy.

> The Acute Medicine clinician should keep in mind the many functions of the pituitary, and the effects on the patient when the 'master gland' malfunctions or is injured. A thorough differential diagnosis and the appropriate gathering of information from laboratory testing and imaging can be life-saving and remain a challenge in effective patient care.

Hypothalamic-pituitary investigations

Unless the endocrine condition is felt to be relevant to the acute medical presentation, many of the laboratory tests related to the hypothalamic-pituitary axis should be deferred to the non-acute ambulatory setting (Box 23.2).

Cortisol deficiency

> - Morning (or random) serum cortisol levels exceeding 400–450 nmol/l assure sufficient adrenocortical function (although stress hormone levels in acute and critical illness should be higher).

Box 23.2 Basic hypothalamic-pituitary-target hormone evaluation

Identify hormone excess
- Measure fasting (preferred) serum prolactin. If there are obvious clinical features or suspicion, investigate for specific condition (e.g. acromegaly, Cushing syndrome).

Identify hormone deficiency
- Measure baseline (8 am) levels.
  - Anterior pituitary hormones: serum cortisol (± ACTH); free thyroxine (FT4), thyroid-stimulating hormone (TSH); testosterone (male), oestradiol (female), luteinising hormone (LH), follicle-stimulating hormone (FSH); insulin-like growth factor-1 (IGF-1); prolactin.
  - Posterior pituitary hormones to exclude central diabetes insipidus (DI): 24-hour urine volume or timed urine output; urine and plasma osmolality; urea and electrolytes. Measuring antidiuretic hormone (ADH) levels is of *no value* in this setting.

Establish the anatomy and diagnosis
- Image the pituitary and hypothalamus by magnetic resonance imaging (MRI, preferred) or computed tomography (CT). CT examinations can be particularly helpful in demonstrating bony erosions, sellar calcifications or acute intrasellar haemorrhage.
- Consider visual field (VF) testing. Classic VF defect with suprasellar enlargement is bitemporal hemianopia.

> • If morning cortisol is <150 nmol/l, patient should be referred urgently to endocrinology and started on glucocorticoids (steroids).

In the acute care setting, morning serum cortisol levels below 200 nmol/l or random <100 nmol/l make adrenal insufficiency possible (context dependent). The serum cortisol cut-offs described are designed to ensure patient safety and err on initiating hydrocortisone therapy if there is any possibility of cortisol deficiency (e.g. patient with pituitary macrolesion, i.e. ≥10 mm). Referral to endocrinology services is advised in all cases.

> Intermediate cortisol levels that are considered non-diagnostic (as well as those that need additional confirmatory testing) require a short ACTH stimulation test. This investigation directly evaluates adrenocortical responsiveness and is quite accurate in the diagnosis of *primary* adrenal insufficiency. However, the diagnostic accuracy of this test in patients with *secondary* hypoadrenalism of *recent onset* is lower, as it takes 4–6 weeks or longer after endogenous corticotropin (i.e. ACTH) secretion is blunted for the adrenals to become atrophic and lose responsiveness to exogenous ACTH stimulation.

Hypopituitarism

> Hypopituitarism is deficiency in pituitary hormone secretion. It can either be complete (panhypopituitarism) or partial deficiency and includes:
> • central (or secondary) hypoadrenalism (i.e. ACTH deficiency)
> • central (or secondary) hypothyroidism (i.e. TSH deficiency)
> • central (or secondary) hypogonadism (i.e. FSH/LH deficiency)
> • growth hormone (GH) deficiency (i.e. GH and IGF-1 deficiency)
> • central (or neurogenic) DI (i.e. ADH deficiency).

Hypopituitarism may be caused by a variety of conditions that either reduce or destroy secretory function of the pituitary and/or interfere with the hypothalamic secretion of pituitary-releasing hormones.

• Enlarging pituitary tumours and pituitary tumour apoplexy. Pituitary adenomas are the most common cause of hypopituitarism in adult patients.
• Radiation therapy to the sella is associated with a lifelong risk of anterior hypopituitarism that becomes more prevalent over time, affecting ~60% at 10 years after therapy.
• Following head trauma due to damage to the pituitary stalk and the blood supply of the pituitary. It has been estimated that ~25% of patients with traumatic brain injury (TBI) severe enough to require hospitalisation develop one or more pituitary hormone deficiencies.
• During or after pregnancy from Sheehan syndrome (infarction of the normal hypertrophied pituitary following a major obstetric bleed).
• As a result of metastatic cancers involving the pituitary gland, its infundibulum or the hypothalamus.
• Other primary inflammatory and infectious processes can also result in the abrupt onset of hypopituitarism. These include lymphocytic and other forms of hypophysitis (e.g. due to immune checkpoint inhibitor treatment of cancer, or post pregnancy) and granulomatous disease (e.g. sarcoidosis or tuberculosis).

> Immune checkpoint inhibitors (ICIs) have gained a revolutionary role in management of many advanced malignancies. However, immune-related endocrine events (irEEs) have been associated with their use in around 10% of patients and often have non-specific clinical presentations and variable timelines, making their early diagnosis challenging.
> • Patients with ICI-related hypophysitis usually present with multiple anterior pituitary hormone deficiencies, including central hypoadrenalism and/or central hypothyroidism. In the acute setting, *primary* (e.g. caused by adrenalitis) and *secondary* (e.g. caused by hypophysitis) cortisol deficiency are treated identically.
> • Thyroid-related adverse events – overall incidence of hyperthyroidism has been reported as 3% and hypothyroidism 8%.
> • ICI-related diabetes mellitus appears to result in complete permanent destruction of insulin secretory capacity (i.e. beta-cell failure) and a need for long-term insulin and is characterised by:
>   ○ rapid onset of hyperglycaemia
>   ○ swift progression of endogenous insulin deficiency
>   ○ high risk of DKA if not detected and treated promptly with insulin therapy.

Investigation of acutely ill patient with suspected hypopituitarism

> Anterior pituitary hormone loss due to destructive pituitary tumors or radiotherapy may take many years to lead to hypopituitarism.
> - The stereotypical sequence of loss of pituitary hormones can be remembered by the mnemonic 'Go Look For The Adenoma' for GH (GH secretion typically first to be lost), followed by LH (results in sex hormone deficiency), FSH (can cause subfertility or infertility), TSH (leads to secondary hypothyroidism) and ACTH (usually the last to become deficient, results in secondary adrenal insufficiency).
> - The sequence of hormone loss with TBI, ICIs or pituitary apoplexy can occur in any order and combination of deficiencies.

- When considering the diagnosis of hypopituitarism, it is essential to measure both *pituitary* and *target organ* hormone levels for investigation of central hypoadrenalism (e.g. ACTH plus cortisol) and central hypothyroidism (e.g. TSH plus FT4).
- Pituitary imaging is recommended in all patients with biochemical evidence of hypopituitarism in order to identify the underlying cause (such as pituitary adenoma, craniopharyngioma, hypophysitis and others).

Emergency treatment of hypopituitarism

> Potentially life-threatening manifestations of hypopituitarism include central hypoadrenalism, central DI or, rarely, central hypothyroidism (i.e. myxoedema coma). In contrast, gonadotropin (LH/FSH) and/or GH deficiency are not life-threatening.

- Glucocorticoid (steroid) replacement should be administered *without* awaiting the results of confirmatory diagnostic testing; this can be subsequently performed.
  - Acutely ill, hospitalised patients with central hypoadrenalism should be given stress dose glucocorticoid coverage, most often intravenous (IV) with a stat dose of IV hydrocortisone 100–200 mg, followed by a hydrocortisone IV infusion at a rate of 2–4 mg/hour, or 50–100 mg

intramuscular (IM) or IV hydrocortisone every six hours. If the patient is hypotensive, resuscitation with IV normal saline is indicated.
- Levothyroxine (synthetic thyroxine) replacement should only be administered *after* glucocorticoid replacement or HPA axis is confirmed to be normal to avoid precipitating adrenal crisis.
- Judicious administration of synthetic ADH and monitoring of fluid balance and serum sodium are essential in the management of central DI.
- Treat the underlying aetiology (e.g. pituitary macroadenoma, pituitary apoplexy, hypophysitis).

Pituitary tumours

Pituitary tumours account for approximately 10–15% of all intracranial tumours.

- The pathogenesis of most pituitary adenomas remains unknown, although genetic causes include multiple endocrine neoplasia (MEN) 1– typically *3 Ps* (i.e. *p*ituitary, *p*arathyroid and *p*ancreas).
- Pituitary adenomas are divided by size on MRI or CT imaging into:
  - microadenomas (<10 mm) – most common.
  - macroadenomas (≥10 mm) – Figure 23.1.

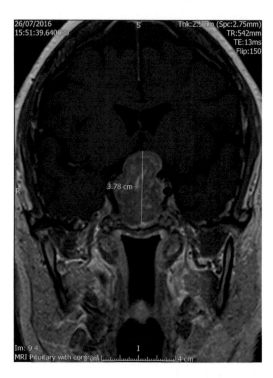

Figure 23.1 MRI pituitary coronal view showing large macroadenoma (non-functioning pituitary tumour).

- Pituitary carcinomas with distant metastases are rare, occurring in 0.1–0.2% of cases.
- Pituitary adenomas may:
  - hypersecrete hormones (i.e. 'functioning' tumour: ~two-thirds). Non-secreting adenomas are 'non-functioning'
  - cause local mass effects (i.e. headache, hypopituitarism, VF defects).
- If an MRI shows the tumour impinging on the optic chiasm, then formal VF testing is indicated to rule out VF defect.
- An evaluation for hypopituitarism should be carried out in all patients with macroadenomas and even large (6–9 mm) microadenomas.
- Central DI is rarely seen with pituitary adenomas (although it may occur as a result of treatment).
- Treatments include medical therapies (e.g. dopamine agonists), transsphenoidal surgery and radiotherapy.

Prolactinomas

Prolactinomas account for ~40–50% of pituitary adenomas overall.

- Present with amenorrhoea, loss of libido, galactorrhoea and infertility in women and loss of libido, erectile dysfunction and infertility in men.
- Only ~5–10% of microprolactinomas enlarge over 10 years; macroprolactinomas more commonly enlarge.
- Investigations.
  - Serum prolactin.
  - Always rule out pregnancy (pregnancy test).
  - Rule out hypopituitarism and visual field defects depending on size of the adenoma.
  - Rule out excessive co-secretion of other pituitary hormones (e.g. GH).
  - Pituitary imaging.
- The treatment of patients with microprolactinomas and macroprolactinomas with dopamine agonist therapy is effective in reducing prolactin levels and adenoma size, restoring gonadal function and improving other clinical features. Cabergoline is the dopamine agonist of choice, due to higher effectiveness in normalising prolactin levels and pituitary tumour shrinkage.

Cerebrospinal fluid (CSF) rhinorrhoea can occur when there is a large, invasive, skull-based prolactinoma that serves as a 'cork' in the base of the skull. When the tumour size is reduced substantially through dopamine agonist use, CSF can leak around the tumour into the sphenoid sinus and nasal passages, with a resultant risk of meningitis. Measurement of beta-2 transferrin in the nasal fluid is diagnostic. Surgical repair is usually required.

Pituitary apoplexy

Pituitary apoplexy is an endocrine emergency resulting from catastrophic haemorrhage or infarct of the pituitary gland that typically manifests with headache, nausea and vomiting, visual impairment and reduced consciousness.

- Headache is the most prominent symptom and is usually retro-orbital but can be bifrontal or diffuse and is present in more than 80% of patients. Headache is also generally the initial symptom, with sudden and severe onset described 'like a thunderclap in a clear sky'. It is often associated with vomiting and nausea and can mimic migraine or meningitis. Signs of meningeal irritation or altered consciousness may complicate the diagnosis.
- In most cases, pituitary apoplexy occurs in an undiagnosed, pre-existing pituitary adenoma and the initial diagnosis is often either subarachnoid haemorrhage or bacterial meningitis, until imaging shows the presence of a pituitary adenoma. Diagnosis thus relies on a combination of clinical manifestations (e.g. sudden headache and visual disturbances) and the detection of a pituitary adenoma.
- Patients with suspected pituitary apoplexy require detailed VF, visual acuity and extraocular eye movement examination; pituitary hormone profile assessment; and emergency glucocorticoid treatment. Extensive or deteriorating VF or visual acuity deficits, or reduced consciousness, necessitate emergency surgical intervention.

Fluid and sodium balance

Human cells dwell in salt water and their well-being depends on the ability of the body to regulate the salinity of the extracellular environment. By controlling water intake and excretion, the osmoregulatory system normally keeps the plasma sodium concentration (Na^+) between

135 mmol/l and 145 mmol/l. Failure of the system to regulate within this range leads to hypotonic or hypertonic stress.

The term 'tonicity' describes the effect of plasma on cells.

- Hypotonicity makes cells swell – hyponatraemia *usually* indicates hypotonicity.
- Hypertonicity makes cells shrink – hypernatraemia *always* indicates hypertonicity.

Abnormal serum sodium levels (dysnatraemias) are common in the inpatient setting. Both hyponatraemia (<135 mmol/l) and hypernatraemia (e.g. >145 mmol/l) are associated with increased morbidity and mortality in the acute care setting.

Although all cells are affected, clinical manifestations of hyponatraemia and hypernatraemia are primarily neurological, and rapid changes in plasma Na⁺ in either direction can cause severe, permanent and sometimes lethal brain injury. Because the brain adapts to an abnormal plasma Na⁺ level, excessive correction of a *chronic* disturbance can be injurious and should be avoided.

Body fluid compartments

For body fluid compartments, remember the **60-40-20** rule.

- Total body water (TBW): **~60%** body weight in men (~50% body weight in women).
- Distribution of water.
  - Two-thirds in intracellular fluid (ICF) = **~40%** of body weight.
  - One-third in extracellular fluid (ECF) = **~20%** of body weight (i.e. plasma is one-third of ECF, with venous 85% and arterial 15%, and interstitial fluid two-thirds of ECF).

Water balance

- Normal water intake: ~2 l/day.
  - 1500 ml – oral fluids/day.
  - 500 ml – solids or product of oxidation.
- Normal water output: ~2 l/day.
  - 500–1500 ml – urine output per day (>0.5 ml/kg/h).

- 250 ml/day – stool water output.
- 500–900 ml/day – insensible losses.

Factors controlling water balance

Internal balance of water

- Osmolality (number of particles/kg of water, i.e. concentration of particles).
  - Normal plasma osmolality (POsm) 280–295 mOsm/kg H_2O.
  - Calculated plasma osmolality and effective osmolality (Table 23.1). As urea freely crosses between the extracellular and intracellular spaces, it does not exert *any* osmotic effects. Hence, urea is not included in the calculation for *effective* osmolality.
- As osmolality of fluids (ECF or ICF) changes (e.g. hyponatraemia, hyperglycaemia), water will shift freely through the permeable cell membranes to maintain isotonicity, which will lead to changes in the distribution of TBW.
- POsm in a healthy person varies by only 1–2% in physiological conditions (where there is free access to water).

External balance of water

The accurate regulation of POsm is maintained by the homeostatic process of *osmoregulation* (Figure 23.2). Changes in the tonicity of the plasma are detected by specialised osmoreceptor cells in the anterior hypothalamus. The osmoreceptor cells are solute specific, in that they respond to stimulations by alterations in plasma [Na⁺], less so to alterations in blood urea, and not at all to perturbations in plasma glucose.

Stimulation of osmoreceptors leads to the following outcomes.

- *Thirst.* The majority of cases of hypernatraemia arise secondary to inadequate water intake. The likelihood of developing hypernatraemia increases with age and particularly with residence in long-term

Table 23.1 Calculated plasma osmolality and effective osmolality

Plasma osmolality	Effective osmolality
2 × Na⁺ (mmol/l)	2 × Na⁺ (mmol/l)
+ Glucose (mmol/l)	+ Glucose (mmol/l)
+ Urea (mmol/l)	
= POsm (mOsm/kg H_2O)	= POsm (mOsm/kg H_2O)

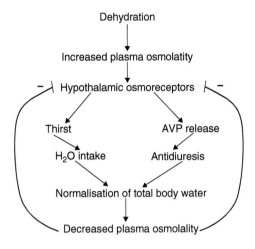

Figure 23.2 The regulation of plasma osmolality – antidiuretic hormone is also known as arginine vasopressin (AVP).

care. Up to 50% of residents of long-term care have been estimated to develop hypernatraemia at some time. The factors which contribute to the excess risk of hypernatraemia in older patients are multifactorial, through a combination of cognitive impairment and osmotically stimulated thirst attenuation in the elderly, which leads to reduced fluid intake.

- *ADH (also known as arginine vasopressin) secretion.* When plasma ADH concentrations rise, there is increased receptor binding in the collecting tubules of the kidneys, generating the synthesis of aquaporin-2 and the insertion of preformed aquaporin-2 into the luminal membrane of the collecting tubules, thus allowing the reabsorption of water and the concentration of urine.

> In addition to osmoregulation, hypovolaemia and hypotension (e.g. >5–10% decrease) can lead to stimulation of baroreceptors, leading to ADH secretion.

Overview of sodium homeostasis

- Na^+ is the major extracellular cation (extracellular $[Na^+]$ is maintained ~140 mmol/l).
- Na^+ regulation is associated with water homeostasis, yet it is regulated by independent mechanisms.
- Changes in *Na^+ concentration* reflect *water* homeostasis. Disturbance of water balance may lead to *hyponatraemia* or *hypernatraemia*.

> **Box 23.3 Sodium balance**
>
> - Na^+_{in} equals Na^+_{out} = Na^+ balance.
> - Na^+ excretion <Na^+ intake = positive Na^+ balance
>   o Can lead to increased ECF volume, with increased blood volume and blood pressure (BP), leading to oedema and possible heart failure.
> - Na^+ excretion >Na^+ intake = negative Na^+ balance.
>   o Can lead to decreased ECF volume, with decreased blood volume and BP, leading to shock.

- Changes in *Na^+ content* (and subsequently ECF volume) reflect *Na^+ homeostasis.* Disturbance of Na^+ balance may lead to *hypovolaemia* or *hypervolaemia* (Box 23.3).

Hyponatraemia

> Hyponatraemia is the most common electrolyte abnormality, present in 15–30% of non-selected emergency admissions to hospital. Approximately 1–3% are severe (e.g. <125 mmol/l).

Classification of hyponatraemia by plasma tonicity, ECF volume status and severity

> Only hypotonic hyponatraemia causes a shift of water from the ECF *into* cells along osmotic gradients. Osmotic water shifts into the brain can lead to significant neurological dysfunction.

Hyponatraemia can be classified in a variety of ways.

1 The first is generally by plasma *tonicity*. Patients with hyponatraemia can be hypotonic, isotonic, or hypertonic in terms of their plasma tonicity. In the most common form, hypotonic hyponatraemia, serum $[Na^+]$ and plasma osmolality are both low. Examples of this form of hyponatraemia include the syndrome of inappropriate antidiuretic hormone (SIADH), heart failure, and cirrhosis.

2 Once it is confirmed that a patient has hypotonic hyponatraemia with a low plasma osmolality, the next level of classification is to determine the

ECF volume status of the patient. Patients with hypotonic hyponatraemia can be:

- Hypovolaemic - with a decreased ECF volume. Hypovolemic patients have typical signs of volume depletion:
  - Low urine Na (<10 mmol/l) — implies increased sodium retention by the kidneys to compensate for *extrarenal* losses of sodium containing fluid (e.g. COVID-19, diarrhoea, vomiting, nasogastric suction, sweating, third-spacing, burns, pancreatitis).
  - High urine Na (>20 mmol/l) — *renal* salt loss (e.g. diuretic excess, decreased aldosterone such as in *acute* primary adrenal insufficiency).
- Euvolaemic - with a normal clinically determined ECF volume.
  - This is the pattern encountered with SIADH; other less common causes include *non-acute* primary adrenal insufficiency and severe hypothyroidism.
- Hypervolaemic - with an expanded ECF volume. Caused by water-retaining states, leading to relative excess of water in relation to sodium:
  - Hypervolaemic hyponatraemia - patients can have oedema, ascites, pulmonary congestion, or oedema-forming disorders that typically include congestive heart failure (CHF), cirrhosis, kidney failure, and the nephrotic syndrome.

3 Finally, hyponatraemia can also be classified by *severity*, which is indicated mainly by neurological symptomatology. Clinical severity depends on balance of several factors:

- Degree of hyponatraemia.
- Rate of Fall in serum [Na$^+$]:
  - Acute hyponatraemia <48 hrs duration.
  - Chronic Hyponatraemia >48 hrs duration.
- Ability of the brain to adapt to osmolar stress.
- Presence of co-morbidities and certain demographic factors (e.g. age, gender).
- Prognosis also dependent on underlying cause of hyponatraemia (e.g. SIADH due to lung cancer).

Severe hyponatraemia

Severe hyponatraemia is generally defined by a lower serum [Na$^+$] (typically <125 mmol/l) and with symptoms indicating significant neurological dysfunction, such as coma, obtundation, seizures, respiratory distress and unexplained vomiting. This is termed *hyponatraemic encephalopathy* and reflects osmotic water shifts into the brain. The typical duration of

Table 23.2 Common clinical causes of symptomatic hyponatraemia in hospitalised patients

Acute hyponatraemia (≤48 h duration)
- Water intoxication from psychogenic polydipsia (typically in schizophrenic patients) or excessive forced water ingestion (student hazing)
- Exercise-associated hyponatraemia (marathons, ultramarathons and similar prolonged endurance exercise activities)
- Postoperative hyponatraemia
- 3,4-Methylenedioxymethamphetamine ('Ecstasy')

Chronic hyponatraemia (>48 h duration)
- SIADH (all aetiologies)
- Drug-induced hyponatraemia (particularly SSRI antidepressants)
- Hypovolaemic hyponatraemia (all aetiologies, but particularly thiazide-induced hyponatraemia)
- Heart failure
- Cirrhosis
- Nephrotic syndrome
- Renal failure

these cases is short and generally represents a more acute form of hyponatraemia (Table 23.2).

In contrast to acute hyponatraemia, chronic hyponatraemia is much less symptomatic. The major reason for the profound differences between the symptoms of acute and chronic hyponatraemia is the process of *brain volume regulation* (Figure 23.3).

> It is important to assess the severity of the hyponatraemia because most treatment algorithms use the severity of hyponatraemia, as determined by the degree of neurological symptoms, to determine the initial therapy.

Specific investigations of hyponatraemia

1 Confirm hyponatremia – [Na$^+$] <135 mmol/l.
2 Measured or calculated plasma osmolality – hypotonic hyponatraemia – POsm <280 mOsm/kg H$_2$O.
3 Urine osmolality (UOsm).
- UOsm low <100 mOsm/kg H$_2$O – the kidneys are responding appropriately by diluting the urine (e.g. psychogenic polydipsia).

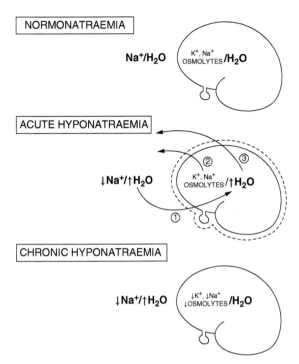

NORMONATRAEMIA

Na^+/H_2O $\underset{OSMOLYTES}{K^+, Na^+}/H_2O$

ACUTE HYPONATRAEMIA

$\downarrow Na^+/\uparrow H_2O$ $\underset{OSMOLYTES}{K^+, Na^+}/\uparrow H_2O$

CHRONIC HYPONATRAEMIA

$\downarrow Na^+/\uparrow H_2O$ $\underset{\downarrow OSMOLYTES}{\downarrow K^+, \downarrow Na^+}/H_2O$

Figure 23.3 Schematic diagram of brain volume adaptation to hyponatraemia. Under normal conditions, brain osmolality and extracellular fluid (ECF) osmolality are in equilibrium (top panel); for simplicity, the predominant intracellular solutes are depicted as potassium (K^+) and organic osmolytes, and the extracellular solute as sodium (Na^+). Following the induction of ECF hypo-osmolality, water moves into the brain (middle panel) in response to osmotic gradients, producing brain oedema (dotted line, #1). However, in response to the induced swelling, the brain rapidly loses both extracellular and intracellular solutes (middle panel, #2). As water losses accompany the losses of brain solute, the expanded brain volume then decreases back toward normal (middle panel, #3). If hypo-osmolality is sustained, brain volume eventually normalises completely and the brain becomes fully adapted to the ECF hyponatraemia (bottom panel).

- UOsm elevated >100 mOsm/kg H_2O – if there are increased levels of ADH (e.g. SIADH, CHF and hypothyroidism).
4 Urine sodium concentration (UNa) – surrogate for the ECF volume (i.e. how much perfusing vital organs).
  - UNa^+ concentration >20 mmol/l – consistent with SIADH, salt-wasting nephropathy or hypoaldosteronism. Diuretics may produce this effect as well.
  - UNa^+ concentration <10 mmol/l – consistent with hypovolaemia.
5 Measure urine electrolytes – if the sum of the urine [Na^+ and K^+] exceeds the serum [Na^+] then fluid restriction as a treatment for SIADH is likely to fail.

SIADH

SIADH is a disorder in which water excretion is impaired by the unregulated secretion of ADH from the posterior pituitary, leading to free water retention and varying degrees of dilutional (hypotonic) hyponatraemia. SIADH is a diagnosis of exclusion, therefore other causes of hyponatraemia must be ruled out (Box 23.4).

Box 23.4 Diagnostic criteria for SIADH

- True plasma hypoosmolality (POsm <280 mOsm/kg).
- Urine concentration inappropriate for POsm (UOsm >100 mOsm/kg).
- Elevated UNa^+ excretion (spot UNa^+ >20 mmol/l).
- Clinical euvolaemia.
- Absence of other causes of euvolaemic hypo-osmolality (e.g. hypothyroidism, hypocortisolism, renal dysfunction, diuretic use within last week).

Common causes of SIADH include the following.

- *Malignancies* (ectopic ADH secretion): small cell lung cancer is the prototypical paraneoplastic tumour, but other malignancies can also cause SIADH.
- *Pulmonary disorders.*
  - Pneumonia, pleural effusion, pneumothorax, etc.
  - Increased intrathoracic pressure (e.g. COPD, non-invasive ventilation [NIV], asthma) activates the baroreceptors, causing non-osmotic release of vasopressin.

- *Central nervous system disorders*: meningitis, encephalitis, brain tumours, etc.
- *Drugs*: selective serotonin reuptake inhibitors (SSRI), antipsychotics, narcotics, tricyclic antidepressants, proton pump inhibitors (PPI).
- *Others*: nausea, pain.

If SIADH is suspected, an extensive evaluation for the aetiology is warranted and should include:

- complete review of medications, e.g. PPI, SSRI
- age-appropriate cancer screening as indicated
- chest X-ray and/or CT-thorax, abdomen and pelvis (CT-TAP) depending on risk factors and clinical scenario
- imaging of the central nervous system with either a CT scan or MRI.

> Hyponatraemia occurs in nearly one-third of patients with COVID-19. The cause of hyponatraemia in COVID-19 may be multifactorial. SIADH and hypovolaemia are equally implicated as the cause of hyponatraemia in most series.

Treatment of symptomatic hyponatraemia

> Correction of hyponatraemia is associated with markedly improved neurological outcomes in patients with severely symptomatic hyponatraemia. Brain herniation, the most dreaded complication of hyponatraemia, is seen almost exclusively in patients with acute hyponatraemia (usually <24 hours).

Severe symptoms associated with hyponatraemia include vomiting, cardiorespiratory arrest, seizures and reduced consciousness/coma (Glasgow Coma Scale [GCS] ≤8). These patients must be treated with IV hypertonic (3%) saline with the aim of increasing serum [Na$^+$] by 6 mmol/l in the *first hour* or until symptoms abate. Acute hyponatraemia, especially when there is a clear timeline of development of hyponatraemia, such as excess hypotonic perioperative fluids, can be rapidly corrected to a normal level quickly because the patient

is not at risk for ODS (i.e. no significant brain adaptation has occurred).

In comparison, chronic hyponatraemia (or when the timeline for development is unclear) must be corrected in a controlled fashion due to *brain adaptation* which can predispose to ODS if corrected too rapidly. This is sometimes referred to as the '*rule of sixes*' – increase serum [Na$^+$] concentration by 6 mmol/l (+/– 2 mmol/l) during the first 24 h but if the patient has severe symptoms/signs, this timing can be preloaded to the first six hours of the first day of correction.

> ODS presents with cognitive, behavioural and neuropsychiatric disorders.
> - ODS is diagnosed clinically and by characteristic MRI changes (hypointense lesions on T1-weighted images and hyperintense lesions on T2-weighted images).
> - The pathophysiology of ODS is not fully understood. The brain loses organic osmolytes very quickly in order to adapt to hyponatraemia. However, neurones reclaim these organic osmolytes slowly during rapid and/or overcorrection of chronic hyponatraemia, resulting in movement of water from brain ICF to ECF, causing *shrinkage* of cerebral cells. This can lead to local brainstem demyelination.

Hypertonic saline

Administration of hypertonic solutions may require special considerations (e.g. placement in the ICU, use of central IV catheters, sign-off by a consultant, etc.), which each clinician needs to be aware of to optimise patient care.

> No other active hyponatraemia therapy (e.g. vaptans) should be administered until at least 24 hours *following* successful increases in serum [Na$^+$] using hypertonic saline.

Hypertonic saline can be given by IV infusion or by administration of a 100 ml bolus of 3% NaCl, repeated twice if there is no clinical improvement at 10-minute intervals. Injecting this amount of hypertonic saline IV raises the serum [Na$^+$] by an average of 2–4 mmol/l, which is well below the recommended maximum daily rate of change to prevent ODS. Because the brain can only accommodate an average increase of approximately 8% in brain volume before herniation occurs, quickly increasing the serum [Na$^+$] by as little as 2–4 mmol/l in severely symptomatic hyponatraemia can effectively reduce brain swelling and intracranial pressure.

Active treatment with hypertonic (3%) or isotonic (0.9%) saline in symptomatic chronic hyponatraemia should be stopped when the patient's symptoms are no longer present, a safe serum [Na$^+$] (usually >120 mmol/l) has been achieved, or the rate of correction has reached maximum limits of 12 mmol/l within 24 h; or 18 mmol/l within 48 hours to avoid precipitating ODS; or 8 mmol/l over any 24-h period in patients at high risk of ODS (i.e. serum [Na$^+$] ≤105 mmol/l; hypokalaemia; alcoholism; malnutrition; and advanced liver disease).

> It is imperative that all patients undergoing active treatment for symptomatic hyponatraemia should have frequent monitoring of serum [Na$^+$] and ECF volume status to ensure that the serum [Na$^+$] does not exceed the limits of safe correction. Monitoring urine output is also important. If this rate of correction is exceeded, especially in patients with high risk of ODS, re-lowering serum [Na$^+$] with hypotonic fluids should be considered. Seek expert help.

Conservative management options for hyponatraemia

- Fluid restriction: mainstay of treatment – 0.5–1 l/day. Restrict *all* intake that is consumed by drinking, not just water. Aim for a fluid restriction that is 500 ml/day *below* the 24-hour urine volume.
- Demeclocycline: induces nephrogenic DI, increases free water excretion.
- Furosemide *plus* oral or IV salt loading.
- Vaptans (V2R antagonists): specifically antagonise the V2 receptors in the principal cells of the kidney (mediate the renal tubular ADH response) leading to reduced renal reabsorption of water (i.e. 'aquaretic'). Vaptans are also used in autosomal dominant polycystic kidney disease (ADPKD).

> The treatment of choice for depletional hyponatraemia (i.e. hypovolaemic hyponatraemia) is isotonic (0.9%) saline to restore ECF volume and ensure adequate organ perfusion. This initial therapy is appropriate for patients who either have clinical signs of hypovolaemia or in whom a spot urine [Na$^+$] is <20–30 mmol/l.

Hypernatraemia

> Hypernatraemia is common in the emergency setting and is associated with significant morbidity and mortality, primarily caused by cell shrinkage due to extracellular movement of water.

Usually occurs due to inadequate water intake and/or excessive water loss, leading to inappropriate plasma hyperosmolality. Clinical features of hypernatraemia are predominantly a consequence of the shrinkage of brain cells, and include lethargy, drowsiness and altered mental status, progressing to seizures, coma and death if left untreated.

Understanding the disorders which cause hypernatraemia is essential to enable prompt, correct management. It is extremely important to note that the severity of symptoms is strongly influenced by the rapidity of the development of hypernatraemia: those with acute hypernatraemia (<48 hours) are at far higher risk than those with chronic hypernatraemia (>48 hours).

Management of hypernatraemia

When hypernatraemia is acute and severe neurological symptoms are present, immediate treatment is indicated with normalisation of plasma sodium within 24 hours of commencement of therapy.

In circumstances where the onset of hypernatraemia is unknown or is chronic, a more conservative recommended rate of correction of plasma sodium with hypotonic fluids would be a maximum of 1 mmol/l/h to a maximum of 10–12 mmol/l/day.

When a patient with hypernatraemia is hypotensive, treatment should start with isotonic IV fluids (either crystalloids or colloids) in order to restore haemodynamic stability. In all other settings, hypernatraemia can be treated with hypotonic fluids administered either orally or IV.

In patients at risk of thrombotic episodes, prophylactic anticoagulation should be considered.

Diabetes insipidus (DI)

Central DI

> Diabetes insipidus which results in inappropriate hypotonic polyuria rarely causes hypernatraemia, as the intact thirst mechanism generates sufficient drinking to replace renal water losses. However, if DI is associated with adipsia (i.e. no thirst response), diminished conscious levels or vomiting, severe hypernatraemia may occur.

Diabetes insipidus rarely occurs in patients with pituitary adenomas but can manifest in patients with inflammatory or infiltrative pituitary lesions, or after surgery or radiation, typically because of hypothalamic or infundibular involvement. Tumours metastatic to the pituitary area may often present clinically with fluid and electrolyte disturbances from DI, the theory being that the network of portal vessels feeding the neurohypophysis may trap circulating tumour cells which then proliferate into a mass lesion.

- In patients with acute pituitary insults affecting the posterior pituitary, including TBI and pituitary surgery, central DI typically presents within 24–48 hours and is characterised by polyuria (urine output exceeding 200 ml/h for >2 h) with inappropriately dilute urine (urine osmolality <300 mOsm/kg) despite the presence of hypernatraemia/hyperosmolality.
- A sequence of events termed the 'triple phase response' may occur.
  - Early polyuric phase: transient central DI due to 'shock' of neurohypophyseal axons with decreased ADH release.
  - Antidiuretic phase: hyponatraemia as a result of SIADH due to degeneration of neurohypophyseal axons releasing preformed stored ADH which generally resolves within two weeks.
  - Late polyuric phase: recurrent central DI due to persistent damage of ADH secretion.
- DI is best managed acutely by vasopressin (shorter-acting) rather than desmopressin (longer-acting) synthetic ADH formulations, as SIADH can quickly follow (as part of the 'triple phase response'). If DI is permanent, desmopressin is the preferred therapy.

- Central DI can be masked by ACTH or TSH deficiency; therefore DI can become apparent with initiation of glucocorticoid and/or thyroxine treatment.

Nephrogenic DI

Nephrogenic DI occurs when the kidney is unable to respond properly to ADH. The defect may be due to an inherited disorder or acquired aetiology. In the Acute Medicine setting, classic reversible causes include hypercalcaemia, hyperglycaemia, hypokalaemia and lithium toxicity. Treatment is aimed at managing the underlying cause.

Thyroid disorders

The normal thyroid gland produces two principal hormones – thyroxine (T4) and tri-iodothyronine (T3). Thyroid hormones are bound to thyroxine-binding globulin (TBG) and other plasma proteins for transport in the blood. Only the free hormone is able to enter cells and also regulate the pituitary feedback mechanism. Thyroid hormones influence cell differentiation, growth and metabolism of all major systems in the body. TSH stimulates thyroid hormone production, secretion and thyroid growth. TSH is regulated by the negative feedback action of T4 and T3.

> Thyroid hormones
> - T4 is the primary secretory product of the thyroid gland, which is the only source of T4.
> - T3 is derived from two processes.
>   - About 80% of circulating T3 comes from deiodination of T4 in peripheral tissues.
>   - About 20% comes from direct thyroid secretion.
> - T4 is biologically inactive in target tissues until converted to T3 by deiodinases. T4 is therefore a *prohormone* – activation occurs with 5' deiodination of the outer ring of T4.
> - T3 then becomes the biologically *active* hormone.

Common thyroid disorders

> Thyroid disorders affect approximately 750 million people worldwide.

Common thyroid issues include the following.

- Thyroiditis – inflammation of the thyroid.
  - Autoimmune thyroiditis: it is estimated that 10% of most populations have antithyroid antibodies. Many will remain biochemically euthyroid. The most common cause of thyroid enlargement (goitre) and hypothyroidism in developed countries is chronic autoimmune thyroiditis (Hashimoto thyroiditis). For patients with elevated TSH, thyroxine (T4) therapy is prescribed.
  - Postpartum: affects about 10% women after pregnancy. One in 10 of these cases can result in permanent hypothyroidism.
  - Drug induced, e.g. ICIs, amiodarone.
  - De Quervain (subacute) thyroiditis: usually related to viral infection. Painful.
- Hypothyroidism – underactive thyroid: affects 4–5% of the population. Much higher prevalence in women. The spectrum of hypothyroidism ranges from asymptomatic subclinical disease to a life-threatening metabolic crisis characterised by multisystem dysfunction and high mortality warranting IV use of thyroxine and supportive therapy (i.e. myxoedema coma).
- Hyperthyroidism – overactive *thyroid* leading to excessive thyroid hormone production. In contrast, thyrotoxicosis is excessive thyroid hormone from *any source* including the thyroid gland, such as excessive *oral* thyroxine replacement or struma ovarii (ovarian teratoma comprises >50% thyroid tissue) directly secreting T4 from the *ovary*. The spectrum of thyrotoxicosis ranges from asymptomatic subclinical disease to a life-threatening metabolic crisis characterised by multisystem dysfunction and high mortality (i.e. thyroid storm).
- Graves' disease (GD) – an autoimmune condition and most common cause of hyperthyroidism in the UK. Management options include antithyroid drug (ATD) therapy (e.g. carbimazole or propylthiouracil), radioactive iodine (RAI) therapy or surgical thyroidectomy. Treatment should be individualised.
  - Graves' ophthalmopathy: an autoimmune condition with heterogeneous expression ranging from mild ocular discomfort to severe and potentially sight-threatening disease. Almost half of all patients with hyperthyroidism due to GD can be identified as having some degree of orbital involvement. The disease progresses in approximately 20% of patients who may experience eye pain, frequent diplopia, severe periorbital erythema and swelling or excessive proptosis (protrusion of the eyeball, also known as exophthalmos). In 3–5%, sight-threatening corneal breakdown or compressive optic neuropathy may develop. Treatments include glucocorticoids, rituximab, tocilizumab (interleukin-6 inhibitor), teprotumumab (human monoclonal antibody inhibitor of the IGF-1 receptor) and surgical intervention.
- Thyroid nodular disease – discrete lesion within the thyroid gland due to an abnormal focal growth of thyroid cells.
  - Very common, ~5% palpable and up to ~30–50% by ultrasound exam (depends on age). Nodular goitre is more common in women, in the elderly, with iodine deficiency, and in populations exposed to external radiation.
  - While nodules are common, they are usually benign (>95%). Risk factors for malignancy include age, worrisome imaging phenotype, size (usually >1 cm, although 25% cancers <1 cm); 'cold' nodule on RAI scan; past radiation exposure; and positive family history of thyroid cancer. Thyroid fine-needle aspiration biopsy (FNA) and cytology is the best method for differentiating benign from malignant thyroid nodules.
- Thyroid cancer – <5% thyroid nodules are cancerous. The incidence of thyroid cancer has increased in the past 50 years, mostly due to the widespread use of sensitive imaging and thyroid FNA in clinical practice. Despite this significant increase in prevalence, mortality remains stable.
- Non-thyroidal illness – constellation of low plasma T3 concentrations and elevated reverse (r)T3 (inactive T3), with decreased, normal or increased TSH, generally referred to as *euthyroid-sick syndrome* or *non-thyroidal illness*.
  - Very common with no obvious clinical sequelae or specific treatment needed. Thyroid function tests (TFTs) improve on recovery of underlying illness.
  - This is a good example of why you should not routinely measure TFTs (and many other endocrine tests) in the acute care setting unless clinically indicated.

> Persons with autoimmune thyroid disease may have other concomitant autoimmune disorders (i.e. part of autoimmune polyglandular syndrome, APS).

Thyroid disorders - basic clinical features

The typical symptoms and signs of hypothyroidism and hyperthyroidism are shown in Table 23.3.

Table 23.3 Symptoms and signs of hypothyroidism and hyperthyroidism

Thyroid state	Symptoms	Signs
Hypothyroidism	Weight gain, constipation, lethargy, dry skin/hair, aching muscles, husky voice, cold intolerance and menorrhagia	Myxoedema (accumulation of a hydrophilic mucopolysaccharide substance in the connective tissues), pale and puffy skin, periorbital oedema, goitre, thin and dry hair, large tongue (macroglossia), slow relaxation tendon reflexes, slow thought and movement, and loss of lateral 1/3 of eyebrows
Hyperthyroidism	Anxious/nervous, sweating, palpitations, fatigue, weight loss, diarrhoea, altered appetite and weakness	Tachycardia, tremor, thyroid bruit, eye signs (GD), goitre (diffuse or nodular), atrial fibrillation, clubbing/pretibial myxoedema (GD) and proximal myopathy

GD, Graves' disease.

Classification of hypothyroidism and hyperthyroidism

- Primary hypothyroidism (thyroid gland failure).
  - Clinical hypothyroidism: obvious symptoms/signs; low FT4, TSH >4.5 (elevated, usually >10). Treat with thyroxine.
- Secondary hypothyroidism (hypothalamic-pituitary-thyroid failure).
  - Clinical hypothyroidism: obvious symptoms/signs; low FT4, TSH low or inappropriately normal. Treat with thyroxine (after ruling out cortisol deficiency).
- Primary hyperthyroidism (thyroid gland excess).
  - Clinical hyperthyroidism: obvious symptoms/signs; high FT4 and/or high FT3, TSH <0.5 (suppressed). Treat with beta-blockers for symptomatic relief; ATD, RAI or surgery for definitive therapy.
- Secondary hyperthyroidism (i.e. TSHoma – functioning pituitary adenoma secreting TSH, stimulating the thyroid gland to secrete excess thyroid hormone).
  - Clinical hyperthyroidism: obvious symptoms/signs; high FT4 and/or high FT3, TSH inappropriately normal or high. Will need initial treatment directed at thyroid with definitive treatment targeting pituitary tumour.

Common causes of thyrotoxicosis include the following.
- Graves' disease.
- Toxic nodular or multinodular goitre.
- Painful subacute thyroiditis (e.g. COVID-19).
- Silent (i.e. painless) thyroiditis (e.g. Hashimoto or postpartum).

- Iodine and iodine-containing drugs (e.g. amiodarone) and radiographic contrast agents.
  - Jod–Basedow effect: excess iodine intake in people who have pre-existing thyroid abnormalities can lead to increased thyroid hormone synthesis/secretion.

Investigation of thyroid disorders

- TSH – first thing you assess (normal range 0.5–4.5 µU/ml).
  - Suppressed = hyperthyroid (primary only).
  - Elevated = hypothyroid (primary only).
- FT4 and FT3.
  - Elevated = hyperthyroid (FT3 can be elevated alone – T3 toxicosis – especially with toxic nodule).
  - Low = hypothyroid.
- Thyroid autoantibodies.
  - Antithyroid peroxidase (TPO) and antithyroglobulin (TG) antibodies – Hashimoto disease.
  - TSH-receptor stimulating antibodies: Graves' disease.
- Thyroid ultrasound scan – can detect nodules >3 mm; colour Doppler – blood flow (e.g. increased in Graves' disease). Other imaging, e.g. CT, MRI: masses, retrosternal expansion and tracheal compression.
- FNA cytology – cytology and cancer genetic profiling.
- Isotope scan and uptake – radioactive material administered (e.g. I^{123}). Measures the ability of the thyroid gland to remove and concentrate iodine from the blood.

Table 23.4 Basic treatment of hypothyroidism and hyperthyroidism

Thyroid state	Treatment

Hypothyroidism	• Levothyroxine (T4) is the treatment of choice for the routine management of hypothyroidism.
	   ○ Adults: about 1.6 µg/kg body weight/d (e.g. start 50–100 µg/day).
	   ○ Elderly: <1.0 µg/kg body weight/d (start 'low and go slow' in elderly, e.g. start 12.5–25 µg/day).
	• Clinical and biochemical evaluations at 6–8-week intervals until the serum TSH concentration is normalised.
	• Must exclude co-existing adrenal failure prior to T4 treatment.

Hyperthyroidism	• ATD – carbimazole or propylthiouracil (PTU). Inhibit synthesis of T4 and T3; PTU also decreases T4 to T3 conversion. Treat for 12–24 months; >50% relapse rate usually within two years of stopping drug. Agranulocytosis 0.2% – warn about stopping drug if sore throat or fever – go to emergency department for full blood count. • RAI – takes about six months to work. Significant number develop hypothyroidism requiring lifelong T4 treatment. Can exacerbate Graves' eye disease, especially in smokers (should stop). • Surgery – if patient choice, or poor adherence to or failed ATD. Risk of hypocalcaemia and vocal cord damage.

○ Thyroid radioactive iodine scan (30 min post iodine – 'structure'), e.g. size, 'hot' or 'cold' nodules.
○ Thyroid radioactive iodine uptake (RAIU, hours-24 hours post iodine – 'function') – useful in defining cause of thyrotoxicosis (i.e. increased uptake with Graves' or decreased uptake with thyroiditis).

Treatment of hypothyroidism and hyperthyroidism

This is outlined in Table 23.4.

Thyroid emergencies

Thyroid emergencies are complex and rare and associated with significant morbidity and excess mortality. General axioms related to thyroid emergencies include the following.

• Having a high index of clinical suspicion.
• General supportive care is critical (e.g. oxygen, vasopressors).
• Treatment before diagnosis is confirmed (treatment is rarely harmful and can be modified or discontinued as more clinical information is acquired).
• Search for precipitating cause or accompanying illness.
• Always seek immediate expert advice and escalation.

Once thyroid emergency is recognised, the patient should be managed in an appropriate emergency setting such as an acute medical unit (AMU), enhanced care unit (ECU), coronary care unit (CCU), high-dependency unit (HDU) or intensive care unit (ICU). Effective, early management of acute medical emergencies requires prompt recognition, immediate correction of life-threatening physiological abnormalities, the methodical application of the Airway, Breathing, Circulation, Disability, and Exposure (ABCDE) approach, and rapid diagnosis and treatment of the underlying condition.

Thyroid storm

Thyroid storm (also known as thyroid crisis) is a critical presentation of severe thyrotoxicosis, requiring urgent ATD and supportive therapy (including iodine; beta-blockers; glucocorticoids; active cooling; sedatives; and seek and treat precipitants).

Definition of thyroid storm.

• Thyroid storm is a rare, life-threatening condition characterised by severe uncontrolled thyrotoxicosis.
• Usually an exacerbation of previously existent thyrotoxicosis with a dramatic clinical picture and fatal outcome in the absence of aggressive management.

Clinical features.

- General features are consistent with thyrotoxicosis.
- Those typical of storm but worse than usual thyrotoxicosis include fever; tachyarrhythmias including atrial fibrillation; congestive heart failure (CHF); abdominal pain; nausea; vomiting; diarrhoea; jaundice; dehydration; cachexia; delirium; and coma.

Precipitating events.

- Poor ATD treatment adherence; Sepsis; non-thyroid and thyroid surgery; radioiodine therapy; iodine loading (e.g. contrast, amiodarone); labour/delivery; psychosis; acute medical problems such as acute coronary syndromes (ACS), DKA.

Diagnosis.

- Thyroid storm is mostly a clinical diagnosis.
- Biochemical thyrotoxicosis – degree is not more profound than in typical thyrotoxicosis.
- Scoring systems are helpful (i.e. Burch–Wartofsky).

Treatment.

- When treating thyroid storm, one should consider the '5 Bs' (Box 23.5).
- General supportive care.
  - Manage in appropriate setting.
  - Treat sepsis, and seek and treat precipitants and co-morbidities.

Box 23.5 The 5 Bs for the treatment of thyroid storm

Block synthesis (i.e. ATD).

- PTU 200–250 mg every 4 h oral (1200 mg/d). *Usual dose for treating GD ~200–400 mg/d.*
- Carbimazole 20–25 mg every 4 h oral (120 mg/d). *Usual dose for treating GD ~20–40 mg/d.*

Block hormonal release.

- Iodine (Note – give iodine one hour *after ATD* or can precipitate worsening, i.e. Jod–Basedow).

Block T4 to T3 conversion (i.e. high-dose PTU, propranolol, glucocorticoid).

- Hydrocortisone 100 mg every 6–8 h IV.

Beta-blocker (e.g. propranolol or esmolol).

- Propranolol 60–80 mg every 4–6 h orally.
- Esmolol IV (short-acting).

Block enterohepatic circulation.

- Cholestyramine or remove excess thyroid hormone (e.g. plasmapheresis or dialysis).

- Treat anxiety and agitation (e.g. chlorpromazine).
- Treat hyperthermia (i.e. cooling, paracetamol).
- Correct dehydration (e.g. fluids, electrolytes), glucose, vitamins.
- Oxygen; vasopressors.

Prognosis: mortality is 15–30%.

Myxoedema coma

Myxoedema coma is a decompensated state of hypothyroidism resulting from severe and prolonged depletion of thyroid hormones leading to altered mental status and other clinical features related to widespread multiorgan dysfunction.

Definition of myxoedema coma.

- The most extreme, critical, life-threatening presentation of severe hypothyroidism.
- Common pathway often is respiratory decompensation with carbon dioxide (CO_2) narcosis leading to coma and fatal outcome in the absence of aggressive management.
- Does not require a *comatose* state for diagnosis.

Clinical features.

- General features consistent with hypothyroidism.
- Those typical of myxoedema coma but worse than usual hypothyroidism include hypothermia; oedema, dry/coarse skin, hair loss; abdominal/bladder distention; impaired pulmonary ventilation with respiratory acidosis; hyponatraemia, hypoglycaemia; bradycardia, CHF and pericardial effusion; and shock.
- Causes of coma or altered mental status include reduced cardiac output and cerebral blood flow; hypoxia; hypercapnia; hyponatraemia; hypoglycaemia; hypothermia; TBI (e.g. falls); effects of drugs, infection, etc.
- Direct effects of hypothyroidism on pulmonary function include depressed ventilatory drive; pleural effusion(s); upper airway obstruction (e.g. goitre, macroglossia); and sleep apnoea syndrome.

Precipitating events.

- Infection; medications (e.g. sedatives, narcotics); surgery; cardiovascular (ACS, CHF, stroke); hypothermia; hypoglycaemia; CO_2 narcosis; poor adherence with thyroid replacement therapy; and co-existing Addison disease.

Diagnosis.

- Myxoedema coma is mostly a clinical diagnosis (more common in women and during winter months).
- Biochemical hypothyroidism.

Treatment.

- Hormone replacement therapy.
  - Thyroid hormone: e.g. thyroxine 7 mcg/kg (350–500 mcg) IV. Then 50–100 mcg IV or oral daily. Alternatively, treat with T3 (liothyronine) or combination of T4 + T3.
  - Hydrocortisone: 50–100 mg every 6 h IV initially.
- General supportive care.
  - Manage in the HDU or ICU.
  - Treat sepsis, and seek and treat precipitants and co-morbidities.
  - Treat hypothermia (i.e. gentle rewarming).
  - Correct fluids (volume expansion), electrolytes, glucose and vitamins.
  - Oxygen (including NIV and mechanical ventilation); vasopressors.

Prognosis: mortality is 30–40%.

Amiodarone-related thyroid dysfunction and emergencies

> Amiodarone has multiple antiarrhythmic effects that justify its use in supraventricular and ventricular tachyarrhythmias, atrial fibrillation (when other therapies are poorly effective) and in preventing sudden cardiac death in selected patients.

Amiodarone is a benzofuranic iodine-rich drug structurally similar to thyroid hormones. Using a standard dose of amiodarone (200 mg per day), patients are exposed to a 75 mg daily iodine load, which greatly exceeds the recommended daily iodine intake (150–200 µg). This excess iodine load can result in thyroid dysfunction in 15–20% of patients, with either deficiency (amiodarone-induced hypothyroidism, AIH) or thyroid hormone excess (amiodarone-induced thyrotoxicosis, AIT).

Amiodarone-induced thyrotoxicosis occurs in 5–10% of all patients on amiodarone. They are divided clinically and pathophysiologically into two types (although both can co-exist in the same patient).

- Type 1 AIT – a form of iodine-induced true hyperthyroidism, in which iodine load reveals the underling thyroid autonomy or latent GD and triggers the occurrence of hyperthyroidism (Jod–Basedow). Type 1 AIT is best treated by ATD but the iodine-replete thyroid gland of AIT patients is less responsive to ATD. Thus, very high daily doses of the drug (40–60 mg/d carbimazole or equivalent doses of PTU) for longer than usual periods of time are needed before euthyroidism is restored.
- Type 2 AIT – direct drug- (and/or iodine-) induced cytotoxic damage of thyroid follicular cells is considered to be the cause (destructive thyroiditis). Type 2 AIT currently is the predominant form (~90%). It is best treated by glucocorticoids.

> Amiodarone-induced thyrotoxicosis occurs in patients with pre-existing serious cardiac disease and should be managed without delay, because the late resolution of thyrotoxicosis is associated with a high mortality rate. Differentiation of the two main forms of AIT is crucial, although challenging, because treatment and outcome differ. Many clinicians pragmatically treat AIT with combination carbimazole 40 mg and prednisolone 40 mg daily (i.e. '40 and 40') and if the patient responds within a few weeks, it is likely that type 2 AIT is the predominant form and is responding to glucocorticoid.

Calcium and metabolic bone disorders

> The skeleton is the major store of calcium. Approximately 99% of total body calcium (1 kg) is found in bone. Most of the remainder is in the intracellular compartment, with only a small amount present in extracellular fluid.

Calcium is required for the mineralisation of bone and is a key regulator of many body processes. Calcium ions play critical roles in intracellular signalling, in the regulation of events at the plasma membrane, and in the function of extracellular proteins such as those involved in blood coagulation.

- In blood, virtually all the calcium is found in the plasma with a narrow reference range 2.1–2.6 mmol/l. Adjusted calcium (ACa) levels (i.e. corrected for albumin concentration) are generally reported.

- The free (ionised) calcium is the physiologically important ion and is tightly regulated. The importance of the tight regulation of free calcium is underscored by the recognition that skeletal health is allowed to suffer markedly to allow physiological processes in other organs to be maintained.
- Calcium homeostasis is regulated through multiple interactions between dietary intake of bone minerals and serum levels of homeostatic hormones – principally parathyroid hormone (PTH), vitamin D metabolites and phosphaturic agents, such as osteocyte-secreted fibroblast growth factor 23 (FGF23), acting principally on bone, intestine and kidneys.
- PTH is secreted by the chief cell of the parathyroid glands. A unique calcium receptor on the cell membrane – extracellular calcium-sensing receptor (CaSR) – responds rapidly to changes in serum free (ionised) calcium.

Clinical disorders of calcium metabolism and metabolic bone diseases

> Hypoparathyoridism is the last of the classic endocrine deficiency diseases for which the replacement hormone has become available.

- Osteoporosis – the most prevalent metabolic bone disease and a disorder of skeletal microstructure, usually typified by reduced bone mineral density (BMD), leading to an increased risk of fragility fracture. The therapeutic landscape of osteoporosis continues to evolve, with new antiresorptive and osteoanabolic agents, and is discussed in Chapter 13.
- Disorders of the parathyroid glands – hyperparathyroidism.
  - Primary hyperparathyroidism (PHPT): relatively common disorder characterised, classically, by *hypercalcaemia* and elevated levels of PTH. Even if the PTH is not frankly elevated, its measurable presence is abnormal in the setting of hypercalcaemia.
  - Secondary hyperparathyroidism (SHPT): occurs when the parathyroid glands respond appropriately to a lowering of the serum calcium with increased PTH secretion. The resulting calcium level will be *hypocalcaemic* or low-normal. Most commonly, secondary hyperparathyroidism is associated with chronic kidney or gastrointestinal disorders (e.g. malabsorption of vitamin D).
  - Tertiary hyperparathyroidism (THPT): prolonged secondary hyperparathyroidism can eventually lead to autonomous parathyroid gland PTH secretion resulting in *hypercalcaemia.*
- Disorders of the parathyroid glands – hypoparathyroidism.
  - Hypoparathyroidism occurs when the parathyroid glands are no longer functional because they have all been removed or they have been irreversibly damaged. This is due most commonly to their removal during parathyroid, thyroid or other neck surgery. Less commonly, autoimmune destruction of the parathyroid glands is responsible for the disease. The co-presence of hypocalcaemia and levels of PTH that are undetectable or very low helps to establish the diagnosis. The resultant hypocalcaemia can present as a medical emergency with life-threatening neuromuscular irritability such as laryngeal spasm and seizures. Recent advances in the therapeutic use of PTH in hypoparathyroidism have led to the approval of rhPTH (1-84) as a replacement therapy.
- Vitamin D sufficiency – key physiological requirement for normal bone and mineral metabolism. Vitamin D (calciferol) is used to encompass both its D3 (cholecalciferol) and D2 (ergocalciferol) forms, which undergo a similar metabolism to 25-hydroxyvitamin D (calcidiol) and 1,25 dihydroxyvitamin D (calcitriol). Calcidiol is transported to the kidney, where it is transformed into active calcitriol.
  - Sufficient vitamin D helps to optimise calcium and phosphate absorption. When the vitamin D level is insufficient, for whatever reason, the serum calcium will tend to be in the lower range of normal and the PTH level will rise (i.e. *secondary* hyperparathyroidism). The serum phosphate will also be low/low-normal.
  - The definition of vitamin D insufficiency continues to be a matter of debate, but most experts agree that 25-hydroxyvitamin D levels <75 nmol/l (30 ng/mL) are deficient and should be corrected.

Hypocalcaemia

> Hypocalcaemia (low total plasma calcium, which may be due to a reduction in albumin-bound calcium, the free fraction of calcium, or both)

represents a serious disruption of calcium homeostasis, in which the normal homeostatic mechanisms have been overwhelmed by specific pathological state(s). Chronic hypocalcaemia may be asymptomatic even at very low levels of serum calcium, but severe or acute hypocalcaemia is associated with predictable symptoms and signs.

It is crucial to identify the clinical manifestations of hypocalcaemia, because if present, they indicate symptomatic patients who may require urgent corrective measures.

Vitamin D deficiency has the greatest contribution to hypocalcaemia in the community (although rarely causes symptomatic hypocalcaemia). Hypocalcaemia is a common electrolyte disturbance complicating approximately 15–26% of hospital admissions and up to 88% of critically ill patients admitted to an ICU.

There are many recognised causes in the inpatient setting, such as anterior neck surgery (including thyroid and parathyroid surgery), acute pancreatitis, blood transfusions and numerous medications. However, multiple other drugs and aetiologies can interact to amplify the impact of any principal pathological process. Although much of the acute management is generic, the overall quality of management is greatly enhanced by an appropriate diagnosis.

Diagnostic considerations

Measurement of PTH level is crucial in identifying the underlying cause, as undetectable or inappropriately low levels in the setting of *hypocalcaemia* suggest hypoparathyroidism, whereas high levels confirm physiological PTH response to hypocalcaemia arising from other aetiology (i.e. secondary hyperparathyroidism).

Hypocalcaemia is defined as an ACa level of less than 2.1 mmol/l or a free (ionised) calcium level of less than 1.1 mmol/l. While not delaying the emergency treatment, the finding of acute hypocalcaemia should always prompt biochemical testing to elicit a cause, comprising renal function, PTH, phosphate, alkaline phosphatase, magnesium, bicarbonate and vitamin D levels (Figure 23.4).

Clinical manifestations of hypocalcaemia

The severity of signs and symptoms depends on both the absolute degree of hypocalcaemia (especially free calcium decrease) and the rapidity of its onset, with most features relating to neuromuscular dysfunction.

- Perioral tingling and acral paraesthesia (regions of relative ischaemia/hypoxia) are the earliest symptoms and almost always present in symptomatic cases. In more severe cases, intense, painful spasm of the fingers and toes develops (tetany) and may be sustained for several minutes. In the most severe cases, life-threatening laryngospasm may occur.
- Manoeuvres to detect possible hypocalcaemia include the following.
  - Chvostek's sign describes ipsilateral twitching of the facial muscle groups including the perioral, nasal and ocular regions, when the facial nerve is tapped 2 cm anterior to the earlobe beneath the zygomatic bone. However, perioral twitching is also seen in up to 25% of normal individuals.
  - Trousseau's sign is more sensitive and specific for hypocalcaemia and describes flexion of the wrist and metacarpophalangeal joints, hyperextension of the fingers and flexion of the thumb producing a characteristic deformity known as *main d'accoucheur*. It is elicited by occluding the brachial artery 20 mmHg above systolic pressure for three minutes and is positive in only 1% of normocalcaemic patients.
- The electrocardiographic (ECG) hallmark of hypocalcaemia is prolongation of the corrected QT interval (QTc), the duration of which is proportional to the degree of hypocalcaemia. The more prolonged the QTc interval, the more likely an arrhythmia. The most common arrhythmia associated with prolonged QTc is *torsade de pointes* which, if untreated, can progress to ventricular fibrillation and cardiac arrest.

A full medical history and 'head-to-toe' examination may not only elicit signs of hypocalcaemia, but also help differentiate acute from chronic, syndromic from non-syndromic hypocalcaemia, and will usually signpost other underlying diagnoses.

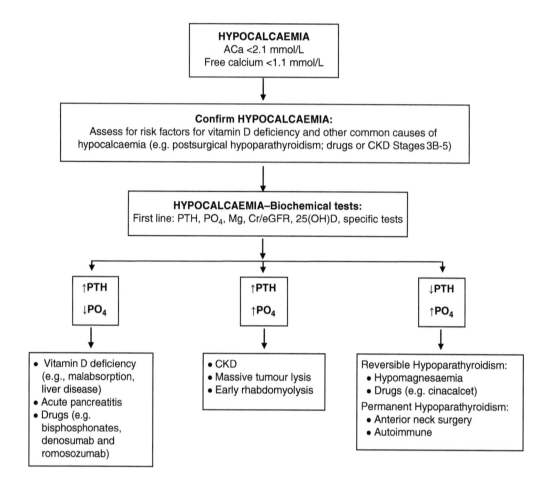

Figure 23.4 Clinical approach to investigation of causes of hypocalcaemia. 25(OH)D, 25-hydroxyvitamin D; ACa, adjusted corrected calcium; CKD, chronic kidney disease; Cr, creatinine; eGFR, estimated glomerular filtration rate; Mg, magnesium; PO_4, phosphate; PTH, parathyroid hormone.

Acute intervention

> Hypocalcaemia with neurological, muscular or cardiac dysfunction is associated with significant morbidity and mortality and should be managed as a medical emergency.

Once severe hypocalcaemia is recognised, the patient should be managed in an appropriate emergency setting such as an AMU, ECU, HDU or ICU. Prompt assessment and management of the ABCDEs should occur.

- Symptomatic patients (e.g. tetany, seizures, laryngospasm or cardiac arrhythmias or dysfunction) or those with ACa <2 mmol/l or free (ionised) calcium <1 mmol/l should prompt emergency intervention with IV calcium replacement (with ECG monitoring). Calcium levels should be carefully monitored (usually at least 4–6 hourly). IV calcium should be continued until the patient is receiving an effective regimen of oral calcium and vitamin D.

It is important to evaluate and treat the underlying cause(s).

- In postoperative parathyroid-related hypocalcaemia (e.g. total thyroidectomy, parathyroid surgery or anterior neck surgery for cancer) and other cases of hypoparathyroidism, undetectable or inappropriately low PTH levels in the context of hypocalcaemia are consistent with the diagnosis (e.g. PTH levels are usually checked 4–24 hours post thyroid surgery to assess the risk of permanent hypoparathyroidism developing). Treatment consists of calcium and vitamin D analogues (e.g. alfacalcidol or calcitriol) acutely. PTH (1-34) and PTH (1-84) therapies also have an evolving role in this setting.

- Hypomagnesaemia should always be corrected as it causes inhibition of PTH secretion as well as resistance to its action; correction of hypocalcaemia may be difficult with uncorrected hypomagnesaemia. The underlying cause(s) of hypomagnesaemia should also be diagnosed and managed (e.g. PPIs should always be stopped if possible and a diuretic replaced with alternative agents wherever feasible).

> Effective chronic care of the hypocalcaemic patient is an important opportunity to prevent/reduce further acute presentations related to both hypocalcaemia and iatrogenic hypercalcaemia.

Hypercalcaemia

> Hypercalcaemia (serum calcium >2.6 mmol/l, measured on at least two occasions) affects about 0.5% of hospitalised patients. It is usually well tolerated if ACa levels are <3.0 mmol/l. ACa above this threshold is associated with nephrogenic DI, increasingly severe volume contraction, neurological, cardiac and gastrointestinal dysfunction, and requires urgent treatment to prevent life-threatening consequences. Severe hypercalcaemia is defined as a total serum calcium >3.5 mmol/l.

Primary hyperparathyroidism and malignancy are the aetiologies in 90% of cases of hypercalcaemia. At least one of the following mechanisms is involved in the pathophysiology of hypercalcaemia.

- Increased intestinal calcium absorption.
- Increased bone resorption.

- Increased renal calcium reabsorption or decreased calcium excretion.

The final common pathway for many types of severe hypercalcaemia is increased mobilisation of calcium from bone due in part to activation of osteoclasts by the RANK/RANKL pathway.

Diagnostic considerations

> Measurement of intact PTH level is pivotal in the differential diagnosis of calcium disorders. The causes of hypercalcaemia can be conveniently divided into those associated with an elevated or inappropriately normal PTH level, and those where PTH output is appropriately suppressed.

In an ambulatory population, PHPT accounts for most detected hypercalcaemia (>90%). PHPT is often characterised by increased secretion of PTH that results in hypercalcaemia.

- Inappropriate autonomous PTH secretion is found in the context of parathyroid adenomas which may be solitary (80–85% of cases) or multiple. Parathyroid adenomas are most commonly sporadic but may be part of an endocrine neoplastic syndrome, especially if numerous or found in the young, such as multiple endocrine neoplasia type 1 (MEN1), MEN2A (MEN2) and MEN4. Hereditary forms of PHPT occur in 5–10% overall, including syndromic (i.e. associated with other glands and systems) and non-syndromic types, but can be even higher in younger patients or with atypical features (e.g. age less than 45 years, multi-gland involvement, parathyroid carcinoma).
- Parathyroid hyperplasia without an obvious physiological stimulus can also occur, and usually involves all four glands (~15% of PHPT).
- Rarely, parathyroid carcinoma may occur (<1% of PHPT cases).

Hypercalcaemia of malignancy (HCM) complicates 5–30% of malignancies and is the most common cause of inpatient hypercalcaemic crises (>50%). Hypercalcaemia secondary to malignancy usually presents in the context of advanced, clinically obvious disease and portends an ominous prognosis with survival typically in the order of months (see Chapter 26).

Between 5% and 15% of patients with hypercalcaemia and malignancy have co-existing primary hyperparathyroidism.

Acute intervention

Once severe hypercalcaemia is recognised, the patient should be managed in an appropriate emergency setting such as an AMU, ECU, HDU or ICU. Prompt assessment and management of the ABCDEs should occur.

- The acute management of hypercalcaemia will depend on a number of factors, including severity of symptoms, co-morbidities that may affect treatment options, and the patient's prognosis.
- For treatment of severe hypercalcaemia, the underlying cause should be identified and multitargeted therapies should be started as soon as possible.
- In malignancy-related severe hypercalcaemia, it may be appropriate to adopt a palliative approach that will emphasise comfort care and symptom control.

General supportive care

- The cornerstone of acute management of hypercalcaemia is fluid resuscitation with correction of the volume state. Appropriate fluid administration should depend on an assessment of volume depletion, but in most situations of hypercalcaemic crises, 500–1000 ml of IV 0.9% saline should be given over the first hour, and 3–6 litres (i.e. 125–250 ml/h) over the first 24 hours. This regimen should be continued for 1–3 days with careful monitoring of cardiac status and total body hydration.
- Any possible agents causing hypercalcaemia should be discontinued as soon as possible.
- Immobilisation promotes osteoclastic bone resorption so early ambulation should be encouraged whenever possible.
- Dietary calcium restriction is only rarely warranted in patients with vitamin D/vitamin D metabolite/vitamin D analogue-dependent hypercalcaemia.

Calcium-specific treatments

- The most effective antiresorptive agents are as follows.
  - Bisphosphonates (e.g. zoledronate): IV bisphosphonates should be administered as soon as possible following rehydration. Due to the long duration of effect of these agents, second doses are usually not required for some time (at least 7–14 days).
  - Denosumab: very effective, including for bisphosphonate-resistant HCM.
- Glucocorticoids can also be used for vitamin D-related hypercalcaemia (e.g. vitamin D overdose, granulomatous disorders) and in certain malignancies (e.g. myeloma).
- If the diagnosis is PHPT, then surgical removal of parathyroid adenoma(s) should be planned. If surgical intervention is not an option or is delayed, a calcimimetic (cinacalcet – stimulates the CaSR) can be used to lower calcium levels.
- For HCM, further therapy will be determined by the diagnosis, extent of the disease and overall prognosis. Definitive treatment of a primary solid tumour with expression of PTHrP may prevent further hypercalcaemic events.
- Consider dialysis in refractory cases with/without renal failure or fluid overload.

Adrenal disorders

The adrenal glands are small, bilateral structures that weigh approximately 5 g each and lie retroperitoneally at the apex of each kidney.

- The medulla or inner portion of the gland (which constitutes approximately 10% of each adrenal) secretes epinephrine (adrenaline) and norepinephrine (noradrenaline) and is part of the sympathetic nervous system.
- The cortex forms the bulk of the adrenal gland (approximately 90%) and is responsible for secreting three types of hormones: glucocorticoids, mineralocorticoids and adrenal androgens.
- Because adrenaline and noradrenaline can also be derived from non-adrenal sources (e.g. noradrenaline from the sympathetic nervous system and mesentery), adrenal medullary function is not essential for life, but adrenal cortical function is.

If untreated, the total loss of adrenal cortical function is fatal in 4–14 days.

Adrenal hormones

> Cortisol (principal glucocorticoid), aldosterone (principal mineralocorticoid) and adrenal androgens constitute the major hormones produced by the adrenal cortex.

The secretion of both glucocorticoids and adrenal androgens is controlled by ACTH secreted by corticotrophs in the anterior pituitary gland, as part of the HPA axis. The glucocorticoid hormones, mainly cortisol, are synthesised in the zona fasciculata and zona reticularis of the adrenal cortex. Both ACTH and cortisol display a circadian variation, with peaks before awakening in the morning and troughs late at night. In the circulation, about 80% of cortisol is bound to cortisol-binding globulin (CBG) and nearly 15% to albumin, with only around 5% being free and bioavailable.

Glucocorticoids influence a vast array of cellular activities in different cell types. They orchestrate responses to stress and are key mediators of physiological and behavioural adaptations to injury and illness. Cortisol and other glucocorticoids stimulate gluconeogenesis (glucose production) by the liver. They also have anti-inflammatory and immune functions.

The mineralocorticoids play an essential role in regulating potassium and sodium levels and water balance. They are produced in the zona glomerulosa (outer layer of cells) of the adrenal cortex. The mineralocorticoids are controlled predominantly by the renin-angiotensin system.

Common adrenal disorders

- Adrenal insufficiency – there are two forms: primary and secondary.
  - Primary adrenal insufficiency (also termed Addison disease) is caused by the inability of the adrenal cortex to produce enough glucocorticoids and/or mineralocorticoids (e.g. due to autoimmune-mediated or other destruction of adrenocortical tissue).
  - Secondary adrenal insufficiency (central hypoadrenalism) results from deficient adrenal glucocorticoid production (mineralocorticoid axis intact), because of ACTH deficiency due to impairment of HPA (i.e. hypopituitarism). The most common cause of secondary adrenal insufficiency is chronic exogenous glucocorticoid treatment.

- Acute adrenal insufficiency (also termed adrenal crisis) is a life-threatening endocrine emergency.
  - Adrenal crisis is brought about by lack of production of the adrenal hormone cortisol and/or mineralocorticoids.
  - It presents with marked symptoms and signs and characteristic laboratory abnormalities, and requires immediate treatment.
  - The severity of this condition is related to the central role of these hormones in energy, salt and fluid homeostasis.
- Cushing syndrome is defined by long-standing exposure to supraphysiological levels of circulating glucocorticoids.
  - The most common cause of Cushing syndrome is the exogenous administration of glucocorticoids for medical reasons. Glucocorticoid-induced adverse drug reaction with secondary (sometimes called tertiary) HPA suppression now contributes to morbidity and premature mortality in the 1–3% or so of Western populations taking exogenous steroids.
  - Endogenous Cushing syndrome can be divided into:
    - *ACTH-dependent* types – Cushing disease (ACTH-secreting pituitary adenoma) is more prevalent (80–85%) compared to ectopic Cushing syndrome (usually caused by a neuroendocrine tumour secreting ACTH)
    - *ACTH-independent* types – unilateral or bilateral cortisol-secreting adenomas are most common (60%), compared with cortisol-secreting adrenocortical carcinoma (40%).
- Phaeochromocytoma – rare neuroendocrine tumour.
  - Traditionally, phaeochromocytomas were known by the 'rule of 10', as 10% were thought to be inherited. Currently, we think that about one-half (50%) of all cases of phaeochromocytomas are hereditary, meaning that the tumours form because of an underlying inherited alteration in a single gene.
  - Recommended tests for diagnosis of phaeochromocytoma include plasma or urinary fractionated metanephrines and normetanephrines. Biochemical testing for phaeochromocytoma is indicated not only in symptomatic patients, but also in patients with adrenal incidentalomas or identified genetic predispositions (e.g. MEN2 and 3).
  - Most common presentation is with paroxysmal episodes of headaches, sweating, palpitations and hypertension (including hypertensive urgencies and emergencies).

o Emergencies arising from hypertensive crises due to phaeochromocytoma can be particularly dangerous. Although the overall mortality rate of a phaeochromocytoma crisis is 15%, patients presenting with acute cardiovascular complications have even a higher mortality rate. Hypertensive emergencies in patients with phaeochromocytoma are best treated with IV infusions of rapidly acting alpha-adrenergic receptor antagonists such as phentolamine, but sodium nitroprusside or nicardipine are reasonable alternatives. Clevidipine, an ultra-short-acting IV dihydropyridine calcium channel blocker, is also an option.

Adrenal incidentalomas – previously unsuspected adrenal lesion (≥1 cm in diameter) discovered on an imaging study for an unrelated reason – occur in 5% of people. The important questions to ask are as follows.

- Is this lesion malignant?
  - o Best answered with CT adrenal imaging phenotype or MRI chemical shift analysis and size (if <4 cm less likely).
  - o If adrenal incidentaloma >4 cm or worrisome imaging phenotype (e.g. >20 Hounsfield units on unenhanced CT), surgical removal may be indicated after further investigations (including ruling out phaeochromocytoma) and shared decision making with patient.
- Is it functioning (i.e. secreting hormones)?
  - o Exclude phaeochromocytoma with plasma or urinary metanephrines/normetanephrines.
  - o Exclude Cushing syndrome with overnight 1 mg dexamethasone suppression test (DST). Mild autonomous cortisol secretion (MACS) is found in up to 50% of patients with incidentaloma. Possible when serum cortisol >50 nmol/l post 1 mg DST and *no* clinical features of Cushing syndrome. Need further testing such as midnight salivary cortisol or 24-hour urine cortisol. Close follow-up important as associated with frailty and increased cardiometabolic morbidities.
  - o Exclude Conn syndrome (primary hyperaldosteronism) if hypertensive. Measure plasma renin/aldosterone ratio (ideally off certain antihypertensive medications).
- If benign imaging phenotype (e.g. <4 cm and an attenuation of 10 Hounsfield units or less on CT evaluation) and biochemical results negative – generally does not warrant intervention or long-term follow-up.
- All other adrenal incidentalomas with indeterminate features on imaging may warrant additional imaging and follow-up.

Other endocrine incidentalomas.

- Pituitary incidentaloma – 10% of unselected pituitaries (meaning those from individuals without suspected pituitary disease) examined at autopsy have an unknown pituitary lesion. Can also be discovered on an imaging study for an unrelated reason (e.g. head trauma).
- Thyroid incidentalomas – commonly detected during routine and emergency imaging for non-thyroidal presentations (e.g. CT chest for suspicious lung lesion). The work-up is similar to other incidentalomas.
  - o Is it malignant? First step would be to get a thyroid ultrasound to confirm lesion and imaging phenotype. If worrying imaging phenotype, get FNA and cytology.
  - o Is it functioning or causing local damage? Get TFTs (i.e. TSH, FT4 and FT3).

Adrenal insufficiency

A National Patient Safety Alert (NatPSA) to support early recognition and treatment of adrenal crisis in adults was implemented across England in 2021. This was prompted by deaths and incidents of severe harm affecting patients with adrenal insufficiency deemed 'preventable in most, if not all, cases'.

Acute adrenal insufficiency, also termed adrenal crisis, is a life-threatening endocrine emergency brought about by lack of production of the adrenal hormone cortisol, the major glucocorticoid. It is either *primary*, due to loss of function of the adrenal gland itself, or *secondary* due to hypopituitarism. However, pituitary regulation of cortisol production is also switched off in patients who receive chronic exogenous glucocorticoid treatment (i.e. doses ≥5 mg prednisolone daily or equivalent for more than four weeks).

Clinical assessment

It is crucial to recognise clinical features suggestive of adrenal insufficiency, because if present, they identify symptomatic patients who may require urgent corrective measures. The severity of signs and symptoms depends both on the absolute degree of glucocorticoid and mineralocorticoid deficiency and the rapidity of its onset.

It is important to ask patients, relatives or healthcare providers about any relevant history, including any exposure to steroid therapy in any formulation, including over-the-counter (OTC) agents. Any previous HPA disorders and treatment should also be explored. Family history may also be useful (e.g. autoimmune conditions and rarer disorders). It is also imperative to elicit any signs of previous steroid exposure resulting in Cushingoid phenotype that may result in HPA suppression. Check for MedicAlert® jewellery (or tattoos!) and steroid emergency cards, and medication reconciliation is also valuable. Manifestations of the primary pathological disorder can also be present (e.g. vitiligo in autoimmune disorders).

The clinical findings of primary adrenal insufficiency are mainly based on the deficiency of glucocorticoids and mineralocorticoids and the resultant weight loss, abdominal tenderness and guarding; fever; orthostatic hypotension with dizziness due to dehydration (≥20 mmHg drop in BP from supine to standing position) and in severe cases hypovolaemic shock; confusion, somnolence, delirium and coma; electrolyte changes; and hypoglycaemia (Table 23.5). Enhanced secretion of ACTH and other pro-opiomelanocortin-derived peptides (e.g. melanocyte-stimulating hormone, MSH) often leads to the characteristic hyperpigmentation of the skin and mucous membranes. The skin looks bronzed or suntanned in exposed and unexposed areas, and the normal creases and pressure points tend to become especially dark (Figure 23.5). The gums and oral mucous membranes may become bluish-black.

Hyperpigmentation occurs in more than 90% of persons with Addison disease and is helpful in distinguishing the primary and secondary forms of adrenal insufficiency.

Table 23.5 **Clinical findings of adrenal insufficiency**

Finding	Primary (%)	Secondary (%)
Anorexia and weight loss	Yes (100)	Yes (100)
Fatigue and weakness	Yes (100)	Yes (100)
Gastrointestinal symptoms, nausea, vomiting	Yes (50)	Yes (50)
Myalgia, arthralgia	Yes (10)	Yes (10)
Orthostatic hypotension	Yes	Yes
Hyponatraemia	Yes (85–90)	Yes (60)
Hyperkalaemia	Yes (60–65)	No
Hyperpigmentation	Yes (>90)	No
Secondary deficiencies of gonadal, GH, thyroxine and ADH may occur	No	Yes
Associated autoimmune conditions	Yes	No

The numbers are representative; some symptoms and signs can be subtle. In acute adrenal crisis, these symptoms and signs can be more common and pronounced (e.g. abdominal pain ~90%, with abdominal rigidity or rebound tenderness in ~20%).

(a)

(b)

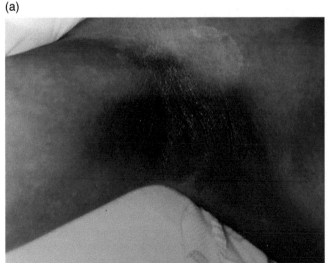
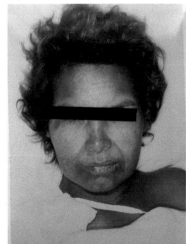

Figure 23.5 Clinical features in primary adrenal insufficiency. (a) Hyperpigmented axilla with no axillary hair (due to loss of adrenal androgens). (b) Hyperpigmented facies.

The clinical findings of secondary adrenal insufficiency due to central hypoadrenalism may lead to dehydration, hyponatraemia (due to dilution and *not* mineralocorticoid deficiency) and shock, unresponsive to fluid resuscitation and vasopressor therapy before glucocorticoid replacement is administered. Vasopressin deficiency causes central DI, which may become clinically apparent only after the initiation of glucocorticoid replacement therapies as a result of improvements in renal haemodynamics, glomerular filtration rate and free water clearance. Notably absent are skin and mucosal hyperpigmentation as well as hyperkalaemia (in contrast to patients with Addison disease). Other features of hypopituitarism may be apparent.

Diagnostic testing of adrenal insufficiency

> The increased requirements for cortisol during physiological stress make it crucially important not to miss a diagnosis of adrenal insufficiency in acute and critically ill patients. However, *diagnostic measures should never delay prompt treatment of suspected adrenal crisis.*

The initial laboratory evaluation of patients should include a determination of plasma glucose, urea, creatinine, electrolytes, urinalysis, full blood count with differential and CRP (if indicated). TFTs should be performed (acute adrenal insufficiency can increase TSH, so do not replace with thyroxine if TSH ≤10 mU/l – and only then *after* glucocorticoid is started). An ECG, chest X-ray, and urine and blood cultures should also be considered where co-morbidity is possible (sepsis is the most common precipitant, although poor adherence to chronic glucocorticoid therapy and failure to observe 'sick day rules' are also common). Other investigations are performed as warranted by the clinical situation (e.g. cardiac troponins, serum lactate, appropriate imaging).

Specific investigations targeting the HPA axis for suspected adrenal insufficiency or adrenal crisis are only needed in patients *without* a prior diagnosis of adrenal insufficiency; those with a pre-existing diagnosis should have general investigations as needed and be treated promptly.

The acute laboratory assessment of the HPA axis is generally limited to measuring cortisol and ACTH. The short ACTH stimulation test (IV or IM 250 μg synthetic ACTH) is used to assess only the adrenal response (of the HPA axis). A cortisol of >450 nmol/l either 30 min or 60 min after short ACTH stimulation testing excludes adrenal insufficiency. A baseline plasma ACTH >2-fold the upper limit of normal is consistent with primary adrenal insufficiency.

Diagnosing the underlying cause in all patients with confirmed primary adrenal insufficiency should include a validated assay of autoantibodies against 21-hydroxylase. In autoantibody-negative individuals, other causes should be sought. Young males and males without autoantibodies should be screened for adrenoleucodystrophy by measuring very long chain fatty acids. Adrenal insufficiency may be the only presenting sign of adrenoleucodystrophy. In antibody-negative cases, CT scan of the adrenals should be performed to identify infectious diseases such as tuberculosis and tumours.

Diagnosing the underlying cause in all patients with confirmed secondary adrenal insufficiency should be as per the hypopituitarism work-up already described.

Treatment of acute adrenal insufficiency

This could be in the ambulatory setting (e.g. same-day emergency care) for selected cases of mild adrenal insufficiency/crisis. However, most patients will be hospitalised and managed in an emergency care setting. Prompt assessment and management of the ABCDEs should occur.

Supportive care includes inserting large-bore IV cannulae and starting appropriate IV fluid resuscitation, electrolyte replacement, nutritional support including monitoring and maintaining blood glucose (BG) levels, continuous cardiac monitoring and pulse oximetry. Co-morbidities should be treated appropriately. It is also imperative to exclude unknown pregnancy by performing a pregnancy test in appropriate patients. All patients with adrenal crisis should receive low molecular weight heparin (LMWH) or similar for the full duration of admission unless contraindicated.

For acute adrenal insufficiency or crisis, the '5 Ss' of management should be followed: (a) **S**alt replacement (i.e. normal 0.9% saline); (b) **S**ugar replacement (i.e. 5% or 10% dextrose); (c) **S**teroid replacement (i.e. glucocorticoid +/- mineralocorticoid); (d) **S**upportive care; and (e) **S**eek and treat precipitants (e.g. infection is the most common precipitant). Where available, the endocrine inpatient team should be involved as early as is practical after admission.

Treatment of adrenal crisis requires immediate bolus injection of 100 mg hydrocortisone IV or IM followed by continuous IV infusion of 200 mg hydrocortisone per 24 h (alternatively 50 mg hydrocortisone IM or IV injection every 6 h). Rehydration with rapid IV isotonic saline infusion followed by further IV rehydration as required (usually 4–6 l in 24 h; monitor for fluid overload).

Oral hydrocortisone replacement therapy can be resumed once the saline infusion has been discontinued and the patient is taking food and fluids by mouth. Mineralocorticoid therapy is not required when large amounts of hydrocortisone are being given, but as the dose is reduced, it usually is necessary to add fludrocortisone (primary adrenal insufficiency only).

Patients should be educated about stress dosing and equipped with a steroid emergency card and glucocorticoid preparation for parenteral emergency administration.

All adults with adrenal insufficiency should be evaluated by an endocrinologist at least annually for symptoms and signs of over- and underreplacement. For those patients with autoimmune primary adrenal insufficiency, screening for other autoimmune diseases known to be more prevalent in this population should also occur.

Diabetes mellitus

> Diabetes mellitus is traditionally viewed as a chronic, *progressive* disease characterised by hyperglycaemia in the absence of treatment. More recently, a paradigm shift has occurred with new treatment approaches to type 2 diabetes, such as nutritional (e.g. very low calorie diet), novel glucose-lowering therapies (e.g. glucagon-like peptide-1 receptor agonists and dual glucose-dependent insulinotropic polypeptide/glucagon-like peptide-1 receptor agonists), and bariatric (metabolic) surgery – all leading to potentially *reversible* diabetes (i.e. induction of *diabetes remission*).

Diabetes is a common disorder, with 90–95% designated as type 2 diabetes mellitus (T2DM), 5–10% as type 1 diabetes mellitus (T1DM) and about 2–3% as rarer types of diabetes. Most T2DM cases (>90%) are linked to obesity ('diabesity'). In 2021, the International Diabetes Federation estimated that approximately 537 million adults (20–79 years) are living with diabetes, and this is projected to rise to 783 million by 2045. More than 5 million people in the UK have diabetes.

The increasing prevalence is a particular issue for in-hospital care as the prevalence of diabetes in the inpatient setting is even greater than in the community. People with diabetes account for nearly one-fifth of all inpatients in English and Welsh hospitals (in some hospitals over a quarter of beds are used by people with diabetes); of these, up to 90% are admitted as an emergency. Most are admitted for a reason other than diabetes, with only ~10% requiring admission for a diabetes-specific cause.

Hyperglycaemia in hospitalised patients is associated with adverse outcomes, including increased mortality, morbidity, length of stay, infections and other complications. Numerous studies have shown that improved in-hospital glycaemic control decreases the rate of complications across all acute care settings.

Insulin administration is generally the preferred way to control hyperglycaemia in hospitalised patients (Endocrine Society 2022 guidelines). However, hypoglycaemia is the main limiting factor of insulin therapy and improving glycaemic control. As with hyperglycaemia, inpatient hypoglycaemia is also associated with poor inpatient outcomes and healthcare costs. Thus, the overall goal of inpatient glycaemic management focuses on treating hyperglycaemia to individualised glycaemic targets associated with reduction/prevention of complications while avoiding hypoglycaemia and its associated morbidity. This may include continuing non-insulin glucose-lowering agents which are widely used but require close monitoring, especially in unwell patients where insulin is usually preferred.

The NHS spends at least £10 billion a year on diabetes, which is about 10% of its entire budget. Almost 80% of the money the NHS spends on diabetes is on treating complications (Table 23.6). With declining mortality from vascular disease, which once accounted for more than 50% of deaths amongst people with diabetes mellitus, cancer and dementia now comprise the leading causes of death in people with diabetes mellitus in some countries or regions.

Criteria for the diagnosis of diabetes

> Glucose should be measured in *all unwell* patients presenting to Acute Medicine services.

Table 23.6 Complications related to diabetes

Acute.
- Severe hyperglycaemia, DKA and hyperosmolar hyperglycaemic state (HHS).
- Hypoglycaemia.
- Other related issues such as infection (including worse severity and increased mortality with COVID-19), electrolyte disturbance and acute kidney injury.

Chronic (up to 50% of persons with diabetes may have already developed at least one diabetes complication by the time they are diagnosed).
- Macrovascular (>50% of T2DM patients die of macrovascular complications).
  - Coronary artery disease (CAD)
  - Cerebrovascular disease (stroke)
  - Peripheral arterial disease (PAD)
  - Heart failure
- Microvascular.
  - Nephropathy
  - Retinopathy
  - Neuropathy
- Combined – diabetic foot disease and amputation
- Many others (examples)
  - Cancer
  - Non-alcoholic fatty liver disease (NAFLD)
  - Dementia

Box 23.6 Diagnostic criteria for diabetes

Fasting plasma glucose (FPG) ≥7.0 mmol/l

OR

2-h plasma glucose ≥11.1 mmol/l during 75 g oral glucose tolerance test (OGTT)

OR

Glycosylated haemoglobin (HbA1c) ≥6.5% (≥48 mmol/mol)

OR

Classic diabetes symptoms + random plasma glucose ≥11.1 mmol/l (or hyperglycaemic crisis)

Diagnostic criteria for diabetes are outlined in Box 23.6. Typical symptoms of uncontrolled hyperglycaemia include the '3Ps' – polydipsia, polyuria and polyphagia; weight loss, fatigue, blurred vision (due to osmotic effects of sorbitol accumulation in lens), and frequent infections due to white cell and other immune dysfunction.

Stress hyperglycaemia

Hyperglycaemia in patients presenting to Acute Medicine can be seen in three main scenarios: (a) patients with previously known diabetes; (b) patients with undiagnosed diabetes at presentation; and (c) patients with stress-induced hyperglycaemia. The latter two groups can be differentiated by measuring HbA1c on admission; group (b) will have HbA1c ≥6.5% (≥48 mmol/mol) whereas group (c) will have HbA1c <6.5% (<48 mmol/mol). The risk of mortality and complications correlates with the severity of hyperglycaemia, with higher risk in patients *without* a history of diabetes, i.e. groups (b) and (c).

Inpatient hyperglycaemia is often defined as a BG ≥7.8 mmol/l at any time during the hospitalisation in patients with or without diabetes (Endocrine Society 2022 guidelines). Stress-induced hyperglycaemia refers to a transient elevation of BG occurring during acute illnesses (e.g. surgery, infections), that resolves spontaneously after the acute insult dissipates (Figure 23.6). Although stress hyperglycaemia typically resolves as the acute illness or surgical stress abates, it is important to identify and follow these patients as the majority will convert to confirmed diabetes within a few years. Individuals who develop stress-induced hyperglycaemia should be treated just as aggressively as people with known diabetes, because their risk of complications is even higher than those with prior diagnosis.

Classification of diabetes

- Type 1 diabetes (5–10% of all diabetes): beta-cell failure due to autoimmune beta-cell destruction leading to *absolute* insulin deficiency (i.e. need insulin to survive).
- Type 2 diabetes (90–95% of all diabetes): progressive insulin secretory defect (beta-cell dysfunction) associated with insulin resistance (i.e. impaired biological response to insulin).
- Secondary types of diabetes.
  - Genetic defects in beta-cell function or insulin action (1–3% of all diabetes).
  - Diseases of the exocrine pancreas (e.g. pancreatitis; cystic fibrosis-related diabetes).
  - Drug or chemical induced (e.g. glucocorticoids).
- Gestational diabetes mellitus (GDM): diabetes diagnosed in the second or third trimester of

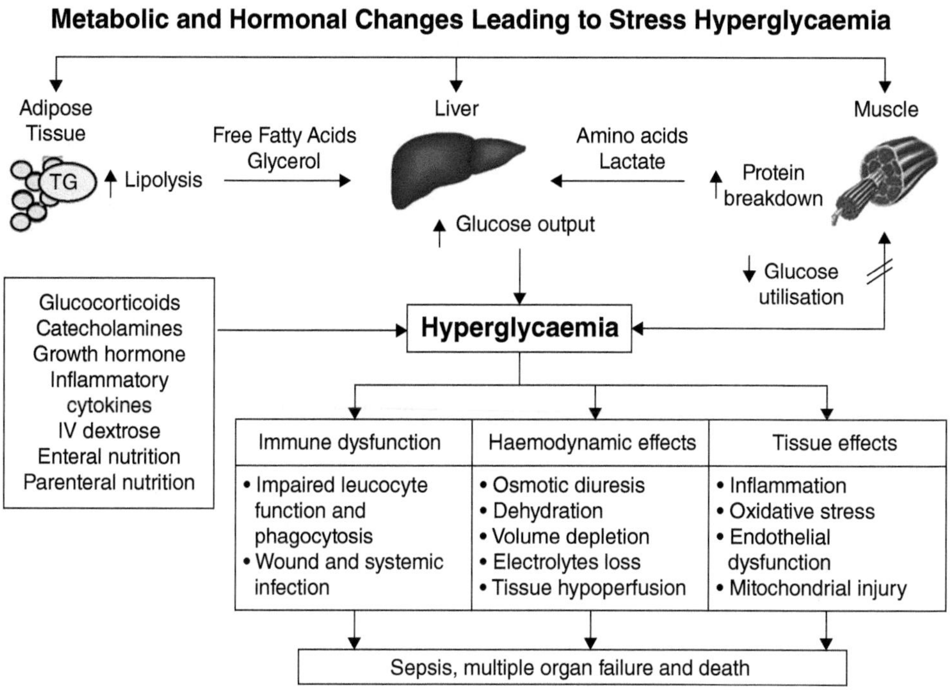

Metabolic and Hormonal Changes Leading to Stress Hyperglycaemia

Figure 23.6 Pathophysiology of hyperglycaemia and its complications in hospitalised patients. Source: Matfin G. Endocrine and Metabolic Endocrine Emergencies, 2nd edn. Chichester: Wiley, 2018.

pregnancy that was not clearly overt diabetes prior to gestation and that is not clearly other forms of diabetes (e.g. T1DM or T2DM).

Differentiating T1DM from other types of diabetes in the acute care setting

Make an initial diagnosis of T1DM on clinical grounds in adults presenting with hyperglycaemia. Although T1DM in children and young adults is usually straightforward to diagnose, misdiagnosis occurs in ~40% of adults with new T1DM.

Consider the **AABBCC** approach.

- **A**ge (e.g. <35 years think T1DM).
- **A**utoimmunity (personal or family history of autoimmune disease or polyglandular autoimmune syndromes).
- **B**ody habitus (e.g. body mass index <25).
- **B**ackground (e.g. family history of T1DM).
- **C**ontrol – is glucose poorly controlled on non-insulin therapies?
- **C**o-morbidities (e.g. if patient has cancer treated with ICIs, this can cause acute autoimmune T1DM).

> **Box 23.7 Severe hyperglycaemia**
>
> - Significant hyperglycaemia, e.g.:
>   - HbA1c ≥9–10% (75–86 mmol/mol) and/or
>   - FPG >14 mmol/l and/or
>   - random plasma glucose >16.7 mmol/l.
> - Catabolic symptoms: sudden persistent weight loss, 3Ps.

Whenever a patient presents with severe hyperglycaemia (Box 23.7), treat with insulin if there is diagnostic confusion about whether it is T1DM or T2DM or other rarer forms of diabetes such as maturity-onset diabetes of the young (MODY). Severe hyperglycaemia can escalate into the potentially fatal complications of DKA and HHS. The diagnosis can be revisited at subsequent clinical reviews. Carry out further investigations if there is uncertainty. Measure at least two different diabetes-specific autoantibodies – such as islet cell cytoplasmic autoantibodies (ICA), glutamic acid decarboxylase autoantibodies (GAD65), insulinoma-associated-2 autoantibodies (IA2), or zinc transporter-8 autoantibodies (ZnT8). Seek expert advice.

For people aged ≥60 presenting with weight loss and new-onset diabetes, follow recommendations on assessing for *pancreatic cancer*.

Glycaemic control

> Intensive glucose-lowering therapy with improved glycaemic control can lead to reduced microvascular (and to a lesser degree macrovascular) complications. Glycaemic goals should be individualised, less tight goals may be reasonable based on a benefit–risk assessment (e.g. age of patient, life expectancy, co-morbidities such as cardiovascular disease, chronic kidney disease, dementia).

Hypoglycaemia is a significant cost burden and the major limiting factor for short- and long-term improved glycaemic control in persons with diabetes. Subsequently, BG goals should be modified in patients with frequent hypoglycaemia or hypoglycaemia unawareness (i.e. threshold for initiation of counterregulatory hormone responses to hypoglycaemia is reduced to a lower BG level and hormone responses become blunted).

Intensive glycaemic control (if it can be achieved safely) is important shortly after diagnosis to take advantage of the *legacy effect* (metabolic memory). The legacy effect is the long-term beneficial effect of the *initial* good glycaemic control on subsequent disease outcomes or complications, even after a long duration of more mediocre glycaemic control (potentially decades). It is probably related to epigenetic effects.

Monitoring glycaemic control

> Glycaemic control is assessed by the HbA1c measurement, continuous glucose monitoring (CGM) using either time in range (TIR) and/or glucose management indicator (GMI), and BG monitoring (BGM). In stable patients, measurement of HbA1c or GMI and TIR should take place at least twice yearly. In poorly controlled patients or when therapies are changing, glucose monitoring should be performed more often. BGM and CGM can be monitored at any time by the person with diabetes and shared virtually or otherwise with the healthcare professional.

Glycaemic control is assessed by the following methods.

- BGM – usually measured pre-meal and bedtime although can be measured at any time.
  - BG target: generally between 4 and 7 mmol/l pre-meals. Higher at bedtime.
  - In-hospital BG target: 6–10 mmol/l for most patients (and acceptable up to 12 mmol/l) in medical and critical care settings.
- HbA1c measurement – reflects average glycaemia over preceding ~2–3 months (i.e. lifespan of red blood cell). Limitations to the use of HbA1c for making therapeutic decisions.
  - Red blood cell issues: anaemia, haemoglobinopathies.
  - Ethnic differences (HbA1c ~0.4% higher in black people due to increased biological glycosylation irrespective of ambient BG levels).
  - Does not provide a measure of glycaemic variability (associated with increased risk of complications and hypoglycaemia), postprandial glucose (PPG) or hypoglycaemia.
- CGM using either:
  - TIR *and/or*
  - GMI: reflects average glycaemia over last ~2–4 weeks (like a HbA1c but shorter time-frame).

Continuous glucose monitoring

Continuous glucose monitoring consists of a sensor, transmitter and receiver (i.e. pump, phone, handheld receiver). The sensor measures glucose levels in interstitial fluid, whereas BG meters measure glucose in blood. CGM usage leads to fewer highs and fewer lows. CGM comes in two forms.

- Real-time CGM (rtCGM) – system automatically transmits data to the receiver and/or smartphone.
- Intermittently scanned CGM (isCGM) – system requires a person to 'swipe' the receiver and/or smartphone close to the sensor to obtain current and historical sensor glucose data ('flash glucose monitoring').

Continuous glucose monitoring provides continuous estimates, direction and magnitude of glucose trends that allow persons with diabetes to achieve their overall glycaemic targets as they avoid the acute complications of hypoglycaemia and hyperglycaemia. The National Institute for Health and Care Excellence (NICE 2022) has recommended offering *all* adults with T1DM a choice of rtCGM or isCGM, based on individual preferences.

Standardised glucose reports with visual cues such as the ambulatory glucose profile (AGP) facilitate more rapid, better informed decision making. Consider the **DATAA** approach to reviewing AGP data (**D**ownload data – is it adequate to make decisions?; **A**ssess safety – focus on hypoglycaemia initially; **T**IR – focus on positives; **A**reas to improve; **A**ction plan – collaborative, shared decision making). TIR is the key measure which is being widely adopted (Box 23.8).

Glycaemic monitoring in the acutely unwell patient

Measurement of HbA1c is recommended in all patients with diabetes who have not had one within the last three months, and in patients without diabetes with persistent hyperglycaemia (e.g. BG >7.8 mmol/l) presenting to the Acute Medicine service.

HbA1c levels provide the opportunity to differentiate patients with stress hyperglycaemia from those with diabetes who were previously undiagnosed, as well as to identify patients with known diabetes who would benefit from intensification of their glycaemic management during hospitalisation and after discharge. However, clinicians should be aware that HbA1c testing in the hospital has significant limitations in the presence of haemoglobinopathies, recent transfusion, severe hepatic, renal and liver disease, and iron deficiency anaemia.

Blood glucose should frequently be measured using an appropriate POC device to allow early detection of any alterations in metabolic control. CGM provides continuous estimates, direction and magnitude of glucose trends, which may have an advantage over POC glucose testing in detecting and reducing the incidence of hypoglycaemia. Although not widely used in the in-hospital setting, monitoring using CGM has increased because of the COVID-19 pandemic (less need to have repeated close contact with infected patients) and is recommended in the Endocrine Society (2022) guidelines for the in-hospital management of individuals with diabetes who are at high risk of hypoglycaemia.

Remote inpatient glycaemic management is also evolving. The Endocrine Society (2022) guidelines also recommend *inpatient glycaemic surveillance* with specific hospital staff utilising glycaemic data collected within the electronic medical record (from *all* admitted patients) to identify those at risk for and those having hypoglycaemic and hyperglycaemic episodes, and then utilising that data to develop strategies for individually managing these adverse outcomes.

Treatment of diabetes

Management should be patient centred, with shared decision making and individualised treatment strategy and glycaemic targets.

T1DM treatment

Insulin has now been around for more than 100 years. Basic insulin nomenclature is as follows.

Human insulin

- Biosynthetic human insulin for clinical use is manufactured by recombinant DNA technology.
  - Short-acting human insulin is referred to as 'regular' insulin.
  - Intermediate-acting human insulin is referred to as 'isophane' or 'NPH' (neutral protamine Hagedorn) insulin.

Analogue insulin.

- Several analogues of human insulin are available. These insulin analogues are closely related to the human insulin structure and were developed for managing specific aspects of glycaemic control in terms of either faster action (e.g. rapid-acting insulins) or longer action (i.e. basal insulins).

Insulin time action profile.

- Basal insulin – intermediate-, long- or ultralong-acting insulin used to provide a background level of insulin throughout the day and night.
- Bolus insulin – short-, rapid- or ultrafast-acting insulin used to provide an increased level of insulin for a short period.

o Prandial insulin: bolus insulin administered prior to a meal to limit postprandial BG level elevation. Can be given immediately *before* meals, *with meals* or *even after meals* (e.g. in children or unwell adults who are reluctant to eat).

o Correction insulin: bolus insulin administered to lower a high BG level (due to whatever cause).

Concentrated insulins.

- A unit of insulin is the most basic measure of insulin.
- U100 is the most common concentration of insulin and means there are 100 units of insulin/ml of liquid. Insulin has been designated U100 since the 1970s.
- However, newer insulin formulations include more concentrated insulins, e.g. U200, U300. Can result in a modified pharmacokinetic (PK)/ pharmacodynamic (PD) profile, e.g. U300 glargine (Toujeo®) acts longer and has a flatter action profile than U100 glargine (Lantus®).

Insulin treatment should be started as soon as possible after T1DM diagnosis in children/adults with hyperglycaemia to prevent further metabolic decompensation and DKA. The basal-bolus concept trying to mimic normal insulin secretion has been shown to give the best results in terms of glycaemic control and long-term complications (Box 23.9).

- Basal insulin (~50% dose). Controls glucose production between meals and overnight. Near-constant levels of insulin, *plus*
- Bolus insulin (~50% dose). Limits hyperglycaemia after meals. Immediate rise and sharp peak post meal.

Box 23.9 Example of starting dose for T1DM

Starting dose based on weight, e.g. 80 kg adult.

- Range: 0.3–0.5 units/kg per day, e.g. 0.5 units of insulin/kg body weight = 0.5 × 80 = **40 units/day.**
  - o Basal: 50% total daily dose (TDD), e.g. give 50% of this dose as long-acting basal insulin = **20 units.** Given as single injection of basal analogue.
  - o Prandial: 50% TDD in divided doses given ±15 min each meal = 20/3 = **7 units per meal.** Can spread depending on size of respective meals, e.g. breakfast 4 units; lunch 6 units; evening meal 10 units (largest meal).

Administer insulin by either:

- multiple daily injections (MDI) by vial and syringe or insulin pen
- continuous subcutaneous insulin infusion (CSII) – also known as 'insulin pump'.

T2DM treatment

Various therapies are available for T2DM (Box 23.10).

Using glucose-lowering agents that target specific pathophysiological defects of T2DM may be a reasonable approach based on clinical phenotypic findings (Figure 23.7) and facilitates choice of agents for effective combination therapy (i.e. choose agents with complementary actions).

Early T2DM management

The cornerstone of T2DM treatment is lifestyle with weight management and physical therapy (Figure 23.8). All patients from initial diagnosis should start on metformin monotherapy (unless contraindicated). Starting GLP-1 receptor agonists or SGLT2 inhibitor monotherapy is an option depending on context (e.g. can they tolerate metformin or is it contraindicated?) and clinician/patient choice. Initial combination therapy is also an option.

Box 23.10 Glucose-lowering therapies and major adverse effects

- Metformin – gastrointestinal, lactic acidosis, B12 deficiency.
- Sulfonylureas/glinides (insulin secretagogues) – hypoglycaemia, weigh gain, fluid retention.
- Pioglitazone (glitazones) – fluid retention, weight gain, fragility fractures, bladder cancer(?).
- Glucagon-like peptide (GLP)-1 receptor agonist – gastrointestinal, pancreatitis, medullary thyroid cancer.
- Dual glucose-dependent insulinotropic polypeptide (GIP)/GLP-1 receptor agonist – gastrointestinal, pancreatitis, medullary thyroid cancer.
- Dipeptidyl peptidase-4 (DPP-4) inhibitors (gliptins) – heart failure (saxagliptin/alogliptin), pancreatitis.
- Sodium glucose co-transporter-2 (SGLT2) inhibitors (gliflozins) – dehydration with associated issues (e.g. acute kidney injury), *Candida* infections, ketosis including DKA.
- Insulin – hypoglycaemia, weight gain, fluid retention.

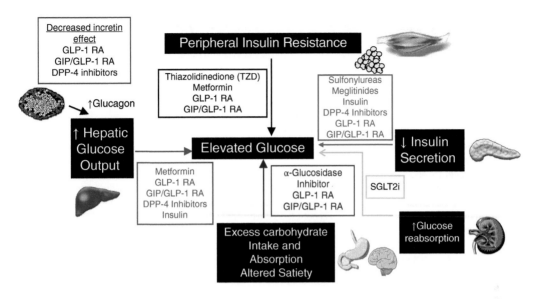

Figure 23.7 Matching T2DM pathophysiology with pharmacological agents.

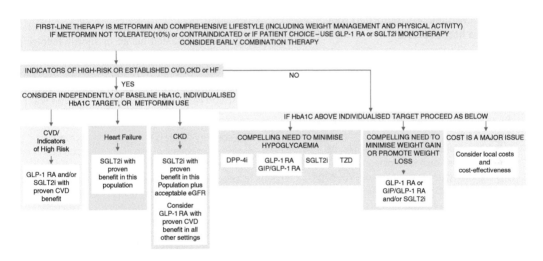

Figure 23.8 Early T2DM treatment pathways. If there are features of severe hyperglycaemia with catabolic symptoms, consider insulin therapy.

After metformin, the key decision pathway is whether the person with T2DM has cardiovascular disease (CVD) risk factors or existing CVD complications, chronic kidney disease (CKD) or Heart Failure (HF). If any of these conditions are present, treatment with a GLP-1 receptor agonist (Box 23.11) or SGLT2 inhibitor (Box 23.12) that has proven benefit in these populations should be added irrespective of degree of glycaemic control (i.e. even if well controlled, these agents do not cause hypoglycaemia). If none of these conditions are present, the choice of the next therapeutic agent should be based on whether the goal is to minimise hypoglycaemia, lose weight or cost. If there are features of severe hyperglycaemia with catabolic symptoms (see Box 23.7), consider insulin therapy.

Hyperglycaemia management in the acute care setting

As a standard of care, every patient with known diabetes presenting to the acute care setting, regardless

---

Box 23.11 Incretins are insulinotropic substances released by the gastrointestinal tract

- Incretins account for approximately 20–70% of insulin secretion after a meal.
- ~90% incretin activity is due to:
  - glucagon-like peptide-1 (GLP-1)
  - glucose-dependent insulinotropic polypeptide (GIP).
- GLP-1 and GIP are inactivated by DPP-4 within minutes.
- In T2DM incretin-based therapies are now widely used.
  - DPP-4 inhibitors: oral, weight neutral, no hypoglycaemia, modest glucose reduction. No CVD or renal benefits.
  - GLP-1 receptor agonists: injectable or oral, excellent weight reduction (up to 15–20%), no hypoglycaemia, best glucose reduction. First choice for injectable agent before basal insulin. CVD benefits (primary and secondary prevention including stroke) which are probably due to antiatherosclerosis effects (e.g. anti-inflammatory). Renal benefits – no eGFR cut-off contraindication for human GLP-1 based therapies, and albuminuria benefits.
  - Dual GIP/GLP-1 receptor agonists: injectable – even better effects than GLP-1 receptor agonists on glucose and weight loss (up to 22%). CVD data awaited. Multireceptor agonists demonstrate additive effects, in part, by engaging a broader range of activities. These agents are termed *unimolecular polypharmacy*.

Box 23.12 Kidney has important role in glucose homeostasis

- The kidney filters ~162 g of glucose every day.
  - 90% reabsorbed by SGLT2.
  - 10% reabsorbed by SGLT1.
- SGLT2 inhibitor drugs are available for treatment of T2DM with and without CVD (e.g. empagliflozin, dapagliflozin).
  - SGLT2 inhibitors decrease renal glucose reabsorption, leading to increased non-insulin-dependent glucose excretion of ~70–80 g/day (~280–320 kcal/day), reducing ambient glucose levels (modest and dependent on baseline eGFR) with potential weight loss. No hypoglycaemia. Early and sustained CVD benefits which are probably due to haemodynamic and myocardial metabolic fuel effects.
- SGLT2 inhibitor drugs are also available for treatment of CKD and HF in people with and without diabetes. They have transformed the CKD and CHF treatment landscape.

(e.g. basal or basal-plus) or IV route (i.e. variable-rate insulin infusion, VRII). Other glucose-lowering therapies should be initiated before or shortly following discharge, depending on circumstances (e.g. has patient had recurrent hypoglycaemia?). Arrange appropriate review by the inpatient diabetes specialist nurse and early follow-up with the diabetes team.

The corollary of this is that when we decrease or stop interventions that can *cause* or *exacerbate* *hyperglycaemia* in the in-hospital setting, such as glucocorticoid (GC) or enteral/parenteral feeding, we must *modify* the dose of glucose-lowering therapy to prevent hypoglycaemia. For example, management of patients with GC-associated hyperglycaemia requires ongoing BG monitoring with adjustment of insulin dosing. All therapies require safeguards to avoid hypoglycaemia when doses of GCs are tapered or abruptly discontinued.

Basic insulin prescribing in the acute care setting

Insulin regimen = pattern of subcutaneous insulin administration through the day and night.

---

of the major reason for presentation, should have a proactive plan for hyperglycaemia management, rather than a reactive response to elevation of BG.

If you have to *hold* or *stop* glucose-lowering therapies – e.g. due to adverse effects, changes in physiology (renal function), need for contrast agents – you must monitor BG closely, and consider starting insulin as needed by either the subcutaneous

Although insulin treatment is generally not the first-choice injectable therapy in T2DM, it is still widely used. Usual insulin regimens include the following.

- Background only (basal) –10 units or 0.1–0.2 units/kg usually given at bedtime and titrate dose as per FPG; add 1 unit per day (patient's preference) or 1–2 units every three days (clinician's preference). Decrease insulin dose (e.g. 10% or 2–4 units) if unexpected hypoglycaemia occurs.
- Background (basal) plus one mealtime (basal plus). If HbA1c is > individualised target despite normal FPG or >0.5 units/kg, add prandial insulin. Add 4 units (or 10% basal dose) prandial insulin to *largest meal* or meal with *largest PPG* excursion and titrate accordingly.
- Stepwise increase to basal-bolus regimen (i.e. MDI) as needed.
- If a T1DM or T2DM patient is already on insulin, take an accurate medication history – full name, dose and timing of each insulin dose. Also ask about adherence. Check recent BG log or download and HbA1c if available.
- Generic insulin is not generally available so insulin is always prescribed by brand name (e.g. 'NPH insulin' cannot be dispensed or administered; for example, prescribe INSUMAN BASAL®).
- Write insulin names and brand name in block capitals, e.g. INSULIN ASPART (NOVORAPID®) – some prescribers just write the brand name. Take great care, there are many sound-alike names.
- Write units in full (e.g. '8 units') – do not abbreviate.
- If specific insulin prescription chart is used, write 'Insulin' in main chart and then under dose write 'As Charted'.
- Concentrated insulin formulations (e.g. U200, U300, U500) should only be prescribed by diabetes specialists – most common insulins are U100.
- It is important to understand how the different types of insulin work – understand basic insulin nomenclature and PK/PD profiles.
- Insulin dosing changes should usually be in the context of the last 48 hours BG levels e.g. alter insulin dose by at least 10% (sometimes greater) when BG is consistently out of target.
- Fix the lows first and highs later. Once the lows are gone, rebound hyperglycaemia (due to overcorrection with carbohydrate) is often eliminated.
- Do not omit insulin due to mild hypos, e.g. if FPG 3.8 mmol/l, give breakfast and normal morning breakfast insulin if on MDI. Consider dose adjustment of long-acting insulin (causing low FPG), depending on recent trends.
- Generally, fix *one insulin* at a time.

If unexplained morning hyperglycaemia is occurring, determine the cause *before* adjusting therapy. Ask the patient to check the BG at 3 a.m. for several nights.

- If 3 a.m. BG is <4 mmol/l, this suggests a Somogyi effect (unrecognised nocturnal hypoglycaemia that the patient sleeps through, resulting in rebound hyperglycaemia due to counterregulatory response).
- If 3 a.m. BG is >4 mmol/l, this suggests:
  - dawn phenomenon (fasting hyperglycaemia due to GH being released in the early hours of the morning) *or*
  - insufficient dose of basal insulin *or*
  - inadequate coverage of evening meal *or*
  - excessive bedtime snacking.

Acute complications related to diabetes

Hypoglycaemia represents one of the most common endocrine emergencies that clinicians are likely to encounter. It usually affects individuals with diabetes mellitus and mainly those taking insulin and/or sulfonylurea agents or prandial regulators (glinides). Hypoglycaemia in non-diabetic individuals is rare. In both persons with and without diabetes, acute hypoglycaemia is associated with increased morbidity and in some individuals even death. The initial emergency management of hypoglycaemia is similar in both those with/without diabetes. However, the evaluation of individuals without diabetes is more complex and requires a careful history and investigation to discern the underlying aetiology.

Emergency admissions due to *hyperglycaemic crises* remain some of the most common and challenging metabolic conditions to deal with. DKA and HHS are biochemically different conditions that require different approaches to treatment. They often occur in different age groups, and there is a need for co-ordinated care from the multidisciplinary team to ensure the timely delivery of the correct treatments.

Over the last few years, the management of these conditions has changed. With DKA, it remains important to ensure that the diagnosis is made only when all three components (the 'D', the 'K' and the 'A') are present. In addition, the use of bedside monitoring of plasma ketone levels now drives treatment. With HHS, the treatment now focuses on the use of fluid rehydration in the initial phases rather than insulin treatment as the means by which BG lowering should be achieved, with insulin only being introduced when the rate of glucose lowering levels off.

Prevention of both hypoglycaemic and hyperglycaemic states is always preferred, and this requires appropriate education of patients, carers and healthcare practitioners on an ongoing basis. With the ongoing COVID-19 pandemic, it is important to highlight 'sick day' rules for a person with diabetes through education on symptoms of high glucose and encouraging them to check their BG and ketones more frequently when unwell. If treated with SGLT2 inhibitors and unwell with diarrhoea, vomiting, fever and unusual drowsiness, advise the patient to *stop* the SGLT2 inhibitor as there is a risk of DKA and not to restart until feeling better and eating/drinking fluids normally. This advice is similar across the acute care setting.

Hypoglycaemia

> No single BG concentration categorically defines hypoglycaemia in *all* individuals *at all* times.

Hypoglycaemia is generally defined as BG low enough to cause symptoms and/or signs, including impairment of brain function (neuroglycopenia).

- Plasma glucose ≤3.9 mmol/l and ≥3 mmol/l – considered a glucose alert value (level 1), indicating a need for correction with fast-acting carbohydrates and/or dose adjustment of glucose-lowering medications.
- Plasma glucose <3.0 mmol/l – considered to be the threshold for clinically significant hypoglycaemia (level 2), indicating serious, clinically important hypoglycaemia.
- Severe hypoglycaemia – defined as hypoglycaemia characterised by altered mental and/or physical status resulting in the requirement of assistance from another individual to administer rescue therapy (level 3).

Most recommend documentation of Whipple's triad (i.e. low plasma glucose, symptoms or signs consistent with hypoglycaemia, and resolution of those symptoms/signs after the plasma glucose has been raised) to confirm hypoglycaemia, especially in persons *without* diabetes.

Clinical features of hypoglycaemia

> In healthy humans, multiple mechanisms have evolved to defend against falling BG.

A co-ordinated interplay of insulin inhibition and release of the powerful counterregulatory hormones, including glucagon and adrenaline, form the acute defence against hypoglycaemia. Sympathetic nervous system responses are also important. Consequently, hypoglycaemia manifests as an array of autonomic (i.e. palpitations, tremor, sweating, pallor, anxiety) and neuroglycopenic (i.e. behavioural changes, fatigue, seizure, loss of consciousness) signs and symptoms. The glucose threshold for the generation of autonomic signs and symptoms is plastic in nature but is typically ~3.3 mmol/l.

Failure of these protective sympathoadrenal mechanisms can lead to severe, unimpeded hypoglycaemia. In cases of recurring episodes of hypoglycaemia, the threshold for initiation of counterregulatory hormone responses is reduced to a lower BG level and hormone responses become blunted. Patients also develop hypoglycaemia unawareness, in which symptoms are delayed and blunted and may be unrecognisable to the individual.

Collectively, the reduction of hormonal and symptom responses to recurring episodes of hypoglycaemia is part of a disorder termed hypoglycaemia-associated autonomic failure (HAAF), the presence of which further increases the risk of severe hypoglycaemia.

Hypoglycaemia has been associated with adverse CV outcomes, such as prolonged QT intervals, ischaemic ECG changes/angina, arrhythmias, sudden death and increased inflammation. In addition, acute hypoglycaemia creates a prothrombotic state, with increased platelet aggregation, endothelial dysfunction and vasoconstriction, abnormal cardiac repolarisation and catecholamine-induced CV changes, such as increase in heart rate, angina and myocardial infarctions, all contributing to increased mortality.

Acute management of hypoglycaemia

Most cases of hypoglycaemia in patients with diabetes are self-diagnosed and addressed at home, without intervention from a medical provider (Figure 23.9). Initial treatment generally consists of the 'Rule of 15' – 15–20 grams of simple carbohydrate to ameliorate the symptoms of mild hypoglycaemia with repeat BG measured 15 minutes after consuming carbohydrate. This sequence can be repeated up to three times. Additional carbohydrate should be ingested if hypoglycaemia or hypoglycaemic symptoms persist. For a measured BG of <2.8 mmol/l, 20–30 grams of carbohydrate should be considered.

Glucagon kits can be prescribed to patients with diabetes, and friends, family members or co-workers

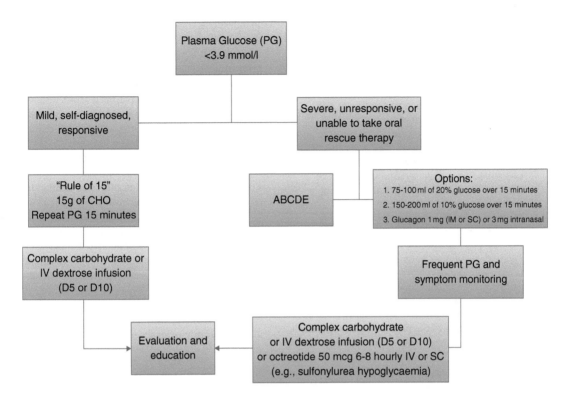

Figure 23.9 Algorithm for acute management of hypoglycaemia.

can be trained to administer glucagon (1 mg) subcutaneously (SC) or intramuscularly (IM), if the patient is unable or unwilling to ingest glucose orally. More recently, intranasal 3 mg glucagon has become available and is easier to administer than an injection. The effects of glucagon, which acts through stimulation of hepatic glycogenolysis, are delayed by approximately 10 minutes from time of administration and are only inducible in those with available glycogen stores (may be ineffective if malnourished).

After resolution of hypoglycaemia, a full meal or complex snack should be consumed as the glucose-lowering agent (e.g. insulin) may still be active and to restore glycogen stores.

Acute management of severe hypoglycaemia

Consideration should always be given to other acute medical conditions that may mimic or coincide with hypoglycaemia (e.g. ACS, acute ischaemic stroke, sepsis, shock). However, rapid recognition of a low BG is imperative as prolonged severe hypoglycaemia can result in irreversible brain damage, CV strain and death.

Severe hypoglycaemia should be assessed and addressed emergently. Initial assessment and management should begin with the ABCDEs (see Figure 23.9).

D10 (10% dextrose) or D20 (20% dextrose) is less irritating than D50 (50% dextrose) and can be administered via a peripheral vein in a proportionally larger volume. Glucagon can also be considered. In cases of sulfonylurea-induced hypoglycaemia, glucose administration can actually stimulate continued insulin secretion, and the somatostatin analogue octreotide, 50–100 mcg administered IV or SC every 6–8 hours, can be used to inhibit insulin secretion and prevent recurring hypoglycaemia in this setting.

As in self-treated patients, once euglycaemia is attained, a meal or a complex snack including carbohydrate and protein should be taken to prevent a recurrent episode of hypoglycaemia. If oral intake is not an option, D5 (5% dextrose) or D10 can be infused to maintain euglycaemia.

Blood glucose measurements should be repeated every 15–30 minutes for at least two hours, or longer depending on the aetiology, following resolution of hypoglycaemia. Symptoms and signs of hypoglycaemia should resolve once euglycaemia is achieved and maintained. However, alternative diagnoses (i.e. stroke, delirium, drug overdose) should be considered if neurocognitive symptoms persist despite biochemical euglycaemia.

> People with hypoglycaemia on sulfonylureas or ultra-long-acting insulins, and in particular the frail, older person with other co-morbidities (especially severe CKD and endstage renal disease, where sulfonylureas and insulin are not cleared effectively), those who live alone or people who have sustained an injury should be admitted to hospital as they are at high risk of further hypoglycaemic episode in the next 48 hours because these glucose-lowering agents are slow to be excreted.

Cause of hypoglycaemia – diabetes related

- Evaluate the cause of hypoglycaemia (e.g. lifestyle changes, treatment changes, worsening renal function, co-existent autoimmune coeliac disease or adrenal insufficiency in T1DM).
- Beware of the low HbA1c and ensure that sulfonylureas are not used in frail, older people and those who have prefilled medicine trays/pill organisers. They and/or their carers may be unable to detect which drug is the sulfonylurea, which must be given with food.
- HAAF may be reversible in 2–3 weeks with scrupulous avoidance of hypoglycaemia. Glycaemic targets should be reviewed to prevent severe hypoglycaemia and preserve awareness. The use of CGM with alarms warning of impending hypoglycaemia is valuable.
- In the in-hospital setting, glycaemic goals should be tailored to the patient, surgical versus medical status and level of acuity. CGM may also be useful. Consult diabetes and/or perioperative team.
- Structured education (e.g. DAFNE training) is key to prevention.

Cause of hypoglycaemia – non-diabetes related

In the case of non-diabetes-associated hypoglycaemia, the goal is to ultimately identify and treat the underlying condition.

- For example, as many as 30% of individuals in the postbariatric surgery population may experience asymptomatic hypoglycaemia; however, a small group are hospitalised (~1%).

- In individuals without historical or physical findings that elucidate the aetiology of hypoglycaemia and who satisfy Whipple's triad, it is reasonable to perform diagnostic differentiation of *endogenous* and *exogenous* hyperinsulinaemia from other causes. At the time of hypoglycaemia, plasma glucose, insulin, C-peptide, proinsulin, beta-hydroxybutyrate (beta-HBA) and an oral sulfonylurea screen that includes glinides should be obtained.
  - ○ Elevated insulin, C-peptide and proinsulin document *endogenous* hyperinsulinism.
  - ○ Low beta-hydroxybutyrate indicates mediation of the hypoglycaemia by insulin (exogenous or endogenous).
- Obtaining insulin antibodies will identify those with insulin autoimmune-mediated hypoglycaemia (i.e. one of the mechanisms of hypoglycaemia is insulin antibodies directly stimulating the insulin receptor).
- Some patients may require a formal 72-hour inpatient fast. If insulinoma is confirmed biochemically, appropriate localising imaging should be pursued.

> Evaluation of an otherwise healthy individual with hypoglycaemia requires some consideration of malicious or surreptitious abuse of insulin or insulin secretagogue therapy or accidental inappropriate medication administration. This may be as simple as sending the urine sulfonylurea screen or close inspection of pills (medication reconciliation).

Hyperglycaemic emergencies

Diabetic ketoacidosis and HHS are acute severe metabolic complications of uncontrolled diabetes mellitus. A mixed picture of HHS and DKA may occur in individual patients. These conditions demand immediate recognition and early, aggressive treatment. Mortality rates for DKA are now <1%. In comparison, HHS is rare but mortality attributed to HHS is considerably higher, with recent rates of 5–20%.

The main causes of mortality in the adult population include cerebral oedema in young adults, severe hypokalaemia (and related cardiac dysrhythmias), adult respiratory distress syndrome (ARDS) and co-morbid states such as pneumonia, ACS and sepsis.

Diabetic ketoacidosis and HHS can be precipitated by various conditions (which can easily be remembered by the letter **I**), including **I**nsulin deficiency (i.e. new diabetes presentation or failure to take enough insulin) – check treatment adherence and persistence;

Iatrogenic (e.g. glucocorticoids, thiazides, atypical antipsychotic drugs, and SGLT2 inhibitors); Infection (the most common precipitating factor for both DKA and HHS; includes COVID-19); Inflammation (e.g. acute pancreatitis, cholecystitis, acute diabetic foot); Ischaemia or Infarction (e.g. ACS, stroke, bowel); and Intoxication (e.g. alcohol, cocaine). The traditional drivers of DKA in T1DM are insulin omission or concurrent illness, or both.

The process of HHS usually evolves over several days to weeks, whereas the evolution of the acute DKA episode tends to be much shorter (typically <24 hours). For both DKA and HHS, the classic clinical picture includes a history of polyuria, polydipsia, weight loss, visual changes, vomiting, dehydration, weakness and mental status change.

Physical findings may include increased rate and depth of respiration in DKA (i.e. Kussmaul breathing) with the odour of acetone, tachycardia and hypotension. Assessment of fluid status encompasses subjective observations (skin turgor, mucous membranes, cerebral dysfunction), objective measurements (BP, pulse, postural measurements, body weight) and laboratory measurements (serum [Na^+], serum osmolality, urea, haematocrit, urine osmolality). Severe hypovolaemia may manifest as tachycardia (pulse >100 bpm) and/or hypotension (systolic BP <100 mmHg). Mental status can vary from full alertness to profound lethargy or coma, with the latter more frequent in HHS. Because HHS usually occurs in older people, the neurological findings may be mistaken for a stroke.

Nausea, vomiting and diffuse abdominal pain are frequent in patients with DKA (>50%) but are uncommon in HHS. Further evaluation is necessary if this complaint does not resolve with resolution of dehydration and metabolic acidosis.

Successful treatment of DKA and HHS requires the correction of dehydration, hyperglycaemia and electrolyte imbalances; identification of co-morbid precipitating events; and above all, frequent patient monitoring.

DKA

Not all patients with ketoacidosis have DKA. Starvation ketosis and alcoholic ketoacidosis are distinguished by clinical history and by plasma glucose concentrations that range from mildly elevated (rarely >11.1 mmol/l) to hypoglycaemia. A clinical history of previous alcohol abuse and intoxication should be sought.

Diabetic ketoacidosis is a complex disordered metabolic state which requires the combined presence of three biochemical abnormalities: (a) ketonaemia ≥3 mmol/l or significant ketonuria (≥2+ urine ketones on standard urine sticks); (b) BG >11.1 mmol/l or known diabetes; and (c) venous (or arterial) blood bicarbonate <15 mmol/l and/or pH <7.3.

Diabetic ketoacidosis primarily affects persons known to have T1DM and may be the initial manifestation of previously undiagnosed T1DM in up to 25% of cases. DKA most frequently results from increased insulin requirements during situations that increase the release of counterregulatory hormones (i.e. glucagon, cortisol, adrenaline, GH). This type of hormonal imbalance enhances hepatic gluconeogenesis and glycogenolysis, resulting in severe hyperglycaemia. Enhanced lipolysis increases serum free fatty acids that are then metabolised as an alternative energy source in the process of ketogenesis. This results in the accumulation of large quantities of ketone bodies and subsequent metabolic acidosis. Acetone is a ketone, while beta-HBA is a hydroxy acid and acetoacetate a ketoacid. The predominant acid in DKA is beta-HBA.

When hyperglycaemia initially presents in the presence of ketones or other signs of metabolic decompensation, the diagnosis of T1DM is generally straightforward. However, ketonaemia can also be found in individuals with T2DM (i.e. ketosis-prone hyperglycaemia, especially in persons of African descent), with 5–25% having DKA. There is also increased risk of developing DKA, especially euglycaemic DKA, in persons with T1DM and T2DM taking SGLT2 inhibitors. More recently apparent, however, is the increased risk of DKA with COVID-19 infection which may present in patients with T1DM and T2DM. In one large study in England of patients with COVID-19, the significant increases in DKA admissions were in people with T2DM and people with newly diagnosed diabetes, which were offset by a concurrent significant reduction in people with T1DM presenting with DKA.

COVID-19 infection is more common and severe in people with diabetes (plus confounding effects for social determinants of health). Severe COVID-19 infection is treated with steroid medication, which can exacerbate hyperglycaemia, potentially leading to DKA/HHS. Overall, this combination results in immune dysfunction, allowing some commonly found pathogens to become more harmful. Mucormycosis ('black fungus') is one type of opportunistic infection caused by fungi belonging to the Mucorales family. Diabetes is the most prominent risk factor for mucormycosis.

HHS

Hyperosmolar hyperglycaemic state is characterised by marked hyperglycaemia (BG >30 mmol/l); no significant ketonaemia (<3 mmol/l); no acidosis (pH>7.3, bicarbonate >15 mmol/l); hypovolaemia; and osmolality usually >320 mOsm/kg. HHS is seen most frequently in persons with existing T2DM, but approximately 20% of cases have no history of this diagnosis.

Unlike DKA, which is a condition most frequently associated with *absolute* insulin deficiency, in HHS there is *sufficient* insulin to prevent ketogenesis but *insufficient* insulin to either prevent hepatic gluconeogenesis and/or stimulate cellular glucose uptake. If a counterregulatory hormone excess is also present (e.g. concomitant illness), then this leads to a further rise in BG and a subsequent osmotic diuresis. If sufficient water is not available or taken, this leads to dehydration and the resultant impaired renal function. The high BG causes a raised serum osmolality. The impaired renal function then leads to a further inability to excrete glucose, thus perpetuating the hyperglycaemia, osmotic diuresis, volume depletion and dehydration. Alterations in mental status are common with serum osmolality >320 mOsm/kg.

Management of DKA and HHS

Once DKA or HHS is recognised, the patient should be managed in an appropriate location. This could be in the outpatient setting (e.g. SDEC) for selected cases of mild DKA. However, the majority of patients will be hospitalised and managed in an emergency care setting such as emergency department, AMU, ECU, HDU or ICU. As with all acute medical patients, prompt assessment and management of the ABCDEs should occur.

The initial laboratory evaluation of patients should include a determination of BG, urea and creatinine, electrolytes, serum osmolality, serum ketones, urinalysis, baseline venous (or arterial) blood gases, full blood count with differential and CRP. An ECG, chest X-ray, COVID-19 testing, and urine and blood cultures should also be considered where co-morbidity is possible. Other investigations are performed as warranted by the clinical situation (e.g. cardiac troponins, serum lactate, appropriate imaging, toxicology screen).

Point-of-care testing equipment should be used to measure the plasma concentrations of beta-HBA, because this is the direct marker of disease severity. The anion gap is calculated by subtracting the sum of chloride [Cl⁻] and bicarbonate [HCO3⁻] concentration from the uncorrected measured [Na⁺]: $(Na^+) - (Cl^- + HCO3^-)$. An anion gap >12 mmol/l indicates the presence of increased anion gap metabolic acidosis. While arterial blood gas (ABG) is the most accurate method of assessing ventilation status, venous blood gas (VBG) is preferred to ABG for bicarbonate and pH measurements because the differences in arterial and venous pH, bicarbonate and potassium measurements are not large enough (in either direction) to alter management.

Supportive care includes inserting large-bore IV cannulae and starting appropriate IV fluid resuscitation, electrolyte replacement, nutritional support, continuous cardiac monitoring and pulse oximetry. Co-morbidities should be treated appropriately. It is also imperative to exclude unknown pregnancy by performing a pregnancy test in appropriate patients.

Hyperglycaemia bundle for treatment.

- Due to the increased risk of arterial and venous thromboembolism (VTE), all patients with DKA or HHS should receive LMWH for the full duration of admission unless contraindicated.
- HHS and some DKA patients are also at high risk of pressure ulceration. An initial foot assessment should be undertaken and heel protectors applied in those with neuropathy, PAD, a history of previous ulceration or lower limb deformity. The feet should be re-examined daily.
- Consider an NG tube with airway protection to prevent aspiration if GCS is <12 or the patient is excessively vomiting.
- Consider urinary catheterisation if the patient is incontinent, if there is difficulty monitoring urine output (minimum urine output should be no less than 0.5 ml/kg/h) or if the patient is anuric (i.e. not passed urine by 60 minutes).

Specific management of DKA is outlined in Box 23.13, and HHS in Box 23.14.

Box 23.13 Management of DKA

Overall goals are to improve circulatory volume and tissue perfusion, decrease BG, correct electrolyte imbalances, correct the acidosis, prevent other complications (e.g. cerebral oedema), and seek and treat precipitants.

- An initial loading dose of short- or rapid-acting insulin may be needed if there is a delay in setting up an IV insulin infusion, followed by a fixed rate insulin infusion (FRII), e.g. 0.1 units per kg per hour.
- SC injections of long-acting insulin should be continued if the patient is already using these agents.
- Frequent POC tests should be used to monitor BG, venous pH and beta-HBA concentrations.
- Frequent laboratory measurements of creatinine and serum electrolyte levels should be done to guide fluid and electrolyte replacement. It is important to replace fluid and electrolytes and correct pH while bringing the BG concentration to a normal level.
- Hypokalaemia is common (about 50%) during treatment of hyperglycaemic crises, and severe hypokalaemia (<2.5 mmol/l) is associated with increased inpatient mortality. Serum potassium levels often fall as glucose and acidosis are corrected and potassium moves from the ECF into the ICF compartment. Thus, it is usually necessary to add potassium to the IV infusion.
- During treatment of DKA, hyperglycaemia is corrected faster than ketoacidosis. Too rapid a drop in BG may cause hypoglycaemia. A sudden change in the osmolality of ECF can also occur when BG levels are lowered too rapidly, and this can cause cerebral oedema. Once the plasma glucose is <14 mmol/l, 10% dextrose should be added to replacement fluids to allow continued insulin administration until ketonaemia is controlled while at the same time avoiding hypoglycaemia.
- Identification and treatment of the underlying cause, such as infection, are also important.
- Continue IV fluids if the patient is not eating and drinking. If the patient is not eating and drinking and there is no ketonaemia, move to a VRII.
- Transfer to SC insulin if the patient is eating and drinking normally. Ensure that the SC insulin is started usually with a meal before the IV insulin is discontinued. If the patient is newly diagnosed with T1DM, make sure basal insulin is given several hours prior to discontinuing IV insulin.
- The diabetes inpatient team should be involved as early as is practical after admission.

Box 23.14 Management of HHS

Overall goals of treatment are to gradually and safely normalise the osmolality; replace fluid and electrolyte losses; normalise BG; prevent arterial or venous thrombosis; prevent other potential complications including foot ulceration; and seek and treat precipitants.

- Measure or calculate osmolality frequently to monitor the response to treatment.
- The aim of the initial therapy is expansion of the intra- and extravascular volume and restoration of peripheral perfusion. The fluid replacement of choice is 0.9% sodium chloride. Measurement or calculation of osmolality should be undertaken every hour initially and the rate of fluid replacement adjusted to ensure a positive fluid balance sufficient to promote a gradual decline in osmolality.
- The aim of treatment should be to replace approximately 50% of estimated fluid loss within the first 12 hours and the remainder in the following 12 hours, although this will, in part, be determined by the initial severity, and the degree of renal impairment and associated co-morbidities such as CHF, which may limit the speed of correction.
- If significant ketonaemia is present (beta-HBA >1 mmol/l), this indicates relative hypoinsulinaemia and insulin should be started at time zero.
- If significant ketonaemia is not present (beta-HBA <1 mmol/l), insulin should not be started initially. Fluid replacement alone with 0.9% sodium chloride will result in a drop in BG.
- Lack of appropriate decline in BG with rehydration should prompt reassessment. Insulin may be started at this point, or if already in place the infusion rate increased (e.g. by 1 unit/hour). The recommended insulin dose is an FRII given at 0.05 units per kg per hour (e.g. 4 units/hour in an 80 kg person).

- Avoid hypoglycaemia. A BG target of between 10 and 15 mmol/l is a reasonable goal in the first 24 hours. If the BG falls below 14 mmol/l, commence 10% dextrose at 125 ml/h and continue the 0.9% saline.
- Potassium replacement. This is the same as DKA.
- Complete normalisation of electrolytes and osmolality may take up to 72 hours or longer.
- Assess for any complications of treatment (e.g. fluid overload, cerebral oedema, ODS, such as a deteriorating conscious level).
- IV insulin can usually be discontinued once the patient is eating and drinking but their fluids may be required for longer if intake remains inadequate.
- Many patients may require conversion to SC insulin treatment. For patients with previously undiagnosed diabetes or those who were well controlled on other glucose-lowering agents, switching from insulin to the appropriate non-insulin therapy should be considered after a period of stability. Check for treatment adherence and persistence.
- Discharge planning – because many of these patients have multiple co-morbidities, recovery will largely be determined by their previous functional level and the underlying precipitant of HHS. Involve the acute frailty team.
- The diabetes inpatient team should be involved as early as is practical after admission.

Diabetic foot complications

Foot problems are among the most common and feared complications of diabetes mellitus, as well as the major cause of lower extremity amputations. Diabetic foot problems have a significant financial impact on healthcare systems, increased in-hospital occupancy and length of stay. All persons with diabetes should be screened for risk of foot problems on at least an annual basis; those with risk factors require regular podiatry, patient education and instruction in foot self-care.

The most common foot complication is skin ulceration, which is usually secondary to diabetes-related peripheral neuropathy (with loss of protective sensation) and less often related to PAD, or both.

- A diabetic foot ulcer can be defined as a localised injury to the skin and/or underlying tissue, below the ankle, in a person with diabetes.
- The lifetime risk of a person with diabetes developing a foot ulcer is 10–25%.
- About half of diabetic foot ulcers are clinically infected at presentation. Infection is best defined as an invasion and multiplication of micro-organisms in host tissues that induce a host inflammatory response, usually followed by tissue destruction. Infection is usually the final precipitating cause of lower extremity amputations.
- Up to 85% of lower limb amputations are preceded by foot ulcers. Across the globe, it is estimated that a limb is amputated every 30 seconds due to diabetes.

- Most foot ulcers should heal if pressure is removed from the ulcer site, the arterial circulation is sufficient, and infection is managed and treated aggressively.
- Persons with diabetes who have an amputation have a five-year survival rate of only 30%. Most of the excess morbidity and mortality in these patients is related to CVD, and emphasises the need for good diabetes and cardiovascular risk management.
- Any person with diabetes with a warm unilateral swollen foot without ulceration should be presumed to have an acute Charcot neuroarthropathy (CN) until proven otherwise. CN is a non-infectious condition affecting bone, joints and soft tissues of the foot and ankle. In the acute phase, a Charcot foot is erythematous, indurated and painful and may be mistaken for gout, deep venous thrombosis, cellulitis or a sprain. In the chronic phase, CN is associated with subluxations and fractures, especially of the midfoot (Lisfranc injury), causing substantial deformity leading to high pressures, recurrent ulcerations and potentially lower extremity amputation. The estimated prevalence of CN among persons with diabetes is 7.5%.

Pathophysiology of diabetic foot problems

Macrovascular complications, such as PAD, and microvascular complications, such as peripheral and autonomic neuropathy, are common, and both are important in the pathophysiology of diabetic foot problems. For example, motor nerve dysfunction results in disturbances in posture and balance that

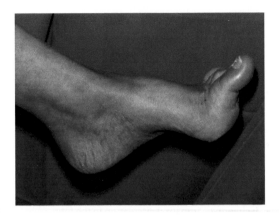

Figure 23.10 High-risk neuropathic foot demonstrating high-arch, prominent metatarsal heads, clawing of toes, and callus under first metatarsal head. The characteristic clawing seen in motor nerve dysfunction is due to the differential loss of strength between the extensor muscles and flexor muscles leading to areas of high plantar pressures (leading to callus and increased risk of ulcer) and an increased risk of the dorsal aspects of the toes rubbing against the inside of the toe box of a shoe. Source: Matfin G. Endocrine and Metabolic Endocrine Emergencies, 2nd edn. Chichester: Wiley, 2018.

> **Box 23.15 Ipswich touch test**
>
> Ask the patient to close their eyes.
> - Confirm right and left sides with patient.
> - Inform patient that you will touch their toes and they should say 'left' or 'right' when they feel the touch.
> - VERY LIGHTLY touch tips of toes for 1–2 seconds.
> - Toe sequence: 1. Right big, 2. Right little, 3. Left big, 4. Left little, 5. Right middle, 6. Left middle.
> - Record the results – **Yes** if touch was felt and **No** if not.
> - **Two or more negatives = abnormal sensation = HIGH RISK.**

---

can lead to increased pressures within the foot (Figure 23.10); loss of sensory perception results in inability to feel pain, thus inhibiting any preventive action from being taken; loss of autonomic function in the lower limbs leads to loss of sweating and hence dry skin that can predispose to infection; and autonomic dysregulation can alter microvascular flow, leading to arteriovenous 'shunting,' with resultant tissue hypoxia and paradoxically warm feet. The other major pathology in addition to neuropathy and ischaemia is infection. Infection can proceed rapidly and the endstage of tissue death is quickly reached. Thus, the window of opportunity for intervention is limited and often missed.

Screening for diabetic foot problems

Most foot complications are potentially preventable. The first step in prevention is identifying the 'at-risk' population during the comprehensive foot evaluation. Detailed foot assessment may occur more often in these 'at-risk' patients. In addition, all patients with diabetes should have their feet (and shoes) inspected at every visit (including acute care settings).

The risk of ulcers or amputation is increased in people with the following risk factors: poor glycaemic control; peripheral neuropathy with loss of protective sensation (LOPS); cigarette smoking; foot deformities; Charcot foot; preulcerative callus or corn; PAD; history of foot ulcer; previous amputation; visual impairment; and diabetic kidney disease (DKD), especially patients on dialysis.

Foot examination should include general inspection of skin integrity and musculoskeletal deformities. Vascular assessment should include inspection and palpation of pedal pulses, capillary refill, foot temperature and ankle-brachial pressure index (as indicated).

Neurological exam is designed to identify LOPS rather than early neuropathy. LOPS (large-fibre function) indicates the presence of distal sensorimotor polyneuropathy and is a risk factor for diabetic foot ulceration and amputation. The 10 g monofilament is used to diagnose LOPS. At least one other assessment, e.g. pinprick or temperature (small-fibre function), vibration or ankle reflexes (large-fibre function), should be performed. One or more abnormal tests would suggest LOPS, while at least two normal (and no abnormal) tests would rule out LOPS. In the UK, the Ipswich touch test is preferred to identify at-risk feet (Box 23.15).

Management of high-risk patients

All patients with diabetes and particularly those with high-risk foot conditions (i.e. history of ulcer or amputation, deformity, LOPS, and/or PAD) and their families should be educated about risk factors and appropriate management. Appropriate footwear (including orthotist review) and footwear behaviours at home (and also in the hospital setting) should be outlined. Regular podiatry review as needed is important and clear instructions on how and when to access urgent/emergency foot care is critical.

Optimal management of glycaemic control, hypertension, dyslipidaemia, smoking cessation, weight management, use of antiplatelet agents and addressing other modifiable risk factors are important to prevent or slow any progression of microvascular and macrovascular complications.

Diabetic foot evaluation across the acute care setting

The general principles for acute medical foot care in people with diabetes should apply to all patients, not just those with active foot disease. These measures include taking a specific foot history and an inspection of the feet, looking for evidence of neuropathy, ischaemia, ulceration, inflammation and/or infection, deformity or CN.

The feet of persons with diabetes should be inspected daily during the hospital stay and new problems that are identified should be managed in conjunction with the specialist diabetic foot multidisciplinary team (or equivalent). Appropriate ongoing education of patients and healthcare providers about the importance of prevention and early recognition of diabetes-related foot problems is critical.

> The acute diabetic foot includes any foot wound present at presentation; any newly acquired foot wound picked up on daily whole-foot checks; suspected CN; any unexplained erythema, discolouration or swelling; and a cold pale foot.

Admission criteria for diabetic foot problems

Consider admitting the following patients with diabetic foot problems.

1 All patients with a life-threatening/limb-threatening problem such as foot ulceration with fever or signs of sepsis.
2 Patients with a moderate infection with complicating features (e.g. severe PAD or lack of home support), or who require urgent surgical debridement (e.g. deep collections usually indicated by a grossly swollen foot with shiny skin) or are unable to comply with the required outpatient treatment regimen.
3 Patients with critical limb ischaemia.
4 Dialysis patients (risk of rapid progression and systemic infection).
5 Patients who do not meet any of these criteria, but are failing to improve with outpatient therapy, may also need to be hospitalised.
6 Patients whose glycaemic control has decompensated to the point that it is now an acute problem in its own right.

Classification of diabetic foot ulcers

Ulcer severity is recorded using the SINBAD scoring system (recommended by the UK NICE), which scores an ulcer between 0 (least severe) and 6 (most severe) depending on how many of the six SINBAD elements are present.

- **Site** (on hindfoot) – ulcer penetrates the hindfoot (rear of the foot).
- **Ischaemia** – impaired circulation in the foot.
- **Neuropathy** – LOPS in the foot.
- **Bacterial infection** – signs of bacterial infection of the foot (e.g. redness, swelling, heat, discharge).
- **Area** ($\geq 1\,cm^2$) – ulcer covers a large surface area (1 cm² or more).
- **Depth** (to tendon or bone) – ulcer penetrates to tendon or bone.

An ulcer with a SINBAD score of ≥ 3 is classed as severe. An ulcer with a SINBAD score of <3 is classed as a less severe ulcer.

Management of diabetic foot ulcer/infection

> When assessing a patient presenting with a diabetic foot ulcer/infection, consider the problem at three levels: (a) the whole patient (e.g. cognitive, metabolic and fluid status); (b) the affected limb (e.g. presence of neuropathy and vascular insufficiency); and, finally, (c) the wound.

The clinician should measure the vital signs, palpate for pedal pulses, check for peripheral neuropathy and debride and probe any open wounds. Special attention should be paid to detecting crepitus, bullae, new-onset tenderness or anaesthesia, rapidly advancing cellulitis or gangrenous tissue (Figure 23.11). The presence of any of these findings should prompt rapid consultation with an experienced foot surgeon.

In addition to basic haematology and blood chemistry tests, virtually all patients with a foot wound should have a plain X-ray of the foot to look for the presence of gas, a foreign body or bone lesions. Where clinical circumstances or the findings on plain X-ray suggest a more sensitive or specific imaging test is needed, MRI is generally best.

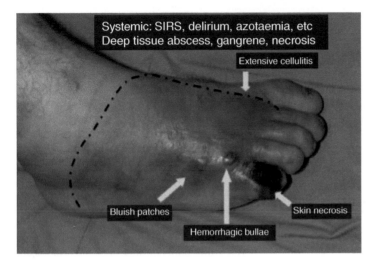

Systemic: SIRS, delirium, azotaemia, etc
Deep tissue abscess, gangrene, necrosis

Extensive cellulitis

Bluish patches

Hemorrhagic bullae

Skin necrosis

Figure 23.11 Diabetic foot infection with rapidly spreading soft tissue infection demonstrating characteristics of a serious soft tissue infection requiring urgent surgical exploration. Source: Matfin G. Endocrine and Metabolic Endocrine Emergencies, 2nd edn. Chichester: Wiley, 2018.

Classifying the severity of a diabetic foot ulcer/infection (e.g. using SINBAD) is important as it helps determine which patients may require hospitalisation and broad-spectrum, IV antibiotic therapy, which is usually required for severe infections but rarely for mild (or many moderate) infections. Initial empiric antibiotic choices may need to be adapted based on the results of culture and sensitivity tests. Antibiotic therapy need only be given until resolution of the infectious signs and symptoms and not prolonged until the complete healing of the wound. The usual duration needed for soft tissue infection is 1–2 weeks.

A severe diabetic foot infection requires rapid evaluation (especially for vascular status), attention to any metabolic disorders and consideration for appropriate surgical procedures. Similarly, the presence of a deep soft tissue abscess or osteomyelitis also requires surgical evaluation.

Discharge planning for people admitted with diabetic foot problems

Prior to being discharged, a patient with a diabetic foot problem should be clinically stable; have had any urgently needed surgery performed; have achieved acceptable glycaemic control; be able to manage (on his/her own or with help) at the designated discharge location; and have a well-defined plan that includes an appropriate antibiotic regimen to which he/she will adhere; total contact casting which is a specially designed cast designed to take weight off the foot (off-loading) in patients with diabetic foot ulcers (if needed); specific wound care instructions; and appropriate outpatient follow-up.

> Safety netting – remind the patient to come back or contact emergently if the infection worsens or other foot complication develops.

Microvascular complications

> The level of chronic hyperglycaemia is the best-established concomitant risk factor associated with *microvascular* complications. This is best understood by the fact that nerve, retinal and kidney cells do not require insulin for glucose entry, so even with insulin deficiency (absolute or relative), these cells are still exposed to elevated ambient glucose levels and subsequent risk of complications.

Neuropathy

Somatic and autonomic nervous system neuropathies are common in diabetes.

- Somatic neuropathic complications have already been discussed in the context of diabetic foot problems. A distal symmetrical polyneuropathy, in which loss of function typically occurs in a 'glove and stocking' pattern, is the most common form of peripheral neuropathy. Somatic sensory involvement usually occurs first, is often bilateral and symmetrical, and is associated with diminished perception of vibration, pain and temperature, particularly in the lower extremities (longest nerves are affected first). In addition to pain and diabetic ulcer risk, the loss of feeling, touch and position sense increases the risk of falling.

- Autonomic neuropathies involve disorders of sympathetic and parasympathetic nervous system function. There may be disorders of vasomotor function, decreased cardiac responses, inability to empty the bladder, gastrointestinal motility problems and sexual dysfunction (e.g. erectile dysfunction).

Renal

Diabetes is the leading cause of CKD and endstage renal disease (ESRD). CKD due to diabetes is also known as DKD or diabetic nephropathy. Unfortunately, the combination of diabetes and CKD is also associated with increased morbidity and mortality, mainly due to increased CVD risk.

Our current understanding of DKD includes the following factors.

- Perform renal evaluation from diagnosis of diabetes – measure albumin/creatinine ratio (ACR) or protein/creatinine ratio for proteinuria assessment, creatinine and derived eGFR (calculated using the 2021 NICE CKD-EPI Race-free formula which discontinued adjustment for ethnicity when calculating eGFR) for CKD stages.
- Natural history of diabetes on the kidney – *microvascular* aetiology.
  - Hyperfiltration stage (eGFR increased).
  - Followed by increased protein excretion: microalbuminuria first (e.g. ACR 30–299 mg/24 h). Over eight years follow-up of people with microalbuminuria (Joslin studies): 40% remission (i.e. normoalbuminuria); 40% remain microalbuminuric; and 20% progress to macroalbuminuria (e.g. ACR >300 mg/24 h). Only macroalbuminuria can be detected on regular urinary protein dipsticks.
  - eGFR starts to decline through the various CKD stages to ESRD.
- Natural history of diabetes on the kidney – *macrovascular* aetiology.
  - DKD with decreased eGFR can occur *without* progression through albuminuria stages (i.e. 'non-albuminuric' pathway) – more common in T2DM and occurs in ~25% of DKD.
- Intensive glucose control is critical in the early natural history of diabetes to prevent or stop progression of DKD (i.e. induces legacy effect or 'metabolic memory').

- Glycaemic targets and management should be individualised and not 'one size fits all'. Glycaemic targets are fluid and should be reviewed regularly, especially in more advanced CKD and definitely in ESRD (increased risk of hypoglycaemia).
- Blood pressure control is critical – with angiotensin-converting enzyme inhibitors (ACE-I) or angiotensin receptor blockers (ARB) as part of the mix.
- CVD is a major cause of morbidity and mortality in CKD – the highest CVD risk occurs in patients with decreased eGFR *and* albuminuria.
  - Requires multifactorial CVD risk factor interventions such as good glycaemic control with agents with proven CVD/renal/HF benefits (i.e. SGLT2 inhibitors and/or GLP-1 RA), weight loss, smoking cessation, statins and other lipid-lowering agents, antihypertensives and antiplatelet treatment.
  - SGLT2 inhibitors are now indicated for the treatment of CKD to preserve and halt progression of eGFR deterioration and albuminuria, as well as reducing CVD outcomes (e.g. CVD events and death, HF hospitalisation) in patients *with* and *without diabetes.*
  - Finerenone (mineralocorticoid antagonist) also reduces CVD outcomes (e.g. CVD events and death, HF hospitalisation) and the risk of CKD progression.
- Consider medication dose adjustment (e.g. many DPP4 inhibitors) or discontinuing agents which are contraindicated in CKD (e.g. metformin should be used cautiously in CKD stage 3B and is contraindicated in stages 4 and 5).
- Metformin should be used cautiously in the in-hospital setting because of possible fluctuations in renal function and cardiorespiratory compromise during an acute hospital admission. Adverse events include nausea, vomiting, diarrhoea and contrast-related complications. The most serious adverse effect is the development of metformin-associated lactic acidosis (MALA).
- Many diabetes medications (including insulin and sulfonylureas) are primarily cleared by the kidneys and can lead to hypoglycaemia. Multiple other factors also predispose to hypoglycaemia, such as impaired renal gluconeogenesis and poor appetite in advanced kidney disease.
- Many insulin-treated patients with T2DM and CKD stop or need less insulin as kidney disease progresses (known as 'burnt out' T2DM). Similarly, insulin total daily dose in persons with T1DM may also decrease dramatically. A specific approach for

insulin dosing in this population of patients is needed to minimise the incidence of hypoglycaemia and takes precedence over meeting strict BG targets. The aims of insulin therapy in diabetes patients on maintenance haemodialysis are to improve the quality of life and avoid the extremes of hypo- and hyperglycaemia.

- Glycosylated haemoglobin values are often unreliable in patients with CKD/ESRD because of anaemia of renal disease; close monitoring by capillary BG testing is recommended during hospitalisation and dialysis. CGM may be of value if available.
- Appropriate referral to a nephrologist (e.g. CKD stage 4 for preparation for ESRD or unusual presentation/progression).

Lactic acidosis has been divided into two categories.

- Type A lactic acidosis results from the accumulation of lactate via glycolysis in the absence of oxygen.
- Type B lactic acidosis occurs when lactate production is increased at a time when clearance of lactic acid by oxidation or gluconeogenesis is reduced. MALA is a form of type B (non-hypoxic) lactic acidosis and is generally characterised by blood pH <7.35, very high lactate levels (>15 mmol/l), large anion gap (>20 mmol/l) and renal insufficiency (eGFR <30 ml/min). Mortality ~50%.

Retinopathy

Diabetic eye disease is the leading cause of blindness in working-age adults.

Diabetic retinopathy (DR) occurs in one-third of diabetes patients and is the leading cause of vision loss.

- DR is classified into non-proliferative and proliferative stages.
  - Non-proliferative DR (NPDR) involves progressive intraretinal microvascular alterations.
  - PDR is characterised by the growth of newly formed vessels on the retina or optic disc.
- Diabetic macular oedema refers to retinal thickening in the posterior pole and may occur in either NPDR or PDR.
- Regular eye checkups from diagnosis are required in T2DM (can wait five years in T1DM).

- Intensive glucose control is critical in the early natural history of diabetes to prevent or stop progression of DR (i.e. induces legacy effect or 'metabolic memory').
- Glucose and BP control are critical.
- Smoking cessation is important.
- Women planning pregnancy or already pregnant should have a prompt eye exam with regular follow-up (i.e. risk of DR progression with rapid initiation of intensive glycaemic control needed for good pregnancy outcomes).
- ACEs/ARBs slow progression of DR.
- Statins decrease DR and fenofibrate may slow progression of DR (30–40%).
- Laser treatment is the gold standard for PDR.
- Intravitreal anti-vascular endothelial growth factor (VEGF) agents with prompt or deferred laser treatment for diabetic macular oedema.
- Glitazones (i.e. pioglitazone) can exacerbate diabetic macular oedema.

Macrovascular complications

Increased CVD morbidity and mortality related to diabetes.

- More extensive atherosclerotic CVD.
  - Multivessel disease.
  - Distal disease – more difficult to revascularise.
  - Multivascular bed disease (i.e. polyvascular disease).
- CAD – silent ischaemia/infarction (partly due to autonomic neuropathy).
- Younger people affected. Die ~12 years prematurely.
- Women lose oestrogen protection.
- Worse outcomes despite revascularisation – restenosis more likely.

The importance of CVD in diabetes mellitus is well established. Metabolic syndrome is a constellation of traditional (e.g. hypertension, hypercholesterolaemia, diabetes, obesity) and non-traditional (e.g. dyslipidaemia, endothelial dysfunction, albuminuria) CVD risk factors within a given individual. Metabolic syndrome imparts a 2–3-fold increased risk of CVD and 3–5-fold increased risk of T2DM (if non-diabetic). The underlying pathophysiology is insulin resistance and central obesity (intra-abdominal obesity). Insulin resistance is one of the two key pathophysiological causes of T2DM present in 90–95%. It is defined as an impaired biological response to insulin and results in:

- decreased peripheral utilisation of glucose by skeletal muscle and adipose tissue
- increased hepatic glucose production – especially related to FPG elevation.

Management of CVD risk in people with diabetes

Cardiovascular disease is a common cause of morbidity and mortality in persons with diabetes. The modern multifaceted management of T2DM (Box 23.16), with a focus on the treatment of hypertension and the use of statins, has reduced the prevalence of atherosclerotic CVD, and where previously this was increased 4–6-fold compared to non-diabetic subjects, it is now around double.

Several glucose-lowering therapies have shown benefit at reducing further CVD events (secondary prevention). One of these agents, the GLP-1 RA dulaglutide, has also demonstrated *primary prevention* of CVD. These agents – certain SGLT2 inhibitors and GLP-1 RA – are preferred for the management of glucose lowering in people with diabetes and at high risk of or with established CVD, CKD or HF.

Coronary artery disease

> ACS is a spectrum of disorders including ST elevation myocardial infarction (STEMI), non-ST elevation myocardial infarction (NSTEMI) and unstable angina.

People with diabetes are more likely to have a NSTEMI than non-diabetic subjects. The clinical presentation in people with diabetes is more likely to be atypical or painless (related to autonomic neuropathy), leading to delays in presentation and treatment. All the modern cardiology treatments used for the initial management of ACS are of proven benefit in people with diabetes, including percutaneous coronary intervention (PCI), dual antiplatelet therapy, LMWH or fondaparinux, ACEI or ARB, beta-blockers and high-dose statin therapy. Serious complications such as reinfarction and CHF are more common in people with diabetes, and despite the use of modern treatments, the mortality is doubled. The increased mortality has been attributed to factors present before the acute event, such as more widespread and distal coronary artery disease (as well as microvascular disease), impaired fibrinolysis, autonomic neuropathy and diabetic cardiomyopathy.

Stroke

> Definition of stroke is acute dysfunction lasting more than 24 hours, or of any duration if CT or MRI shows infarction or ischaemia relevant to the symptoms. Transient ischaemic attack (TIA) is defined as focal dysfunction lasting less than 24 hours with no evidence of infarction on imaging. The risk of stroke is more than doubled in people with diabetes, mortality is increased and functional outcomes are worse than non-diabetic subjects with stroke.

Patients with hyperglycaemia following an acute stroke have worse outcomes than patients whose glucose remains in the normal range, including an increase in mortality, worse stroke severity and greater functional impairment. This occurs both in subjects treated with thrombolytic therapy and those who do not receive this treatment. However, intensive

---

Box 23.16 T2DM patients with high CVD risk or established CVD, and/or CKD and/or HF

Address the following *concurrently*.

- Guideline-driven multifactorial CVD risk factor interventions.
  - Hypertension: include ACE-I/ARB, mineralocorticoid receptor antagonist (finerenone).
  - Lipids: moderate or high-dose statins.
  - Antiplatelet agents (generally only used in *secondary* prevention).
  - Smoking cessation.
  - Weight management including nutritional measures, GLP-1 RA, GIP/GLP-1 RA, metabolic surgery.
  - Glucose-lowering treatments with proven CVD/ renal/HF benefits (e.g. SGLT2 inhibitors and GLP-1 RA).
  - Individualise glycaemic goals (to reduce hypoglycaemia).
- 'Residual risk', e.g.:
  - TZD (pioglitazone).
  - PCSK9 inhibitors, ezetimibe, fibrates, small interfering RNA (inclisaran) and omega 3 fatty acids.

insulin therapy following an acute stroke has not demonstrated any reduction in mortality or disability and is not routinely recommended as it increases hypoglycaemia. Patients with acute stroke can be treated to maintain a BG concentration between 5 mmol/l and 15 mmol/l, with close monitoring to avoid hypoglycaemia.

> Pioglitazone reduced events in non-diabetic subjects with insulin resistance following a recent stroke, but is not widely used because of fluid retention and an increase in fractures. GLP-1 RA have demonstrated benefits at reducing stroke and should be more widely used.

Heart failure (HF)

> HF, T2DM, and CKD are interrelated.
> - HF occurs in 35–45% of persons with diabetes.
> - 35–45% of persons with CHF have CKD.
> - 60% of patients with CHF and diabetes have CKD.

The current definition of HF is based on left ventricular ejection fraction (EF).

- Normal 50–75%.
- HF with reduced EF (HFrEF, EF ≤40%).
- HF failure with preserved EF (HFpEF, EF ≥50%). Also termed *diastolic dysfunction*.
- HFpEF, borderline (EF 41–49%).

Heart failure is a common endstage vascular complication of diabetes, particularly in people who have survived previous myocardial infarctions. It is also common for patients with HF to develop diabetes, related to the counterregulatory hormone increases and insulin resistance that accompany HF.

- Cardiology treatment builds on the same principles as in people without diabetes and includes ACEI or ARB, angiotensin receptor–neprilysin inhibitor (ARNI) – sacubitril/valsartan (Entresto®), beta-blockers, mineralocorticoid antagonists, SGLT2 inhibitors, ivabradine if heart rate is raised, and diuretics for symptom relief.
- Metformin should be withheld during acute HF episodes, then restarted once the patient is stable. Metformin appears safe in patients with CHF, and may be of some benefit. Clinically, it would be prudent to avoid the DPP-4 inhibitors saxagliptin or

alogliptin in patients with previous HF. Pioglitazone should be avoided due to associated fluid retention.

> The SGLT2 inhibitor empagliflozin was the first agent to be approved to reduce the risk of CV death and HF hospitalisation in adults with HF with *reduced* or *preserved* EF regardless of whether they have *diabetes* or *not*.

Discharge planning for people with diabetes

Transition to the ambulatory and community setting requires planning and co-ordination. Patients with acceptable preadmission diabetes control may be discharged on their prehospitalisation treatment regimen. Patients with suboptimal glycaemic control should have more intensified therapy and be reviewed by the diabetes specialist team.

> If the person drives, they must be informed of the appropriate Driver and Vehicle Licensing Agency (DVLA) regulations regarding being started on insulin or other glucose-lowering therapies (depending on licence type) or if they had a severe hypoglycaemia. This advice can be found at www.gov.uk/diabetes-driving.

Obesity

> Obesity is defined as abnormal *fat distribution* (e.g. ectopic fat within liver, skeletal muscle) or *function*, and/or excessive *fat accumulation* that may impair health (i.e. 3 Ms – metabolic, mechanical and mental).

Globally, ~39–49% of the world's population (2.8–3.5 billion people) are overweight or obese (2017 figures). Almost two-thirds (63%) of adults in England are overweight or obese. Body mass index (BMI) is the most common measure of overweight and obesity.

- Overweight is defined as a BMI of between ≥25 kg/m² and <30 kg/m².
- Obesity is classified as a BMI of ≥30 kg/m².
- Severe obesity is classified as a BMI of ≥40 kg/m².

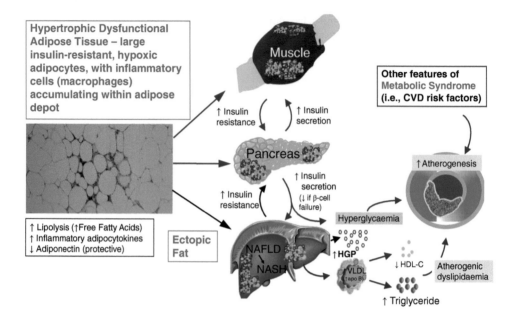

Figure 23.12 Role of lipotoxicity in obesity-associated complications. Lipotoxicity is caused by elevated free fatty acids released by dysfunctional adipocytes leading to ectopic fat storage and inhibition of insulin action, as well as adversely affecting insulin secretion. HDL-C, high-density lipoprotein-cholesterol; HGP, hepatic glucose production; VLDL, very low-density lipoprotein (triglyceride-rich).

Measures of fat distribution are also used (central obesity or intra-abdominal adiposity).

- Waist circumference.
- Waist:hip ratio.

Some ethnic groups have a disproportionate ability to lay down harmful central visceral fat at lower BMIs (i.e. BMI and waist circumference diagnostic cut-offs for Asian and certain other ethnicities are lower), a location that contributes to insulin resistance and a higher risk of T2DM and CVD. Diabesity is a term used to describe the combined adverse health effects of the twin epidemics of obesity and diabetes in an individual. The majority of T2DM cases globally are linked to excess weight.

Obesity is associated with a plethora of other sequelae, including cancer (11–12 cancers are increased related to proinflammatory and insulin resistance states), hypertension, obstructive sleep apnoea, pulmonary thromboembolism, atrial fibrillation (obesity may account for one-fifth of atrial fibrillation cases), pulmonary hypertension, NAFLD, cholelithiasis, degenerative joint disease, oligomenorrhoea/infertility (polycystic ovaries), erectile dysfunction, male obesity-related hypogonadism and cognitive impairment. Obesity also increases vulnerability to more severe COVID-19 infection and increased death.

Traits associated with *unhealthy* obesity include increased intra-abdominal fat, high liver fat (ectopic fat) and abnormal adipose tissue function (Figure 23.12). An ectopic fat depot is generally considered a lipid deposit that is not physiologically stored in adipose tissues such as when in the liver, pancreas, heart and skeletal muscle.

Management of overweight/obesity

Obesity is related to genetic and epigenetic factors, microbiome, medications that cause weight gain (e.g. insulin, steroids), environmental factors (e.g. inactive lifestyle; poor food choices and insecurity; climate; racial, social and healthcare disparities; psychological factors, endocrine-disrupting chemicals; COVID-19 related lockdowns).

The best treatment of overweight/obesity is prevention. Maintaining energy balance is important; it is estimated that on average, adults in England consume 200–300 excess calories per day. Lifestyle changes are important to lose and maintain weight loss. In general, there is no ideal diet for weight loss and no superiority for any particular diet. Thus, choosing a diet composition based on the patient's preferences and health status is best, with the assistance of a dietician when possible. For weight loss maintenance, face-to-face or telemedicine-delivered weight loss maintenance programmes that provide regular contact with a trained interventionist are evidence based, and a high level of physical activity (i.e. 3–5 hours/week) is recommended. Aiming for at least 5–10% weight loss can have health benefits. Further benefits occur with even more weight loss (e.g. diabetes remission can occur with >15% weight loss depending on factors such as 'personal fat threshold' for improvements in NAFLD).

For severe obesity or a BMI ≥35 kg/m² with co-morbidities, a surgical procedure may be best. Currently, metabolic surgery is the only obesity therapy proven to prolong life, a benefit attributable to reductions in cancer as well as CVD-related mortality. Increasing evidence also indicates the value of metabolic surgery in treating patients with T2DM, with many patients free of diabetes medications and some postoperative patients rendered non-diabetic (i.e. *diabetes remission*).

However, so-called *second-generation* weight loss agents (which are also glucose-lowering agents) are transforming the weight loss management landscape. These therapies include the GLP-1 RA semaglutide 2.4 mg once weekly and the once-weekly GIP/GLP-1 RA tirzepatide, which can lead to 15–20% weight loss and reductions in NAFLD which can lead to cardio-metabolic benefits, including diabetes remission.

> Affecting about 25% of adults worldwide, NAFLD is the leading driver of chronic liver disease globally and is the main cause of endstage liver disease in the Western world. NAFLD progresses to non-alcoholic steatohepatitis (NASH) in about 20% of cases, which is a major cause of progression to cirrhosis and hepatocellular carcinoma. NAFLD is closely related to obesity and T2DM. Excess fat within the liver (see Figure 23.12) results in increased hepatic glucose production, leading to fasting hyperglycaemia and artherogenic dyslipidaemia (decreased protective high-density lipoprotein cholesterol and increased triglycerides). The increased triglycerides lead to *ectopic* fat accumulation in other tissues and organs, leading to dysfunction (e.g. beta-cell dysfunction, increased skeletal muscle insulin resistance). The major cause of death in NAFLD is CVD.

Inherited metabolic disorders

> Inherited metabolic diseases (IMDs) are clinically heterogeneous, individually rare disorders that can present at any age, and typically, but not always, are associated with abnormal biochemical tests (usually specialist rather than routine laboratory testing).

Broadly speaking, IMDs can be divided into three groups.

1 Disorders of intoxication give rise to an acute or progressive intoxication secondary to the accumulation of toxic compounds proximal to a metabolic block; for example, disorders of amino acid metabolism such as phenylketonuria (PKU), the organic acidurias and the urea cycle defects such as ornithine transcarbamylase deficiency.

2 Disorders of energy metabolism result in an energy deficiency in tissues such as liver, muscle, brain or heart; for example, mitochondrial respiratory chain defects, fatty acid oxidation defects and glycogen storage disorders.

3 Disorders of complex molecules causing disturbance in the synthesis or catabolism of complex molecules. Symptoms tend to be progressive and not dependent on dietary/energy intake; for example, the lysosomal storage disorders and peroxisomal disorders.

Most adults with an IMD will already have a known diagnosis, usually made in childhood. They may bring with them specific guidelines for emergency management of their condition. Nationally agreed guidelines are also accessible via the internet (e.g. the British Inherited Metabolic Disease Group guidelines, www.BIMDG.org.uk), However, affected adult individuals can also present for the first time. It is important for Acute Medicine clinicians to be aware of these disorders, not only to manage survivors of childhood but also to recognise patients presenting in adulthood.

- The possibility of an underlying IMD should always be considered in patients presenting with encephalopathy (which can be a psychiatric presentation in adults), disturbances of acid–base balance, atypical stroke, psychiatric features or rhabdomyolysis, particularly if these episodes are recurrent and there is no other obvious underlying cause.

- Hypoglycaemia is a fairly unusual initial presentation in adulthood. Adults can maintain their BG levels despite significant metabolic disturbance and thus presentation with hypoglycaemia often represents a late event in a severe metabolic decompensation.
- IMD should also be considered if events are recurrent and where acute decompensations are triggered by metabolic 'stress', such as fasting, intercurrent infection, major surgery, gastrointestinal illness and excessive alcohol or exercise. However, it is not always possible to identify a precise precipitating factor.

As they are genetic diseases, missing the diagnosis may have implications for both the affected individuals and their families. Not all diagnostic tests are readily available in the emergency setting, so appropriate samples should be collected during the acute event. Seek expert help from chemical pathology.

Basic clinical genetics.

- Pathogenic variants: change in gene sequence that cause disease (previously called mutations).
- Penetrance: how likely a pathogenic variant is to cause a disease.
- Polymorphisms/benign variants: genetic variant that does not cause disease in itself.

Classic clinical genetics was largely focused on pathogenic variants that caused diseases with high penetrance. Nowadays, with better, cheaper and more widely available genetic testing, a more accurate diagnosis with *specific* treatment can be offered to some of our patients and their families. However, it is always important to consider the psychosocial implications of having a genetic diagnosis.

24

People with neurological disorders

Hani Ben Amer

 KEY POINTS

- Neurological disorders account for 10–20% of acute medical admissions.
- Most acute neurology patients are managed by Acute Medicine clinicians, and only a small minority are reviewed by neurologists.
- However, acute neurology patients benefit from early neurology expertise, ideally working closely with emergency departments and Acute Medicine services to deliver specialist care at the front door.
- Around 50% of acute neurological presentations are headache and episodes of loss of consciousness (e.g. syncope and seizures).
- There is good evidence that 'neurophobia' is common among non-specialists and can lead to poorer outcomes for patients with neurological presentations.

Introduction

Neurological disorders account for 10–20% of acute medical admissions.

Most acute neurology patients in the UK are managed by Acute Medicine clinicians, with only a small minority being reviewed by neurologists. However, acute neurology patients benefit from early neurology expertise, ideally working closely with the emergency department (ED) and Acute Medicine services to deliver specialist care at the front door (including rapid-access clinics).

Disorders of the neurological system present with a wide range of symptoms and signs, reflecting numerous pathological mechanisms. Around 50% of acute neurological presentations are headache and episodes of loss of consciousness (e.g. syncope and seizures). Patients presenting with possible stroke are assessed and managed by the stroke team, often in collaboration with Acute Medicine depending on local set-up. Hyperacute stroke units (HASUs), operating 24/7, provide better outcomes when available.

There is good evidence that 'neurophobia' is common among non-specialists, leading to the well-established reputation of neurology being a difficult subject. One of the reasons for this is the ease with which non-specialists can get lost in unnecessary details. Therefore, it is important to develop a logical and systematic approach to the clinical history and examination based on knowledge of the underlying anatomy and physiology and concentrating on the most common and important neurological presentations and disorders. The key is to focus on the presenting problem without losing sight of the patient's wider medical and social context and delivering appropriate advice and care when patients need it most.

Acute Medicine: Lecture Notes, First Edition. Edited by Glenn Matfin.
© 2023 John Wiley & Sons Ltd. Published 2023 by John Wiley & Sons Ltd.

Basic neuroanatomy

The nervous system is divided into the:
- central nervous system (CNS)
- peripheral nervous system (PNS).

Although some basic neuroanatomy is needed, comprehensive knowledge of neuroanatomy is not required for everyday Acute Medicine clinical practice.

The CNS

- There are 12 cranial nerves.
- The function of different lobes of the brain is as follows.
  - Frontal: contains the precentral gyrus which controls motor function on the opposite side of the body (motor cortex). Also, the dominant hemisphere contains the Broca's area (inferior frontal gyrus) that controls speech output. The frontal lobe controls the emotions.
  - Parietal: contains the postcentral gyrus which controls sensory function on the opposite side of the body (sensory cortex).
  - Temporal: controls the memory. Also, the dominant hemisphere contains the Wernicke's area (superior temporal gyrus) that controls the comprehension of speech.
  - Occipital: controls the vision.
  - Brainstem (midbrain, pons and medulla).
  - Basal ganglia.
- The following are important tracts.
  - Corticospinal tract (motor pathway) (Figure 24.1): starts at the motor cortex (precentral gyrus), descends through the anterior part of the internal capsule, crosses to the other side in the medulla, traverses the spinal cord in the lateral column and terminates in the ventral horn motor neurones.
  - Spinothalamic tract (pain and temperature) (Figure 24.2): pain and temperature fibres enter the spinal cord at the dorsal horn and cross to the opposite side and ascend through the lateral column to the thalamus. They then project through the posterior part of the internal capsule to the sensory cortex, the postcentral gyrus.
  - Dorsal column (position and vibration) (see Figure 24.2): position and vibration sensory fibres enter the spinal cord at the dorsal horn and ascend through the posterior (dorsal) column to the medulla, then cross to the other side to project

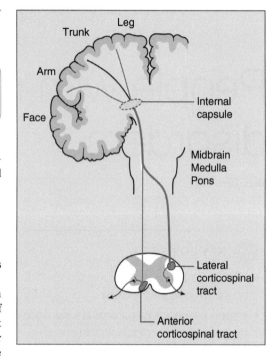

Figure 24.1 Motor pathways. Source: Bradley JR. Lecture Notes: Clinical Medicine, 8th edn. Chichester: Wiley, 2018.

through the posterior part of the internal capsule to the sensory cortex, the postcentral gyrus.
  - It is important to remember that the body is represented upside down in both the sensory and motor cortex. Both the sensory and motor cortex function are contralateral (controlling the opposite side of the body).
- Spinal cord (usually ends at the level of the L1 vertebra).

The PNS

- Nerve roots including the cauda equina (the nerve roots from the lower end of the spinal cord).
- Plexus (brachial and lumbosacral).
- Nerves.
- Neuromuscular junction.
- Muscles.

Basic clinical neurology

The acute care setting is under tremendous pressure, including time. This makes it necessary to conduct an efficient neurological assessment. Most neurological

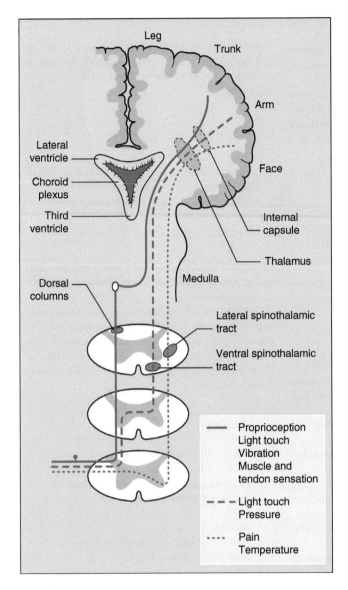

Figure 24.2 Sensory pathways.
Source: Bradley JR. Lecture Notes: Clinical Medicine, 8th edn. Chichester: Wiley, 2018.

diagnoses rest on the history (direct and collateral). The temporal aspects of presentation (e.g. hyperacute or chronic, stable or progressive) are especially useful in making a diagnosis. Develop an examination routine to rapidly screen for neurological deficits. Target investigations to define aetiology. Agree on a timely, patient-centred, shared decision-making management plan. Involve the multidisciplinary team. Decide whether the patient needs admission or can be managed in an ambulatory or home setting.

Neurological consultation

The neurological consultation usually has the following stages.

- Greeting – introduce yourself to the patient/carer.
- History.
  - Opening: start by asking 'tell me about your symptom' rather than 'your doctor referred you because of. . . (headache, etc.), tell me about it'. The patient's agenda may differ markedly from that of the referring doctor.
  - Exploring: ask direct questions to explore the possible cause of the patient's symptoms: 'How often do you have headache?'.
  - Generating a diagnosis or differential diagnosis: by the end of the history taking, you should have a clear idea about the possible explanation(s) of the patient's symptoms.

- Examination – no neurologist does a full and detailed neurological examination on any one patient. Contrary to general belief, neurological examination rarely provides a diagnosis alone, but usually supports the history findings.
- Conclusions – formulating a plan which may include investigations. Explain the plan to the patient. Ask the patient if he/she would like to ask any questions.

History

Some of the major acute neurological presentations (e.g. headache, loss of consciousness) are diagnosed mainly on the history. Patients with such presentations often have very few clinical signs and the investigations may be normal. Therefore, history taking in neurology carries greater importance compared with many other medical specialties.

- It is important to obtain a precise understanding of the patient's symptoms. For example, dizziness could mean lightheadedness, vertigo or even loss of consciousness.
- The onset of the symptoms could help in determining the pathological processes.
  - Sudden onset (hyperacute or acute) – e.g. vascular.
  - Gradual onset – e.g. degenerative.
  - Paroxysmal – e.g. epilepsy or migraine.
- Other components of the history could be helpful in making the diagnosis.
  - Excess alcohol intake in peripheral neuropathy, withdrawal seizures.
  - Drug history such as antipsychotic agents in (drug-induced) parkinsonism.
  - Adherence to medications such as antiepileptics.
- Handedness is important, especially in patients with speech symptoms.

Examination

The examination in the Acute Medicine setting is usually *focused* and guided by diagnosis or differential diagnosis generated from the history.

Practise a neurological screening examination. Extend the assessment appropriately if the history dictates so.

Mental state examination

The mini-mental test is widely used as a screening tool for mental state. Normal cognitive function is 24–30/30; <24/30 is the cut-off score for cognitive impairment.

Coma (unconsciousness)

Unconsciousness or coma is defined as a sleep-like state, due to a diverse range of aetiologies and pathologies, from which the patient cannot be aroused.

Consciousness depends on the intact reticular activating system in the brainstem and includes both arousal and awareness.

The Glasgow Coma Scale (GCS) is vital in assessing and reporting a patient's level of consciousness. The patient's scale and score should be recorded. The Alert, Confusion, responsive to Voice, Pain, or Unresponsive (ACVPU) tool is also widely used in Acute Medicine.

The causes of coma include the following.
- Infection (meningitis and encephalitis).
- Electrolyte abnormalities.
- Metabolic causes such as hypoglycaemia, diabetic ketoacidosis, hypoxia, liver and renal failure.
- Seizures.
- Cerebral haemorrhage (intracerebral and subarachnoid haemorrhage).
- Poisons and drug overdose such as alcohol and opiate toxicity.
- Tentorial herniation and coning – a mass lesion in the brain could push the cerebral hemisphere through the tentorial hiatus (tentorial herniation), causing the brainstem and cerebellum to be pushed downward and impacting in the foramen magnum (coning).
- Head injury.

Speech

- The cortical area of speech is in the dominant hemisphere (left hemisphere in right-handed people and in 60–70% of left-handed people).

- Speech has four components – comprehension of language, production of language, articulation of speech, and phonation (sound and volume).
  - Dysphasia is the impairment of comprehension or production of language.
  - Dysarthria is the impairment of articulation.
  - Dysphonia is the impairment of phonation.
- The anatomy of speech includes the following aspects.
  - Superior temporal gyrus (Wernicke's area).
  - Inferior frontal gyrus (Broca's area).
  - Arcuate fasciculus (perisylvian region) which connects the superior temporal gyrus with the inferior frontal gyrus.
  - Motor input from the corticobulbar pathway, cerebellum and basal ganglia.
  - Cranial nerve input such as 10th nerve (supplies the larynx), 12th nerve (supplies the tongue).
- The two most important aspects in examination of speech are comprehension (understanding) and fluency (spontaneous speech). This should be examined together by the following methods.
  - Ask questions, e.g. What is your address? What do you do for a living?
  - Give commands, e.g. start with simple commands (close your eyes) and increase the complexity as appropriate.
  - Assess repetition, e.g. ask the patient to repeat a simple word such as 'pen' or 'watch'; try a full sentence, 'it is very cold today', and try a complicated phrase, 'no ifs, ands or buts'.
  - Receptive (sensory, fluent, Wernicke's, posterior) aphasia (dysphasia): the patient's comprehension is impaired. However, the speech is very fluent but does not make any sense (unintelligible), hence receptive aphasia. If it is an isolated finding, the patient could be mislabelled as confused. Repetition is impaired. Receptive aphasia is due to a lesion in the superior temporal gyrus in the dominant (left) hemisphere.
  - Expressive (motor, non-fluent, Broca's, anterior) aphasia (dysphasia): the patient's comprehension is preserved but the speech is not fluent. Repetition is impaired. Expressive aphasia is due to a lesion in the inferior frontal gyrus in the dominant (left) hemisphere.
  - Many patients usually have a combination of both types of aphasia (global aphasia).
  - Naming is impaired in all forms of aphasia so it is not usually of any localisation value.
  - Isolated impairment in repetition is called conductive aphasia and is usually due to a lesion in the arcuate fasciculus.
- Causes of the aphasia are usually stroke and brain tumours.

Cranial nerves

Traditionally, examination of the cranial nerves is conducted according to their numerical order. However, it is a lot easier and more practical if the cranial nerves are examined together (Box 24.1).

Neurological motor limb examination

Neurological motor examination for both upper and lower limbs should include inspection, tone, power, reflexes and co-ordination.

It is important to use the Medical Research Council scale when describing muscle weakness.

Grade 0: no *visible* contraction.

Grade 1: flicker of contraction.

Grade 2: movement with gravity.

Grade 3: movement against gravity.

Grade 4: movement against partial resistance.

Grade 5: normal power.

Remember the following points.

- Inspection – check for muscle wasting or fasciculation. Look at the patient's back for spinal scar.
- Ask the patient to place their upper limbs outstretched in front of them with their eyes closed and palms facing upward (pronator test). This will give you a quick idea about any problems with power (drifting down), position sense (fingers move up and down – pseudo-athetosis) or cerebellar disease (arms move up).
- Take time in explaining to the patient each step of the examination (e.g. heel-shin test). This will save time and ensure correct technique.
- Grade the power according to the maximum power achieved.
- When examining muscle power, test each side and then compare.
- When reflexes are absent, do the reinforcement by asking the patient to clench the teeth or hold the fingers of both hands together and pull them against each other.
- Grade the reflexes as absent, normal or brisk.
- Remember that asymmetry of reflexes is usually significant.
- CNS lesions usually cause upper motor neurone (UMN) signs.

Box 24.1 Cranial nerve examination

Inspection

- Reduced forehead wrinkles (7th).
- Ptosis (3rd).
- Wasting of the temporalis muscles (5th).
- Absence of the nasolabial folds (7th).

Ask the patient to:

- raise the eyebrows (7th)
- shut the eyes tightly; you should try to force them open (7th)
- blow out the cheeks (7th)
- show the teeth or smile (7th).

Examine the eyes

- Be sure that the patient can see by checking their visual acuity using a (pocket) Snellen chart, with glasses. Or, if a Snellen chart is not available, a newspaper or something similar could be used (2nd).
- Look at the size of the pupils and their reaction to light, direct and indirect responses (2nd/3rd).
- Do the eye movements and ask if there is double vision (3rd, 4th, 6th).
- Examine the fundi mainly looking at the optic discs (2nd).

Examine the face

- Test pinprick sensation in the upper, middle and lower parts of the face (the three divisions of the 5th).
- Palpate the masseter and temporalis muscles by asking the patient to clench the teeth (5th).

Examine the mouth

- Ask the patient to open the jaw against your hand (5th).
- Inspect the tongue inside the floor of the mouth (12th).
- Ask the patient to protrude the tongue (12th).
- Ask the patient to move the tongue from side to side and look for any slowness (12th).
- Ask the patient to say 'Ah' and assess the movement of the soft palate and uvula (10th).

Examine the neck and shoulders

- Ask the patient to twist the head to one direction against your hand. Palpate the opposite sternomastoid (11th).
- Ask the patient to shrug the shoulders against resistance (11th).

Others (occasionally needed in clinical practice)

- Examine the visual field by confrontation. Use a white hat pin, sit at the same level as the patient, about 1 metre away, and compare your field to the patient and test the four quadrants. A red pin is used to test for central scotoma.
- Test the reaction of the pupils to convergence by asking the patient to look straight ahead and then at the tip of the nose.
- If you find evidence of 5th nerve impairment, test the corneal reflex. Remember to stimulate the cornea, not the sclera.
- If the patient has hearing problems, test for evidence of sensorineural deafness (8th).
  - Rinne's test: hold a 256 or 512 Hz tuning fork in front of the external auditory meatus and then against the mastoid. In the affected ear, air conduction < bone conduction in conductive deafness; and air conduction > bone conduction in sensorineural deafness.
  - Weber's test: place a 256 or 512 Hz tuning fork in the middle of the forehead. The sound will be louder in the affected ear in conductive deafness, and in the normal ear in sensorineural deafness.

  - Increased tone (spasticity).
  - Weakness with no wasting.
  - Brisk reflexes and clonus.
  - Upgoing plantars.
- Peripheral nervous system lesions usually cause lower motor neurone (LMN) signs.
  - Reduced tone (hypotonia).
  - Weakness, wasting and fasciculation.
  - Reduced or absent reflexes.
  - Downgoing (normal) plantars.

Sensory examination

The main purpose of the sensory examination is to:
- identify any sensory level
- identify any evidence of 'glove and stocking' distribution
- determine any dermatomal impairments.

Remember the following points.

- Always teach the patient first by starting at the sternum or the forehead. The patient needs to recognise normal sensation!
- Test the pain sensation by using the sharp end of a neurotip.

- Start from the hand and work up, in the case of upper limb examination, or feet and go up in the lower limb examination. Test random points covering the outer and inner aspects of the hands, forearms and upper arms, that should cover all dermatomes of the upper limbs, and outer and inner aspects of the feet, calves and thighs, that should cover all dermatomes of the lower limbs.
- Do the joint position sense. Hold the distal interphalangeal joint of the middle finger between your two fingers from the sides and move it up and down. Make only a small movement (2–3 mm) and avoid putting the joint in extreme positions. First, show the patient what you are going to do and then get the patient to do it with their eyes closed. Do the same in the lower limbs by holding the big toe at the sides and moving it up and down.
- Test for vibration sense. Start with the wrist; if abnormal, move to the elbow and shoulder in the upper limbs or start with the ankle (medial malleolus) and if abnormal, move to the knee and iliac crest in the lower limbs.
- When you examine pinprick sensation, ask the patient 'Does the pin feel as sharp as it did on your chest or forehead?', *not* 'Do you feel it?' as the answer will probably be yes!
- There is no need to ask the patient to close their eyes during the pinprick examination. It serves no purpose.
- If there is dermatomal impairment of pinprick, map the abnormality (e.g. L5/S1).
- Test the vibration sense with a 128 Hz tuning fork.
- Light touch examination does not usually add anything.

Gait examination

- Look very carefully at the gait base (e.g. wide or narrow), the steps, the arms (do they swing?), posture (e.g. stooped) and the ability to turn.
- Ask the patient to do the tandem walk (heel to toe). Demonstrate this to the patient first.
- If you think the patient is ataxic, do Romberg's test.
  ○ Ask the patient to stand with feet together, arms by the side, and then ask the patient to close their eyes.
  ○ Romberg's sign tends to be overrated. All patients with ataxia tend to get worse when they close their eyes. Romberg's sign should only be considered positive if there is a significant degree of worsening of the ataxia after closing the eyes, which indicates sensory ataxia.
- Always stand close to the patient when examining the tandem gait or Romberg's test. You do not want the patient to fall during the examination.

Classic gait abnormalities

- Hemiplegic gait – the lower limb moves in a semicircle, the toe scraping the floor with each step, and the arm is held in a flexed position close to the chest.
- Spastic gait – a stiff, scissor gait with the legs crossing in front of each other while walking.
- Ataxic gait – patient's gait is wide-based with difficulty performing the heel-to-toe test – 'drunken gait'. Patients with sensory ataxia usually have severe impairment of joint position and vibration. Patients usually stamp their feet on the floor when walking.
- Parkinsonian gait – patient walks with small steps and shuffles. He/she stoops with lack of arm swing. The arms are held in flexed positions.
- Steppage gait – patient lifts the foot high during walking to avoid scraping the toes and foot slapping. This is due to foot drop.
- Waddling gait – patient's legs are held wide apart. Lumbar lordosis. Trunk moves from side to side with pelvis dropping usually due to hereditary muscular dystrophies.

Neurological investigations

In general, if clinical assessments indicate an UMN lesion, the patient may need neuroimaging studies, and if they indicate a LMN lesion, the patient may need a neurophysiological study.

Neuroradiology

- Computed tomography (CT) scan – easily available and commonly used in emergencies. However, it exposes the patient to a relatively large dose of radiation. CT is useful in detecting intracranial bleed, but not helpful in detecting demyelinating plaques or spinal cord pathology. CT angiography (CTA) and CT venography (CTV) are useful in demonstrating abnormalities in intracranial blood vessels such as arterial aneurysm or venous thrombosis.
- Magnetic resonance imaging (MRI) scan – does not involve doses of radiation but some patients find it claustrophobic. MRI cannot be used in patients with metallic foreign bodies such as cardiac pacemakers because of the effect of the magnetic field (although this situation can be reviewed by the pacing department in non-acute setting). MRI is useful in detecting various brain and spinal cord pathology. MR angiography (MRA) and MR venography (MRV) are also widely used to demonstrate abnormalities in intracranial blood vessels.
- Angiography – still considered as the 'gold standard' for imaging the intracranial blood vessels.

However, it is mainly used as a treatment tool (interventional radiology) in coiling aneurysms, for example.

- Single-photon emission computed tomography (SPECT) and positron emission tomography (PET) have limited use in routine clinical practice.

Neurophysiology

- Electroencephalogram (EEG) – useful for epilepsy evaluation.
- Nerve conduction study (NCS) – by electrical stimulation of different peripheral nerves, it is possible to measure both sensory and motor function of these nerves. Usually used in assessment of peripheral neuropathy to differentiate between axonal and demyelinating neuropathy and nerve entrapment.
- Electromyography (EMG) – a fine needle inserted directly into a muscle to look for spontaneous activity and motor unit potential. EMG can be helpful in:
  - assessment of peripheral neuropathy to differentiate between axonal and demyelinating neuropathy
  - neuromuscular disorders such as myasthenia gravis (MG)
  - demonstrating fibrillation potentials, for example in motor neurone disease (MND).

Lumbar puncture

- Lumbar puncture (LP) is one of the most commonly used investigations in neurology. It is usually indicated in acute settings such as acute headache or patients with possible diagnosis of meningitis or encephalitis. Also used in investigating patients with possible multiple sclerosis (MS) or any other inflammatory diseases.
- LP is contraindicated in patients with symptoms or signs attributable to raised intracranial pressure as this could lead to tentorial herniation and coning.
- Document the opening pressure with the patient in the lateral position.
- Routinely, the cerebrospinal fluid (CSF) is analysed for protein, cells and glucose (a blood sample for glucose should be sent with the CSF). If infection is suspected, perform CSF Gram stain, routine culture and molecular tests that detect the genetic material of any microbes present. Spectrophotometry looking for blood breakdown products is indicated in suspected subarachnoid haemorrhage (SAH). Checking for oligoclonal bands is used to help diagnose MS.

- The most common complication of LP is 'post-LP headache' which results from reduction in intracranial pressure. The headache is worse on sitting or standing and usually resolves spontaneously within 7–10 days.

Common cranial nerve disorders

Optic (2nd) nerve

The optic nerve disorders can be divided as follows.

- Pupil abnormalities.
- Visual field defects.
- Optic disc disorders.

Pupil abnormalities

- The optic nerve carries the afferent limb of the pupillary light reflex.
- Relative afferent pupillary defect (RAPD) is tested by the light swing test (swing the light from one pupil to the other every second or two). Normal pupils constrict every time they are exposed to light. In afferent pupillary defect, the pupil dilates instead when exposed to light. RAPD indicates optic nerve disease, usually optic neuritis in patients with MS.
- Horner syndrome is another pupil abnormality encountered in clinical practice. However, Horner syndrome is *not* due to an optic nerve lesion but to a lesion in the sympathetic pathway. Clinically, patients present with unilateral incomplete ptosis with no evidence of abnormal eye movement. The pupil is small and reactive to light and accommodation. Other features include enophthalmos (eye appears sunken) and lack of sweating of the face on the side of the lesion. The lesion in Horner syndrome could occur at any level from hypothalamus, medulla, cervical cord or sympathetic chain. Causes of Horner syndrome include idiopathic, Pancoast syndrome because of apical lung malignancy, and trauma or surgery such as thyroid surgery.
- Other pupillary defects not related to optic nerve (the site of pathology is not known) are as follows.
  - Argyll Robertson pupil: rare classic neurological sign. It is a small irregular pupil reacting to accommodation but not to light due to syphilis or diabetes.

o Adie's pupil: a unilateral dilated pupil not reacting to light (or sluggish reaction) in young or middle-aged women. Holmes–Adie syndrome is a combination of Adie's pupil and reduced or absent tendon reflexes.

Visual field defects

- The visual pathway includes the following (Figure 24.3).
  o Retina and optic nerve.
  o Optic chiasm.
  o Optic tract reaching lateral geniculate body.
  o Optic radiation through parietal and temporal lobes.
  o Visual cortex in the occipital lobe.

- Bitemporal hemianopia – visual field assessment showing evidence of impairment of both temporal fields because of a lesion in the optic chiasm. Causes of optic chiasm lesion are usually pituitary tumours (Figure 24.4). Other causes include craniopharyngioma, meningioma and large internal carotid artery aneurysm.
- Homonymous hemianopia – visual field assessment showing evidence of impairment of the temporal field on one side and the nasal field on the other side as a result of an optic tract lesion (behind the optic chiasm). The visual field defect in this case is on the contralateral side to the lesion (e.g. a lesion in the *right* posterior optic tract causes *left* homonymous hemianopia). Causes of optic tract lesion include cerebrovascular disease, such as

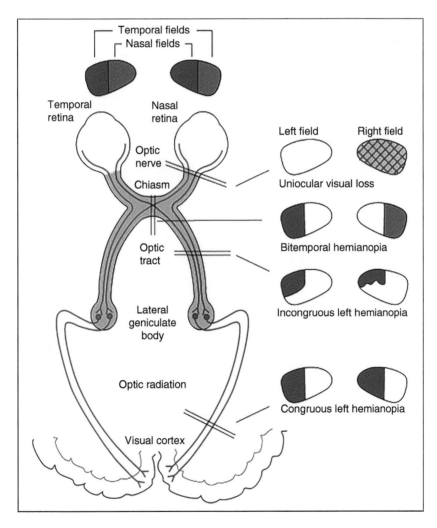

Figure 24.3 Anatomy of the optic pathway and the field defects produced by lesions at different sites.
Source: Bruce J, et al. Lecture Notes: Ophthalmology. Chichester: Wiley, 2016.

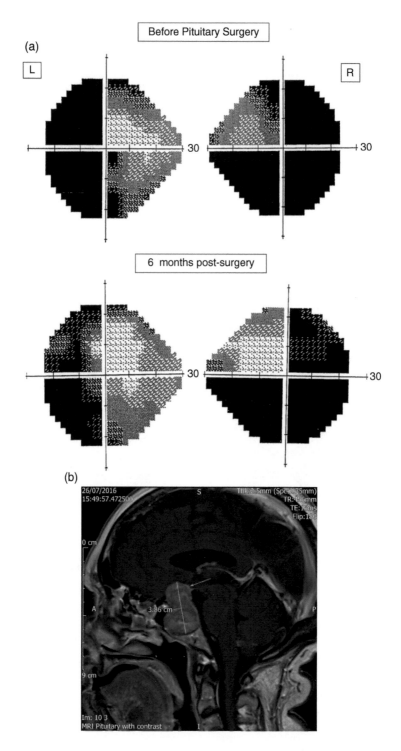

Figure 24.4 (a) Humphrey visual fields before and six months after transsphenoidal surgery. Eyesight was much improved following surgery with some improvement on formal visual field testing. (b) MRI pituitary sagittal views of the same patient at baseline showing a large macroadenoma (gonadotropin staining non-functioning pituitary tumour). Elevated and compressed optic chiasm not seen on sagittal view but probably in vicinity of arrow.

(a)

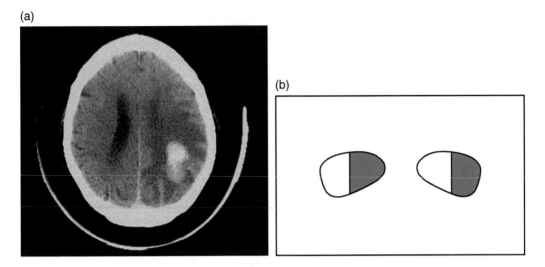

(b)

Figure 24.5 (a) A CT scan showing a left cortical infarct. (b) The complete congruous right homonymous hemiano-pia produced by the infarct. Source: Bruce J, et al. Lecture Notes: Ophthalmology. Chichester: Wiley, 2016.

occipital infarction or haemorrhage (Figure 24.5), and tumours. The visual loss could be only in the quadrant of the visual field if the lesion is in the temporal lobe (superior quadrantanopia) or pari-etal lobe (inferior quadrantanopia).

Optic disc swelling (papilloedema)

- Papilloedema is an optic disc swelling due to raised intracranial pressure. Therefore, optic disc swelling is a more correct term.
- Papilloedema causes absent venous pulsation and blurring of the optic disc margin with or without haemorrhages or exudates.
- Causes of papilloedema include the following.
  o Increased intracranial pressure due to brain tumours, cerebrovenous sinus thrombosis and cerebral abscess.
  o If the patient is a young obese female, then the likely diagnosis is idiopathic (benign) intracra-nial hypertension.
  o Other rare causes include malignant hyperten-sion and cavernous sinus thrombosis.
- Optic neuritis (papillitis) is another cause of optic disc swelling and is defined as acute inflammation of the optic nerve. MS is a common cause of optic neuritis. Retrobulbar optic neuritis causes inflam-mation of the optic disc with acute visual loss and normal-looking optic disc.
- Optic neuritis causes visual loss, central scotoma, retro-orbital pain and RAPD, whilst papilloedema causes peripheral visual field constriction (visual acuity

is usually normal until a very late stage); patients may report headache and pupils are normal.

Optic atrophy

- Optic disc is pale with sharp margins.
- Causes of optic atrophy.
  o MS in young patients.
  o Ischaemic optic neuropathy in older people.
  o Other causes include optic nerve compression, Leber hereditary optic neuropathy, toxins (tobacco and methyl alcohol) and nutritional deficiencies (vitamin B1 and B12).
- Secondary optic atrophy is due to long-standing papilloedema. The discs appear pale with ill-defined disc margins.

Oculomotor (3rd) nerve

- The oculomotor nerve supplies all muscles of the eye (medial rectus, superior rectus, inferior rectus and inferior oblique) except the lateral rectus (6th nerve) and superior oblique (4th nerve). It also supplies the levator palpebrae muscle and carries the parasympathetic fibres to the pupil (efferent limb of the pupillary light reflex).
- Patient usually presents with partial or complete ptosis with eye deviation laterally (down and out), with or without pupillary dilation and impaired response to light and accommodation.
- Causes of 3rd nerve palsy include the following.

- Ischaemic (microvascular): usually painless with pupillary sparing in patients with diabetes and/or hypertension. Spontaneous recovery is the usual outcome within several months.
- Surgical causes: such as posterior communicating artery aneurysm (painful) or brainstem tumour.
- Local lesions such as metastasis, meningioma, nasopharyngeal carcinoma, aneurysm, infection (tuberculosis or fungal) or cavernous sinus thrombosis.
- Tentorial herniation and coning.

Trigeminal (5th) nerve

- The 5th nerve provides sensory supply to the face.
  - Ophthalmic (V1): supplies the forehead to the vertex and the cornea.
  - Maxillary (V2): supplies the cheek.
  - Mandibular (V3): supplies the lower jaw but not the angle of the jaw.
- The motor component of the 5th nerve supplies the masseter and temporalis muscles.
- Any pathology affecting the brainstem, cerebellopontine angle or cavernous sinus could lead to sensory abnormalities on the face with absent corneal reflex.

Abducens (6th) nerve

- The 6th nerve supplies the lateral rectus muscle.
- Patients usally present with horizontally separated double vision (diplopia) on looking to the side (right or left), with limitation of abduction of the eye.
- Causes of 6th nerve palsy include the following.
  - Ischaemic (microvascular): usually in patients with diabetes and hypertension. Spontaneous recovery is the usual outcome within months.
  - The 6th nerve is vulnerable to an increase in intracranial pressure due to the long peripheral course of the nerve leading to false localising signs.
  - Brainstem lesions such as tumour or demyelination (MS).

Facial (7th) nerve

- The facial nerve is primarily motor. The nerve leaves the pons in the cerebellopontine angle to enter the internal auditory meatus and the facial canal. It provides supply to the stapedius muscle before emerging from the skull through the stylomastoid foramen to supply the facial muscles. The facial nerve also supplies taste to the anterior two-thirds of the tongue.
- Due to the bilateral cortical innervation of the facial nerve nucleus, there are two types of 7th nerve palsy: UMN type (contralateral weakness of the lower part of the face with forehead and eye closure relatively spared) and LMN type (ipsilateral weakness of the whole side of the face).
- The most common cause of UMN 7th nerve palsy is hemisphere stroke.
- Bell's palsy is a common cause of LMN 7th nerve palsy. Patients usually present with facial weakness involving the whole side of the face. Examination shows difficulty with raising the eyebrow, inability to shut the eye fully, Bell's phenomenon (turning of the eye upwards when the patient is asked to shut the eyes), difficulty with cheek blowing, obliteration of the nasolabial fold and droopy mouth. No investigation is usually required to diagnose Bell's palsy. Spontaneous full recovery occurs in more than 80% of patients with Bell's palsy. The role of steroids and aciclovir is still controversial. However, steroids are commonly used, especially if the patient is seen within 72 hours from the onset of the palsy. Protection of the cornea by using artificial tears is essential.
- Other causes of LMN 7th nerve palsy include cerebellopontine angle lesion such as acoustic neuroma, middle ear infection, parotid tumour, parotid gland or ear surgery, pontine lesion such as tumour and Ramsey–Hunt syndrome due to herpes zoster infection affecting the geniculate (facial) ganglion. COVID-19 infection and post-COVID syndromes may also be related.
- Hyperacusis (sound heard abnormally loudly) could be a feature of 7th nerve palsy.
- Bilateral LMN lesion of the 7th nerve could be tricky to detect due to the absence of asymmetry. Causes of bilateral LMN 7th nerve include Guillain–Barré syndrome, neurosarcoid and Lyme disease.

Vestibulocochlear (8th) nerve

- The 8th nerve nucleus is located in the pons. The nerve exits at the cerebellopontine angle and enters the internal auditory meatus. It connects the cochlea (cochlear nerve) and labyrinth, also known as vestibular body (vestibular nerve), with the CNS. The function of the nerve consists of maintaining balance and equilibrium (vestibular nerve) and hearing (cochlear nerve).
- Lesions in the cerebellopontine angle such as acoustic neuroma could present with deafness and loss of balance.
- Patients with hearing loss usually present to the ENT clinics. Ménière's disease includes deafness, tinnitus and episodic vertigo and vomiting.

- Other relatively common problems that could present to both neurology or ENT clinics are acute labyrinthitis or vestibular neuronitis and benign paroxysmal positional vertigo (BPPV).
  - Acute labyrinthitis or vestibular neuronitis is a sudden onset of rotatory vertigo, vomiting and losing balance to the extent that the patient may not be able to walk. The severe symptoms usually resolve within days but full recovery could take several weeks.
  - BPPV: episodes of short-lived vertigo, usually seconds, in certain positions such as turning in bed. Spontaneous resolution of symptoms is the norm.
- Any brainstem pathology such as vascular or demyelination could impaire the function of the 8th nerve.

Glossopharyngeal (9th), vagus (10th) and hypoglossal (12th) nerves

- The 9th nerve supplies the palate and pharynx, the 10th nerve supplies the pharynx and larynx and the 12th nerve supplies the tongue muscles.
- Bulbar palsy (bilateral LMN lesion of the lower cranial nerves): wasted and atrophic tongue with fasciculation. Causes of bulbar palsy include MND, syringobulbia, skull base lesion, which is usually due to cancer, and brainstem tumour.
- Pseudobulbar palsy (bilateral UMN of the lower cranial nerves): small, slow-moving spastic tongue. Causes of pseudobulbar palsy include extensive cerebrovascular disease, causing bilateral ischaemia, and MND.
- Mixture of bulbar and pseudobulbar palsy is usually caused by MND and leads to a slow-moving, wasted and atrophic tongue with fasciculation.
- A brisk jaw reflex, spastic slurring dysarthria and emotional lability are indicators of pseudobulbar palsy.
- A depressed jaw reflex and nasal speech are features of bulbar palsy.
- Swallowing is usually impaired in both bulbar and pseudobulbar palsy.
- Unilateral LMN lesion of the 12th nerve usually presents with unilateral wasting and fasciculation of the tongue and deviation of the tongue to one side. The tongue deviates towards the side of the lesion. Causes of unilateral LMN lesion 12th nerve palsy include cancer, lymphoma, tuberculosis and sarcoidosis.

Common neurological patterns

Monoplegia/hemiplegia

There is unilateral arm and/or leg weakness with increased tone and brisk reflexes. There is possible impairment of pinprick sensation over the affected side and facial weakness (ipsilateral UMN lesion of 7th nerve).

The causes of monoplegia and/or hemiplegia are as follows.

- Cerebrovascular disease (sudden onset).
- Brain tumour (gradual onset).
- Spinal cord lesion (gradual onset).

The investigation of monoplegia/hemiplegia could include the following.

- Brain CT and/or MRI.
- Spinal MRI.
- Assessment of vascular risk factors such as blood glucose and cholesterol.
- If there is loss of joint position and vibration on the monoparetic side and loss of pain and temperature on the opposite side to a certain sensory level (e.g. T10), then the diagnosis is Brown–Séquard syndrome which is usually caused by spinal cord tumour or MS.

Spastic paraparesis/ quadriparesis

Bilateral increased (spastic) tone with brisk reflexes, and upgoing plantars in the lower limbs. There is (possible) weakness, ankle clonus and sensory level. The upper limbs may show signs of UMN lesion.

Common causes include MS in younger patients; cervical spondylotic myelopathy in middle-aged and elderly patients; spinal trauma; spinal tumours (primary or metastatic); vascular causes such as spinal arteriovenous malformation and spinal ischaemia (anterior spinal artery syndrome). MND and B12 deficiency are less common causes.

The investigation of spastic paraparesis/quadriparesis could include the following.

- Brain MRI.
- Spine MRI.
- CSF looking particularly for oligoclonal bands (MS).
- Other specific investigations if there is clear indication of the cause (e.g. NCS/EMG in MND, checking vitamin B12).

Peripheral neuropathy

> Predominantly sensory peripheral neuropathy: there is reduction in pinprick sensation in the glove and stocking distribution. There is also impairment in vibration and joint position sense. Ankle jerks may be absent.

The causes of predominantly *sensory* peripheral neuropathy are as follows.

- Diabetes.
- Vitamin B deficiency (thiamine and B12), especially in alcoholics.
- Paraneoplastic neuropathy.
- Drugs such as antituberculosis (isoniazid and ethambutol) and chemotherapeutic agents (cisplatin and vincristine).
- Others such as amyloid and chronic kidney disease.
- Idiopathic, especially in elderly patients.
- Paraproteinaemic neuropathy (mixed sensory and motor neuropathy).

> Predominantly motor peripheral neuropathy: bilateral generalised weakness more marked distally with absent jerks and mild impairment of pinprick, joint position and vibration sense.

The causes of predominantly *motor* peripheral neuropathy are as follows.

- Guillain–Barré syndrome.
- Chronic inflammatory demyelinating polyneuropathy (CIDP).
- Charcot–Marie–Tooth disease.
- Porphyria.
- Lead poisoning.

Investigations could include the following.

- NCS/EMG – important to confirm the diagnosis and to determine whether there is axonal neuropathy or demyelinating neuropathy.
- CSF, looking particularly for high protein (demyelinating neuropathy).
- Blood glucose.
- Full blood count (FBC), erythrocyte sedimentation rate (ESR) or C-reactive protein (CRP).
- Liver function test (LFT).
- Vitamin B12.

- Vasculitis screen.
- Paraprotein screen.
- Special investigation such as paraneoplastic antibodies, genetic tests and sural nerve biopsy may be needed in some patients.

Ataxic

The patient usually presents with loss of balance. Examination may show ataxic gait (wide-based gait), difficulty performing heel-to-toe test (drunken gait), nystagmus, dysarthria, abnormal finger-to-nose test, abnormal heel-to-shin test, intention tremor (worse on approaching the target), dysdiadochokinesia (breakdown of rhythmic, rapid alternating movements such as rapid pronation and supination movements of one hand on the other one).

The causes of ataxic syndrome include MS; alcoholic cerebellar degeneration (usually gait ataxia); drugs such as anticonvulsants (phenytoin and carbamazepine) and lithium; stroke such as ischaemic or haemorrhage; paraneoplastic syndrome (usually with lung and breast cancer); spinocerebellar ataxia (genetic ataxia); idiopathic cerebellar ataxia; Friedreich's ataxia (pes cavus, absent ankle jerks, upgoing plantars, scoliosis); posterior fossa tumours; and hypothyroidism.

The speed of the onset of ataxia, the age of onset and family history could give a clue about the cause.

Investigation of ataxic syndrome could include the following (according to the likely cause).

- Brain MRI.
- CSF analysis looking particularly for oligoclonal bands.
- Anticonvulsants blood level.
- Paraneoplastic antibodies.
- Genetic testing for spinocerebellar ataxia or Friedreich's ataxia.
- NCS/EMG.

Common neurological problems – the Big Five

1. Headache

Headache is the most common neurological problem that neurologists deal with in outpatient clinics. Also common in the inpatient setting.

- You could think of causes of headache in the following way.
  - Benign (green light!): most causes of headache are benign (tension headache, migraine, medication

overuse headache, cluster headache, trigeminal neuralgia and posttraumatic headache).

- o Serious (amber light!): headache could be the main symptom of some serious diseases. Missing or delaying the diagnosis could lead to permanent complication such as loss of vision (giant cell arteritis and idiopathic intracranial hypertension).
- o Dangerous (red light!): headache could be a symptom of dangerous diseases such as SAH or meningitis. However, contrary to general belief, brain tumours rarely present with headache only.
- The classic teaching indicates that morning headaches which increase with coughing and are associated with vomiting are due to raised intracranial pressure. However, in clinical practice, migraine tends to be more associated with such symptoms while patients with raised intracranial pressure usually have new-onset, mild and short-lived featureless headaches. Focal symptoms and signs may or may not present.
- Patients could have more than one type of benign headache, e.g. tension *and* migraine headache.
- The diagnosis of benign headaches is based on good history taking. Examination and scans rarely help apart from reassuring the patient and doctor!

Tension headache

- Tension headache is the most common type of headache.
- The headache is usually generalised and daily. Patients may describe it as a tight band around the head or as the head being in a vice. There are no gastrointestinal or visual symptoms associated with the headache.
- Headache does not interfere with sleep.
- Patients could have underlying anxiety or depression.
- Patients need reassurance that nothing sinister is causing the headache. Amitriptyline is widely used. Although brain scan is not indicated, it is increasingly being used for reassurance.

Migraine headache

More than 1 billion people worldwide suffer from migraine.

- Migraine headache is more common in women and young people.
- The headache is episodic and usually lasts from several hours to three days.

- The unilateral throbbing headache could be preceded by aura which can last for 20–30 minutes. Pain behind the eye is common. Headache is made worse with movement.
- The most common type of aura is visual where patients could experience flashing lights or zigzag lines. Other types of aura, such as paraesthesia in the hand spreading upward to involve the lips and the tongue, unilateral weakness or speech difficulties, are less common.
- Nausea, vomiting, photophobia (dislike of light) and phonophobia (dislike of sound) are associated with migraine. Sleep helps in relieving the headache.
- Contrary to general belief, finding a specific trigger factor for migraine, such as eating cheese, is not common in clinical practice. However, menstruation is commonly reported as a trigger factor.
- Patients need full explanation about the diagnosis and different treatment strategies. Reassurance that nothing sinister is causing the headache is important. Again, brain scan is not indicated in most cases, but it is increasingly being used for reassurance.

Migraine treatment

- Avoiding trigger factors (if you find one). The 'SEEDS' mnemonic, which stands for 'Sleep, Exercise, Eat, Dairy, Stress' reminds clinicians and patients to pay attention to these key lifestyle triggers.
- Treating acute attacks with simple analgesia such as paracetamol or aspirin, or simple analgesia combined with antiemetics such as Migraleve™. If these fail, triptans ($5HT_1$ agonists) are commonly used and available as tablets, nasal spray and subcutaneous injections. Calcitonin gene-related peptide (CGRP) antagonists (e.g. gepants such as rimagepant) are a new type of acute treatment for migraine. They are well tolerated and are given orally. At the start of the migraine process, CGRP is released by the nerves, and this helps to prolong and sustain the migraine attack. Gepants bind to the CGRP receptor and block this effect. Triptans, on the other hand, suppress the release of CGRP and act on different receptors. Gepants (unlike triptans) do not cause vasoconstriction and may be more useful in people with cardiovascular disease.
- Preventive treatment should be considered if patients experience frequent attacks, such as more than two per month. Propranolol, amitriptyline, pizotifen and topiramate are commonly used. CGRP antagonists (monoclonal antibodies and oral formulations) are a new type of preventive treatment for migraine. They are well tolerated. The injectable formulations are given either

monthly or every few months. Oral rimegepant is approved for prophylaxis of episodic migraine in adults who have at least four migraine attacks per month.

Medication overuse headache

- Medication overuse headache is a chronic headache (dull or throbbing pain) resulting from taking analgesia (especially those that contain codeine) almost on a daily basis to treat tension or migraine headache. The headache is transiently relieved by analgesia.
- It is important to explain to the patient the harmful effects of overusing the analgesia. Preventive treatment for headache such as amitriptyline should be introduced, and the analgesia should be stopped gradually or abruptly.

Cluster headache

- Cluster headache is uncommon, affects men and occurs in clusters (once or twice daily, for 4–8 weeks, once every year or two).
- The headache usually lasts from half an hour to two hours, mainly at night. It tends to occur at the same time each day, for example at 1 am each day for the whole length of the cluster.
- It is a unilateral excruciating pain around the eye associated with watering red eye, nasal blockage and, occasionally, Horner syndrome.

> The treatment of cluster headaches includes the following.
> - Treating the acute attacks with sumatriptan subcutaneous injection (5HT$_1$ agonist) or by high-flow oxygen.
> - Preventive treatment could be given until the cluster is over. Pizotifen, verapamil, topiramate and steroids are used.

Trigeminal neuralgia

- Trigeminal neuralgia usually affects people above the age of 40 years. It is believed that trigeminal neuralgia is caused by irritation of the 5th nerve by an ectatic blood vessel. However, in younger patients it may be associated with MS.
- Patients present with severe unilateral pain lasting for seconds (like an electric shock or needle stabs) over the area supplied by one of the branches of the 5th nerve, usually the maxillary or mandibular.

- Patients usually experience several attacks a day and may complain of dull aching pains between the episodes.
- Talking, eating, drinking, shaving and washing the face may trigger the attacks.

> The treatment of trigeminal neuralgia includes the following.
> - Anticonvulsants: carbamazepine is the usual first choice. Phenytoin, lamotrigine and gabapentin are also used.
> - Surgical treatment includes glycerol injection of the 5th nerve and microvascular decompression.

Posttraumatic headache

- Following any type of head injuiry, including minor ones, patients may experience headaches for several weeks or months.
- The headache usually starts within two weeks of the injury.
- The headache could be part of a posttraumatic (concussion) syndrome where patients could experience other symptoms such as lack of concentration, poor memory and dizziness.
- Patients need reassurance, and maybe a brain scan. Amitriptyline is widely used.

Giant cell (temporal) arteritis

> Giant cell arteritis (GCA) is a medical emergency as it can lead to sudden, permanent blindness.

- GCA is a disease that affects older people. Patients present with pain and tenderness on the temple. Patients find it difficult to brush their hair. Jaw claudication is a classic symptom. Non-specific symptoms such as feeling generally unwell are common and may be related to overlap with polymyalgia rheumatica. Ophthalmic features include transient monocular loss of vision (amaurosis fugax) and transient or persistent diplopia, usually preceding permanent loss of vision. Examination could show tenderness around the temple and lack of pulsation of the temporal artery.
- ESR (usually >60) and/or CRP, and temporal artery biopsy are the investigations of choice. European guidance has recommended the first-line investigation of colour Doppler ultrasound of

the temporal arteries. PET/CT is beneficial in terms of visualising the inflammation in the arterial tree (aortic disease).
- Patients should be treated immediately with oral (or IV) steroid to avoid permanent loss of vision due to infarction of the optic nerve. Headache settling within a day from starting treatment is diagnostic (but can also occur with mimics). Patients will normally need a maintenance dose of steroid for some years. Monitoring for side-effects of steroids is important (e.g. hyperglycaemia, osteoporosis, gastritis). The dose will need weaning slowly under expert guidance. Relapse is common and other steroid-sparing agents (e.g. methotrexate) may be useful.

Idiopathic intracranial hypertension

- The patient is typically an obese young woman presenting with headache and blurred vision.
- Examination shows bilateral papilloedema.
- Brain scan is normal and CSF pressure is high but with normal constituents. CTV or MRV to exclude cerebrovenous sinus thrombosis is essential.
- Patients should be treated promptly to avoid permanent loss of vision due to infarction of the optic nerve.

The management includes the following.
- Full and regular visual assessment, including visual fields.
- Weight loss.
- Diuretics such as acetazolamide.
- If the vision deteriorates, neurosurgical intervention is needed (lumboperitoneal shunting).

2. Epilepsy

Seizure is defined as an abnormal function of the brain as a result of abnormal paroxysmal neuronal discharge. Clinically, epilepsy is defined as a tendency to have recurrent seizures (more than one unprovoked seizure).

- Epilepsy is common (0.8% of population).
- Epilepsy has a bimodal age of onset with higher incidence in children and the elderly.
- Males and females are similarly affected.

Causes

- Seizure is considered to be a symptom, not a disease. In 25% of epilepsy patients, a specific cause would be identified. Brain tumour, cerebral infarction, cerebral haemorrhage, cerebral venous thrombosis and arteriovenous malformation could present with seizures. Head injury is an important cause of posttraumatic epilepsy. Seizures might be associated with other neurological diseases such as meningitis, encephalitis and neurodegenerative diseases. Alcohol, drugs, toxins, immune, metabolic and biochemical disorders could all lead to seizures.
- Genetic factors also contribute to the aetiology of epilepsy either as a single major locus or interaction of several loci with environmental factors.

Seizure types

Seizures are broadly classified as partial-onset (focal) or generalised. In partial seizures, the seizure discharges originate from a localised part of the cerebral hemisphere while in generalised seizures the discharges are simultaneous and involve both cerebral hemispheres. Partial-onset seizures may spread to involve the whole brain, leading to secondary generalisation.

Partial-onset seizures

- Partial-onset seizures may present with the following symptoms.
  - Motor: rhythmic twitching or jerking of one part of the body opposite to the epileptic focus, such as fingers, toes or face, may spread to the rest of the body part (Jacksonian). Sustained tonic or dystonic movement of one limb and the head with eyes turning could be another feature. This can last for seconds or minutes.
  - Sensory: tingling or numbness could affect one part of the body. Visual symptoms such as flashing lights may occur.
  - Psychic: dysphasic symptoms, disturbance of memory in a form of flashbacks, and *déjà vu* are well-recognised symptoms. Being in dreamy states, fear, anger, irritability, illusions of size, shape, weight, distance or sound may be features of a seizure. Visual, auditory, gustatory or olfactory symptoms can occur.
- Partial-onset seizures are called *simple* if consciousness is not impaired and *complex* when consciousness is impaired.
- Complex partial-onset seizures consist of three components.
  - Aura: these are simple partial seizures as described above (motor, sensory and psychic). They can be very short so that patients would not be able to recall them.
  - Automatism: automatism is aco-ordinated involuntary motor activity that occurs either

during or after the seizure. This includes fiddling movements with hands, lip smacking, chewing, emotional expression, humming, grunting and whistling.

○ Impaired consciousness could be in the form of absence or motor arrest. The patient may appear vacant or glazed.

- The most common type of partial-onset seizure is temporal lobe epilepsy (60%) that usually presents with an epigastric sensation that rises up to the throat, psychic manifestations, auras, altered consciousness and automatism.
- Frontal lobe epilepsy represents 30% of partial seizures and usually presents initially with deviation of the head and eyes to one side and is associated with jerking of the arm on the same side. This may be followed by paralysis of the arm (Todd's paralysis). Also, it can cause complex or bizarre automatisms.
- Parietal lobe seizures can present with sensory symptoms, and occipital seizures may cause visual symptoms such as visual hallucinations with impairment in sensations of colours, shapes and patterns. Both parietal and occipital epilepsy are uncommon.

Generalised seizures

Generalised seizures can be divided into three main types.

- Tonic-clonic seizures – patients may cry out then fall, becoming rigid with jaw clenching, breath holding and frothing coming from the mouth (tonic phase). This is followed by the clonic phase – rhythmic clonic jerking of the limbs, neck and back followed by tongue biting and urinary incontinence. On coming round, patients are usually confused, irritable and drowsy with headaches and muscle pain and tend to go to sleep in what is called the postictal stage. As a result of the seizures, patients may sustain injuries. The tonic phase could last for seconds and the clonic phase for minutes, while the postictal stage could go on for hours. Sometime there is no tonic phase (clonic seizures) or no clonic phase (tonic seizures). Also, patients may suddenly collapse as a result of losing muscle tone that is associated with loss of consciousness (atonic seizures).
- Absence seizures – usually occur in children; there are two types: typical and atypical. In typical absences, there is a sudden, momentary loss of contact with the surroundings, possibly with some minor jerking in the eyelids. These attacks may occur several times a day without the child's awareness and may present as learning difficulties.

Atypical absences, which are more common, tend to occur in children with brain damage. They tend to be prolonged and are associated with dropping to the ground, leading to injuries.

- Myoclonic seizures – these are sudden, brief jerks, which affect the upper limb with or without loss of consciousness. They may precede a generalised tonic-clonic seizure, often in the morning, and occur in late childhood. This can form part of what is called juvenile myoclonic epilepsy.

Differential diagnosis

Syncope

- Syncope is the most common cause of loss of consciousness.
- Syncope results in an abrupt and transient drop in blood pressure, leading to a reduction in the brain's blood flow.
- A typical attack starts with the presyncopal phase when the patient feels nauseated, clammy and sweaty combined with blurring and loss of vision, dizziness, lightheadedness and tinnitus. The patient appears pale and sweaty which is followed by loss of consciousness and falling to the floor. The patient usually looks floppy with eyes rolled up. When the patient regains consciousness, they become flushed and may feel unwell, drowsy and slightly confused for a short time. Urinary incontinence is uncommon but could happen, especially if the bladder was full at the time. Tongue biting is rare. Syncopal attacks commonly occur in a standing position but could also occur in a sitting position. The patient may appear stiff, and a few myoclonic jerks could lead to confusion with epileptic seizure.
- Vasovagal syncope and postural hypotension are common causes of syncope. Cardiac disorders such as arrhythmias or structural lesions could present with syncope. Cardiac syncope tends to occur at any position, during exercise and emotional situations.

Non-epileptic attack disorder

- Non-epileptic attack disorder or psychogenic non-epileptic seizure (previously known as pseudoseizure) is commonly misdiagnosed as epilepsy. It is more common in females and usually starts in adolescence or early adulthood.
- A history of emotional trauma such as sexual abuse is common, as well as a history of abnormal illness behaviour such as a recurrent unexplained abdominal pain.
- The attacks can be divided into two types: fall down, lie still and unresponsive; and convulsive – fall

down with coarse alternating movement (usually) or thrashing (less common). Pelvic thrusting is characteristic but rather uncommon. Patients may resist any attempts to open their eyes during the attacks. Patients may recover rapidly from the attacks or after a prolonged period of time, and they may be very tearful.

Others

Panic attacks, hyperventilation, transient ischaemic attacks, hypoglycaemic episodes, migraine and movement disorders such as tics and chorea could all be misdiagnosed as epilepsy.

Diagnosis

The diagnosis of epilepsy is a *clinical* one and taking a proper history is crucial. Every effort must be made to get an eyewitness account (e.g. call or virtually). Video recording on smartphones or other devices can also be useful. Examination rarely helps but should be carried out to look for any abnormal neurological signs. Cardiological assessment and ECG could be essential, especially if syncope is expected. Past medical history, family history of epilepsy and drug history are important.

The steps outlined in Box 24.2 should be followed to obtain a proper history.

Investigation

Patients may need an ECG or a full cardiological assessment if the history or examination is suggestive of a cardiac disorder.

EEG

- EEG is very commonly used (and abused) in clinical practice for patients with suspected epilepsy. The EEG should *only* be used to *support a clinical diagnosis* of epilepsy.
- A normal EEG does not exclude the diagnosis of epilepsy, as only 30–40% of patients with epilepsy have epileptiform discharges on a routine (interictal) EEG. An abnormal routine EEG is not in itself diagnostic of epilepsy, as up to 4% of subjects with abnormal EEGs do not have a history of epilepsy.
- EEG is usually a poor guide to seizure control or to the likelihood of seizure relapse.
- A routine EEG includes a period of activation by overbreathing for three minutes and photic stimulation. Sleep EEG could show epileptiform discharges in up to 70–80% of patients with a clinical diagnosis of epilepsy and therefore it could be requested when a routine EEG is normal or borderline abnormal.

> **Box 24.2 History taking in epilepsy**
>
> *Events before the attack (from the patient)*
> - Number of attacks.
> - The duration of the attacks, the shortest and the longest attack.
> - The gap between the attacks (days, weeks or months).
> - The date of the first and the last attack.
> - General health in the days before and on the day of the attack.
> - Precipitating factors such as changing position, stress and menstrual cycle.
> - Exact position just before the attack.
> - The time of the attack, and whether it occurred during sleep.
> - Warning symptoms such as aura or palpitations.
>
> *Events during the attack (from the eyewitness)*
> - Change in colour.
> - Breathing pattern.
> - Abnormal movements.
> - Tone (rigid or floppy).
> - Duration of the attack.
>
> *Events after the attack (from the patient and eyewitness)*
> - Tongue biting.
> - Incontinence.
> - Confusion.
> - Headache.
> - Muscle aches and pain.
> - Feeling sleepy and drowsy.
> - Any abnormal behaviour.

- The EEG may show focal or generalised spike or spike/wave activity, and therefore helps in localising an epileptogenic focus which, in turn, leads to the classification of the epilepsy such as 3 per second generalised spike-wave discharge in typical absence seziures.
- Continuous or intermittent EEG monitoring is needed in treating patients with status epilepticus both as a diagnostic tool and to monitor the treatment, especially if general anaesthesia was induced.
- Ambulatory EEG and video-EEG telemetry are useful in monitoring prolonged attacks ranging from one day to five days and are especially helpful in patients with frequent attacks and diagnostic difficulties (patients with non-epileptic attack disorders). Also, they are used to localise seizures prior to considering any surgical treatment.

Neuroimaging

- There have been great advances in neuroimaging over the last decade and that has helped identify structural lesions causing seizures and epilepsy syndromes.
- MRI is the scan of choice and its superiority over CT is well established. However, CT brain could certainly help in identifying structural abnormalities such as tumours.

Management

A diagnosis of epilepsy is a major event in patients' lives and could have a huge impact on their social life. Therefore, a full explanation about the diagnosis is essential. Patients should be given information explaining the diagnosis and every effort should be made to reassure the patient and encourage them to lead as normal a life as possible. However, general advice such as avoiding dangerous sport, not to swim without supervision and not to use dangerous and sharp tools should be discussed.

Anticonvulsants

- Anticonvulsants (also known as antiepileptic drugs) are the main treatment of epilepsy. Drug treatment is usually needed for at least 2–3 years and sometime life-long. Therefore, patients should understand the nature of the treatment to increase their compliance. Most clinicians in the UK do not treat patients with a single seizure.
- There are general principles that need to be applied in using antiepileptic drugs (AEDs). The aim of the treatment is freedom from seizures. The chosen drug should be introduced at a low dose and gradually increased to reach the standard dose. If seizures are not controlled, the dose should slowly be increased to the maximum tolerated, before changing to another drug. Patients should be treated with monotherapy if possible. However, combined therapy is needed in 10–15% of patients with epilepsy.
- There are many AEDs that could be used in clinical practice. The choice of medication usually depends on the type of epilepsy although the majority of AEDs could be used in both generalised and partial seizures. Broadly, valproate or levetiracetam is used in patients with generalised-onset seizures and lamotrigine or levetiracetam in those with focal-onset seizures.
- Drug interaction is an important issue to be considered in patients taking anticonvulsants and other drugs such as warfarin.

- Measuring drug levels in the blood is of limited use, mainly to check patient adherence or in case of carbamazepine or phenytoin toxicity.
- Stopping AEDs could be discussed with the patient if they achieve seizure freedom for at least two years. The risk of relapse is up to 40%. The decision to stop AEDs is personal and the majority of the patients prefer to take the medication rather than risk losing their driving licence.

Management of tonic-clonic status epilepticus

- Tonic-clonic status epilepticus is a medical emergency with a mortality rate of 20%, and prompt treatment is required to prevent any long-term cerebral damage.
- Status epilepticus is usually defined as prolonged or recurrent tonic-clonic seizures persisting for 30 minutes or more. However, in clinical practice, patients should be aggressively treated if they have more than 5 minutes of continuous seizures or two or more discrete seizures between which there is an incomplete recovery of consciousness.
- Status is more common in children, patients with learning difficulties and those with structural brain lesions. Drug withdrawal or non-adherence, intercurrent illness, metabolic disturbance and progression of the underlying disease are the most common factors precipitating status in patients with an established diagnosis of epilepsy.

The following are the general principles of treating status (NICE 2022).

- Follow the standard ABCDE approach; establish intravenous (IV) access; take blood for emergency investigation (e.g. FBC, glucose, renal, LFTs, calcium and magnesium level and AED level).
- Give dextrose if there is a possibility of hypoglycaemia or thiamine if there is a history of alcohol abuse.
- Lorazepam as an IV bolus should be given initially (diazepam IV or rectally could be used), followed by second-line medication if status epilepticus becomes established. Any one of the available IV preparations can be used: phenytoin/fosphenytoin (a precursor drug to phenytoin), levetiracetam, or sodium valproate given by infusion. ECG, blood pressure monitoring and pulse oximetry are also needed.
- If status continues, the patient should be transferred to the intensive care unit and propofol, thiopental or midazolam should be

started after discussion with the intensivist. EEG monitoring is needed in anaesthetised patients.
- If the patient is known to have epilepsy, their regular AEDs should be given orally or through a nasogastric tube. Maintenance AEDs should be started in patients not known to have seizures.

Other aspects of epilepsy

- The diagnosis of epilepsy could have huge social implications due to the stigma attached to it. Employers tend to be reluctant to offer jobs to people with epilepsy, which could encourage social isolation.
- Alcohol may provoke seizures and should be consumed in moderation. Sleep deprivation could also lower seizure threshold.
- In the UK, patients with seizures are not allowed to drive motorcars or motorcycles unless they are seizure free for one year or had attacks only during sleep for three years. For driving large lorries and passenger-carrying vehicles, the requirement is 10 years of seizure freedom without taking AEDs.
- Sudden unexpected death in epilepsy (SUDEP) is becoming increasingly recognised as a major cause of death in patients with chronic epilepsy. It is defined as sudden, unexpected, witnessed or unwitnessed, non-traumatic and non-drowning death in patients with epilepsy, with or without evidence of a seizure, and excluding documented status epilepticus, in which postmortem examination does not reveal a toxicological or anatomical cause for death. The cause of SUDEP is not clear. It is recommended that tailored information and discussion should be part of the counselling of patients.

3. Stroke

Worldwide, one in six people will have a stroke in their lifetime.

Stroke is a common neurological disorder, the second most common overall cause of death and a major cause of disability in survivors. The incidence increases with age.

- Stroke is defined by the World Health Organization as 'a clinical syndrome consisting of rapidly developing clinical signs of focal (at times global) disturbance of cerebral function, lasting more than 24 hours or leading to death with no apparent cause other than that of vascular origin.'
- Transient ischaemic attack (TIA) is defined as stroke symptoms and signs that resolve within 24 hours. However, in the majority of patients the TIA symptoms usually resolve within minutes or a few hours at most.
- A non-disabling stroke is defined as 'a stroke with symptoms that last for more than 24 hours but later resolve, leaving no permanent disability.'

The **FAST** campaign is a UK-wide awareness campaign designed to help detect and enhance responsiveness to the needs of a person having a stroke. The acronym stands for:
- **F**acial drooping
- **A**rm weakness
- **S**peech difficulties
- **T**ime to call emergency services.

Types of stroke

- Ischaemic – the most common type of stroke (80%). Ischaemic stroke is due to reduction of the blood supply to the brain as a result of occlusion of arteries. The ischaemic stroke could be due to:
  - thrombosis: usually at the site of atheromatous plaque
  - embolism: results from ulceration and fragmentation of atheromatous plaque. Less commonly, the heart can be the source of the emboli
  - small vessels disease: due to atheroma of the small penetrating arteries leading to 'lacunar infarction.'
- Haemorrhagic – due to rupture of the arteries causing either intracerebral haemorrhage (ICH) or SAH.

Cerebral circulation

- The cerebral hemispheres are supplied by the:
  - anterior circulation: formed by the internal carotid ateries and its branches the middle cerebral arteries and the anterior cerebral arteries
  - posterior circulation: formed by the two vertebral arteries which join to form the basilar artery which bifurcates into two posterior cerebral arteries.
- The anterior communicating arteries connect the middle cerebral arteries and anterior cerebral arteries, while the posterior communicating arteries connect the middle cerebral arteries and posterior cerebral arteries, forming the circle of Willis.

- The small (penetrating) vessels are branches from all the above-mentioned arteries.
- The anterior circulation supplies the frontal, parietal and temporal lobes and the eyes (hence amaurosis fugax) while the posterior circulation supplies the occipital lobes, cerebellum, brainstem and thalamus.

Clinical patterns of ischaemic stroke

- Anterior circulation ischaemia (carotid territory) is the most common pattern and comprises around 50% of strokes and leads to hemiparesis with or without sensory loss, homonymous hemianopia, dysphagia, dysphasia (dominant hemisphere) and dysarthria.
- Posterior circulation ischaemia (vertebrobasilar territory) comprises around 25% of strokes and leads to vertigo, diplopia, ataxia, cortical blindness, hemiparesis or tetraparesis.
- Features such as hemiparesis, homonymous hemianopia, dysphagia and dysarthria could be due to anterior or posterior circulation ischaemia.
- Lacunar strokes comprise 25% of strokes and present with one of the following four patterns.
  o Pure motor hemiparesis due to lacunar infarction in internal capsule or pons.
  o Hemisensorimotor pattern due to lacunar infarction in internal capsule, pons or corona radiata.
  o Ataxic hemiparesis due to lacunar infarction in internal capsule or pons.
  o Pure hemisensory pattern due to lacunar infarction in thalamus.

Vascular risk factors

- Hypertension.
- Diabetes.
- Hyperlipidaemia.
- Family history of atheromatous diseases (stroke or ischaemic heart disease).
- Smoking.
- Previous history of TIA or stroke.
- Cardiac diseases associated with embolic stroke such as atrial fibrillation, mitral valve disease, mural thrombus following myocardial infarction and bacterial endocarditis.

Haemorrhagic stroke

Intracerebral haemorrhage

- ICH usually presents with sudden onset of severe neurological deficit with headache. However, ICH cannot be differentiated from ischaemic stroke on clinical grounds. Therefore, non-contrast CT brain is essential.
- The most common cause of ICH is hypertension due to rupture of the small penetrating arteries which typically occurs in the basal ganglia. Other sites of bleeding are lobar white matter, pons and cerebellum.
- Anticoagulants and arteriovenous malformations can cause ICH.

Subarachnoid haemorrhage

- Patients present with sudden-onset severe headache associated with vomiting and neck stiffness. The headache peaks within seconds. Patients usually have neurological deficit but may present *only* with acute headache.
- The most common cause of SAH is rupture of an intracranial aneurysm on the circle of Willis.
- Brain CT is essential to diagnosis SAH. However, this could be normal. If the brain CT is normal than a LP should be performed around 6–8 hours after the onset of symptoms, looking for blood-stained CSF (xanthochromia). Spectrophotometry is needed to confirm the xanthochromia.
- SAH could lead to complications such as rebleeding or secondary ischaemia due to vasospasm.

Investigations

- Conditions that may mimic stroke, such as brain tumour, subdural haematoma and cerebral abscess, should be excluded by brain scan. CT brain could be normal in the early stages of ischaemic stroke.
- FBC, biochemical profile including fasting glucose, ECG and chest X-ray should be considered for all patients with stroke.
- If a cardiac source of emboli is suspected, then consider transthoracic or transoesophageal echocardiography and 24-hour ECG.
- If stroke in carotid territory, consider carotid Doppler ultrasound.
- Patients with TIA and non-disabling stroke should be investigated in similar ways to stroke patients.

Management of stroke

- It is important to remember that stroke is a preventable (primary and secondary prevention) and treatable disease. Primary prevention focuses on interventions aimed at reducing the risk of stroke in people who have not yet had a stroke. The major focus is on detecting atrial fibrillation (AF) and starting anticoagulation when safe to do so. Hypertension must also be controlled. Other factors such as obesity, smoking and excess alcohol are also important.

- The premise for acute stroke care is to salvage viable ischaemic brain tissue (ischaemic penumbra) surrounding the irreversibly injured core through reperfusion.

- Ensuring that appropriate information is available to clinicians receiving the patient at the hospital enables quicker decision making and timely access to imaging and treatment upon arrival. Pre-alert refers to the sharing of information about a patient with the hospital during transfer by an ambulance crew.

- People with suspected acute stroke should be assessed immediately to determine the best approach to treatment. This is particularly important for identifying people who would benefit from specific hyperacute stroke treatments such as thrombolysis and/or thrombectomy. Senior stroke decision maker and senior leadership involvement is needed at the front door to minimise door-to-needle times for thrombolysis (e.g. straight to CT protocols). In locations where specialist clinicians are not available on site, telestroke services should provide access to specialist assessment and decision making.

- If the patient presents within 4.5 hours from the onset of stroke symptoms, an urgent non-contrast brain CT is needed to exclude cerebral haemorrhage followed by thrombolysis with IV alteplase (if not contraindicated). The earlier the treatment is given, the better the potential outcome for the patient ('time is brain').

- The most severe 10–20% of acute ischaemic strokes are due to a large vessel occlusion (LVO). Restoring blood flow with early thrombectomy, sometimes referred to as clot retrieval, significantly reduces dependency. In some cases, thrombolysis is given prior to the thrombectomy procedure. Generally, mechanical thrombectomy for acute ischaemic stroke can be considered less than six hours after the onset of stroke symptoms. Outside this window, perfusion-based imaging techniques such as CTA rapid protocol or MRA may identify other candidates for endovascular treatment. This includes the 15–25% of stroke patients who will not have a recognised time of stroke onset, with patients frequently waking from sleep.

- The majority of patients with acute stroke will not be eligible for thrombolysis or thrombectomy. The key focus for these patients is ensuring access to the stroke bundle (UK National Guideline 2023). There are four components to the bundle.

  o Swallow screen (before any food, fluids or oral medication are administered): reduces the risk of aspiration pneumonia, dehydration, malnutrition and death.

  o Brain imaging (accepting that hyperacute patients require a scan as soon as possible after arrival), since confirmation of the stroke diagnosis and distinguishing strokes due to ischaemic and bleeding has wide-reaching effects on management from the earliest stages.

  o Clopidogrel 300 mg and/or aspirin 300 mg loading dose for those with ischaemic stroke. This is reduced to 75 mg daily for 21 days, and then secondary prevention options are reviewed.

  o Admission to stroke unit ('multidisciplinary well-organised stroke service') which reliably provides a wide range of targeted interventions. This reduces the risks of complications, improves the patient's experience and is known to improve functional outcomes and reduce mortality. Involvement of physiotherapists, speech therapists and occupational therapists is essential.

- Early mobilisation of the patient with stroke is essential to prevent complications such as deep vein thrombosis, bed sores and contractures.

- A period of rehabilitation may be needed. Social services involvement may be required.

- About one in 20 people with acute stroke will be receiving end-of-life care within 72 hours of onset, and one in seven people with acute stroke will die in hospital. If required, appropriate end-of-life care for patients with stroke, and the avoidance of harm and unintended limitations of care should be ensured by timely senior-level decision making regarding advanced care planning.

- Secondary prevention aims to reduce the risk of a recurrent stroke and includes the following measures.

  o Long-term clopidogrel 75 mg daily (NICE 2022). If the patient cannot tolerate it then aspirin or dipyridamole could be used.

  o Anticoagulation is indicated in patients with AF.

  o Control blood pressure (usually permissive hypertension initially with gradual lowering).

  o Statins even if the patient's serum cholesterol level is normal.

  o Manage any other modifiable risk factors such as diabetes (certain glucose-lowering therapies have benefit in primary and secondary cardiovascular prevention such as pioglitazone, glucagon-like peptide-1 receptor agonists, and sodium-glucose transporter-2 inhibitors) and smoking.

- o Patients who have made a reasonable recovery and are found to have a significant internal carotid artery stenosis (>70%) should benefit from carotid endarterectomy.
- Measures of secondary prevention also apply to patients with TIA and non-disabling stroke.
- Young patients with severe middle cerebral artery infarction may need decompressive hemicraniectomy for malignant stroke syndrome. Large, space-occupying, hemispheric, ischaemic brain infarcts (described as malignant infarcts) are associated with the development of massive brain oedema, which may lead to herniation and early death. Decompressive hemicraniectomy has been shown to prevent fatal internal displacement of brain tissue (and subsequent herniation) in cases of malignant MCA infarction within 48 hours of stroke, with a potential trigger for such consideration being a decline in the level of consciousness.
- ICH is usually treated conservatively. However, surgical evacuation of the haematoma may be indicated if the neurological status of the patient deteriorates or they develop hydrocephalus. Treating hypertension is the best way to prevent ICH. Rapid anticoagulant reversal protocols may be warranted as up to 20% of ICH cases occur in patients taking anticoagulant medication.
- Once a diagnosis of SAH is confirmed, the patient should be transferred to a neurosurgical unit to determine the source of bleeding by CTA, MRA or cerebral angiogram. Nimodipine and IV fluids should be given to reduce the risk of secondary ischaemia. Surgical clipping or coiling of the aneurysm is the main treatment.

Other types of stroke

Cerebrovenous sinus thrombosis (CVST)

- Thrombosis in the cerebral venous system is relatively uncommon.
- Patients may present with headache, seizure and focal neurological signs. They could also present with headache and papilloedema mimicking idiopathic intracranial hypertension.
- CVST may be associated with pregnancy and the oral contraceptive pill. Hypercoagulability disorders need to be excluded and therefore full thrombophilia screen is essential. Otitis media and mastoiditis can cause CVST. More recently, it has been associated with adenoviral-based COVID-19 vaccines.
- Brain CT could identify venous infarction. CTV or MRV is usually diagnostic although cerebral angiography with venography may be needed in some cases.
- The mainstay of treatment is anticoagulation.

Dissection of the cervicocerebral arteries

- Dissection of internal carotid or vertebral arteries is relatively rare.
- Trauma, even trivial, is a well-known cause of dissection.
- Headache or neck pain is common. Horner syndrome is another feature. Dissection usually leads to thromboembolic stroke affecting the carotid or posterior circulation tertiary.
- CTA or MRA is usually diagnostic although cerebral angiography may be needed in some cases.
- There is no clear agreement about the best treatment for dissection although antiplatelet agent(s) or anticoagulants are commonly used.

Prognosis

The prognosis depends on the type and severity of the stroke. However, generally:

- 30% die at one year and 60% at five years.
- 30% are dependent at one year.
- 30% have a further stroke before five years.

4. Parkinson disease

- Parkinson disease (PD) is a common progressive neurogenerative disorder which was first described by James Parkinson in 1817.
- It is a disease of the basal ganglia (extrapyramidal). The basal ganglia include the following nuclei which have a rather complicated interconnection.
  - o Putamen.
  - o Caudate.
  - o Globus pallidum.
  - o Substantia nigra.
- The combination of bradykinesia (slowness of movement), rigidity (increased resistance to passive extension and flexion), tremor (mainly resting) and postural abnormalities is called *parkinsonism*. PD is the most frequent cause of parkinsonism.
- The prevalence of the disease increases with age and about 2% of people >65 years have PD.
- The mean age at onset of PD is 55–65 years, with a slight male predominance of 60%.

Pathology

- PD is characterised pathologically by loss of pigment from the substantia nigra with neuronal loss and the presence of Lewy bodies in the surviving neurones.

- Lewy bodies are eosinophilic intracytoplasmic inclusions. They are not specific for PD and are reported in other neurodegenerative disorders.

Aetiology

- The exact cause of PD is not known. It is possible that the disease is a result of interaction between several environmental and genetic factors.
- PD is a sporadic disease. However, up to 20% of patients have a positive family history, with only 1–2% having the familial form of PD. Gene mutations implicated in the development of PD have been described (i.e. PARK genes numbering approximately 20). However, most of the heritability is polygenic.

Clinical features

- The onset of disease is usually asymmetrical.
- Patients usually present with non-specific aches and pains, stiffness, reduced handwriting size, general slowing down or depression and sleep disturbance.
- Tremor is the presenting feature in 70% of patients. Some patients have tremor with minimal bradykinesia or rigidity, hence the name benign tremulous PD.
- Examination usually shows loss of arm swing when walking, tendency to drag a leg, difficulty with hand movements, stooped posture and loss of facial expression. Also, reduced voice volume, lead pipe rigidity or cogwheel rigidity if tremor is superimposed, and the pill-rolling resting tremor are typical features.
- In the late stages of PD, patients develop speech and swallowing difficulties. Other features of the late stages of the disease are falls, gait problems, autonomic dysfunction and dementia.

Differential diagnosis

Essential tremor

- Essential tremor (ET) is the most common movement disorder. Men and women are equally affected.
- ET is a familial disorder and around 50% of patients report a positive family history. There are no specific pathological features of ET.
- Typically, the tremor is postural, occurring while voluntarily maintaining position against gravity. This mainly involves the hands and forearms, starting intermittently and progressing to become permanent, rarely remitting and usually worsened by emotion. Tremor of the head, voice, tongue and legs may follow. No rigidity or bradykinesia.

- Treatment is mainly with beta-blockers, particularly propranolol. Up to 60% of ET patients report an improvement in their tremor after consuming alcohol.

Vascular parkinsonism

- Common in elderly patients with a history of hypertensive disorder, who usually present with gait difficulty, symmetrical rigidity, absent tremor and no or some response to levodopa therapy.
- There are no generally accepted clinical criteria to diagnose vascular parkinsonism. Also, there is no specific treatment but a trial of levodopa is worth considering. Manage cardiovascular risk factors.

Drug-induced parkinsonism

- Drug-induced parkinsonism can occur with neuroleptics such as phenothiazines and butyrophenones. This occurs in 10–15% of psychotic patients treated with these drugs.
- Antiemetic drugs such as prochlorperazine and metoclopramide can cause parkinsonism. Other drugs have also been reported to cause parkinsonism.
- Stopping the offending drug is obviously the treatment of choice in drug-induced parkinsonism. However, this can be difficult, especially with neuroleptic drugs.
- Anticholinergics and amantadine may help in reducing the parkinsonian symptoms in patients with drug-induced parkinsonism.

Parkinson Plus syndromes

- This is a group of neurodegenerative disorders which share some features with PD but have different pathological features and do not respond to dopaminergic therapy.
- Progressive supranuclear palsy includes postural instability and falls, symmetrical bradykinesia and rigidity, cognitive impairment, dysarthria and speech changes and vertical gaze palsy.
- Multiple system atrophy includes symmetrical bradykinesia and rigidity, features of autononmic dysfunction, cerebellar and pyramidal signs.

Wilson disease

- Wilson disease is a rare but treatable disease. Therefore, it should not be missed. It is an autosomal recessive disorder due to impairment in the copper transport system and deficiency of the copper-carrying plasma protein caeruloplasmin, leading to copper deposition in all the body's tissues.
- PD rarely affects young people, therefore any patient below the age of 40 presenting with parkinsonism should be screened for Wilson disease.

- Serum caeruloplasmin is almost always low which is associated with low serum copper and high urinary copper excretion.
- Kayser–Fleischer rings (deposition of copper in the Desçemet membrane of the cornea which appears brown or grey) is present in all patients with neurological features of Wilson disease, so slit-lamp examination is essential.
- Several medications can be used in treating Wilson disease. Chelating agents, such as penicillamine, are effective treatments.

Management

- PD is a chronic progressive disease and establishing a good relationship between the patient and the treating physician is essential. Patients should be realistically informed about the prognosis and expectation from treatment. Every effort should be made to support patients throughout the course of the disease. Patient-oriented leaflets, booklets and websites help patients to understand the nature of their disease.
- Dopamine agonists are widely used as the first choice, in the hope of reducing the long-term motor complications of levodopa, especially in younger patients.
- There is no drug that is proven to slow the progress of the disease.
- Multidisciplinary team input and effective management of non-motor symptoms are important at all stages of Parkinson disease.

Dopamine agonists

- Dopamine agonists act directly on the postsynaptic dopamine receptors. Drug-induced motor complications are less frequent and less severe than with levodopa. Therefore, dopamine agonists have been advocated as the drugs that delay the introduction of levodopa. They are used as monotherapy or adjuvant therapy.
- Some patients experience dizziness, hypotensive reactions, nausea and vomiting initially. Adding domperidone during the initiation phase can counteract this.
- Currently, non-ergot derivative dopamine agonists such as pramipexole, ropinirole, rotigotine (self-adhesive patches) and apomorphine are used.
- Apomorphine hydrochloride is indicated in patients with refractory motor fluctuations. It can only be given as a subcutaneous injection or continuous subcutaneous infusion.
- Patients must be counselled about the risk of impulse control disorder when taking dopaminergic therapy, especially dopamine agonists.

Levodopa

- Levodopa was introduced in the late 1960s and is still the most effective drug treatment in PD – the 'gold standard' therapy. It is metabolised to dopamine by aromatic amino acid decarboxylase and is then stored in and released by the nigrostriatal neurones. Levodopa is always given with a peripheral decarboxylase inhibitor, either carbidopa or benserazide, to prevent peripheral dopamine formation and reduce side-effects such as nausea and vomiting.
- Initially, patients respond very well to levodopa ('honeymoon period') but after around 3–5 years of treatment, levodopa-related motor complications usually emerge.
  - Wearing off: the beneficial effect of levodopa wears off quickly and patients may need more frequent doses.
  - On-off phenomena: the patient's condition fluctuates from good treatment effect ('on') to severe parkinsonian state ('off') with no relation to levodopa dosing regime.
  - Dyskinesia: drug-induced purposeless involuntary movements which affect upper or lower limbs as well as the neck and trunk.
- These levodopa-related motor complications can be mild and cause no major disability. However, as the disease progresses, it becomes more troublesome and difficult to manage.
- Duodopa®, which is levodopa as a concentrated intestinal gel, could be used in patients with refractory motor fluctuations. However, it requires insertion of a percutaneous gastrostomy tube.

Catechol-O-methyl transferase (COMT) inhibitors

- Levodopa is metabolised by catechol-O-methyl transferase (COMT) to inactive products in both the peripheral blood and the brain. COMT inhibitors increase the amount of dopamine available by reducing the metabolism of levodopa. They are used to reduce wearing-off effects. Nausea, vomiting, abdominal pain, constipation and diarrhoea are possible side-effects with COMT inhibitors.
- Entacapone is widely used and a single preparation combining levodopa, carbidopa (peripheral decarboxylase inhibitor) and entacapone is available (Stalevo®).

Monoamine oxidase B (MAOB) inhibitors

Intracerebral MAOB metabolises dopamine. Blocking this process increases the amount of endogenous dopamine. Selegiline and rasagiline are used as both monotherapy and adjuvant treatment. MAOB inhibitors can cause constipation, nausea, postural hypotension and hallucinations as side-effects.

Anticholinergics

Anticholinergics such as trihexyphenidyl hydrochloride and orphenadrine hydrochloride can help in treating tremor. They may cause dry mouth, confusion, hallucinations and urinary retention, especially in elderly patients, and therefore are of limited use.

Other therapies

The antiviral agent amantadine was found by chance to improve the symptoms of PD, although it is not widely used nowadays except to treat dyskinesias.

Surgical treatment

Bilateral subthalamic nucleus stimulation has replaced pallidotomy as the operation of choice in patients with PD. It is indicated in patients with motor complications not responding to medical treatment. The patients have to be levodopa responsive with no significant neuropsychiatric problems.

Treating non-motor symptoms

Depression is common and should be treated with antidepressants such as the selective serotonin reuptake inhibitors. Hallucinations and psychosis can be difficult to manage and are best treated with atypical antipsychotics. There is some evidence that cholinesterase inhibitors may help PD dementia. Physiotherapy, occupational therapy and speech therapy can be of help to some patients, especially if they have falls.

Inpatient management of Parkinson disease

Patients with PD are often admitted to hospital for other reasons. PD-related complications include constipation, delirium and falls. It is essential that antiparkinsonian medications are given on time and in the correct dosage, as sudden reduction or withdrawal of medication can lead to severe morbidity or even mortality due to *parkinsonism-hyperpyrexia syndrome* (pyrexia, muscle rigidity, reduced level of consciousness and autonomic instability). Dopamine-blocking drugs such as certain antipsychotic agents should be avoided, and antiemetics such as metoclopramide and prochlorperazine must not be given. Other routes of administration may be needed if unable to take

PD drugs orally (e.g. equivalent dosage given via nasogastric tube or via transdermal route – rotigotine patch). Use local guidelines or OPTIMAL calculator. Seek expert help.

Prognosis

- The effect of PD on survival is not clear; however, the disease has a greater effect on younger patients because of their greater life expectancy.
- Tremor-dominant patients have a better prognosis than those without tremor (akinetic – rigid presentation).
- Patients with endstage PD usually die from infections such as bronchopneumonia.

5. Multiple sclerosis

- Multiple sclerosis is a chronic inflammatory demyelinating disease of the brain and spinal cord (CNS), and one of the most common disabling neurological diseases amongst young people in developed countries.
- MS usually presents at an age range of 20–40 years.

Pathology

- MS is characterised pathologically by loss of myelin (inflammatory process) with possible secondary axonal damage (degenerative process).
- The hallmark of MS is white matter lesions affecting the CNS which commonly include the periventricular areas, corpus callosum, optic nerve, brainstem, cerebellum and cervical spine.
- The immune system is involved in MS pathogenesis, with autoimmune attack on myelin.

Aetiology

- The exact cause of MS is not known. It is possible that the disease is a result of interaction between environmental (e.g. EBV) and genetic factors.
- There are geographic and latitude effects on the prevalence of MS; increased distance from the equator increases the prevalence of the disease. Also, migration from a high- to a low-risk area before the age of 15 reduces the MS risk and vice versa.
- There is an association between MS and HLA types.
- There is an increased incidence of MS in first-degree relatives.

Clinical features

Optic neuritis

- Common presentation of MS.
- Painful eye (especially with eye movements) and visual impairment (varies from mild to severe).
- There are two types of optic neuritis.
  - ○ Retrobulbar (posterior): common form of optic neuritis. The optic disc appears normal.
  - ○ Papillitis (anterior): less common form of optic neuritis. The optic disc is usually red and swollen with exudate and haemorrhages.
- Examination shows reduced visual acuity, central scotoma, loss of colour vision and RAPD.
- Complete or near complete visual recovery over a period of weeks or months is the usual outcome.

Sensory and motor features

- Sensory symptoms such as numbness, pins and needles are common and could affect any part of the body.
- Weakness affecting the lower limbs is more common than the upper limbs. The motor deficit is of UMN type usually leading to spastic paraplegia.

Brainstem and cerebellum

- Dizziness and vertigo.
- Double vision usually due to a lesion in the pathways that maintain conjugate eye movement rather than a specific cranial nerve abnormality.
- Internuclear ophthalmoplegia: when the patient looks to the right/left, there is ataxic nystagmus in the abducted eye and failure to adduct the other eye due to a lesion in the medial longitudinal fasciculus which connects the 3rd nerve nucleus on one side with the 6th nerve nucleus on the other side.
- Limbs or gait ataxia.
- Dysarthria.

Other features

- Fatigue is common (up to 80%).
- Bladder and bowel dysfunction.
- Sexual problems.
- Depression, euphoria and cognitive impairment.

Types of MS

- Relapsing-remitting MS (the most common presentation) – neurological episodes with variable recovery but stable in between the episodes.
- Relapsing-remitting with secondary progressive MS – neurological episodes superimposed on progressive course, usually starts as relapsing-remitting disease.
- Primary progressive MS – gradual development of neurological deficits from the onset without any relapses.

Diagnosis

- MS is a clinical diagnosis, but brain MRI and CSF analysis are important.
- The occurrence of lesions in the CNS (clinically and radiologically) should be disseminated in time and place (at least two separate episodes).
- Brain MRI is abnormal in 95% of patients with MS. The multiple white matter lesions are characteristically seen in periventricular areas, corpus callosum, brainstem and cerebellum. Active lesions are enhanced with gadolinium.
- Routine CSF anaylsis is usually normal. Oligoclonal bands are positive in CSF but not in the blood; in 95% of patients with MS, they indicate intrathecal immunoglobulin synthesis.
- Remember that multiple white matter lesions on brain MRI are also seen in other disorders such as cerebral ischaemia, neurosarcoid and vasculitis. Oligoclonal bands in CSF are positive in other inflammatory conditions such as autoimmune disorders and neurosarcoid.
- The neurophysiological test for visual evoked responses could be delayed in patients with MS. However, this is not widely used.

Management

- Explaining to newly diagnosed patients about the nature of MS is vital, emphasising that the disease could follow a benign course. Although severe disability (ending up in wheelchair) is a possibility, it is not an eventuality.
- Always encourage patients to live a normal life!

Symptomatic treatment

- Baclofen and tizanidine are used to treat spasticity.
- Fatigue is difficult to treat. Fluoxetine, amantadine and modafinil are used with very limited success.
- Pain is common and should be treated with amitriptyline or gabapentin.
- Depression is treated with the usual antidepressants.
- A full urinary bladder assessment by a urologist may be needed. Anticholinergic drugs such as oxybutynin help with bladder instability. Laxatives help in constipation. Patients with sexual problems will need help from the sexual dysfunction clinic.

Treating relapses

- IV methylprednisolone (1 g daily for three days) is commonly used to shorten the duration of relapse without any influence on the long-term outcome. Although it can be used in patients with progressive disease, the response is usually limited.
- A short course of rehabilitation is useful especially after a relapse.

Disease-modifying treatments

- Disease-modifying treatments such as beta-interferons and glatiramer acetate have been shown to reduce the number of relapses by one-third. In the UK, several disease-modifying treatments are available. The progression of MS will increase significantly if left untreated, which supports beginning treatment as early as possible after diagnosis. As these agents are immunomodulatory, increased risk or reactivation of infection can occur (e.g. COVID-19, HSV/varicella zoster, TB, PML, hepatitis B).

Prognosis

- The prognosis is variable but male gender, high number of relapses, motor or cerebellar presentations and progressive course are poor predictive signs.
- Probably one-third of patients have a mild form of MS. However, life expectancy is reduced by 5–10 years and there is a 50% chance of patients losing their ability to walk independently after 15 years.

Other demyelinating diseases

Neuromyelitis optica (NMO, Devic disease)

- This is a monophasic disease of a combination of optic neuritis and myelitis (inflammation of the spinal cord) occurring simultaneously or in succession.
- Brain MRI is normal while spinal MRI shows demyelination lesions extending over three or more vertebral segments. Oligoclonal bands are usually negative in the CSF. NMO-IgG may be detected in the patient's serum.
- The disease is usually aggressive, and patients are left with several disabilities. IV methylprednisolone, IV immunoglobulin and immunosuppressive agents are used in treating NMO.

Acute disseminated encephalomyelitis (ADEM)

- ADEM is a monophasic fulminant demyelinating syndrome, more common in children (after immunisation).

- It usually presents with encephalopathy (seizures, meningism) and features of myelitis, cerebral or cerebellar involvement. Half of the patients report a preceding infectious illness.
- Brain and spinal MRI show demyelination lesions and oligoclonal bands are positive in the CSF in around one-third of patients.
- The disease is treated with IV methylprednisolone and/or IV immunoglobulin.

Other common neurological disorders

Infections of the CNS

- Meningitis is inflammation of the meninges while encephalitis is inflammation of the brain.
- Different microbes (bacteria, viruses, fungi, parasites) can cause acute meningitis while certain viruses can lead to encephalitis. However, there is always a degree of overlap between meningitis and encephalitis (meningoencephalitis). The infective process could involve a local area of the brain (cerebritis) leading to cerebral abscess.
- COVID-19 infection can lead to central or peripheral neurological complications, possibly due to viral invasion of the central nervous system, inflammatory response, vascular and immune dysregulation.
- Infection with human immunodeficiency virus (HIV) can result in numerous neurological complications including direct viral effects, opportunistic infections and tumours.

Aetiology

- Acute bacterial meningitis is usually caused by:
  - *Streptococcus pneumoniae*
  - *Neisseria meningitidis*
  - *Haemophilus influenzae.*
- The most common cause of viral meningitis is enteroviruses.
- Herpes simplex virus is a well-recognised cause of encephalitis.
- Cerebral abscess is usually a result of spread of local infection (sinuses or middle ear infection) or traumatic head injury and can occur in immunocompromised patients.
- *Listeria monocytogenes* (listeriosis) manifests most commonly as meningoencephalitis or septicaemia in high-risk groups including people aged over 60 years, pregnancy, immunocompromised and alcoholism.

Clinical features

- Non-specific features such as fever and rigors.
- Features related to meningeal irritation such as headache, photophobia and neck stiffness (positive Kernig's sign).
- Features of raised intracranial pressure such as headache, vomiting, impairment of consciousness and papilloedema.
- Encephalitic features such as focal neurological deficit, seizures and impairment of consciousness.
- Cerebral abscess tends to present with fever, headache, focal neurological deficit and seizures.
- Viral meningitis is a benign disease and presents with headache and fever with no impairment of consciousness.
- Meningococcal purpuric rash may be seen with meningococcal meningitis.

Investigations

- FBC may show a high white cell count.
- High ESR or C-reactive protein.
- Blood cultures could help in identifying the organism in bacterial infection.
- CT brain is normal in meningitis. MRI brain may show temporal lobe changes in herpes simplex encephalitis. Ring-enhancing lesion with surrounding oedema points to cerebral abscess.
- CSF analysis is vital to confirm the diagnosis and identify the organism. CT brain must be done before LP in any patient with contraindications to initial LP (e.g. focal features, papilloedema). If a head CT is indicated, blood cultures should be obtained immediately, and dexamethasone and empiric antimicrobial therapy should be started once blood cultures have been obtained and *prior* to head CT.
- Bacterial meningitis leads to high white cell counts in the CSF (>200/mm³), mainly polymorphs with high protein and low glucose. Viral meningitis, on the other hand, causes raised white cell counts in the CSF (<200/mm³), mainly lymphocytes with slightly raised protein and normal glucose. CSF lactate is usually low in viral meningitis and can help differentiate from bacterial causes. Partially treated bacterial meningitis could alter the CSF analysis. Herpes simplex encephalitis leads to high white cell counts in the CSF (up to 500/mm³), mainly lymphocytes with slightly raised protein and normal glucose. Polymerase chain reaction (PCR) for herpes virus in CSF is positive in the majority of patients with herpes simplex encephalitis. Multiplex PCR is gold standard for viral meningitis and also useful for bacterial causes. LP is not indicated in cerebral abscesses.

Management

- IV treatment with a broad-spectrum antibiotic (third-generation cephalosporin such as ceftriaxone) and aciclovir (if concerns about encephalitis) should be started immediately until the diagnosis is clear. The antibiotic regimen can be altered if certain risk factors are present (e.g. add vancomycin if suspicion of penicillin-resistant pneumococci or amoxicillin if Listeria risk factors) or once the organism and sensitivities are identified.
- IV dexamethasone can be effective in reducing unfavourable outcomes in acute bacterial meningitis. The first dose of dexamethasone should be given with the first dose of antibiotic. If pneumococcal meningitis is confirmed, dexamethasone should be continued for 4 days.
- Antimicrobial treatment and surgical intervention are needed to treat cerebral abscesses.
- No specific treatment is needed for viral meningitis as it is a self-limiting disease.
- Acute complications such as hydrocephalus should be treated.
- Patients with acute CNS infections may need intensive supportive measures in high-dependence or intensive care units (e.g. GCS ≤12).

Prognosis

- Acute CNS infections still carry a high mortality rate (around 20%), especially if there is a delay in starting treatment.
- Patients may have long-term sequelae such as epilepsy and cognitive impairments.

Other infections of the nervous system

Tuberculous meningitis (TBM)

- Certain ethnicities (e.g. Asian), immigrants and immunocompromised patients are at higher risk of developing TBM.
- Onset is usually subacute and patients could have non-specific symptoms such as headaches, fever and weight loss. Patients may develop seizures and cranial nerve abnormalities.
- CSF is vital in making the diagnosis. There is usually high protein (>1.0 g/l), lymphocytes (50–500/mm³) and low glucose (<50% of the blood glucose). Ziehl–Neelsen stain is usually negative and cultures are positive in 60% of cases and usually take several weeks to obtain results.
- Brain CT/MRI may show basal meningeal enhancement. Hydrocephalus, ischaemic infarction or tuberculomas (slow-growing granulomas) could

be seen. Chest X-ray may show evidence of pulmonary tuberculosis.

- Treatment with antituberculous drugs should be started as soon as possible. Dexamethasone is widely used. Seek expert help regarding drug-resistant strains.

Cryptococcal meningitis

- Fungal infection is usually seen in immunocompromised patients (e.g. HIV).
- Cryptococcal meningitis could present with non-specific headache, fever, cranial nerve palsies and seizures resembling TBM.
- Brain CT/MRI may show mass lesions (cryptococcomas).
- CSF shows high protein, lymphocytosis and low glucose. A CSF India ink is positive in 50% of cases.
- Antifungal therapy such as fluconazole or amphotericin B should be started as soon as possible.

Guillain–Barré syndrome

Guillain–Barré syndrome (GBS) is the most common cause of acute flaccid paralyis in the Western world.

Clinical features

- Patients present with rapidly progressing ascending paralysis with sensory symptoms (over a week or two).
- GBS is predominantly a motor peripherial neuropathy.
- The neurological examination shows generalised weakness (tetraparesis) more marked distally with absent reflexes and minimal sensory signs.
- Facial weakness (LMN lesion of 7th nerve) and bulbar involvement are common.
- There is usually a history of antecedent upper respiratory tract infection or diarrhoea (especially *Campylobacter jejuni*).

Investigations

- NCS/EMG – important to confirm the diagnosis and usually shows evidence of demyelinating neuropathy.
- CSF analysis shows high protein.

Management

- IV immunoglobulin is the treatment of choice.
- Regular monitoring of forced vital capacity (FVC) as patients at risk of respiratory failure.
- Regular monitoring of blood pressure and heart rhythm as patients at risk of autonomic neuropathy.
- Thromboprophylaxis needed to prevent venous thromboembolism.

- Intensive care support as ventilation may be needed.
- Neurorehabilitation.

Prognosis

Around 80% of patients make a complete recovery after one year. About 5% die and 15% of patients are still unable to walk unaided after one year.

Myasthenia gravis

- Myasthenia gravis is an uncommon autoimmune disorder affecting the neuromuscular junction.
- MG has a bimodal age of onset, 20–40 years of age (predominantly females) and 50–70 years of age (predominantly males).
- Patients with MG and their family members have increased incidence of other autoimmune diseases such as Graves' disease, pernicious anaemia and rheumatoid arthritis.

Pathophysiology

- Acetylcholine is the transmitter at the neuromuscular junction.
- In normal circumstances, acetylcholine is released from the axon of the LMN to the synapses. Acetylcholine then binds to the postsynaptic receptors on the muscle membrane.
- In MG, autoantibodies (acetylcholine receptor antibodies) block the postsynaptic receptors, causing impaired neuromuscular transmission.
- It is believed that the thymus has a role in the pathogenesis of MG. The precise role of the thymus is not clear.

Clinical features

- Ocular symptoms – double vision and/or ptosis.
- Speech and swallowing difficulties (bulbar symptoms).
- Facial and neck muscle weakness.
- Painless limb weakness, mainly proximal muscle, is a common feature of generalised MG (e.g. patient has difficulty lifting arms above shoulder level).
- Respiratory muscles could be affected, leading to breathing difficulties.
- Fatiguability is very suggestive of MG. The more a muscle is used, the weaker it gets. Therefore, symptoms tend to be worse in the evening and after repeated use of the muscle (e.g. difficulty in swallowing is worse at the end of a meal). In the clinic, fatiguability could be demonstrated by asking the patient to look up for 30–60 seconds as the ptosis

will get worse, and by examining shoulder abduction before and after asking the patient to abduct the shoulder 20 times. The patient's speech may get worse as the medical consultation progresses.

- Distal limb muscle weakness is rare in MG.
- Patients who carry on having only ocular features for two years without developing generalised MG are diagnosed as ocular myasthenia.

Investigations

- Acetylcoline receptor antibody is positive in around 90% of patients with generalised MG and 50% of patients with ocular myasthenia. The detection of this antibody is diagnostic of MG. The titre does not correlate with disease severity.
- EMG – may show decrement on repetitive stimulation.
- Edrophonium (Tensilon®) test rarely used nowadays.
- Once the diagnosis is confirmed, a CT or MRI scan of thorax is needed to look for thymic hyperplasia or thymoma.

Management

- Symptomatic therapy – acetylcholinesterase inhibitors (pyridostigmine) improve patients' symptoms by slowing the breakdown of acetylcholine, thus increasing its availability in the neuromuscular junction. Side-effects such as abdominal cramps and diarrhoea are common, and could be overcome by giving antimuscarinic drugs such as propantheline.
- Immune therapy aims to suppress production of the abnormal antibodies. Prednisolone is commonly used. The patient's condition may deteriorate initially (steroid dip) and therefore close monitoring is needed, and sometime patients need hospital admission to introduce the prednisolone. Azathioprine is used as a steroid-sparing agent but may take 6–18 months to work. Patients with severe disease, acutely ill or not responding to oral therapy should be treated with IV immunoglobulin or plasmapheresis.
- Patients who are acutely ill with respiratory muscle weakness need close montoring in hospital by measuring FVC. Ventilatory support may be needed in patients with FVC <1.5 litres.
- Thymectomy is indicated in patients with thymoma. It should also be considered in young patients (aged <45 years) with generalised MG.
- Some drugs such as aminoglycosides, quinidine, antiarrhythmic drugs, magnesium and benzodiazepines can worsen MG and should be avoided. D-penicillamine can cause MG.

Prognosis

- With modern treatment, the majority of patients with MG do well and lead a normal life but may need long-term treatment.
- The mortality rate is around 4%.
- Long-term and spontaneous remission is well recognised but late exacerbation is possible.

Motor neurone disease

- MND is a progressive degenerative disease of the motor neurones of the brain, brainstem or spinal cord.
- MND is a sporadic disease of unknown aetiology. However, 5–10% of cases are familial.

Clinical features

- There are three forms of MND.
  - Amyotrophic lateral sclerosis: the most common form. The patient presents with weakness mainly in the hands with a combination of UMN signs (brisk reflexes) and LMN signs (wasted muscles and fasciculation). The weakness and wasting progress to other muscles in the trunk and lower limbs.
  - Progressive bulbar palsy: the patient presents with progressive dysarthria followed by swallowing difficulty. There is wasting and fasciculation of the tongue.
  - Progressive muscular atrophy: the patient presents with progressive weakness of LMN type.
- The majority of patients will have a combination of amyotrophic lateral sclerosis and progressive bulbar palsy.
- There are *no* sensory signs or bladder involvement.
- Patients die from respiratory failure due to weakness in respiratory muscles and bulbar palsy.

Investigations

NCS/EMG shows denervation and fasciculations in both wasted and normal muscles.

Management

- Multidisciplinary care is needed to provide full support to patients and their carers.
- Riluzole, a glutamate antagonist, is widely used as a disease-modifying treatment. It may increase survival by a few months.
- Percutaneous endoscopic gastrostomy and non-invasive ventilation (NIV) may be needed.

Prognosis

Motor neurone disease is relentlessly progressive with a survival rate of three years.

Intracranial tumours

- Primary brain tumours are uncommon in comparison with other tumours such as breast and lung cancer.
- CNS tumours have an annual incidence of around 6 per 100 000 population. The median age of onset is 56 years.

Types of brain tumours

- Meningiomas – benign tumours which arise from any part of the meninges.
- Gliomas – can be benign or malignant. Histologically, they are graded from I to IV, I being benign and IV very malignant (glioblastoma multiforme). However, grade I gliomas may progress to malignant ones over time.
- Metastases – usually from lung or breast cancer.
- Pituitary ademomas – most common functioning tumour is prolactinoma. However, non-functioning tumours are also common.
- Acoustic neuromas – also known as acoustic nerve schwannomas. They are benign tumours arising from the 8th cranial nerve at the cerebellopontine angle.

Clinical features

- Features of raised intracranial pressure such as headache, vomiting, papilloedema and false localising signs (6th nerve palsy).
- Seizures which could be focal or generalised.
- Progressive focal neurological deficit such as hemiplegia and speech impairment. The nature of the deficit depends on the site of the tumour.
- Pituitary ademomas may present with visual field defects, usually bitemporal hemianopia, and/or endocrine disturbance (see Figure 24.4).
- Acoustic neuromas usually present with deafness with 5th and 7th nerve impairment.

Investigations

- Brain CT/MRI are the investigations of choice to detect brain tumours.
- If the scans suggest that the tumour could be due to metastatic disease, then the primary tumour should be sought.

Management

- Multidisciplinary care is needed to provide full support to patients and their carers.
- Dexamethasone is used to reduce brain oedema and could help in relieving some of the acute symptoms such as headache. AEDs are important if the patient is having recurrent seizures.
- Partial or complete removal of the tumour is needed in most cases to help in the histological diagnosis. If the tumour is in a part of the brain where attempting even partial removal is dangerous, a biopsy may be needed.
- Sometimes the tumour is small or inaccessible and repeated brain scans in three or six months intervals are needed.
- Depending on the nature of the tumour, radiotherapy and/or chemotherapy may be necessary.
- Prolactinomas respond well to dopamine agonists such as cabergoline.

Prognosis

- Benign tumours such as meningiomas, pituitary adenomas and acoustic neuromas carry a very good prognosis although patients may end up with some residual deficit.
- Patients with low-grade glioma usually survive for many years. However, the progress of the low-grade glioma to a high-grade one is common.
- Metastases and high-grade gliomas have a poor prognosis.

Head injury

- Head injury leading to traumatic brain injury (TBI) is the most common cause of death and disability in young people in Western countries.
- Head injury is more common in men, with a male:female ratio of 2.5:1.
- In the UK, around 1 million patients present to hospital per year following head injury. The majority (90%) have minor or mild head injury.

Causes of head injury

- Road traffic accidents are the main cause of serious head injury.
- Falls cause around 40% of head injuries in the UK. These are common in the inpatient setting.
- Assaults cause around 20% of head injury in the UK.
- Accidents at work, including sports-related injuries.
- Alcohol is a major contributory factor to head injury.

Classification

- Mild head injury – initial score of 13–14 on GCS with no evidence of intracranial pathology. If the GCS is 15, the head injury could be classified as minor.
- Moderate head injury – initial GCS of 9–12.
- Severe head injury – initial GCS of 3–8.

Short-term sequelae of head injury

- Diffuse brain damage.
  - Mild head injury could lead to minimal diffuse damage to the brain.
  - Moderate-to-severe head injury causes diffuse cerebral damage leading to generalised cerebral oedema which could be severe enough to cause tentorial herniation and coning.
- Cerebral haemorrhage such as:
  - intracerebral bleeding
  - subarachnoid haemorrhage
  - acute or chronic subdural haematoma.
  - extradural haematoma.
- Hypotension and hypoxia, as a result of the head injury or associated body injuries, could lead to ischaemic and hypoxic brain damage.
- Skull fractures which could be simple or depressed. Basal skull fractures could cause CSF rhinorrhoea (CSF leaking through the nose).
- CNS infection as a result of open wounds and skull fractures, especially with basal skull fractures.
- Seizures which may aggravate the cerebral hypoxia.

Management

- In the UK, around 20% of patients with head injury require admission for observation and less than 5% are managed in neurosurgical units.
- All patients with head injury need initial neurological assessement which should include GCS, pupil size and any evidence of focal neurological signs. Depending on the severity of the head injury, patients will require neurology observation at regular intervals.
- Patients with minor or mild head injury can be discharged home after a short period of observation with clear safety netting written instructions to return to hospital if they show any signs of deterioration. However, if the patient has an associated medical or social problem, hospital admission may be needed.
- Patients with moderate-to-severe head injury need resuscitation ideally in the prehospital setting (site of the accident). This includes the usual ABCDE approach.
- Patients with altered level of consciousness, focal neurological deficit, suspected skull fracture, vomiting or any associated medical problems (on warfarin or other anticoagulants) will require brain CT.
- The management of patients with moderate-to-severe injury should aim to prevent secondary brain damage as a result of hypoxia, hypotension, infection, cerebral haematoma and increased intracranial pressure. Patients may need transferring to a neurosurgical unit, for evacuation of intracranial haematomas, or to intensive care (ideally neurointensive care).
- Patients who recover from moderate-to-severe injury will need a period of neurorehabilitation.

Long-term sequelae of head injury

- Posttraumatic syndrome – common after minor and mild head injury. Patients experience non-specific symptoms such as headache, dizziness, lack of concentration, memory problems and poor sleep. Symptoms usually resolve within 12 months. It is not clear whether compensation claims could be contributing to the symptoms.
- Posttraumatic epilepsy – head injury is the cause of 2% of epilepsy cases. Early seizures (within the first week of the injury) are more common than late-onset seizures. Depressed skull fractures, intracranial haematoma, prolonged posttraumatic amnesia (>24 hours), dural tear and early seizures increase the risk of posttraumatic epilepsy.
- Loss of the sense of smell (anosmia) as a result of head injury is usually permanent due to damage to the olfactory (1st) nerve.
- Chronic subdural haematoma – usually occurs in elderly people and alcoholics after a minor head injury. Patients present with headaches or drowsiness weeks after the injury. Brain CT is diagnostic and surgical evacuation is needed. If missed, patients develop focal neurological signs and coma and may die as a result of increased intracranial pressure leading to coning.
- After head injury, patients may have behavioural and psychological problems, impairment of memory and permanent neurological deficit (e.g. hemiplegia).
- Chronic traumatic encephalopathy (CTE) – progressive brain condition thought to be caused by repeated blows to the head and repeated episodes of concussion. Associated with contact sports (e.g. boxing, rugby). Definitive diagnosis is made at postmortem.
- Following head trauma due to damage to the pituitary stalk and the pituitary blood supply, it has

been estimated that ~25% of patients with traumatic brain injury severe enough to require hospitalisation develop one or more pituitary hormone deficiencies (i.e. hypopituitarism).

Functional disorders

- Functional disorders are usually defined as patients with neurological symptoms but no disease. They are common in neurological practice.
- Many terminologies have been used such as functional, non-organic, psychogenic, psychosomatic and medically unexplained,
- Patients who *consciously* fabricate symptoms are described as:
  - factitious: if the purpose is to get medical care and attention
  - Munchausen: if a patient with factitious disorder gets medical care (usually in emergency and inpatient departments) in different hospitals (wanders between doctors and hospitals)
  - malingering: factitious disorder for material gain.
- The most common presentations of patients with functional disorders in neurology practice are as follows.
  - Non-epileptic attack disorder.
  - Weakness – usually develops suddenly. There is always a degree of inconsistency (patient able to walk but can't lift the leg up on the bed).
  - Gait disorders – patient could swing from side to side in a very unusual way, sometimes mistakenly labelled as ataxic gait.
  - Tremor – tends to be easily distractable.
  - Sensory symptoms – impairment of sensation in one half of the body (split in half).
- Investigations and overinvestigations with repeated scans are usually inescapable.
- Patients need a full explanation about the problem. Some patients find it difficult to accept that there is no physical cause for their symptoms. The way in which the diagnosis is explained to the patient is vital.
- Further referral to psychiatry, psychology or neuropsychiatry is helpful. However, it is vital that the psychiatrist, psychologist or neuropsychiatrist has an interest in functional disorders otherwise it may make things worse!
- Cognitive behavioural therapy may help.
- Physiotherapy for patients with gait disorders or weakness is useful.
- The earlier the diagnosis is made, the better the outcome.

Muscle diseases

- Muscle diseases are relatively rare in clinical practice.
- Patients usually show signs of proximal myopathy (weakness around the hip and shoulder girdles). Patient has difficulty standing from a sitting position. Muscle diseases could involve the respiratory and cardiac muscles.
- Patients could have a waddling gait.
- The following are causes of muscle diseases.
  - Polymyositis or dermatomyositis: these can occur in isolation or be associated with other autoimmune diseases. Dermatomyositis is associated with skin changes such as heliotrope rash and photosensitive rash. It is also associated with malignancy.
  - Inclusion body myositis, which is the most common form of myopathy after the age of 50. Involvement of finger flexors, foot extensors and quadriceps is an early pointer to the diagnosis.
  - Endocrine causes: Cushing syndrome, diabetes mellitus (amyotrophy) and thyrotoxicosis.
  - Drug-induced myopathies: steroids, amiodarone, lithium, statins.
  - Genetic myopathies: includes muscular dystrophies such as Duchenne and Becker muscular dystrophy and limb girdle dystrophy.
  - Metabolic myopathies such as mitochondrial disorders and inherited metabolic disorders.
  - Alcoholism.
  - Osteomalacia.
- The following investigations are usually needed.
  - Blood tests (such as blood glucose, thyroid function tests, 25-hydroxyvitamin D).
  - Muscle enzymes.
  - Myositis specific antibodies, e.g. antisynthetase autoantibodies are a collection of antibodies that target tRNA synthetase enzymes. They are associated with antisynthetase syndrome (includes myositis, interstitial lung disease, inflammatory arthritis, fever and malaise, mechanic's hands). The most common antisynthetase antibody is anti-Jo-1.
  - EMG.
  - Muscle biopsy.
  - Genetic testing.
- Depending on the type of muscle disease, some disorders are not treatable and only supportive measures are available. Other diseases such as polymyositis and dermatomyositis are treatable usually by corticosteroids and other immunosuppressive agents such as azathioprine and methotrexate.

Narcolepsy

- Patients with narcolepsy present with excessive daytime sleepiness (irresistible urge to sleep).
- Narcolepsy is usually associated with cataplexy (sudden loss of muscle tone without losing consciousness), sleep paralysis (patient is fully awake but can't move) and hypnagogic hallucinations.
- Sleep studies are warranted. CNS stimulants such as modafinil and dexamphetamine are used to treated narcolepsy, while cataplexy, sleep paralysis and hypnagogic hallucinations respond to tricyclic antidepressants and selective serotonin reuptake inhibitors.

25

People with mental health issues

James Bolton

KEY POINTS

- Mental illness is common in the general hospital setting and in the context of physical illness. Patients may present with the physical consequences of mental illness, or physical illness and its treatment may have psychiatric repercussions. Mental and physical illnesses may also be unrelated but coincident in a single patient.
- Staff should be alert to stigmatising attitudes towards mental illness and subsequent discriminatory care, such as physical symptoms being underinvestigated or undertreated.
- Liaison psychiatry services work at the interface of physical and psychiatric healthcare, most often in general hospitals. Such services can assist with the assessment and management of complex cases and those where mental illness places a patient at increased risk.

Introduction

> Although there is a tendency to consider the mind and body as being afflicted by different illnesses, this is an artificial distinction. All illnesses have physical, psychological and social dimensions, and mental health problems are commonly encountered in Acute Medicine.

Mental illnesses are generally considered to be those that affect thinking, emotional state or behaviour to a degree that significantly impairs day-to-day functioning. In Acute Medicine, patients may present with:

- the physical manifestations of mental illness, such as self-harm or severe malnutrition in anorexia nervosa

- the mental health repercussions of physical illnesses and their treatment, such as mood disorder or delirium
- coincident but unrelated mental and physical illness.

The stigma of mental illness is the single biggest obstacle to the provision of effective mental healthcare. Stigmatising beliefs about patients with mental illness include the following.

- They are a danger to others.
- Their illness is self-inflicted.
- They are hard to talk to.

Such beliefs can lead to discriminatory behaviour by hospital staff, who may see patients with mental illness as less of a priority for care. Physical symptoms may be overlooked and physical illness underinvestigated or undertreated. Staff should be alert to, and

---

Acute Medicine: Lecture Notes, First Edition. Edited by Glenn Matfin.
© 2023 John Wiley & Sons Ltd. Published 2023 by John Wiley & Sons Ltd.

challenge, potentially stigmatising attitudes and discriminatory care.

This chapter will discuss the assessment and management of common psychiatric problems and related challenging situations in the acute medical setting. Other relevant topics such as alcohol and substance misuse, delirium and dementia, and learning disability are discussed in other chapters.

Psychological impact of physical illness

Co-morbid physical and mental illness

Compared to the general population, people with physical illnesses are twice as likely to have a co-morbid mental illness. Rates are highest in those with long-term physical health conditions and those with more than one physical illness.

The pain and impact of a physical illness on someone's life can cause depression or make it worse. In turn, depression can worsen the pain, distress and disability associated with physical illness. Someone with both a long-term condition and depression is less likely to adhere to treatment and follow advice for healthy living. Having both a physical and mental illness delays recovery from both and reduces life expectancy.

When someone with a long-term condition has a mental illness, the cost of their physical healthcare increases. For example, patients with depression and long-term lung disease have longer hospital stays. The cost of treating diabetes is over four times higher for those who are depressed compared with those who are not.

What is the psychological impact of a specific illness?

Different illnesses affect different people in different ways, depending upon how various factors interact (Figure 25.1).

- Illness and its treatment – the more stressful illnesses include conditions that involve the brain and those that are life-threatening, chronic or disabling.
- Treatment – unpleasant, invasive and painful investigations and treatments are likely to have a greater detrimental impact on mood. Drug treatments, such as steroids, opiate analgesics and forms of chemotherapy, can have significant

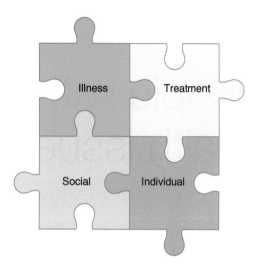

Figure 25.1 The psychological impact of physical illness depends on the interaction of various factors.

psychological adverse effects. Hospital admission itself can be stressful as patients lose their independence and have less access to social support.
- Social support – the quality of an individual's social support is more important than the quantity. A confiding relationship is particularly important in helping patients cope.
- Individual factors – the impact of an illness may be influenced by an individual's:
  - previous experience of illness and care, both personal and in family and friends
  - understanding of their illness, its treatment and prognosis
  - personality, and emotional coping style and resources.

Mood disorders

A transient change in mood is an expected response to a challenging situation. Indications that a hospitalised patient may have a depressive illness include the following.

- Persistent symptoms that do not resolve as expected.
- Mood symptoms that are more extreme or disabling than expected.
- Reduced social interaction with staff or visitors.
- Slower than expected recovery and rehabilitation from physical illness.
- Failure to adjust to physical illness.
- Suicidal thoughts.

Depressive disorder

Around one in 20 people will experience an episode of depressive illness each year. Depressive episodes may be single or recurrent. Individual episodes can be graded as mild, moderate or severe, depending upon the number and severity of symptoms, and their impact on day-to-day functioning.

The aetiology of depressive illness is idiosyncratic and may be due to an interaction of factors, both inherited and environmental. In the majority of cases there is a stressful precipitant to an episode of illness.

Symptoms of a depressive episode include:

- depressed mood or numbing of emotions
- disturbed sleep
- reduced appetite and weight loss, or the reverse
- reduced libido
- reduced energy and increased fatigue
- poor concentration and memory difficulties
- reduced self-esteem and self-confidence
- loss of interest and enjoyment in activities
- negative thinking and pessimism
- guilt
- social isolation
- thoughts of being better off dead.

In the context of physical illness, treatment and hospitalisation, the biological symptoms of depression, such as sleep disturbance, poor appetite and reduced energy, are less reliable.

A simple screening test is to ask a patient whether they have experienced either of the following over the past month.

- Feeling down, depressed or hopeless.
- Having little interest and pleasure in doing things.

Broaching the subject of how someone is feeling may give them the confidence to discuss it further.

Mild-to-moderate depressive episodes may respond to psychological therapy. Moderate-to-severe depression may benefit from antidepressant medication. Sometimes a combination of the two is appropriate.

When choosing an antidepressant, potential interactions with co-morbid physical illness and other medications should be considered. For example, in the context of renal impairment, an appropriate choice would be a drug with low renal clearance. Usually, a selective serotonin reuptake inhibitor (SSRI) is the drug of choice, with sertraline and citalopram having a lower propensity for interactions. SSRIs are associated with an increased risk of bleeding and may not be appropriate in those with a history of gastrointestinal bleeding. A gastroprotective drug can be prescribed for older people who are taking non-steroidal anti-inflammatory drugs (NSAIDs) or aspirin. The hospital liaison psychiatry service or pharmacy can advise on the choice of antidepressant.

Anxiety-related disorders

There are several disorders that have anxiety as a key symptom.

- Generalised anxiety disorder – symptoms of anxiety are present most of the time.
- Panic disorder – sudden, intense and transient attacks of anxiety, that may occur with or without a stressful precipitant.
- Phobic disorder – a disproportionate fear of a situation or object that is not inherently dangerous. Common phobias include agoraphobia – a fear of situations from which there is not an easy escape to a safe place (usually home) – and social phobia – a fear of scrutiny by other people. A blood and injury phobia or a needle phobia may affect a patient's ability to engage with healthcare.
- Obsessive-compulsive disorder – recurrent obsessional thoughts or compulsive acts, which the individual finds pointless and unwanted, but resistance cause severe anxiety.

Anxiety-related disorders are common. As in depressive disorder, the potential aetiology is multifactorial. Treatments include antidepressant medications, which generally have an anxiolytic effect, and psychological therapies, especially cognitive behavioural therapy. In the short term, a benzodiazepine may reduce a patient's anxiety sufficiently to undergo investigation or treatment.

Self-harm and suicidal thoughts

There are over 200 000 attendances at UK emergency departments following self-harm each year. However, many instances, if not the majority, do not come to the attention of health services. Self-harm is one of the most common reasons for medical admission, especially amongst younger people.

Terminology

Terms sometimes used to describe an act of self-harm include 'attempted suicide' and 'deliberate self-harm'. These imply a motivation that is often not the case.

The recommended term is 'self-harm', which the National Institute for Health and Care Excellence (NICE) defines as 'self-poisoning or self-injury, irrespective of the apparent purpose of the act'.

Epidemiology

In patients seen in an emergency department (ED) following self-harm, the most common method is overdose and the drugs most frequently taken are analgesics. The most common form of self-injury is by cutting. Other methods of self-harm include burning, asphyxiation, jumping from a height and ingestion of foreign objects.

An act of self-harm carries a risk of repetition of around 15% over the next year, and a risk of suicide of approximately 1% within the next year and 10% over the next 10–15 years. Suicide is a tragic but relatively rare event. However, self-harm is the single most powerful predictor of suicide. Hence, presentation to health services following self-harm is a golden opportunity to prevent future suicide.

Principles of management

Key steps in the management of a patient following self-harm are to:

- minimise physical harm arising from the act
- assess the risk of self-harm or suicide, at the time of the act, currently and in the future
- detect and assess psychiatric disorder
- explore the stresses that have contributed to the act and the patient's coping resources
- compile a treatment and risk management plan.

Assessing the risk of self-harm or suicide

The assessor should enquire about the following factors.

- The circumstances of the event.
- What the patient did (e.g. what they consumed and when).
- Alcohol consumption before or during the episode.
- How the patient came to the attention of health services. This may provide information about the anticipated outcome and underlying degree of suicidal intent.

Self-harm may occur for many reasons. Often, it is a way of coping with stress with no suicidal intent. However, patients may be ambivalent or unclear about the suicidal intent associated with their self-harm, particularly when they have consumed alcohol.

Epidemiological factors associated with a higher degree of suicidal intent in an episode of self-harm include the following.

- Age and gender – the rate of suicide generally increases with age, with an additional peak in middle age for men. The rate is higher in men than women, but the rates become closer with increasing age.
- Being unemployed or retired.
- Social isolation.
- Physical illness.
- Mental illness.
- Alcohol or substance misuse.

Factors in the individual history of an episode of self-harm associated with high suicidal intent include the following.

- Evidence of planning.
- Preparation for a final act (e.g. writing a suicide note, making a will).
- Being alone at the time.
- The act was unlikely to be discovered for some time.
- Taking precautions to avoid discovery.
- Making no effort to seek help.
- Taking all available drugs in an overdose.
- Having an expectation of a fatal outcome.

Questions to explore current suicidal intent

There is no evidence that asking a patient about suicidal ideation increases the risk that they will harm themselves. By not asking, there is a danger that significant suicidal thoughts will be overlooked or the patient's risk underestimated. The following questions may be helpful.

- Do you still feel the same as you did at the time?
- Do you regret what you did?
- Do you still feel hopeless?
- What would make you try again?
- What would you do if you went home now?
- How do you see yourself in a month's time?

There is obviously a risk in discharging a patient back to the same situation where self-harm occurred. Consider asking: 'Has anything changed as a result of what happened?'. Change may occur in the patient's thinking or emotional state, in their social situation or the availability of practical support with problems. A positive change may indicate a reduction in the risk of self-harm.

Psychiatric disorder

Psychiatric disorders commonly associated with self-harm include depression, anxiety, personality disorder, and alcohol and substance misuse. Rates of suicide are increased in many psychiatric disorders, including affective disorders (e.g. depressive illness, bipolar affective disorder), schizophrenia and personality disorder.

Enquire about past psychiatric history, including previous episodes of self-harm. Examine the patient's mental state for evidence of an ongoing mental health problem. Enquire specifically about 'hopelessness', which is associated with an increased risk of further self-harm.

Stress and coping resources

Assess an individual's coping resources, their level of social support, and any problems that may have contributed to the self-harm, such as relationship difficulties, social isolation, financial problems, housing problems and physical illness. Are there any potential coping resources or strategies that the patient has not considered or tried, such as seeking support from friends or family?

Risk management plan

Even though a referral may be made for specialist mental health assessment, hospital staff will need to assess a patient's risk of further self-harm and suicide at the time of initial presentation and throughout admission. Constant observation may be required for patients judged to be at a high ongoing risk of self-harm.

When estimating the risk of further self-harm or suicide, factors to consider include suicidal intent at the time of the act, ongoing thoughts of suicide or self-harm, background stresses, psychiatric disorder and the availability of social support. Factors which may help to guide such a decision are shown in Table 25.1.

Risk assessment tools should not be used as the sole means of predicting an individual's risk of repetition of self-harm or suicide, or to determine management. If they are used, they should form part of a wider assessment, including the areas described above. The assessment of risk and the management plan should be clearly documented.

Specialist assessment

All patients who attend an ED or are admitted to a general hospita, following self-harm should be offered assessment by a mental health professional, usually a member of the hospital's liaison psychiatry service. This assessment will generally include a more detailed assessment of the patient's ongoing needs and risks, which will inform management during and following hospital admission.

Discharge planning

Management following discharge from an acute hospital may include such measures as:

- emergency psychiatric admission
- referral to community mental health services
- referral to drug and alcohol services
- referral for psychological therapy
- giving advice on seeking help from social services or non-statutory services.

Table 25.1 Risk factors that may inform risk assessment and management following self-harm

Risk factors	Low risk	Medium risk	High risk
Age			65 years or older; middle-aged man
Suicidal thoughts	Fleeting but dismissed	Fleeting	Frequent or fixed
Suicidal plans	None	None	Considered methods or definite plan
Hopelessness	None	None or transient	Present
Mental disorder	None or mild	Present	Significant
Alcohol or drug misuse	None	Present	Significant
Psychosocial situation	Stable	Unstable, but no impending crisis	Unstable with impending crisis
Recent dangerous behaviour	None	Infrequent	Escalating

For patients judged to be at sufficiently low risk to be discharged home, staff should discuss with them contingency plans in the event of thoughts of self-harm recurring – often called a 'crisis plan' or 'safety plan'. Patients can be encouraged to consider self-help strategies in a crisis, such as talking to a friend, listening to music or taking a walk. If these are not successful, the plan may then include contacting psychiatric or emergency services or mental health support lines, such as the Samaritans.

Patients who refuse treatment following self-harm

In the majority of cases, patients who initially decline assessment or treatment following self-harm are eventually persuaded to accept intervention. However, use of mental health legislation, such as the Mental Health Act (MHA) 1983 or the Mental Capacity Act (MCA) 2005 in England and Wales, may be considered if the patient cannot be persuaded to co-operate with the suggested care. Such cases should be discussed with a senior colleague. The decisions made and the reasons for them should be carefully documented.

The MHA in England and Wales allows for the medical treatment of the consequences of self-harm. However, in an emergency situation when waiting for a MHA assessment may result in significant harm, treatment under the MCA may be considered. For this to occur, a patient must be assessed as lacking the capacity to refuse the suggested care.

Instances occasionally arise where there is uncertainty about a patient's capacity to consent to treatment, particularly when they are unco-operative with assessment. The assessor may be uncertain whether to presume that the patient has capacity, recognising that one of the statutory principles of the MCA is that adults are assumed to have capacity unless shown otherwise. Alternatively, the assessor may consider that there is sufficient evidence to indicate that the patient lacks capacity, in which case decisions about care should be made in their best interests. In such circumstances, patients are often judged to lack capacity to refuse treatment, recognising that self-harm is strongly indicative of an altered mental state, either chronic or transient, that would affect an individual's ability to use or weigh up the necessary information.

If the patient is judged to lack capacity and resists treatment, or attempts to leave, it should be considered whether restraint is in their best interests. Bearing in mind the underlying principles of the MCA, the degree of force used should be no more than necessary to control the patient's behaviour and allow the proposed treatment to be carried out.

Psychological reactions to stress and trauma

Acute medical patients experience many stressful and traumatic experiences related to physical injury or illness, and their repercussions. An emotional response is normal in such circumstances and people generally cope with support from families, friends and hospital staff. A minority may experience psychiatric disorder as a consequence and require specific treatment.

Normal psychological reactions

Immediately after a traumatic event, it is common to feel shocked and numb, or to experience a degree of denial. These are normal emotional responses, which gradually dissipate.

Following this, other thoughts and feelings will arise as an individual comes to terms with what has happened. They may experience a mixture of feelings including anxiety, anger, distress and helplessness. They may also experience sleep disturbance and nightmares, tiredness, concentration and memory problems, and minor physical symptoms.

People will react differently and take varying times to recover. Normal ways of coping include:

- using social support, including family and friends
- talking things over
- obtaining information about what has happened
- taking time to engage in normal activities.

Psychiatric disorder

A minority of people may develop a mental illness following significant stress or trauma. The risk of this is increased by the following factors.

- Predisposing – previous mental health problems.

- Precipitating – life-threatening stress or trauma; an early profound emotional response.
- Perpetuating – lack of social support.

The most frequent disorders include:

- adjustment disorder
- depressive illness
- anxiety-related disorder
- alcohol and substance misuse
- posttraumatic stress disorder (PTSD).

Adjustment disorder

Adjustment disorder reflects the emotional adaptation to a significant life change or consequences of stressful life events. The associated emotional disturbance is usually great enough to interfere with an individual's day-to-day functioning, but the symptoms do not reach the diagnostic threshold for another disorder, such as depressive illness.

Adjustment disorder occurs within a month of the precipitating event and is generally self-limiting within about six months. However, if a patient has ongoing stress, such as persistent physical symptoms or disability, the emotional response may be protracted.

There is limited data to support an evidence-based approach to treatment, but brief psychological interventions are preferred.

Posttraumatic stress disorder

Posttraumatic stress disorder is not an inevitable consequence of a traumatic event and not all posttraumatic illness is PTSD. Anxiety, depression and substance misuse are more common. Also, many people experience posttraumatic symptoms that do not reach the threshold for diagnosis of PTSD.

Common symptoms of PTSD include the following.

- Re-experiencing the traumatic event through vivid and distressing memories or dreams.
- Avoiding situations that are reminders of the trauma.
- Feeling numb.
- Hypervigilance – feeling on edge and being alert for danger.

Treatments for PTSD include antidepressant medication and psychological therapies.

Medically unexplained physical symptoms

In clinical practice, bodily symptoms that are disproportionate to any underlying physical pathology are common, occurring in about one in five new presentations to primary care with bodily symptoms, and between a quarter and half of patients in medical outpatient clinics. The most common such symptoms include musculoskeletal pain, headaches, tiredness, feeling faint, chest pain, palpitations and abdominal symptoms. However, patients may experience a wide range of other problems, including neurological symptoms, episodes of collapse and breathlessness.

Diagnosis

The diagnoses for such symptoms are potentially confusing and often not mutually exclusive.

Physicians often recognise recurring patterns of symptoms, such as:

- fibromyalgia – where an individual experiences widespread bodily pain and tenderness
- non-epileptic attack disorder or 'pseudoseizures' – where fits are phenotypically similar to epileptic seizures but are not associated with disordered electrical activity in the brain.

Mental health professionals often use diagnoses that are based on a suggested underlying psychological mechanism, such as:

- dissociative-conversion disorder – where intolerable emotional conflict or stress is 'converted' to a neurological symptom that is easier to bear, and the process is 'dissociated' from conscious awareness
- somatisation or somatoform disorders – where stress is thought to be a significant aetiological factor.

A useful starting point is to recognise that this is a group of patients who have bodily symptoms that are not adequately explained by physical pathology – 'medically unexplained symptoms'. This umbrella term is itself unsatisfactory, as the symptoms *can* be explained, but only by considering how physical, psychological and social aetiological factors interact.

Aetiology

A physical symptom arises when a change or sensation in the body is interpreted as evidence of possible illness. This process is influenced by psychological and emotional factors.

Aetiological factors include the following.

- Predisposing – genetic factors; prior experience of illness in both childhood and adult life; childhood abuse; illness beliefs.
- Precipitating – social stresses, both acute and long term; physical illness and injury, e.g. chronic pain that persists after physical healing.
- Perpetuating – reaction of family and carers; iatrogenic factors, such as overinvestigation; anxiety-related or depressive illness which amplifies the symptoms.

An example of how medically unexplained chest pain may arise and persist is given in Box 25.1.

Management

Management of medically unexplained symptoms can be divided into basic strategies that might be used by any clinician, specialist management that might be undertaken by a mental health professional, and

> **Box 25.1 Aetiological factors in a case of medically unexplained chest pain**
>
> - *Precipitating factors*: Paul is a 53-year-old businessman with a family history of premature ischaemic heart disease. He is under chronic stress from working long hours, which are also having a detrimental effect on his marital relationship.
> - *Precipitating factors*: Paul is late for an important meeting, which causes him to feel anxious. Activation of his sympathetic nervous system leads to an increase in his heart and respiratory rates. He experiences these changes as palpitations and chest tightness, which remind him of his family history of heart disease. This in turn makes him feel more anxious.
> - *Perpetuating factors*: Paul visits an ED where doctors try to reassure him that his physical examination and ECG are normal. However, they also arrange for him to undergo further cardiac investigations. This leaves Paul with the concern that there must be something wrong with his heart. He becomes more aware of sensations and discomfort in his chest, which he interprets as symptoms of heart disease.

techniques to support patients with long-term intractable problems.

Basic management

> Clinicians should screen for alcohol or substance misuse, as the symptoms of intoxication or withdrawal may contribute to medically unexplained symptoms. Screening for mood disorder may identify an anxiety-related or depressive illness that has an aetiological role.

Basic management techniques are most likely to be of help in patients with symptoms of recent onset. When taking a history in a case where the clinician suspects that the symptoms may not be explained by physical pathology, it can be helpful to enquire about the patient's concerns and understanding. This may allow previously unspoken anxieties about a serious underlying physical illness, such as cancer, to be discussed and any misconceptions to be addressed. It is also helpful to ask about any background stresses, such as money, job or relationship difficulties.

Overinvestigation should be avoided as it can reinforce a patient's concern that there must be something physically wrong. It can be helpful to prepare a patient for anticipated negative results of investigations, and to discuss with them what these might mean.

Following assessment, most patients benefit from a combination of reassurance and a positive explanation for their symptoms. An explanation is likely to involve reattribution of their symptoms from a purely physical explanation to one that considers the interaction of physical, psychological and social factors.

In helping a patient appreciate how such factors interact, it can be useful to discuss the physical consequences of emotions. For example, being in certain social situations can cause a psychological feeling of embarrassment and the physical reaction of vasodilation and blushing. When we are upset, we may cry or feel our throat tighten. Feeling anxious or frightened can cause an uncomfortable feeling of 'butterflies in the stomach' as activation of the sympathetic nervous system diverts blood away from the gut to the peripheral muscles. People can also be reminded of the recognised links between long-term stress and physical illnesses, such as peptic ulcers or cardiovascular disease.

The explanation for a specific patient's symptoms may involve discussion of the following possible mechanisms.

- Activation of the body's 'fight or flight' response – the evolutionary response that prepares the body for physical exertion in the face of danger leads to a variety of physiological changes that may be interpreted as symptoms of underlying illness, e.g. palpitations, chest tightness, feeling faint, tremor, indigestion, tension headaches.
- A vicious circle of pain and depression – pain can cause low mood, which then lowers the pain threshold and makes the pain feel worse. Pain and depression thereby reinforce each other.
- Hardware and software – an analogy can be drawn between the nervous system and a computer. The brain and nerves act like the computer 'hardware' running programs or 'software' to control movement and sensation. In medically unexplained neurological symptoms, there is a software rather than a hardware problem. Just as a computer may not function correctly or 'crash' due to a software problem, the nervous system can also malfunction when under psychological or emotional stress.

Additional and specialist treatments

Patients whose problems do not respond to basic management strategies may require additional treatment, or referral to a specialist psychiatry or psychology service. Such patients are more likely to have severe or long-term symptoms.

Antidepressant medication can be effective in treating medically unexplained symptoms. Reasons for this include the following.

- The symptoms may be the somatic or bodily representations of a mood disorder, such as anxiety or depression, which improve with treatment for that disorder.
- Alleviation of a vicious circle between physical symptoms and a mood disorder.
- Some antidepressants are recognised to have an analgesic effect.
- There is evidence of effectiveness for a range of medically unexplained symptoms, even though the mechanism of action is unclear.

Psychological therapy can also be of benefit, with most evidence for cognitive behavioural therapy. Psychodynamic psychotherapy may be of benefit for patients where early life experiences play an important role in the aetiology of their symptoms. Problem-solving therapy can help someone identify and tackle specific problems in their life that may be contributing to their symptoms.

Some patients have chronic, severe and disabling symptoms that do not respond to available treatments. Strategies to help such patients include the following.

- Facilitating communication between health professionals involved in the patient's care to ensure that there is a shared understanding and approach to supporting the patient.
- Limiting unnecessary investigations.
- Reducing frequent emergency consultations by offering regular appointments.

Prognosis

A physician may be concerned about making a misdiagnosis in a case of medically unexplained symptoms. However, research has indicated that rates of misdiagnosis are no greater than in other areas of medicine. Generally, patients with a shorter duration of symptoms have a better prognosis.

Eating disorders

Anorexia nervosa has the highest mortality of any psychiatric condition. Death can be due to a number of causes, especially as anorexia affects every organ system in the body. About 60% of deaths are due to cardiac complications or suicide.

Patients may be admitted to a general hospital for management of the physical complications of an eating disorder. The key clinical features of the two most common eating disorders, anorexia nervosa and bulimia nervosa, are listed in Box 25.2. These may present as sub-threshold disorders or disorders with a mixture of anorectic and bulimic symptoms.

A physical risk assessment of patients with anorexia nervosa is described in the UK MARSIPAN (Management of Really Sick Patients with Anorexia Nervosa) guidelines and is summarised in Table 25.2. Patients can appear deceptively well and active up to the point of physical collapse.

Patients should be transferred to a specialist eating disorders unit where possible. However, the severity

---

Box 25.2 Key features of anorexia nervosa and bulimia nervosa

Anorexia nervosa
- Core psychopathology is a fear of fatness resulting in body image distortion.
- Self-induced weight loss, most often by dietary restriction. Other behaviours may include self-induced vomiting, laxative misuse, excessive exercise, use of appetite suppressants or diuretics.
- Low body weight; body mass index (BMI) ≤17.5 kg/m².
- Endocrine disorder involving the hypothalamic-pituitary-gonadal axis, presenting in women as amenorrhoea and in men as loss of libido. Other endocrine perturbations may include elevated growth hormone, raised cortisol, changes in peripheral thyroid metabolism and abnormal insulin secretion.

Bulimia nervosa
- Core psychopathology is a fear of fatness, with the patient setting themselves an ideal body weight below the normal range. However, patients are generally at or above a normal weight.
- Episodes of overeating, associated with a sense of loss of control, in which a large amount of food is consumed in a short period of time.
- Attempts to counteract the perceived fattening effects of food by one or more of the following behaviours: self-induced vomiting; dietary restriction; laxative or diuretic misuse; use of appetite suppressants. Dietary restriction may lead to hunger, which then triggers further binge-eating.
- Patients with type 1 diabetes may omit their insulin to try and manipulate their weight – so-called 'diabulimia'.

Table 25.2 Risk assessment of anorexia nervosa (summarised from the MARSIPAN guidelines)

Body mass index kg/m²
- Low risk 15–17.5.
- Medium risk 13–15.
- High risk <13, or rapid weight loss of >1 kg/week

Physical examination
- Vital signs: bradycardia <40 beats per minute; hypotension (especially with postural drop); hypothermia
- Reduced muscle power. Sit-up and squat-stand test score of ≤2.
  - Sit-up: patient sits up from lying flat
  - Squat-stand: patient squats down and then rises from squatting
  - Scores: 0, unable; 1, using hands to help; 2, noticeable difficulty; 3, no difficulty

Blood tests
- Hyponatraemia (high risk <130 mmol/l) – suspect water loading or syndrome of inappropriate antidiuretic hormone (SIADH)
- Hypokalaemia (high risk <3.0 mmol/l) – suspect vomiting or laxative misuse. Hypokalaemia may indicate low body potassium which can recur after discharge
- Raised liver transaminases
- Hypoglycaemia – suspect occult infection, especially with raised C-reactive protein or low albumin
- Renal impairment

Electrocardiogram
- Bradycardia.
- Raised QTc (>450 ms)
- Non-specific T-wave changes
- Hypokalaemia changes

of physical complications, or a lack of specialist beds, often mean that patients are treated in acute hospitals The UK MARSIPAN guidelines contain detailed recommendations for the treatment and monitoring of inpatients with anorexia nervosa.

An expert in nutrition should be involved in determining an appropriate refeeding regimen for inpatients with anorexia nervosa. Such patients have a high risk of refeeding syndrome, which is characterised by rapid reductions in certain electrolytes such as phosphate, potassium and magnesium, caused by rapid transit into cells. The resulting cardiac effects can be fatal. Other complications can include respiratory failure, liver dysfunction, abnormalities of the central nervous system, myopathy and rhabdomyolysis. The risk of refeeding syndrome can be reduced by a slow, gradual increase in caloric intake. Patients should also be prescribed thiamine, and vitamin and mineral supplementation.

During a patient's treatment, there should be regular liaison with a psychiatrist, ideally a liaison psychiatrist or an eating disorders psychiatrist. Ward staff should be aware of potential sabotaging behaviours by the patient, such as disposing of food, excessive drinking to manipulate weight, and exercising. Patients may require constant supervision by experienced staff, to ensure their concordance with care. Patients who fail to improve may require treatment under mental health legislation, which can include nasogastric feeding.

Bulimia nervosa may cause serious and sometimes life-threatening acute physical complications that require acute medical treatment and possible admission. These include dehydration, renal failure, electrolyte disturbance (particularly hypokalaemia), cardiac arrhythmias and heart failure.

Severe mental illness

Those with severe mental illnesses, such as schizophrenia and bipolar affective disorder, are at greater risk of poor physical health and have a higher premature mortality than the general population. Major causes of death include chronic physical illnesses such as cardiovascular disease, respiratory disease, diabetes and hypertension.

The stress of physical illness and hospitalisation may increase the risk of a relapse of severe mental illness, which may then jeopardise care. When a patient with severe mental illness is admitted to hospital, their psychotropic medication should be continued, unless contraindicated by their physical illness or treatment.

If there is uncertainty about the appropriate psychotropic regimen, or if mental illness is adversely affecting a patient's physical healthcare, advice should be sought from the hospital liaison psychiatry team or the patient's community mental health team.

Schizophrenia

Schizophrenia is characterised by distortions of thinking, perception and mood, occurring in clear consciousness. It is generally thought of as a 'psychotic' condition, whereby patients have difficulty in distinguishing external reality from mental experiences.

There are two main groups of symptoms.

- Positive symptoms – these can be thought of as an addition to normal mental functioning and include delusions, hallucinations and thought disorder.
- Negative symptoms – these represent diminished mental functioning and include emotional blunting, apathy, poor attention, and a reduced output and content of speech.

The pattern of illness is variable but is most commonly one of acute relapses of positive symptoms against a background of chronic negative symptoms.

Patients with schizophrenia are generally prescribed antipsychotic medication. Common adverse effects include oversedation, weight gain, extrapyramidal movement disorders, hyperprolactinaemia and cardiovascular complications.

Clozapine

Clozapine is an antipsychotic used in the management of treatment-resistant schizophrenia. Clozapine carries a risk of neutropenia or agranulocytosis, hence patients undergo mandatory blood monitoring. Other physical adverse effects that may warrant discontinuation of the medication include:

- severe constipation which can lead to fatal bowel obstruction
- myocarditis and cardiomyopathy
- seizures
- liver dysfunction.

Smoking induces clozapine metabolism, so smoking reduction or cessation following hospital admission may lead to increased plasma levels of the drug with a risk of drowsiness, ataxia, confusion and seizures. Hence, a lower dose of the drug may be required. This should be discussed with the hospital pharmacy.

If clozapine is omitted for over 48 hours, restarting at the previous dose carries a risk of seizures, tachycardia, hypotension and circulatory collapse. Restarting requires discussion with the hospital pharmacy, and a regimen of titration and physical monitoring.

Bipolar affective disorder

Bipolar affective disorder is characterised by repeated episodes of excessively elevated or low mood, with recovery between episodes. Symptoms of depression are described above. Symptoms of a manic episode may include the following.

- Persistent elevation of mood, out of keeping with circumstances.
- Increased energy and overactivity.
- Reduced need for sleep.
- Irritability.
- Poor attention with distractibility.
- Disinhibition.
- Grandiose or overoptimistic ideas, that may be of delusional intensity.
- Speech is fast and difficult to interrupt (pressured).

Lithium

Patients will usually be prescribed a mood-stabilising drug, most often lithium. This has a narrow therapeutic range (0.4–1.0 mmol/l). Levels below this range are ineffective and too high a level is associated with life-threatening adverse effects (Box 25.3). Patients taking lithium should have their lithium blood level checked every three months and, because of potential adverse effects, renal and thyroid function every six months.

An increased risk of lithium toxicity is associated with dehydration, urinary tract infection, diarrhoea, vomiting, excessive sweating, renal impairment and acute physical illness. It is good practice to check a patient's lithium level if they require acute physical healthcare. Ideally, a lithium level is taken 12 hours after the last dose but should be checked urgently if toxicity is suspected.

If there is uncertainty about a patient's drug treatment, or if they appear to be experiencing an acute relapse of bipolar disorder, they should be discussed with the hospital liaison psychiatry service.

> **Box 25.3 Lithium toxicity**
>
> Lithium toxicity usually occurs at levels of ≥ 1.5 mmol/l. Clinical features include:
> - coarse tremor
> - ataxia
> - blurred vision
> - muscle weakness
> - slurred speech
> - vomiting and diarrhoea
> - polyuria (nephrogenic diabetes insipidus)
> - confusion
> - seizures
> - coma.

Personality and healthcare

Aspects of a patient's personality can adversely affect their engagement with healthcare, which may be a source of frustration for clinical staff. Examples of behaviour that may be difficult to understand or manage include:

- use of analgesic medication that appears excessive
- not following the suggested treatment plan
- frequent expressions of dissatisfaction with care
- frequent presentations in crisis
- causing confusion, frustration and conflict in staff and teams.

Personality consists of those enduring characteristics that mark someone out as an individual, including the ways in which they typically think, feel and behave. Key aspects of personality are an individual's abilities to cope with stress, and to make and sustain relationships with others.

Personality develops through an interaction of physical factors, including genetic and intrauterine influences, and early life experiences. Adequate parenting facilitates the development of an individual's ability to control their own feelings, manage stress and make healthy relationships.

If an individual experiences inadequate care and parenting, or childhood abuse, they may develop an adult personality that is ill equipped to manage stress and relationships in a healthy way. When problems are particularly severe or persistent, an individual can be said to have a 'personality disorder'. It is estimated that about one in 20 people have such a condition, with higher rates in those in healthcare.

Different types of personality disorder are recognised where individuals have shared symptoms and behaviours. The following are specific personality disorders that are more likely to be encountered in physical healthcare settings.

Emotionally unstable personality disorder

Individuals tend to have a marked instability in their mood and may easily become distressed or angry. They may act impulsively, without consideration of the consequences of their actions, especially when under stress. They can have trouble making and sustaining relationships, which are often intense, chaotic and unstable. They may also be more sensitive to perceived criticism than others, which can be a cause of conflict.

Patients may have problematic relationships with healthcare staff, and difficulties in following treatment plans, perhaps due to unrealistic expectations of a quick solution. They may sabotage aspects of care. These difficulties can cause frustration in those trying to help them and disruption in clinic teams.

Recommendations for supporting patients include the following.

- Communication.
  - Listen to patients and take an interest. They may be very sensitive to perceived boredom or irritation in others.
  - Keep information clear and unambiguous. Avoid uncertainty, speculation and different opinions.
  - Set clear boundaries and expectations for their involvement in care.
- Team working.
  - Arrange for patients to be seen by the same team members.
  - Hold regular team discussions to agree a consistent and shared treatment plan, and to minimise team divisions or 'splitting'. Allow staff to ventilate difficult feelings that patients' behaviour may arouse.

Paranoid personality disorder

People with paranoid personality disorder have often had experiences that have taught them that people are untrustworthy. Consequently, they may be suspicious of others' intentions, or see others as having malign intent. They can hold a strong sense of their personal rights.

Patients with paranoid personality disorder may easily feel that they are being treated unfairly. They are more likely to request a second opinion, or to raise complaints.

Recommendations for supporting patients include the following.

- Be open about all communication about patients.
- Give patients copies of correspondence and reports.
- Be clear about the purpose of actions taken on their behalf or treatment recommended.
- Avoid discussing their care without them being present.

Dependent personality disorder

People with dependent personality disorder experience a high level of need to be taken care of. This can lead to fears of separation and abandonment.

In healthcare settings, they may request frequent and regular appointments. They often seek reassurance and may have difficulty making decisions for themselves. It can be challenging to discharge such patients from care and when this is attempted, they may report a worsening of their symptoms.

Recommendations for supporting patients include the following.

- Encourage them to make their own decisions.
- Set clear limits to contacts, e.g. the number of appointments.
- Prepare them for discharge.
- Encourage social rather than medical contact.

Managing aggressive behaviour

In a general hospital, challenging behaviour may arise in the context of, and independently from, mental disorder, and may be exhibited by both patients and visitors. This section will focus primarily on patients with co-morbid mental illness.

Risk assessment

Aggression may involve verbal abuse or threats, as well as physical assault. Risk factors for a patient behaving aggressively are both environmental and individual (Table 25.3). The best predictor of aggression is a history of such behaviour.

Examples of early warning signs of aggression are given in Table 25.4.

The risk of aggression cannot be predicted with complete accuracy and contributory factors may

Table 25.3 Environmental and individual risk factors for aggression

Environmental

- A busy ward or department
- Waiting a long time to be seen or treated
- Miscommunication and misunderstanding
- A perceived lack of attention from staff
- Perceived staff attitudes, e.g. uncaring, dismissive, blaming

Individual – illness related

- Organic brain disorder, e.g. delirium, dementia, brain injury
- Psychiatric symptoms, e.g. anxiety, agitation, suspiciousness, hostility
- Alcohol or substance misuse, both intoxication and withdrawal states
- Adverse effects of prescribed drugs, e.g. delirium, disinhibition

Individual – past history

- Previous episodes of aggression
- Previous threats or expressions of intent to harm others

Table 25.4 Early warning signs of aggression

General observation

- A high state of arousal
- Tense, restless, pacing

Interaction

- Withdrawal and refusal to communicate
- Irritability
- Prolonged eye contact
- Physical intimidation
- Blocking exits or escape routes

Speech

- Loud
- Verbal threats
- Lack of clarity in thinking

change, so risk assessment is a dynamic process. Risk management involves trying to ensure the safety of the clinician, the patient, and other staff and patients.

De-escalation

De-escalation techniques are those used to try and calm a situation. Key steps are to contain the situation, clarify the patient's problem, and seek to resolve it. During this process, the clinician should control their own behaviour and demonstrate respect and empathy for the patient.

Contain the situation

- Undertake an initial risk assessment.
- If judged safe to do so, invite the patient to move to a quiet place away from others.
- If necessary, ask other staff to be present.
- Ask the patient to sit and discuss the problem.
- Stay alert and maintain personal safety.
- Ensure you can easily and quickly exit if necessary.

Clarify the problem

- Speak clearly, introduce yourself and use the patient's name.
- Offer to help and ask what is happening, using open questions.
- Seek to understand and clarify any misunderstandings.
- Summarise what the patient has said and check with them that you have understood.

Resolve the problem

- Try to deal with the patient's complaints and apologise for deficiencies in care.
- Be honest, give reasons, and acknowledge fallibility.
- Offer the patient choices and options and outline different potential courses of action. Be flexible, negotiate and avoid a power struggle.

Control yourself

- Try to act calmly and confidently.
- Adopt a relaxed facial expression and body language, for example, by having your arms relaxed at your side with open hands.
- Avoid sudden movements.
- Maintain a safe distance from the patient and respect their personal space.
- If the patient is accusatory or insulting, do not take this personally, or react with anger or criticism.
- Avoid arguing with the patient, making threats or saying that they are right or wrong.

Show respect and empathy

- Show interest and concern and be sympathetic.
- Take time to listen to the patient's problems and try not to talk over them.
- Empathise with their feelings, but not with aggressive behaviour.

Restraint and rapid tranquillisation

If de-escalation techniques are unsuccessful, consider requesting additional support to help manage the situation. This might involve colleagues, hospital security staff and, in extreme situations, the police.

A patient may need to be restrained when this is judged to be a necessary and proportionate response to prevent significant harm to themselves or others. If a patient is judged to lack capacity to consent to or refuse care, restraint may be justified under mental capacity legislation. If it is not possible to assess capacity, then restraint may be justified under common law to prevent significant harm.

Sedative medication may be required if a patient's behaviour poses a risk to themselves or others, and other measures have been ineffective. When making a decision about whether to give psychotropic medication, consideration should be given to potential adverse effects, and interaction with other prescribed drugs. Oral medication should be given, if possible, before considering parenteral administration, often intramuscular. Hospitals should have a protocol that guides use of medication in such situations. First-line treatment will often be a benzodiazepine drug, especially when a patient is antipsychotic naïve, or has cardiovascular disease or a prolonged QTc interval.

Postincident review

Following an incident when a patient has behaved aggressively, the staff involved should be offered support to discuss their experiences and feelings. A review should be undertaken to understand any learning points for the management of future incidents.

Capacity and mental illness

> The assessment of capacity to consent to or refuse treatment and care in patients with mental illness is important in Acute Medicine.

Legislation pertaining to capacity varies between different legal jurisdictions, including within the UK. However, there tend to be shared general principles. The assessment of capacity in patients following refusal of treatment after self-harm, or when restraint is being considered, is discussed above.

Capacity *may* be affected by both chronic and acute changes in mental state, but mental disorder does not automatically make someone incapable of making healthcare decisions. The MHA for England and Wales primarily regulates the treatment of mental disorders, but not unrelated physical health problems. In such circumstances, patients detained under the MHA have the same rights as others regarding decisions about their physical healthcare. The MHA can be used to treat physical disorders that directly cause mental illness, and the physical manifestations of a mental disorder, such as parenteral feeding in anorexia nervosa or the consequences of self-harm.

In most instances, a patient's capacity can be assessed by the treating team. A psychiatric opinion can be helpful when mental illness may be compromising a patient's decision-making ability, especially in complex cases or when there is uncertainty about a patient's capacity following initial assessment.

> Although psychiatric staff may assist with assessment, decisions about a patient's capacity and subsequent treatment rest with those delivering care.

Mental health services

Liaison psychiatry

Liaison psychiatry operates at the interface between physical and psychological health, with most services based in acute hospitals. Hospitals with an ED should have access to a 24-hour liaison psychiatry service.

Most services will assess and manage inpatients as well as those presenting to the ED, and some offer an outpatient service. Services usually adhere to national response time standards, whereby emergency referrals are seen within one hour and urgent referrals within 24 hours.

A liaison psychiatry service will usually accept referrals for adults of all ages, but larger hospitals may have separate services for younger and older adults. A service will generally assess and treat patients with a wide range of mental health problems. A comprehensive service will also accept referrals for patients with alcohol and substance misuse.

Most mental health problems can be managed by ward teams. Liaison psychiatry can assist in the management of complex cases, including the following situations.

- Where there is diagnostic uncertainty.
- When the patient has not responded to first-line treatment.
- Where the benefit or choice of psychotropic medication is uncertain.
- Where mental illness is associated with significant risk.
- To help understand and manage challenging behaviour.

Liaison psychiatry services also have a role in the training of hospital staff in the management of patients with mental health problems.

Other hospital mental health services

Services vary between hospitals, but there will ideally be a mental health service for children and young people. Most often, this will be an in-reach service provided by a community mental health service, but some hospitals have a dedicated paediatric liaison psychiatry service.

There may also be specific in-reach services for patients with learning disability, alcohol or substance misuse, and perinatal mental illness.

The hospital liaison psychiatry team may include a psychologist. Clinical and health psychologists also work within individual hospital departments.

Community mental health services

Community mental health services are generally organised around multidisciplinary teams who have expertise in the management of specific age groups or clinical problems. They work in partnership with non-statutory mental health support services. A local area will also have access to an inpatient psychiatric facility.

When a general hospital patient is also under the care of the community mental health service, it may be helpful for the ward team to contact that service to keep them informed about the patient's care and to raise management queries.

26

Acute oncology

Glenn Matfin

 KEY POINTS

- Advances in cancer management continue to improve patient outcomes, but this has been accompanied by a steady increase in emergency admissions due to tumour-related and treatment-related complications.
- Consequently, a new discipline of acute oncology has emerged that covers the care of these non-elective emergencies. The role of the multidisciplinary acute oncology service is to manage these cancer patients collaboratively with Acute Medicine clinicians.
- Approximately 15% of all urgent care is cancer related. Oncological emergencies are common and prompt treatment often results in good outcomes.
- Patients with cancer attend the emergency department more often than the general population, are more likely to be admitted and have longer lengths of stay.
- Although many patients with cancer may not have curable disease, systemic therapy may be used to improve survival, palliate symptoms and maintain quality of life. For others, prompt referral to palliative and end-of-life care may be most appropriate.
- Always make sure that the acute oncology team are informed of the patient's assessment and/or admission as soon as possible.

Introduction

Cancer is not a single illness but a collection of many diseases that share common features, such as abnormal cells dividing without control and ability to metastasise to other parts of the body (Figure 26.1).

Cancer is a common cause of increased morbidity and mortality. In the UK:

- there are around 375 000 new cancer cases every year, which is around 1000 every day
- there are more than 166 000 cancer deaths every year, which is more than 450 every day
- half (50%) of people diagnosed with cancer survive their disease for 10 years or more.

There are more than 200 different types of cancer, but four of them (breast, lung, colorectal and prostate) account for over half of all new cases in the UK. Representative illness scripts for these cancers are outlined in Table 26.1. In addition, common patterns of metastasis for these four types of cancer are shown in Figure 26.2.

Acute Medicine: Lecture Notes, First Edition. Edited by Glenn Matfin.
© 2023 John Wiley & Sons Ltd. Published 2023 by John Wiley & Sons Ltd.

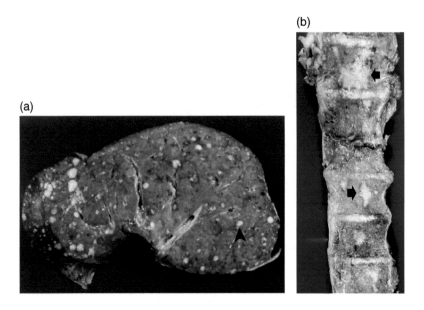

Figure 26.1 (a) Cross-section of the liver showing numerous metastatic pale foci (arrowhead). (b) Cross-section of spine showing numerous metastatic pale foci (arrows).

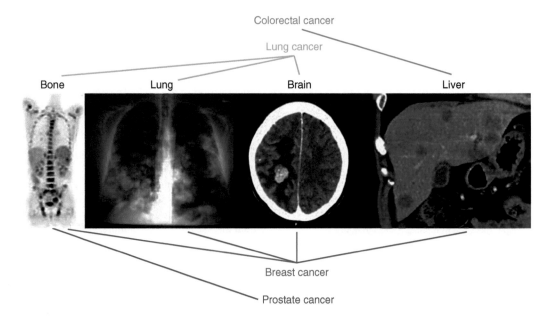

Figure 26.2 Patterns of metastatic spread for the four most frequent cancers in the UK (breast, lung, colorectal and prostate).

Table 26.1 Illness scripts for the four most common UK cancers

	Breast	Lung	Colorectal	Prostate
Epidemiological risk factors	Female, increasing age. Personal/family history. *BRCA1/BRCA2* genes. Previous chest wall irradiation (Hodgkin lymphoma). Obesity. Duration of oestrogen exposure – early menarche, nulliparity, late first pregnancy, hormone replacement therapy.	85% linked to smoking. Other exposures, e.g. asbestos, air pollution.	Increasing age. Family history. *BRCA1* gene, Lynch and polyposis syndromes. Smoking. Dietary factors. Ulcerative/Crohn's colitis.	Increasing age. Family history. *BRCA2* gene. Ethnicity – increased in black men.
Symptoms and signs	Dominant mass, irregular borders, fixation, skin changes, nipple discharge, lymphadenopathy.	Local effects: cough, dyspnoea, chest pain, haemoptysis. Systemic effects: e.g. bone pain, paraneoplastic, clubbing.	Change in bowel habits, blood in stool, weight loss. Signs of iron-deficiency anaemia.	Local effects: urinary symptoms, haematuria. Systemic effects: e.g. bone pain, spinal cord compression.
Time course/ pattern	Chronic, gradual worsening.	Chronic, gradual worsening.	Chronic, gradual worsening.	Chronic, gradual worsening.
Pathophysiology	Oestrogen-related. 10% specific genetic abnormality (e.g. *BRCA1* mutations carry 50–85% lifetime risk).	Tobacco smoke contains carcinogens. Genetic mutations.	Majority develops from adenomatous polyps. Genetic mutations including mismatch repair deficient (e.g. Lynch syndrome).	Androgen-related. Environmental factors
Diagnostics	Mammogram, USS, biopsy with FNA, cytology and histology. Tumour hormone receptor status, *HER2* status. Cancer staging.	Chest X-ray, CT scan, CT/PET scan. Bronchoscopy with tissue diagnosis. Cancer staging.	Faecal occult blood and DNA testing. Endoscopy with tissue diagnosis. CT, MRI. Cancer staging.	PSA. CT, MRI, USS. Biopsy with FNA, cytology and histology. Cancer staging.
Treatment	Surgery. Radiotherapy. Hormonal therapy. Chemotherapy. Immunotherapy. Targeted therapy.	Surgery. Radiotherapy. Chemotherapy. Immunotherapy. Targeted therapy.	Surgery. Radiotherapy (rectal lesions). Chemotherapy. Immunotherapy. Targeted therapy.	Surgery. Radiotherapy. Androgen deprivation therapy. Chemotherapy. Immunotherapy. Targeted therapy.

BRCA, BReast CAncer gene; CT, computed tomography; FNA, fine needle aspiration; *HER2*, human epidermal growth factor receptor 2; MRI, magnetic resonance imaging; PET, positron emission tomography; PSA, prostate-specific antigen; USS, ultrasound scan.

The causes of cancers can be classified into hereditary germline and somatic mutations and environmental factors including radiation, chemical and infectious agents. Many of the causes of cancers are modifiable by lifestyle interventions.

Basic clinical oncology

Clinical presentations of cancer depend on many factors, including the type of cancer, location(s) affected, and associated systemic effects such as presence of paraneoplastic syndromes (remote effects of cancer that occur without local spread).

Treatment of cancer is multifactorial and can result in well-recognised adverse effects, depending on the therapies used. Treatment with radiation, chemotherapy, or both, in addition to definitive surgery is called *neoadjuvant* if administered preoperatively or *adjuvant* if postoperatively.

Precision medicine focuses on identifying effective treatment approaches for patients based on specific aspects of the tumour that can guide clinicians in deciding which therapies to use. Trastuzumab (Herceptin®), a monoclonal antibody against the human epidermal growth factor receptor 2 (*HER2*) on the cell surface, is only active in those breast tumours that overexpress *HER2*. In short, targeted therapy only works if the target is both present and clinically relevant.

Advances in cancer management continue to improve patient outcomes, but this has been accompanied by a steady increase in emergency admissions related to tumour- and treatment-related complications. Consequently, a new discipline of acute oncology has emerged in the UK that covers the care of these non-elective emergencies. The role of the multidisciplinary acute oncology service is to manage these cancer patients collaboratively with Acute Medicine clinicians.

The COVID-19 pandemic has had a detrimental impact on cancer care for both people with a suspected new cancer diagnosis and those with established disease. The knock-on effect of managing COVID-19 has resulted in huge waiting lists for primary and secondary care medical services. Subsequently, many patients with new or established cancer diagnosis may present to Acute Medicine with late cancer presentations, including oncological emergencies.

Initial management of an acute oncology patient presentation

Most oncology decisions can be made utilising three fundamental pieces of information.

- The condition, functional status and co-morbidities of the patient (history and examination).
- The stage of the cancer (cross-sectional imaging). Generally, this is the most accurate prognostic indicator and largely dictates the therapeutic strategy for patients with cancer.
- The type of cancer (histology and other factors, e.g. genetic).

Initial assessment by way of a thorough history and examination with particular emphasis on the patient's cancer pathway is pivotal to their effective acute care management. Determine the patient's cancer history and management.

- Ensure that details of the patient's cancer diagnosis, disease stage, treatment intent, drugs and timings of most recent treatments are ascertained and considered in decision-making processes.
- Review recent investigations if available.
- Contact the patients and/or local oncology team.
- Obtain baseline diagnostic tests, including point-of-care ultrasound (POCUS) as indicated.
- Is the patient for further active treatment, including resuscitation? What is the DNACPR (do not attempt cardiopulmonary resuscitation) status? Reversible toxicities and/or problems can be treated even in the presences of any DNACPR orders; decisions should be made on an individual basis. Do we need palliative care and end-of-life care referral?

Does the patient require enhanced or critical care now? If so, get senior help.

Is this an oncological emergency?

Effective, early management of acute medical emergencies requires prompt recognition, immediate correction of life-threatening physiological abnormalities, the methodical application of the modified ABCDEFG approach, and rapid diagnosis and treatment of the underlying condition.

In acute oncology, the **ABCDEFG** approach is required.

A – airway

B – breathing

C – circulation

D – disability, drugs, dying

E – exposure, endocrine

F – fluid third spacing

G – glucose

A small number of well-defined oncological emergencies exist (Box 26.1). They are all characterised by the possibility of rapid and catastrophic deterioration. Get senior help.

Other important considerations in acute oncology management

- If not an oncological emergency, is this presentation related to any of the following?
  - Anticancer therapy complication.
  - Cancer-related complication.
  - New cancer diagnosis (~20% of previously undiagnosed cancers detected during an emergency admission). Refer to appropriate site-specific specialist cancer team. If cancer of unknown primary, seek acute oncology team advice.
  - Non-cancer related. Acute Medicine team to manage.

- Late effects: the past 40+ years have seen a great improvement in survival of children and young adults treated for cancer. However, the quality of survival is affected by the 'consequences of cancer therapy' which develop continually and cumulatively over a number of years after treatment and lead to a multitude of secondary health complications. These complications are termed 'late effects'.

- Where is the best place to manage this patient?
  - Patient's home: including 'Hospital at Home', virtual ward or telemedicine.
  - Ambulatory care: including rapid-access (hot) specialist clinic, same-day emergency care (SDEC). These ambulatory care settings can manage many acute oncology presentations without inpatient admission, such as those requiring interventions (e.g. paracentesis) or the need for rapid-access diagnostics.
  - Inpatient care: acute medical unit (AMU), specialist ward, enhanced care unit (ECU), high-dependency unit (HDU), intensive care unit (ICU).
  - Hospice.

- Is the patient in a clinical trial? Manage the patient as per usual standard care. However, contact the trial team to get further background information about the clinical study interventions and any advice about known toxicities.

If not done already, refer the patient to the acute oncology team.

Box 26.1 Common oncological emergencies

- Hypercalcaemia of malignancy – severely compromised patient with profound volume depletion and altered sensorium, which may manifest as coma, cardiac decompensation (including dysrhythmias) and abdominal pain that may mimic an acute surgical abdomen. For treatment of severe hypercalcaemia, multitargeted therapies should be started as soon as possible.
- Metastatic spinal cord compression – includes both spinal cord and cauda equina compression. Characteristic pain and neurological signs can occur and rapid treatment by surgical decompression or radiotherapy reduces risk of permanent neurological deficit.
- Tumour lysis syndrome – usually a feature of tumour response to chemotherapy with resulting excessive release of cellular components leading to hyperphosphataemia, hyperuricaemia, hyperkalaemia and hypocalcaemia. Urgent recognition and treatment are life saving.
- Superior vena cava obstruction – causes upper body swelling and bluish skin discoloration with venous distension that may be relieved by radiological vascular stenting. Requires histological diagnosis for decision of optimal treatment.
- Neutropenic sepsis – myelosuppression is a common consequence of treatment for cancer and can cause life-threatening neutropenic sepsis that needs urgent treatment with intravenous broad-spectrum antibiotics and supportive care.

Oncological emergencies

A small number of oncological emergencies exist which require immediate diagnosis and intervention (see Box 26.1).

Hypercalcaemia of malignancy (HCM)

Hypercalcaemia of malignancy complicates 5–30% of malignancies. Hypercalcaemia complicates the course of a variety of cancers when tumour factors overwhelm normal calcium and bone homeostasis.

- Hypercalcaemia, defined as serum calcium >2.6 mmol/l, is usually well tolerated if adjusted calcium (ACa) levels (i.e. corrected for albumin concentration) are <3.0 mmol/l.
- ACa above this threshold is associated with nephrogenic diabetes insipidus, increasingly severe volume contraction, neurological, cardiac and gastrointestinal (GI) dysfunction, and requires urgent treatment to prevent life-threatening consequences.

> The term 'hypercalcaemic crisis' is frequently used to describe the severely compromised patient. Hypercalcaemic crises usually occur when ACa levels are >3.5 mmol/l. HCM is the most common cause of inpatient hypercalcaemic crises (>50%). The diagnosis of hypercalcaemic crisis can sometimes be difficult to make clinically when associated with malignancy. This is because the patient may already be debilitated, anorexic, nauseated, constipated, weak or confused, from the underlying malignancy, concurrent medications, complications of chemo- or radiotherapy, and co-morbid disorders. Clinical vigilance is crucial in this setting to prevent unnecessary morbidity and mortality.

Pathophysiology of HCM

> HCM usually presents in the context of advanced, clinically obvious disease and portends an ominous prognosis with survival typically in the order of months.

Hypercalcaemia of malignancy results from either:

- humoral-mediated bone resorption (>80%). The majority of humoral HCM (>80%) is induced by parathyroid hormone-related peptide (PTHrP), a peptide with significant homology to parathyroid hormone (PTH), or
- direct destruction of bone, either in myeloma or lytic metastatic disease (~20%).

Many solid tumours are associated with HCM and include squamous cell carcinomas of the lung, head and neck, and oesophagus, renal cell carcinoma and breast carcinoma. Humoral-mediated bone resorption stimulated by PTHrP accounts for most of the hypercalcaemia in these malignancies.

> Between 5% and 15% of patients with hypercalcaemia and malignancy have co-existing *primary hyperparathyroidism*.

Emergency management of HCM

> For treatment of severe hypercalcaemia, the underlying cause should be identified and multitargeted therapies should be started as soon as possible.

The cornerstone of acute management of hypercalcaemia is fluid resuscitation with correction of the volume state (rapid-acting). Other treatment options include short-term calcitonin, and in the longer term the most effective antiresorptive agents such as bisphosphonates (e.g. zoledronate) or denosumab should be considered. Steroids can also be used in certain malignancies (e.g. myeloma).

For HCM, further therapy will be determined by the cancer diagnosis, extent of the disease and overall prognosis. In malignancy-related severe hypercalcemia, it may be appropriate to adopt a palliative approach that will emphasise comfort care and symptom control.

> Bisphosphonates may have additional putative benefits in neoplastic disease such as analgesic properties if bone metastases; decreasing the likelihood of pathological fracture; and antitumour effects.

Metastatic spinal cord compression (MSCC)

MSCC is common and in up to half of cases, it is the first presentation of their cancer. Pain is the presenting symptom in 90–95%. Back pain may precede neurological changes by weeks. Thoracic spine is the most common site. Requires *immediate* medical assessment.

Red flags for MSCC are shown in Table 26.2.

Table 26.2 Red flags for MSCC – signs and symptoms

Limb weakness	Thoracic/cervical pain
Difficulty walking	Progressive lumbar pain
Sensory loss	Pain increased by
Bladder/bowel dysfunction	straining
Neurological signs	Nocturnal spinal pain
	Bone tenderness

Emergency management of MSCC

Request urgent whole-spine magnetic resonance imaging (MRI) with or without contrast on anyone with suspected MSCC.

- Start intravenous (IV) dexamethasone 16 mg with proton pump inhibitor (PPI), *before* diagnosis is confirmed. Then continue 4 mg orally every six hours (or local regimen).
- Moving and handling recommendations need to be made for each patient with MSCC.
- Refer for definitive treatment once diagnosis is established.

Tumour lysis syndrome (TLS)

TLS occurs when bulky, rapidly growing tumours with high sensitivity to cytotoxic chemotherapy are treated. Heading the list of these tumours are haematological malignancies such as acute lymphoblastic/cytic and myeloid leukaemias and Burkitt lymphoma. However, treatment of other rapidly growing, chemosensitive tumours can

also result in TLS. Besides tumour bulk and chemosensitivity, a pre-existing decrease in renal function (e.g. serum creatinine >1.4 mg/dl, >123 µmol/l) increases the risk of TLS.

- Rapid cellular destruction releases uric acid and phosphate, both of which are toxic to renal tubules, causing acute kidney injury (AKI). Hyperkalaemia and hypocalcaemia can also occur.
- Prevention of TLS is optimal by recognition of types of tumours which can result in this complication.

Emergency management of TLS

Hydration with IV crystalloid, at least 3 litres per day as long as urine output is adequate, is the recommended treatment for TLS.

There are several agents available to prevent and treat hyperuricaemia associated with TLS.

- Allopurinol is available in oral and IV formulations and may be used for treatment and prevention of hyperuricaemia in TLS. It blocks the conversion of hypoxanthine to xanthine and xanthine to uric acid, resulting in rapid clearance.
- Febuxostat is a selective xanthine oxidase inhibitor that effectively reduces uric acid levels. Its biliary elimination makes it an attractive option for patients with pre-existing nephropathy for both preventing and treating TLS.
- Rasburicase is a recombinant form of urate oxidase which lowers serum uric acid dramatically by converting insoluble uric acid into the more soluble allantoin. Since it is highly effective, rasburicase should be used in patients at high risk for TLS and for treating TLS.
- Most patients at high risk of or with established TLS will be on a regimen of renal-dosed allopurinol and rasburicase.

Complications related to acute hyperphosphataemia include AKI and profound hypocalcaemia with resultant tetany, cardiac arrhythmias, hypotension and seizures. The decision to treat hyperphosphataemia depends on the magnitude of hyperphosphataemia, the rate of rise of serum phosphate, the adequacy of the urine output and the deterioration of renal function. Because

Case study

A 76-year-old man presents confused, with increased thirst, lower back and hip pain, lower limb weakness, no bowel movement for several days, and decreased urine output for 48 hours prior to admission. He has a past history of prostate cancer and had a previous prostatectomy. Investigations reveal prostate-specific antigen (PSA) >100 ng/ml (normal <4), ACa 3.5 mmol/l, PTH suppressed. Widespread osteoblastic lesions on spine and pelvic X-rays (Figure 26.3a).

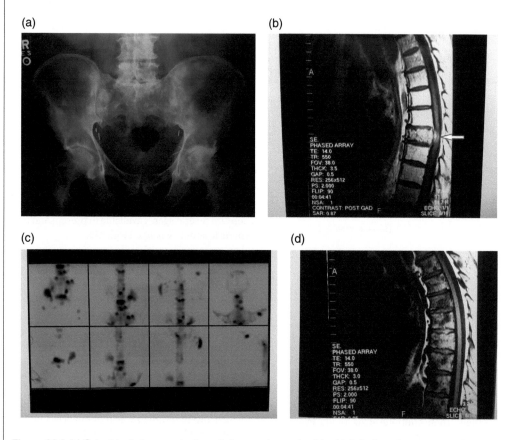

Figure 26.3 (a) Osteoblastic bone metastases in lower spine and pelvis. (b) Spinal cord metastases with obstruction (red arrow shows obstruction). (c) Widespread metastases on bone scanning. (d) Widespread lytic bone metastases, but no spinal cord compression.

What oncological emergency needs to be excluded?

This patient has MSCC (Figure 26.3b, red arrow) secondary to widespread metastatic prostate cancer (Figure 26.3c). He also has hypercalcaemia of malignancy (HCM) with high calcium and appropriately suppressed PTH. He received rehydration, urinary catheter, pain relief, IV zoledronate, high-dose dexamethasone and radiation treatment to the spine. He was reviewed by urology for further management of the prostate cancer. Compare Figure 26.3b showing spinal metastases with spinal cord compression (red arrow) with Figure 26.3d from a patient with widespread metastatic lytic lesions due to lung cancer and HCM but no evidence of spinal cord compression.

phosphate clearance is time dependent, phosphate removal is best accomplished with continuous renal replacement therapy (CRRT) rather than intermittent haemodialysis.

Superior vena cava obstruction (SVCO)

- SVCO occurs in 3–8% of patients with cancer.
- SVCO is caused by a mediastinal mass (usually small cell lung cancer, lymphoma or metastatic breast or germ cell cancer) compressing the vessel with or without intraluminal thrombus.
- The presenting symptoms of SVCO include dyspnoea, swelling of the face and arms, and headaches. The most important clinical sign is loss of venous pulsations in the distended neck veins. This is usually accompanied by facial oedema, plethora and cyanosis.

SVCO is an oncological emergency in the presence of airway compromise, and delays whilst histological findings are confirmed may adversely affect the outcome. In such circumstances, patients are treated empirically with steroids and radiotherapy. In the acute setting, radiologically directed vascular stenting can be effective. Definitive treatment usually is chemotherapy or radiotherapy depending on tumour type.

Neutropenic sepsis

Don't wait for blood results – once neutropenic sepsis is suspected, the goal is a 'door to needle' time of 60 minutes for administration of first-dose IV antibiotics.

- Immunosuppressed state which, if undiagnosed, leads to a mortality rate approaching 20–30%.
- Severe neutropenia defined as an absolute neutrophil count (ANC) of $<0.5 \times 10^9$/l, with a temperature of $>38\,°C$ and/or septic symptoms/signs.
- The primary risk factor is type of chemotherapy.
- An infectious source is identified in a minority of cases. Most cases are bacterial (translocation of gut flora). Gram negatives, *Staphylococcal aureus* and enterococci cause severe illness.

- Undertake immediate assessment with urgent routine bloods including lactate and blood cultures (including from indwelling central lines – seek help if needed). Sign/symptom-directed work-up. If there are additional new signs of organ dysfunction, manage as severe sepsis. Get help now.
- After neutropenic sepsis is confirmed, refer to local antibiotic policy or call a microbiologist for further advice.
- Target specific infection if found. If not, continue the empiric regimen until ANC is $>0.5 \times 10^9$/l.
- Granulocyte colony-stimulating factor (G-CSF), which stimulates the marrow to produce granulocytes, is available. However, G-CSF use is generally not recommended in most patients with suspected or established neutropenic sepsis. Seek expert guidance.
- If neutropenia is excluded, an alternative management plan can be made.

Some very stable patients at low risk of septic complications may be treated in an ambulatory care setting (i.e. SDEC).

Multiple myeloma is a clonal plasma cell neoplasm that secretes monoclonal paraprotein. Subtypes of disease can be dictated by the predominant immunoglobulin (IgG is the most common) and light chain (kappa or lambda). Multiple myeloma can affect people of any age. The presentation of end-organ failure is often referred to by the mnemonic '**CRAB**'.

- **C**: Hypercalcaemia.
- **R**: Renal impairment.
- **A**: Anaemia – normocytic anaemia is a common finding in multiple myeloma due to bone marrow plasma cell infiltration and associated kidney disease. The peripheral blood smear may show rouleaux formation (appearance of erythrocytes stacked on each other).
- **B**: Bone disease (>1 lytic bone lesion of >5 mm on skeletal imaging). Can present with spinal cord compression secondary to vertebral collapse or extraosseous plasmacytoma. Oncological emergency.

Anaemia, kidney disease and bone disease (lytic lesions) leading to hypercalcaemia or spinal cord compression are classic findings requiring therapy.

Anticancer therapy complications

Gastrointestinal symptoms

These are common with chemotherapy and radiotherapy (e.g. mucositis, nausea, vomiting and diarrhoea). Do not assume that GI complaints are the result of the patient's treatment – other common causes in cancer patients should be assessed for. Treat as per standard care and refer to gastroenterology service as needed.

Steroid related

Steroids such as prednisolone, methylprednisolone and dexamethasone are commonly prescribed in oncology patients due to their useful anti-inflammatory, antiemetic and immunosuppressive effects.

- Despite their beneficial effects, steroids are the most common medication class associated with drug-induced hyperglycaemia. Consequently, healthcare providers should anticipate and be ready to treat hyperglycaemia prior to initiation of steroids. There should be a low threshold to initiate insulin in patients who have sustained hyperglycaemia.
- Other common steroid adverse drug reactions include hypokalaemia, altered mental status (e.g. paranoia and psychosis), insomnia, osteoporosis (with long-term treatment) and immunosuppression (including *Pneumocystis jirovecii* pneumonia – consider co-trimoxazole prophylaxis in prolonged high-dose steroid treatment).
- If the patient has had prolonged high doses of steroids, wean doses carefully under specialist supervision. Warn of risk of secondary adrenal insufficiency or crisis (patient should have steroid card and MedicAlert® bracelet).

Immunotherapy

The treatment paradigm for many advanced malignancies has changed with the advent of immune checkpoint inhibitors (ICIs). ICIs produce durable responses in a growing number of patients with metastatic cancer and are being used increasingly in (neo) adjuvant settings.

- ICIs are a group of monoclonal antibody therapies. Over the last 10 years, they have rapidly gained an important role in treating various types of solid cancers and haematological malignancies as both single and combination agent therapies.
- ICIs exert their effect by upregulating the immune response to malignant cells, blocking the usual inhibitory pathways of T-cell regulation (checkpoints). These agents target:
  - programmed death-1 receptor (PD-1), e.g. nivolumab, pembrolizumab
  - programmed death-ligand 1 (PD-L1), e.g. atezolizumab
  - cytotoxic T-lymphocyte-associated protein 4 (CTLA-4), e.g. ipilimumab.
- Despite their promising therapeutic effects, a predicted 60–95% of patients experience ill effects which, if left untreated, may be life-threatening.
- Various severe immune-related adverse events (irAEs) have been reported and may affect almost any organ system and have broad clinical presentations. The mechanism is due to the exaggerated immune response towards non-cancerous cells, causing significant inflammation and destruction.
- The most common irAEs are covered by the 'LEGS' acronym.
  - Liver (e.g. transaminitis)
  - Endocrinopathies (e.g. thyroiditis)
  - GI (e.g. colitis)
  - Skin (e.g. rash, vitiligo).

Other systems affected include respiratory (e.g. pneumonitis) and rheumatological.

- The spectrum of toxicities can be categorised from mild (grade 1) to death (grade 5), with severe symptoms requiring hospitalisation defined as grade 3 and above. Incidence of severe events is reported as 26% for monotherapy and increases to 55% with combination therapy. Fatal toxicities also comprise a diverse set of clinical manifestations and can occur in 0.4–1.2% of patients.
- Acute severe irAEs are managed with reasonable effectiveness by providing symptom management, withholding ICIs and administering high-dose steroids.
- Adverse effects may occur several years after *discontinuing* the therapy.
- Early recognition and management are key, with prompt referral to appropriate organ-specific specialists for ongoing management.

Osteonecrosis of the jaw (ONJ) is defined as exposed necrotic bone in the maxillofacial region, not healing after eight weeks in patients with no history of craniofacial radiation. ONJ has been described in patients receiving chronic bisphosphonate therapy but appears to be much more common in cancer patients receiving bisphosphonates in 10–12 times higher doses than those used to treat osteoporosis.

Cancer-related complications

Brain metastases

These account for the majority of all intracranial tumours. Brain metastases affect 17–25% of the cancer population.

- The most common tumour types which metastasise are lung, breast, cancer of unknown primary, melanoma and colon.
- Symptoms and signs can vary depending on the level and rate of change in intracranial pressure caused by the metastases.
- CT brain is indicated.
- Dexamethasone 8 mg twice daily IV/oral (am and lunchtime) with PPI cover if significant symptoms or mass effect. Refer to neurosurgery and acute oncology to determine best management pathway.

Cancer-related fluid collections

Pleural effusions, pericardial effusions and ascites affect the function of adjacent organs and may be relieved by drains. POCUS is especially useful for diagnosing these complications and aiding intervention. Refer to the appropriate site-specific specialist service.

Cancer-associated thromboses

Rudolf Virchow described three factors that are critically important in the development of venous thrombosis: (1) venous stasis, (2) activation of blood coagulation, and (3) vein damage. These factors are known as the Virchow triad.

Patients with cancer have an increased tendency to thrombosis for all three reasons.

1. Pressure effect, where the primary tumour mass or secondary nodal masses impinge upon the vasculature, producing venous stasis and thrombosis.
2. Procoagulant release from the tumour.
3. Damage to the venous vessel (endothelial) wall by indwelling catheters and related inflammation as well as damage from chemotherapeutic and other agents.

Once cancer has been diagnosed, venous thromboembolic events (VTE) are remarkably common and are described in about 10–20% of all patients.

Management of cancer-related thromboses

- All patients with VTE should receive anticoagulant treatment in the absence of absolute contraindications.
- In patients with acute VTE in the setting of cancer, recommend an oral factor Xa inhibitor (e.g. apixaban, edoxaban, rivaroxaban) over parenteral low molecular weight heparin (LMWH) for the initiation and treatment phases of therapy.
- Edoxaban and rivaroxaban appear to be associated with a higher risk of GI major bleeding than LMWH in patients with cancer-associated thrombosis and a luminal GI malignancy, while apixaban does not. Apixaban or LMWH may be the preferred option in patients with luminal GI malignancies.
- LMWH also has the potential advantages of bypassing the GI system in patients with nausea or mucositis and may be more easily dose-adjusted in patients with thrombocytopenia due to cancer therapy.

Neuroendocrine tumours (NETs)

These constitute a heterogeneous group of malignant solid tumours that arise in hormone-secreting tissues of the diffuse neuroendocrine system.

- NETs of the GI system were initially considered to be rare but currently constitute the second most common GI malignancy.
- All subtypes of NETs can be divided into functioning tumours, which are associated with

hormone-related symptoms, and non-functioning tumours which do not cause any clinically apparent hormone-related symptoms.

- Carcinoid syndrome – occurs in 20–30% of patients with small intestinal NETs with hepatic metastases. Production of serotonin, tachykinins and bradykinin presenting with flushing, abdominal pain, diarrhoea and specific carcinoid heart disease (right-sided).

Somatostatin analogues are currently the most effective drugs inhibiting the secretion of bioactive compounds in most functioning NETs.

> Carcinoid crisis is a life-threatening medical emergency which presents with sudden changes in blood pressure, most often hypotension, sometimes combined with prolonged and excessive flushing, hyperthermia and occasional bronchospasm. Somatostatin analogues are useful to both prevent and treat carcinoid crisis.

Other NET functioning tumours

- Other functioning NETs include hypoglycaemia caused by insulinoma.
- Cytoreductive techniques (i.e. therapy to debulk tumour) should always be considered in refractory functioning syndromes aiming at reducing tumour load and the amount of the secretory component.
- Occasionally, the substances secreted by NETs are not directly related to the tissue of origin, and the corresponding clinical syndromes are related to these *ectopically* secreted compounds. Appreciation of the presence of such paraneoplastic syndromes is highly relevant as, if the clinical presentation is not identified, it may delay diagnosis of the underlying neoplasia and lead to increased morbidity and mortality. For example:

  o hypersecretion of PTHrP by metastatic pancreatic NETs can cause HCM
  o bronchial and thymic NETs can cause Cushing syndrome with marked hyperpigmentation due to ectopic production of adrenocorticotropic hormone (ACTH).

Paraneoplastic syndromes

- Most arise due to secretion by tumours of hormones, cytokines and growth factors. This can result in diverse manifestations such as finger clubbing, acanthosis nigricans (with GI tumours) and dermatomyositis (~10–30% of adult patients have an underlying malignancy).

- Paraneoplastic syndromes also arise when normal cells secrete products in response to the presence of tumour cells. For example, antibodies produced in this fashion are responsible for many paraneoplastic neurological syndromes, including cerebellar degeneration and Lambert–Eaton myasthenic syndrome.

- The most common cancer associated with most paraneoplastic complications is small cell lung cancer, although finger clubbing is most common with squamous cell lung cancer.

- Paraneoplastic complications of cancer can present years before cancer diagnosis, and often regress with successful treatment of the cancer.

Bone metastases

> Of the 44 million people worldwide who are living with treated cancer, 30–80% will experience bone metastases. Metastatic bone disease can lead to pain, loss of function and pathological (low-energy) fractures. Metastatic bone disease is also seen in about a third of patients with cancer of unknown primary presentations and is typically lytic in nature.

- *Red flag* symptoms for cancer-related bone pain include severe progressive pain that is worse on movement or at night, inability to bear weight, signs of hypercalcaemia and pain on direct palpation.

- Metastases may not show up on radiographs until 50–70% of the bone has been destroyed, so initial radiographs may be normal.

- They typically present as an emergency with significant skeletal events such as pathological fracture, MSCC or uncontrolled pain.

- For those patients without a known history of cancer, it is imperative to arrange radiotherapy before any further investigations can be undertaken. Men over the age of 40 should have a digital rectal examination and a PSA checked. All patients with lytic bone lesions should have serum protein electrophoresis and serum light chains checked to rule out myeloma. If the patient presents with a pathological fracture and is scheduled for internal fixation, then ensure that the surgeon sends reamings to the laboratory for histological analysis.

New cancer diagnosis

- Refer to appropriate site-specific specialist cancer team.
- Cancer of unknown primary – represents a very broad spectrum of presentations where evidence of a metastatic malignancy is apparent without a primary tumour identified.
  - Accounts for 3% of adult cancers.
  - Defined as 'metastatic malignancy identified on the basis of a limited number of tests, without an obvious primary site, before comprehensive investigation'.
  - The aim is early identification of patients who would benefit from anticancer treatment and to prevent futile further investigations or treatment in a patient who is approaching the end of their life. Given these factors, early holistic needs assessment and palliative care referral are important considerations.
  - The use of blood tumour markers is not routinely recommended except in a limited number of circumstances (e.g. alpha-fetoprotein with suspected germ cell or hepatocellular tumours; PSA in men >40 with bone metatstases; and CA-125 in women with peritoneal or pelvic metastases, ascites, pleural effusions).
  - CT thorax, abdomen and pelvis (CT TAP) is the staging investigation of choice in most circumstances.
  - Refer to acute oncology advice for expert management advice and appropriate care pathway referral.

Late effects

> The acute presentation of a cancer survivor regardless of time since treatment should prompt the treating clinician to consider the potential implication of previous cancer therapy when formulating diagnoses, as all bodily systems can be impacted, and they are at risk of second primary neoplasms and cardiometabolic complications. Early recognition and treatment of these complications may reduce morbidity and mortality.

- Based on data from childhood cancer survivors in the United States, it has been estimated that nine out of 10 survivors will acquire a chronic health disorder by the age of 45, and a quarter will develop a chronic health disorder that is severe and may be life-threatening or disabling. In the UK, there are currently over 2 million cancer survivors, which is predicted to rise to over 5 million by 2040.
- In the care of cancer survivors, it is also important to be aware of other consequences of cancer therapy that may result in an acute presentation, in particular the risk of second primary neoplasms and cardiovascular disease (CVD).
- CVD is the leading non-malignant cause of death in survivors of cancer. Much of the CVD arises from direct toxicity of cancer therapy, anthracycline chemotherapy or radiotherapy, to either the heart or arteries. CVD risk factors like diabetes mellitus and the metabolic syndrome (clustering of CVD risk factors within a given individual) are also more common in cancer survivors.
- Patients who have had cranial irradiation are at risk of meningiomas or gliomas, cerebrovascular accidents and SMART ('stroke-like migraine attacks after radiation therapy') syndrome. Patients who have had radiation affecting their spleen have a non-functioning spleen and are at risk of overwhelming infection.
- As cancer therapy evolves, ongoing surveillance is required to define consequences of new therapies and follow-up required. For example, chronic irAEs with ICIs are increasingly recognised, and can affect up to 40% of patients.

Acute Medicine best practice approach to acute oncology

- The first principle is that of putting patients first (i.e. person-centred).
- People with cancer should be involved in deciding their own healthcare (i.e. shared decision making).
- Meeting the health needs of people with cancer with respect, dignity and compassion.
- Always make sure that the acute oncology team is informed of the patient's assessment and/or admission as soon as possible.
- Immediate advice is available from the acute oncology service or oncology on call.
- The patient's site-specific specialist team providing cancer treatment must be informed of any admission/assessment, as adjustments to the subsequent cycle may be required.

- Consider drug toxicity as a possible cause of the presenting problem.
  - Systemic anticancer therapy (SACT) includes cytotoxic chemotherapy, monoclonal antibodies, targeted agents, immunotherapy, and new and novel therapies.
  - SACT toxicities can cause acute deterioration but are often reversible if managed rapidly and appropriately.
  - Patients should know what treatment they are receiving and have written information about their SACT and an alert card with a 24-hour advice line telephone number.
  - Always *withhold SACT*, including oral therapy, until you have discussed with the acute oncology or site-specific team.

- If the patient is in a clinical trial, the trials team should be contacted about the admission.
- Consider the involvement of the palliative care team for symptom control advice and end-of-life care.
- Effective communication. Serious illness refers to health conditions that carry a high risk of mortality, poor function and quality of life, and strain on patients, family and caregivers. Advanced cancer is a good example. People with advanced cancer who recognise that they are nearing the end of life generally prefer care focused on quality of life and increased time spent at home. High-quality communication that improves patients' awareness of prognosis and elicits their goals and preferences can improve care quality and patient experiences.
- General medical management is critical, such as adequate pain relief, antiemetics, bowel care, mouth and skin care, IV access, adequate hydration and nutrition, clarifying DNACPR status, and VTE prophylaxis.
- Rectal examination. Due to the risk of damage to rectal mucosa, it is recommended that in patients receiving SACT, rectal examination is *not* performed. If it is deemed necessary to conduct rectal examination, this should be undertaken with caution.
- COVID-19. People with cancer are at increased risk of COVID-19 infection due to the immunosuppressed state caused by the cancer, ill health and anticancer therapy. Response to COVID-19 vaccination may also be inadequate due to the immunosuppression. Regular booster doses are indicated.

Section Three

Common presentations in Acute Medicine

27

Common presentations in Acute Medicine

Glenn Matfin and Aya Akhras

Introduction

The most common Acute Medicine presentations (prior to the COVID-19 pandemic) were listed alphabetically in Table 1.1. A general overview, differential diagnosis and basic management of these presentations will now be outlined.

Clinical reasoning

- Creating a *problem representation* related to the major presenting presentation (i.e. complaints). This is a 'one-sentence' summary (a 'tweet') that highlights the defining features of a case. Effective problem representation allows clinicians to summarise their thoughts and then *hypothesis generate* a provisional *differential diagnosis* (i.e. list of plausible explanations for a patient's presentation) using techniques such as pattern recognition, mnemonics and/or diagnostic schema.
- Clinicians store and recall knowledge as diseases, conditions or syndromes – 'illness scripts' – that are connected to problem representations. Compare and contrast *key* and *differentiating features* (such as MUST HAVE features – without it, the disease can't be diagnosed – and REJECTING features – if present, this diagnosis cannot be made) between the patient's problem representation and illness scripts related to diseases, conditions or syndromes included in the differential diagnosis.

- Once a prioritised differential diagnosis is created, it is important to *first* consider:
  - *red flags* (i.e. clinical features that may implicate serious pathology)
  - *'rule out worst-case scenarios'* (ROWS, i.e. conditions that are both common and can deteriorate rapidly and/or cause fatality).
- Then consider *most likely* and *least likely* diagnoses.
- Perform *diagnostic testing* to help confirm ('rule in') or eliminate ('rule out') various illnesses (i.e. investigative diagnostic reasoning). The decision about which potential diagnoses to investigate initially depends on probability (i.e. starting with the most likely ones), as well as on the severity and acuity of a potential diagnosis (i.e. common ROWS first).
- *Therapeutic reasoning* with *patient-centred*, *shared decision making* to define best individualised management plan.

Abdominal pain

Abdominal pain is a subjective and unpleasant sensation of pain in the abdominal region. It can be acute, subacute or chronic. Peritoneal pain localises to the area affected, whereas visceral pain tends to be felt in the upper abdomen – foregut; central abdomen – midgut; or lower abdomen – hindgut.

Abdominal pain is a common presentation to Acute Medicine. The immediate aim is to identify potentially life-threatening acute abdominal conditions that require early resuscitation, prompt investigation and early intervention. For conditions that are not life-threatening, defining timely and pertinent investigations is essential for appropriate intervention and management. It is highly important not to forget obstetric and gynaecological causes of abdominal pain in women.

Abdominal pain is diagnosed by a combination of history, physical examination, imaging and laboratory results. Characteristics of pain can be evaluated using the mnemonic SOCRATES: Site, Onset, Character, Radiation, Associated features, Time course, Exacerbating and relieving factors, and Severity of the pain. Symptoms associated with the pain are invaluable in further localising the disease process (e.g. fever, weight loss, fatigue, nausea, vomiting, anorexia, bowel alteration, menstrual history). Physical examination includes a thorough general, abdominal (inspection, auscultation, palpation, percussion) and groin, pelvic and rectal examination as indicated.

So-called 'medical' causes of abdominal pain can be diffuse (e.g. acute adrenal insufficiency, diabetic ketoacidosis, hypothyroidism, hypercalcaemia, sickle cell crisis) or localised (e.g. hepatitis, shingles). High-risk medications include non-steroidal anti-inflammatory drugs (NSAIDs), aspirin, antibiotics, steroids and immunosuppressants. The most common cause of chronic abdominal pain is functional.

Determine whether there is a possibly life-threatening cause of the abdominal pain.

- Unstable vital signs.
- Abdominal crises give rise to one or more major symptoms or signs.
  ○ Severe pain.
  ○ Collapse.
  ○ Vomiting.
  ○ Signs of peritonitis (e.g. tenderness, guarding, rebound and rigidity).
  ○ Abdominal distension (i.e. the 'five Fs': Flatus, Fluid, Faeces, Fetus and Fat. To this list should be added a sixth: massive organomegaly or 'Filthy big tumour').
  ○ Red blood per orifice.

The differential diagnosis of abdominal pain is very broad and includes the following possibilities.

- Acute and chronic pancreatitis
- Adhesions

- Appendicitis
- Cholecystitis
- Colitis
- Constipation
- COVID-19
- Diverticulitis
- Gastroenteritis
- Gastro-oesophageal reflux disease (GORD)
- Gynaecological (e.g. ectopic pregnancy, pelvic inflammatory disease, endometriosis)
- Hernia (incarcerated/strangulated)
- Inflammatory bowel disease (IBD)
- Malignancy (e.g. colon, gastric, oesophageal and pancreatic cancer)
- Peptic ulcer (including perforation)
- Renal (colic, pyelonephritis)
- Sickle cell disease
- Vascular (abdominal aortic aneurysm, mesenteric ischaemia/infarction, ischaemic colitis)

The location of the abdominal pain may help identify possible causes (examples).

- Epigastric pain – gastric ulcer/perforation, pancreatitis, perforated oesophagus and myocardial infarction.
- Right upper quadrant (RUQ) – cholecystitis, hepatitis, appendicitis with high appendix (especially pregnant women), perforating duodenal ulcer, renal calculi, pyelonephritis.
- Left upper quadrant (LUQ) – pancreatitis, perforating gastric ulcer, splenic rupture or infarct, renal calculi, pyelonephritis.
- Left lower quadrant (LLQ) – diverticulitis, pelvic peritonitis, pericolitis (inflammation of tissues around the colon), renal calculi, sigmoid volvulus (typically older patients), incarcerated/strangulated hernia.
- Right lower quadrant (RLQ) – appendicitis, inflamed ileocecum (IBD), diverticulitis, inflamed Meckel diverticulum, renal calculi, incarcerated/strangulated hernia.
- Acute central abdominal pain – appendicitis (may radiate to the RLQ), acute mesenteric ischaemia, leaking or ruptured abdominal aortic aneurysm, small bowel obstruction.

Rule out worst-case scenarios (examples): abdominal aortic aneurysm, acute mesenteric ischaemia/infarction, acute pancreatitis, pancreatic cancer, perforated viscus, ruptured ectopic pregnancy.

Initial investigations include a routine battery of tests that would differentiate between gastrointestinal, biliary, pancreatic, renal and/or inflammatory causes of abdominal pain. These would include the following.

- Full blood count (FBC) and differential.
- Liver function tests (LFT) – aminotransferases, alkaline phosphatase, bilirubin (hepatobiliary).
- Lipase and amylase (pancreatitis).
- Urea and electrolytes (U&E), creatinine, blood glucose (BG), thyroid function tests (TFT), calcium (Ca), coagulation profile, arterial blood gas (ABG) or venous blood gas (VBG), lactate level (ischaemic bowel, sepsis).
- Inflammatory markers – C-reactive protein (CRP).
- Cultures – blood, stool, urine: if evidence or suspicion of infection. *Clostridioides difficile* (C-diff) multistep testing. COVID-19 testing.
- All women of childbearing age should have a pregnancy test.
- Urinalysis.
- Electrocardiogram (ECG).
- Other tests as per clinical context (e.g. immunosuppression, recent travel).
- Endoscopy – can be:
  - diagnostic, e.g. oesophago-gastro-duodenoscopy (OGD), sigmoidoscopy, colonoscopy. Can also facilitate biopsy. Special types of endoscopies (e.g. capsular endoscopy – good for small bowel aetiology)
  - therapeutic.
- Basic abdominal imaging (Table 27.1). Chest X-ray (e.g. free gas from perforation, pneumonia).

Initial management includes the following aspects.

- First consider *red flag* features and acute life-threatening causes (i.e. ROWS), Airway, Breathing, Circulation, Disability, Exposure (ABCDE), optimise physiology and supportive care. Monitor vital signs and obtain large-bore intravenous (IV) access. Hypovolaemia should be corrected with fluids and/or blood products as clinically indicated. Your patient may need to proceed to theatre or endoscopy while investigation results are awaited. Close liaison between the medical team, emergency surgeons and critical care is essential.
- Analgesia and antiemetic. Keep nil by mouth (NBM) until patient stability and management plan are clarified. Consider nasogastric (NG) tube (e.g. small bowel obstruction, acute pancreatitis).
- Identify and treat potential causes.
- Treat sepsis as per Sepsis Six care bundle. Prophylactic antibiotics are recommended for

Table 27.1 Basic abdominal imaging

Imaging method	Name
X-ray	Acute abdomen series: erect and supine (bowel gas pattern; fluid levels; pneumoperitoneum – gas under the diaphragm). Vascular calcification (mesenteric ischaemia) and calcified calculi (e.g. gallstones, renal).
	Examples: perforation, small and large bowel obstruction, volvulus, constipation, mesenteric ischaemia/infarction.
Ultrasound scan (USS)	Abdominal USS (e.g. aortic aneurysm, diverticular mass).
	RUQ USS (e.g. cholecystitis, biliary colic).
	Pelvic USS (e.g. ectopic pregnancy, ovarian torsion – with reduced/absent blood flow on colour Doppler).
	Renal USS (e.g. hydronephrosis, renal calculi).
Computed tomography (CT) scan	CT abdomen/pelvis; CT kidney, ureter, bladder (KUB).
	Examples: appendicitis, diverticulitis, abscess, cancer.
Magnetic resonance imaging (MRI)	MRI (abdomen), MR cholangiopancreatography (MRCP).
Others	Angiograms (e.g. mesenteric ischaemia); Positron emission tomography (PET) scan; nuclear scanning.

patients with a perforated viscus, diverticulitis, appendicitis, mesenteric ischaemia or ruptured abdominal aortic aneurysm. These patients can rapidly develop sepsis.
- Withdrawal of precipitating agents. Medication review and deprescribing is important (e.g. gastritis, hepatitis and pancreatitis where drugs are commonly implicated).
- Management of associated complications (e.g. perforation, peritonitis, jaundice, sepsis).
- If ectopic pregnancy is suspected, send blood for blood typing and cross-matching, and obtain an urgent gynaecological consultation. Urgent gynaecology consultation is also important for ovarian torsion as the longer an ovary is torsed, the less likely that it can be salvaged.

Small bowel obstruction (SBO)

Features	Illness script for small bowel obstruction
Epidemiological risk factors	• Can occur at any age. History of previous pelvic or abdominal operations. Most common cause is intra-abdominal adhesions. Also occurs with cancer, Crohn's disease and hernias.
Pathophysiology	• Obstruction due to adhesions from previous surgery or trapped bowel loops/masses causes hyperperistalsis of proximal segments. • Most feared complication is ischaemic or perforated bowel, which presents with signs of peritonitis.
Time course	• Acute, usually progressive unless intervention.
Key symptoms and signs	• Acute onset of colicky abdominal pain, nausea, vomiting (can progress to faeculant vomiting) and obstipation (severe form of constipation where patient cannot pass stool or gas). • Physical examination: diffuse abdominal distension, hyperactive bowel sounds, signs of peritonitis (late sign, surgical emergency).
Diagnostics	• Investigations: FBC with differential, CRP, ABG/VBG, lactate, U&E, creatinine. Blood cultures. • Imaging: abdominal X-ray: dilated (>3 cm) air-filled small bowel loops with air–fluid levels. Abdominal CT – better at differentiating SBO from postoperative ileus.
Treatment	• Uncomplicated SBO – NBM, NG tube decompression, IV fluids, analgesia, antiemetic, electrolyte repletion and antibiotics. Urinary catheter. • Complicated SBO (signs of peritonitis) – Sepsis Six care bundle, emergency exploratory laparotomy.

Diverticulitis

Features	Illness script for diverticulitis
Epidemiological risk factors	• Increasing age (>40 years of age). By the age of 80, ~70% of Western adults have colonic diverticulosis (presence of diverticula). Low-fibre diet, constipation. • Patients who are immunosuppressed have an increased risk of acute and complicated diverticulitis.
Pathophysiology	• Diverticula form when mucosa and submucosa herniate through the muscularis propria layer of the colon wall. • Most common complication of diverticulosis (15% of patients). Infection may be secondary to an impacted faecolith. Micro/macroscopic perforation of the diverticulum, leading to colonic and surrounding tissue inflammation with possible abscess formation. Can also create strictures and fistulas.
Time course	• Acute/subacute/chronic. Recurrent episodes common.
Key symptoms and signs	• LLQ pain, systemic features (fever, increased CRP and leucocytosis), may have peritonism. Typical presentation is like 'left-sided appendicitis'. Patients may develop constipation or obstruction secondary to localised swelling.
Diagnostics	• Investigations: FBC with differential, CRP, U&E, creatinine. Blood cultures. • Imaging: CT abdomen with both oral and IV contrast.

Treatment	• Uncomplicated (non-perforated) diverticulitis:
	  ○ without systemic features: outpatient treatment usually with broad-spectrum oral antibiotics and clear liquid diet.
	  ○ with systemic features: admit and begin bowel rest, analgesics, fluid resuscitation, broad-spectrum antibiotics.
	• Complicated diverticulitis – if signs of abscess or perforation present (may have peritonitis).
	  ○ Surgery and drainage of abscess. Sepsis Six care bundle. Supportive management.

Features	Illness script for diverticulitis
	• Follow-up colonoscopy is indicated (6–8 weeks later): to rule out underlying malignancy (present in ~1–8%). • Follow-up counselling: healthy diet (high-fibre), smoking cessation and probability of recurrent diverticulitis.

Biliary causes of abdominal pain

There is a time-honoured mnemonic that patients with upper abdominal pain and who conform to a profile of 'fair (i.e. white), fat, female, fertile and forty' are likely to have cholelithiasis. However, gallstones are more common in other ethnicities (e.g. in the US, prevalence as high as 60–70% in American Indians). Additionally, as adolescents and young adults become more overweight/obese following the general population trend, the age of 'forty' could easily be 'fourteen'! Family history should be added to the mnemonic.

Most gallstones are asymptomatic. However, they can cause abdominal pain in a variety of conditions.

- Choledocholithiasis – stone in the common bile duct (CBD) causes cholestatic jaundice.
- Ascending cholangitis – infection in biliary tree occurs upstream from CBD blockage (e.g. secondary to gallstone, tumour, parasite). Charcot triad – RUQ abdominal pain, fever, jaundice. Urgent biliary drainage and decompression via endoscopic retrograde cholangiopancreatography (ERCP).
- Biliary colic – gallstone obstructs the cystic duct, causing gallbladder distension. The pain typically builds to a crescendo following a (fatty) meal and then subsides. It does not cause jaundice or deranged LFTs. RUQ USS may demonstrate gallstones.
- Acute and chronic cholecystitis occurs when the gallbladder is inflamed (usually secondary to gallstones).

Features	Illness script for cholecystitis
Epidemiological risk factors	• Risk factors: age, female, pregnancy, obesity (plus weight loss, including around a third of patients developing gallstones in the first six months after bariatric surgery), and conditions/medications leading to gallbladder stasis. • Acalculous cholecystitis (inflammation of the gallbladder in absence of gallstones) can occur in hospitalised and critically ill patients.
Pathophysiology	• Most common complication of gallstone disease. • Stone impacted in cystic duct leading to gallbladder inflammation and infection. • Acalculous cholecystitis: gallbladder stasis and ischaemia.
Time course	• Acute; chronic with acute exacerbations.
Key symptoms and signs	• Cholecystitis presents as a constant pain in RUQ: pain may radiate to the right shoulder or scapula. Associated with fever, nausea and vomiting. May have past medical history of biliary colic or gallstones. • Physical examination: tenderness in RUQ. Positive Murphy's sign – pain/tenderness sufficient to cause an abrupt halt in inspiration (normally occurs toward the end of inspiration) with RUQ palpation.
Diagnostics	• Investigations: FBC with differential, CRP, U&E, LFTs, coagulation studies, amylase and lipase. Blood cultures. • Imaging: RUQ USS.
Treatment	• Initial management: NBM, IV hydration, correction of electrolyte abnormalities, analgesia, antiemetics and IV antibiotics. Acalculous cholecystitis may need percutaneous cholecystostomy. • Definitive management: cholecystectomy.

Acute pancreatitis

Acute pancreatitis is an acute inflammatory process of the pancreas.

Features	Illness script for acute pancreatitis
Epidemiological risk factors	• Most common causes are gallstones (40%) and alcohol (30%). Can be due to many causes – mnemonic I GET SMASHED (the first four causes are the most common): **I:** idiopathic **G:** gallstones, genetic – cystic fibrosis **E:** ethanol (alcohol) **T:** trauma **S:** steroids **M:** mumps (and other infections), malignancy **A:** autoimmune (e.g. IgG4-related disease) **S:** scorpion stings/spider bites **H:** hypertriglyceridaemia (200-fold risk with concentrations above 20 mmol/l) **E:** ERCP **D:** drugs (<5% of cases), diabetes
Pathophysiology	• Autodigestion of the pancreas secondary to inappropriate activation of pancreatic enzymes.
Time course	• Acute, recurrent attacks, can progress to chronic pancreatitis.
Key symptoms and signs	• Acute-onset epigastric pain radiating to back, associated with nausea, vomiting and anorexia. History of cholelithiasis/alcohol abuse. • Physical examination: ecchymotic discolouration may be observed in the periumbilical region (Cullen sign) or along the flank (Grey Turner sign) related to retroperitoneal bleeding in the setting of pancreatic necrosis.

Diagnostics	• Investigations: FBC with differential, CRP, BG, LFT, amylase and lipase, gamma-glutamyl transferase (GGT), lactate dehydrogenase (LDH), U&E, creatinine, Ca (can decrease due to saponification within peritoneal cavity), ABG/VBG, non-fasting triglyceride levels. Blood cultures.
	• Imaging: abdominal USS, CT scan.
	• Diagnostic criteria for acute pancreatitis.
	  1 Epigastric pain radiating to the back.
	  2 Laboratory findings (amylase >3× ULN or lipase elevation).
	  3 Consistent imaging findings on USS, CT or MRI.
	• Risk stratification – Ranson criteria.
	  o Measured at admission and 48 hours after, to predict severity of acute pancreatitis.
	  o If >3 criteria fulfilled (especially those associated with haemoconcentration, such as urea level), this means severe pancreatitis and admit to critical care.

Treatment	Conservative management. • NBM, IV fluids, analgesia and antiemetics. • Once pain has subsided, begin oral or enteral feeding via NG tube with low-fat diet. • Secondary causes should be addressed, and precipitating drugs should be stopped. • Monitor BG levels regularly (i.e. 4–6 hourly) in all patients with acute pancreatitis because of transient or permanent beta-cell failure/destruction. • If patients do not improve within 5–7 days of conservative management, obtain CT with contrast to look for underlying complications (necrotising pancreatitis).

Features	Illness script for acute pancreatitis
	Gallstone pancreatitis – same as above, plus the following. • If gallstone pancreatitis (+/- cholangitis) – urgent ERCP and sphincterotomy within 24 h. • If mild gallstone pancreatitis – early cholecystectomy. • If severe gallstone pancreatitis – late cholecystectomy. Complications. • Patients can develop pancreatic fluid collections including acute pancreatic fluid collections, pancreatic pseudocysts, acute necrotic collections, and walled-off necrosis. Infected abscess. • Fever, abdominal pain and leucocytosis 10–14 days after episode. • Obtain a CT scan of abdomen with contrast. Abscess will appear as non-enhancing area. Treat with empirical antibiotics and occasionally surgical debridement. Pancreatic pseudocyst. • Presents four weeks after episode with abdominal pain, palpable mass and persistently elevated amylase. Obtain CT scan of abdomen. If symptomatic or complications, draining required.

ULN, upper limit of normal.

Intestinal ischaemia

> *Examples of abdominal pain aggravated by eating*
>
> • Gastritis
> • Gastro-oesophageal reflux disease
> • Peptic ulcer (gastric)
> • Gastric cancer
> • Acute and chronic pancreatitis
> • Gallstones (especially fatty meals)
> • Irritable bowel disease
> • Chronic mesenteric ischaemia

Atherosclerotic stenoses of the coeliac (collateral to bowel), superior mesenteric (small bowel and colon) and inferior mesenteric arteries (colon) can occur. However, extensive collateral vessels form between the territories of these major arteries, such that compensatory blood supply is achieved in the setting of single-vessel stenosis. Most cases of symptomatic chronic mesenteric ischaemia therefore occur in the setting of several mesenteric arteries being affected. Mesenteric blood flow normally increases from 10–25% of total cardiac output to 35% or more after a meal. In the absence of sufficient perfusion, ischaemia ensues with anaerobic glycolysis and lactate production by intestinal enterocytes. Classic symptoms are postprandial pain and nausea (i.e. 'intestinal angina') with subsequent anorexia, avoidance of meals and weight loss.

The goals of treatment of chronic mesenteric ischaemia are as follows.

• Symptom relief.
 o Weight restoration (i.e. nutritional support).
 o Prevention of progression to acute mesenteric ischaemia and intestinal infarction (Figure 27.1).
• The treatment of chronic mesenteric ischemia centres around revascularisation (i.e. endovascular or surgical).
• Lifestyle modifications, such as eating small frequent meals and smoking cessation, are only adjuncts.
• Medical therapy, such as antiplatelet agents, statins, blood pressure (BP) control and other cardiovascular disease (CVD) risk factor modifications, is important (also addresses other CVD complications in other cardiovascular beds, i.e. 'polyvascular disease').

(a)

(b)

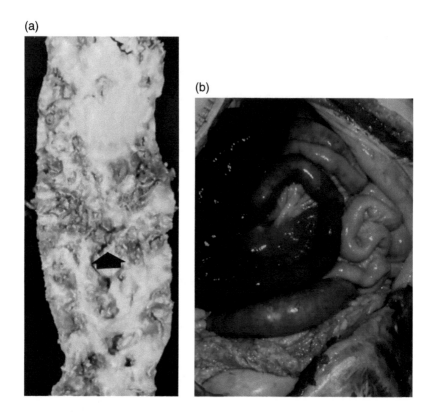

Figure 27.1 (a) Severe aortic atherosclerosis with fissured plaque occluding superior mesenteric artery (arrow). (b) Abdominal organs at autopsy showing well-demarcated loops of infarcted small intestine and associated mesentery.

Ischaemic colitis presents with acute colicky abdominal pain, diarrhoea and haematochezia (bright red rectal bleeding). Examination reveals lower abdominal tenderness. An abdominal CT scan is the initial test to perform if ischaemic colitis is suspected. Colonoscopy is usually performed subsequently to confirm the diagnosis. Urgent management is required because of the risk of perforation. Peritoneal signs and absent bowel sounds suggest perforation or transmural infarction, necessitating urgent laparotomy.

Peptic ulcer disease

The word 'peptic' means that the problem is due to acid. Duodenal ulcers are more common than gastric ulcers.

Features	Illness script for peptic ulcer
Epidemiological risk factors	• Age. Common in both males and females. Long-term NSAID use, steroids and aspirin. Smoking, alcohol consumption.
Pathophysiology	• *Helicobacter pylori* (*H. pylori*) is the most common cause of peptic ulcer. *H. pylori* infection increases acid and decreases protective mucus. Also causes chronic inflammation.
	• NSAIDs inhibit cyclo-oxygenase (COX) which leads to decreased prostaglandin E2, resulting in less protective mucus cover and mucosal erosion and ulcer formation.

Features	Illness script for peptic ulcer
Time course	• Acute, recurrent, or chronic.
Key symptoms and signs	• Dyspepsia, epigastric pain, relief with antacids, proton pump inhibitors (PPI) or histamine type-2 (H2) receptor blockers. • Bleeding presenting with symptoms of anaemia, haematemesis, coffee ground vomitus, melaena or fresh blood per rectum. • Physical examination: tenderness to palpation in epigastrium.
Diagnostics	• Without alarm features: urea breath test for *H. pylori* (test and treat approach). • With alarm features: OGD with biopsy and rapid urease (CLO) test for *H. pylori*.
Treatment	• *H. pylori* positive: eradication therapy. • *H. pylori* negative: PPI 4–8 weeks and follow-up. • Stop NSAID or other precipitating factors if possible. • Surgery (refractory disease).

CLO, *Campylobacter*-like organism.

Upper gastrointestinal (GI) symptoms with alarm features

• New onset >55 years old.
• Progressive dysphagia (difficulty with the act of swallowing solids and/or liquids). Must be distinguished from odynophagia (pain on swallowing) and globus sensation (sensation of a lump in the throat between meals).
• Recurrent vomiting or early satiety.
• Abdominal distension.
• Upper GI bleed or iron deficiency anaemia.
• Weight loss.
• Family history of GI malignancy.

Renal colic

Kidney stones are a common diagnosis, affecting approximately 1 in 11 people at least once in their lifetime.

The term 'renal colic' is widely used to describe the pain resulting from the passage of kidney stones through the urinary tract. This 'colicky' renal pain is among the most common symptoms leading to emergency care presentation, and often prompts extensive differential diagnosis and work-up.

Features	Illness script for renal calculi
Epidemiological risk factors	• Increasing age, male:female ratio of about 2:1. Positive family history. • Low fluid intake, dehydration. Changing dietary practices (including calcium supplementation), migration from cooler rural settings to warmer urban settings, and even global warming. • Obesity, hypertension and diabetes (metabolic syndrome) recognised as important risk factors. • Postcolectomy and/or postileostomy (oxalate stones). • Calcium phosphate stones should lead to consideration of primary hyperparathyroidism.
Pathophysiology	• The most common crystal composition of kidney stones is calcium oxalate. About 20% of calcium stones are predominantly calcium phosphate. Although calcium stones are occasionally secondary to a systemic disease, on most occasions they are idiopathic. • The most common urinary risk factor for calcium stones remains hypercalciuria. In most cases, the aetiology of hypercalciuria remains unexplained and is usually termed *idiopathic hypercalciuria*. • Uric acid stones occur as the result of low urine pH. Uric acid stones are associated with the metabolic syndrome, obesity and diabetes, all of which lead to impaired ammoniagenesis and acid urine. • Struvite stones are composed of 'triple phosphate' crystals made of calcium ammonium magnesium phosphate. They occur exclusively in the presence of very high urine pH (≥ 7.5) as the result of urease-producing organisms, particularly species of *Proteus*.

(*Continued*)

Features	Illness script for renal calculi
Time course	• Acute. Can be recurrent.
Key symptoms and signs	• Sudden-onset colicky flank pain that may radiate to the groin, testes or labia. Associated symptoms: nausea, vomiting, dysuria, frequency and urgency (+/- haematuria). • Physical examination: flank tenderness.
Diagnostics	• Investigations should include a urinalysis, FBC, CRP, U&E, creatinine, LFT, Ca, phosphate. The most important use of the urinalysis is to rule out urinary tract infection. Stone can be sent for biochemical analysis. • Unenhanced, non-contrast CT KUB (kidney, ureter, bladder) is the gold standard imaging modality for the initial evaluation of kidney stones. USS in pregnant women.
Treatment	• Acute management of renal colic consists of pain management, antiemetics and IV fluids. Antibiotics if suspected infection. • Medical expulsive therapy with alpha-blockers (tamsulosin) or calcium channel blockers (nifedipine) for stones 5–10 mm. • For larger stones (>1 cm) or with evidence of obstruction or sepsis, consult urology. • Kidney stone prevention is relatively inexpensive, cost-effective and infrequently practised.

An acute abdomen can occur *without* pain in older people, the immunocompromised and in the last trimester of pregnancy, and often presents atypically. A lower threshold for admission to hospital and cross-sectional imaging is required.

Older people.

• Co-morbid conditions or medications may affect an older patient's ability to mount a characteristic physiological response.
• Higher risk due to decreased immune function.
• Communication problems and decreased peripheral nervous system function can alter perception of pain, making diagnosis and management more difficult.

Pregnant women.

• The enlargement of the uterus, which displaces and compresses intra-abdominal organs, and the laxity of the abdominal wall make it difficult to localise pain and can blunt peritoneal signs.
• Pregnant women may have a mild physiological leucocytosis, so this finding is non-specific in pregnant women presenting with an acute abdomen.

Immunocompromised patients.

• Immunocompromised patients mount an altered inflammatory response and may display atypical features. Abdominal pain is usually non-specific, and physical examination is often inconclusive.
• Immunocompromised patients are susceptible to opportunistic infections, e.g. cytomegalovirus colitis with advanced human immunodeficiency virus (HIV).
• An acute abdomen may occur because of immunosuppressive therapy. Typhlitis (neutropenic enterocolitis) is a complication of chemotherapy that typically presents with fever, neutropenia and right iliac fossa pain 10–14 days after initiation of chemotherapy.

Acute back pain

Acute back pain is often defined as lasting less than four weeks. Subacute back pain lasts 4–12 weeks. Chronic back pain lasts more than 12 weeks.

In 90% of cases of acute back pain, no cause is found (usually labelled 'mechanical'). Lumbar disc herniation is the most common cause of radicular pain (sciatica – pain or numbness that is usually referred below the knee – in contrast to non-radicular pain referred to the upper posterior thigh). Beware of *red flag* features especially bilateral sciatica, saddle anaesthesia, urinary or faecal incontinence, and are-flexia which indicate central cord compression.

The differential diagnosis of acute back pain is broad and includes the following.

- Aortic aneurysm.
- Cauda equina syndrome (compression of nerve roots at base of spine usually caused by central disc prolapse at the L4/5 or L5/S1 level).
- Degenerative disc disease (degenerated disc that protrudes and presses on the spinal cord or nerve roots causing significant pain, weakness, numbness and loss of movement).
- Infection: spinal osteomyelitis, spinal epidural abscess, discitis (infection in the intervertebral disc space), vertebral tuberculosis (TB, known as Pott's spine).
- Inflammatory arthritis (spondyloarthritides) such as ankylosing spondylitis and psoriatic arthritis (pain with stiffness worse in morning and gets better as day goes by).
- Lumbar spinal stenosis (associated with neurogenic claudication).
- Malignancy: metastatic carcinoma (e.g. breast, lung, prostate), multiple myeloma.
- Mechanical: muscular strain or tear.
- Sickle cell crisis.
- Vertebral compression fracture (usually osteoporotic but could be malignancy).

ROWS (examples): cauda equina syndrome (cord compression), compression fracture, ruptured aortic aneurysm, sickle cell crisis.

Initial investigations include the following.

- FBC, blood film, CRP, Ca, phosphate, alkaline phosphatase and infectious screen as needed. Other tests as needed (e.g. myeloma screen, osteoporosis investigations, TB).
- Spinal imaging.
  - MRI of spine and specialist consultation are warranted if there is a history of trauma, cancer, presence of *red flag* features, signs of cauda equina syndrome or progressive neurological deficits.
  - If suspicion of osteoporotic fracture or 'mechanical' pain, plain spinal X-ray is the initial choice of investigation.

Initial management includes the following.

- First, consider *red flag* features and acute life-threatening causes (i.e. ROWS), ABCDE and supportive care (analgesia). Neurosurgical consultation if signs of cord compression present.
- Identify and treat potential causes.

- Management of associated complications (e.g. hypercalcaemia with myeloma or bone metastases, osteoporosis).
- If serious causes are ruled out (negative neurological exam, no signs of compression or focal tenderness) and suggestive of muscular strain, no imaging is indicated (although it is often performed). Management is primarily composed of NSAIDs, analgesia and physiotherapy with encouragement of activity as tolerated.

Red flag features for acute back pain
- History or high risk of malignancy/infection
  - Fever.
  - Unexplained weight loss.
  - Pain at night.
- Symptoms/signs of cauda equina syndrome.
  - Any alteration in the sensation of a full bladder, desire to pass urine, or awareness of passing urine.
  - Urinary retention.
  - Neurological symptoms: progressive bilateral numbness or weakness localising to a single nerve root (e.g. L5, S1), areflexia.
  - Saddle anaesthesia: numbness or pins and needles around the anus ('numb bum') or genitals, reduced anal tone.
- Fractures.
  - Trauma.
  - Immunosuppression (e.g. chronic steroid use).
  - Osteoporosis.

Cauda equina syndrome (CES)
- The spinal cord ends at L1/2 level, so the nerve roots from lumbar and sacral segments of the spinal cord have to travel a relatively long distance before exiting the spinal canal, forming a structure that looks like a horse's tail, called the *cauda equina*.
- The nerve fibres in the cauda equina supply saddle, bladder and rectal sensation; sensation and motor control of the external urethral and anal sphincters; and fine-calibre parasympathetic fibres of the pelvic viscera.
- CES is a rare condition in which the lumbosacral nerve roots that extend below the spinal cord itself are compressed within the lumbosacral spinal canal. Usually, the cause is a central disc prolapse at the L4/5 or L5/S1 level.
- CES is diagnosed when both of the following are present.

o Clinical features of CES (e.g. acute or chronic low back pain: disturbance of urinary function, disturbance of saddle sensation, reduced anal tone, and possibly bilateral sciatica).

o Evidence of compression of the cauda equina on MRI.

- If a patient who is developing CES but is *not yet* incontinent undergoes surgery, there is a reasonable chance of avoiding the potentially catastrophic consequences of urinary incontinence, faecal incontinence, loss of sexual function, saddle anaesthesia, neuropathic pain and sometimes paralysis of the legs. It is critical to diagnose CES before the patient becomes incontinent.
- CES is a *neurosurgical emergency* and patients undergo surgical decompression.

Acute confusion/delirium

The National Early Warning Score 2 (NEWS2) adds 3 points for new confusion or delirium. Alert, Confusion, responsive to Voice, Pain, or Unresponsive (ACVPU) tool: 'New onset of confusion' or 'V' or 'P' = Delirium. Use 4AT tool (or similar) to confirm (Figure 13.2).

Delirium very common. On average: >150 people in 1000-bed hospital; 20% in Acute Medicine patients; 25–60% hip fracture patients; 40–60% intensive care unit; ~50% palliative care settings.

Confusion is clouding of consciousness characterised by an impaired capacity to think, understand and respond to and remember stimuli. Delirium is a more profound state of confusion associated with an acute onset and fluctuating course and tends to worsen at night. Delirium may be hyperactive or, more dangerously, hypoactive which can be overlooked. Other symptoms include impaired memory, disorientation to time and place, disordered thought, hallucinations and mood swings with agitation. Dementia is a risk factor for confusion and delirium and is defined as an acquired disease with *persistent* loss in many cognitive domains, which is severe enough to interfere with everyday functioning.

The differential diagnosis of delirium is broad and includes the following.

- Acute metabolic: electrolyte disturbances, acid–base disturbances, hypo/hyperglycaemia, hypercalcaemia.
- Acute vascular: shock, hypertensive encephalopathy.
- Central nervous system (CNS) pathology: stroke, tumour, seizures or postictal state, haemorrhage or infection.

- Hypoxia: anaemia, cardiac/pulmonary failure, hypotension.
- Infection: sepsis, encephalitis.
- Medications: steroids, anticholinergics, psychotropics, opiates.
- Traumatic brain injury.
- Vitamin deficiency: thiamine deficiency (Wernicke syndrome).
- Withdrawal: alcohol, benzodiazepines, sedative-hypnotics.

ROWS (examples): hypoxia, seizure, sepsis, shock, withdrawal.

Initial investigations include FBC and film (consider B12 level if deficiency suspected), CRP, BG, U&E, creatinine, Ca, phosphate, LFT, TFT, ABG, blood cultures. Toxicology screen. ECG. Urinalysis and culture. Imaging: chest X-ray. Head CT not routine but consider in new focal neurology, reduced Glasgow Coma Scale (GCS), history of recent fall(s), head injury, anticoagulants. Electroencephalogram (EEG): if seizures, including if non-convulsive status suspected. Lumbar puncture (LP): not routinely performed, only if relevant CNS cause suspected.

Initial management includes the following aspects.

- First, consider *red flag* features and acute life-threatening causes (i.e. ROWS), ABCDE, optimise physiology and supportive care. Always check BG.
- Identify and treat potential causes (e.g. Sepsis Six care bundle if bacterial infection likely, antivirals if herpes encephalitis suspected).
- Withdrawal of precipitating agents (including medication review and deprescribing).
- Management of associated complications.
- Detect and treat agitation and distress.
- Pharmacology – routine treatment for delirium *not* recommended.

Delirium is discussed fully in Chapter 13.

Acute kidney injury (AKI) and chronic kidney disease (CKD)

Acute kidney injury (AKI) can be differentiated from chronic kidney disease (CKD) based on the following factors.

- Previous U&E, creatinine and estimated glomerular filtration rate (eGFR) results.
- Evidence of CKD-mineral and bone disorders (especially increased parathyroid hormone [PTH]).

- Bilateral small kidneys on ultrasound scan.
- Gradual onset of oedema over weeks to months.

Treat as AKI, at least initially if none of these features are present or other clear evidence. If *de novo* presentation, perform full diagnostic work-up.

Acute kidney injury

AKI is a very common condition that can occur in up to 35% of acute medical admissions.

Acute kidney injury, previously known as acute renal failure, encompasses a wide spectrum of injury to the kidneys. The definition of AKI is constantly evolving but usually involves sudden and temporary loss of kidney function resulting in the retention of urea and other waste products. Presenting symptoms are secondary to renal functional decline, including decreased urine output or anuria (if severe), oedema and hypertension. Further evaluations reveal elevated urea, potassium and hyponatraemia (if fluid overloaded). The diagnosis of AKI currently focuses on monitoring serum creatinine levels and derived eGFR, with or without urine output (e.g. RIFLE criteria).

The majority of causes of AKI are secondary to sepsis and hypotension. AKI occurs most commonly in at-risk patients, who either are acutely ill or have had major surgery. Most patients with AKI will be managed (at least initially) by a non-renal specialist. AKI should be regarded as a spectrum of injury that may progress to organ failure and the need for renal replacement therapy (RRT), with associated increased mortality. AKI tends to be underdiagnosed and underreported, yet is associated with recurrent AKI hospitalisation (~30% within one year) and increased mortality rate. AKI is now recognised as a major risk factor for the development of CKD.

Differential diagnoses of AKI can be narrowed down based on the site of kidney injury (i.e. diagnostic schema based on pre-renal, renal and postrenal causes).

Pre-renal AKI – decreased renal perfusion.

- Hypovolaemia – e.g. cardiorenal syndrome, hepatorenal syndrome, diuretics, vomiting/diarrhoea.
- Hypotension.

- Oedematous states (decreased effective circulating volume).
- Renal ischaemia – e.g. NSAID, angiotensin converting enzyme (ACE) inhibitors/angiotensin receptor blockers (ARBs) use.
- Sepsis.

Renal AKI (most common) – damaged tubules, interstitium, glomeruli or blood vessels.

- Acute tubular necrosis (ATN) – e.g. iodinated contrast agents, nephrotoxins (e.g. NSAID), rhabdomyolysis.
- Acute interstitial nephritis.
- Atheroemboli.
- Glomerulonephritis (e.g. proteinuria due to podocyte damage; haematuria due to inflammation, reactive cell proliferation and breaks in glomerular basement membrane).
- Vasculitis.

Postrenal AKI (least common) – obstruction of urinary outflow tracts.

- Obstructive nephropathy – e.g. prostate hypertrophy, tumours, renal calculi.

ROWS (examples): ATN, cardiorenal syndrome, hepatorenal syndrome, postrenal obstruction.

Initial investigations include FBC – if platelets low, request blood film/LDH (to diagnose haemolytic uraemic syndrome/thrombotic thrombocytopenic purpura), CRP, BG (diabetes mellitus), U&E, creatinine, eGFR, bicarbonate, Ca, phosphate, LFT (diagnose hepatorenal syndrome), ABG/VBG, creatine kinase (CK, rhabdomyolysis), coagulation studies, autoantibodies (including antiglomerular basement membrane antibodies), complement levels, antineutrophil cytoplasmic antibody (ANCA)-associated vasculitis, other vasculitides screen, myeloma screen, COVID-19, and blood cultures if sepsis suspected. ECG (hyperkalaemia).

Urinalysis – if blood, protein, leucocytes or nitrites, send midstream urine. Urine microscopy (casts, red blood cells) and spot urine albumin/creatinine ratio (ACR) or protein/creatinine ratio. Consider measuring fractional excretion of sodium to differentiate prerenal and renal causes of AKI. KUB USS (e.g. bilateral small kidneys consistent with CKD, hydronephrosis, and postvoid bladder volume). Consider renal biopsy.

Initial management includes the following.

- First, consider *red flag* features and acute lifethreatening causes (i.e. ROWS), ABCDE, optimise physiology and supportive care (consider urinary catheterisation, strict input/output monitoring).
- Identify and treat potential causes.
- Treat sepsis as per Sepsis Six care bundle.

- Withdrawal of precipitating agents – it is critical to discontinue/hold/review any nephrotoxic drugs, such as gentamicin, ACE inhibitors, ARBs, mineralocorticoid antagonists, diuretics and NSAIDs for patients presenting with AKI or CKD/endstage renal disease (ESRD). Be careful with radiocontrast agents.
- Fluid resuscitation and hold BP medications.
- Management of associated complications, e.g. fluid overload (loop diuretics when eGFR <30 ml/min), hyperkalaemia (all hospitalised patients with a serum K$^+$ level ≥6.0 mmol/l should have an urgent 12-lead ECG performed and be assessed for changes of hyperkalaemia). Acute management of hyperkalaemia – ABCDE *plus*:
  - protect the heart (e.g. calcium gluconate)
  - shift K$^+$ into cells (e.g. glucose/insulin infusion; nebulised beta-2 agonist)
  - remove K$^+$ from body: oral potassium binders can be considered as a therapy option if K$^+$ level ≥6.5 mmol/l or remains raised but their use must be initiated by the renal team. Sodium zirconium 10 g three times a day for up to 72 hours should be first line (onset of action approximately one hour). If unsuitable, consider alternatives (e.g. patiromer 8.4 g once daily though longer onset of action, 4–7 hours). Dialysis option for severe hyperkalaemia (or when other indications for dialysis present)
  - monitor K$^+$ levels
  - prevent recurrence (e.g. review medications).
- Monitor electrolytes and kidney function.
- Evaluate for multisystem disease (e.g. rash, joint disease, haemoptysis).
- Consult nephrology if renal transplant patient, AKI stage 3, CKD stage 4 and 5, diagnostic uncertainty, inadequate response to treatment, if complex management anticipated (e.g. vasculitis, glomerulonephritis), or patient has complications that may need RRT.
  - Severe electrolyte abnormalities (e.g. hyperkalaemia).
  - Persistent anuria or oliguria despite adequate fluid resuscitation.
  - Metabolic acidosis (pH <7.25) unresponsive to bicarbonate therapy.
  - Fluid overload refractory to diuretics.
  - Uraemic pericarditis or encephalopathy.
  - Poisoning (e.g. lithium, salicylates).
- Follow-up should be initiated for *all* patients who have experienced significant AKI.

Chronic kidney disease

> AKI and CKD can co-exist in the same patient, resulting in acute-on-chronic deterioration in renal function. In the in-hospital setting, the general approach to CKD management is very similar to AKI.

Chronic kidney disease (also known as chronic renal failure/insufficiency) is much more prevalent than AKI (e.g. affecting 13% of the UK adult general population, but >30% aged >75). The definition of CKD also focuses on serum creatinine levels and derived eGFR calculated using the 2021 National Institute for Health and Care Excellence (NICE) CKD-EPI Race-free formula, which discontinued adjustment for ethnicity when calculating eGFR in people from black ethnic groups. Other kidney damage is detected predominantly through urinary albumin excretion estimated by urine ACR, although other renal abnormalities on pathological, urine, blood or imaging tests can be included (Table 27.2). In addition, persistence of abnormalities in the eGFR and/or ACR for at least three months or longer is required for CKD diagnosis.

Development of CKD is characterised by a progression from stages 1 to 5 (see Table 27.2). Advanced CKD usually relates to CKD stages 4–5 (although stage 3B can also have significant metabolic and other systemic consequences). CKD stage 5 occurs when eGFR is <15 ml/min, and is further sub-divided into:

- endstage renal disease (ESRD) for those patients treated with dialysis or transplant
- kidney (renal) failure for the remainder not treated with these modalities.

The progression of CKD is often variable and non-linear, but person-centred intervention can delay progression of CKD, reduce morbidity and mortality, and allow time for preparation for RRT, ultimately providing the best possible personalised care.

- Monitor eGFR (using the 2021 NICE CKD-EPI Race-free formula) and creatinine regularly.
- Proteinuria is the strongest predictor of renal risk and is associated with adverse patient outcomes. Urine ACR is preferred to urine protein:creatinine ratio (PCR) for monitoring protein – especially low levels.
- Counsel on dietary modifications for CKD.
- 'Sick-day rules' are important if patient has nausea, vomiting, diarrhoea with decreased oral intake.

Table 27.2 Stages of CKD

Stage	Estimated GFR (eGFR)	Description
1	> 90 ml/min	Kidney damage[a] with normal or increased eGFR
2	60–89 ml/min	Kidney damage[a] with mildly decreased eGFR
3A	45–59 ml/min	Mildly to moderately decreased eGFR
3B	30–44 ml/min	Moderately to severely decreased eGFR
4	15–29 ml/min	Severely decreased eGFR
5	<15 ml/min or renal replacement therapy (i.e. transplant or dialysis)	Kidney failure or endstage renal disease

[a] Kidney damage is defined as persistent micro- or macroalbuminuria or other abnormalities on pathological, urine, blood or imaging tests.

- People with CKD have a substantially increased risk of CVD, requiring a multifactorial approach.
  - Good BP control, good glycaemic control, consider ACE inhibitors or ARBs, sodium glucose co-transporter 2 (SGLT2) inhibitors (with or without diabetes), mineralocorticoid antagonists (finerenone), statins, stop smoking, and antiplatelets (secondary prevention) to prevent progression.
- Patients with CKD are not only at higher risk of thrombosis, they are also at increased risk of bleeding. Consider anticoagulant treatment carefully in CKD. Seek expert help.
- Treat anaemia. Approximately 75% of stage 5 CKD patients will have Hgb <110 g/l. Hepcidin is a major regulator of iron, increased in anaemia of renal disease leading to functional iron deficiency. Patients should be iron replete before receiving erythropoietin (erythropoietin-stimulating agent). Causes of iron deficiency should be considered, such as poor appetite and GI blood loss. IV iron is the first-line therapy for those patients treated with haemodialysis. The target haemoglobin for people with CKD receiving erythropoietin is 100–120 g/l.
- Metabolic acidosis – associated with poor nutritional status, muscle wasting and loss of bone density, and may contribute to progression of renal disease. Aim to correct this using oral sodium bicarbonate in people with CKD stage 4/5 and a serum bicarbonate of <20 mmol/l.
- Patients with chronic hyperkalaemia, especially when using renin-angiotensin-aldosterone system inhibitors, may benefit from long-term potassium-binding therapy, initiated at the recommended dose and titrated according to serum K+ levels. Choices include sodium polystyrene sulfonate and the newer agents: patiromer and sodium zirconium.
- CKD-mineral and bone disorders – serum Ca, phosphate, PTH and vitamin D levels should be routinely measured in people with a GFR <30 ml/min.
  - Cholecalciferol or ergocalciferol should be offered to treat vitamin D deficiency in people with CKD and vitamin D deficiency. If vitamin D deficiency has been corrected and symptoms of CKD-mineral and bone disorders persist, alfacalcidol or calcitriol (agents already 1-alpha hydroxylated which normally occurs in the kidney) should be offered to people with a GFR <30 ml/min. Serum Ca and phosphate concentrations should be monitored regularly in people receiving these drugs.
  - Hyperphosphataemia: phosphate is usually excreted by the kidneys and reduction leads to hyperphosphataemia. Patients may require a phosphate binder with their meals to reduce absorption of dietary phosphate.
- Medications – beware drugs normally cleared by the kidneys (e.g. insulin, sulfonylureas).
  - Altered pharmacokinetics and pharmacodynamics make frail older patients with CKD/ESRD particularly susceptible to drug–drug interactions; polypharmacy should therefore be avoided.
- Gout – ~70% of adults with gout have an eGFR of <60 ml/min, and almost a quarter of people with CKD stage 3 or worse have gout. Gout in people with CKD also may have more atypical presentations. Corticosteroids have been generally accepted as the safest option in most people with gout flares and concomitant CKD; reduced-dose colchicine and interleukin (IL)-1 inhibitors may also be used, while NSAIDs are contraindicated.
- Avoid untreated urinary outflow obstruction, especially in the elderly male population.

- Preparation for ESRD – consider initiation of dialysis or transplantation. Use the four-variable (age, sex, eGFR, urine ACR) Kidney Failure Risk Equation instead of eGFR threshold for referral.
  - Refer adults with CKD and a five-year risk of needing RRT of >5% (measured with the Kidney Failure Risk Equation) for specialist assessment.
- Be mindful that a patient with advanced CKD may require fistula formation and avoid repeated venepuncture or cannulation of the forearm veins (the dorsum of the hand is the preferred site).

> Diabetes remains the leading cause of CKD and accounts for ~50% of ESRD in the developed world. Consequently, many individuals with CKD also have diabetes (~40%). Hypoglycaemia is a common problem in persons with diabetes receiving haemodialysis.

Blackout/collapse

> The term 'collapse query cause' refers to one or more episodes of transient *loss of consciousness* before a thorough evaluation has been made. The major causes of this presentation are as follows.
>
> - Acute illness causing syncope.
> - Syncope – generally divided into four subtypes.
>   - Arrhythmia related.
>   - Cardiac (e.g. massive pulmonary embolus, severe aortic stenosis).
>   - Orthostatic: due to failure of homeostatic maintenance of BP on *standing*.
>   - Reflex vasodilation and/or bradycardia secondary to a 'trigger' (e.g. vasovagal episode).
> - Non-syncopal attacks – include seizure, hypoglycaemia, functional disorders.

Syncope is a transient loss of consciousness (T-LOC) due to impaired cerebral blood flow. It is characterised by rapid onset, short duration and spontaneous complete recovery. Presyncope is defined as a light-headed feeling of impending syncope.

The differential diagnosis of T-LOC is broad and includes the following.

- Cardiac arrhythmias.
- Cardiogenic shock/outflow obstruction.
- Hypoglycaemia.
- Hypoxia.

- Massive pulmonary embolism (PE).
- Myocardial infarction (MI).
- Orthostatic hypotension.
- Seizure.
- Vasovagal syncope.

ROWS (examples): cardiac arrhythmias, cardiogenic or obstructive shock, seizure and status epilepticus.

Initial investigations include BG, FBC, CRP, troponin, Ca, magnesium (Mg), U&E, creatinine, LFT, TFT, D-dimer, COVID-19. ECG and cardiac monitoring, echocardiogram. Consider urgent neuroimaging in seizure; anticoagulation; recent head injury; headache preceding T-LOC; known malignancy; and if focal signs, decreased GCS, confusion >30 minutes post T-LOC. Consider LP if meningism suggestive of infection or subarachnoid haemorrhage (SAH).

Initial management includes the following.

- First, consider *red flag* features and acute life-threatening causes (i.e. ROWS), ABCDE, optimise physiology and supportive care. Get eyewitness account.
- Identify and treat potential causes.
- Withdrawal of precipitating agents (e.g. antihypertensive agents).
- Management of associated complications.
- Consider using San Francisco Syncope rule (see Table 8.2) to determine whether the patient is in the low-risk group and can be managed in an ambulatory setting (e.g. same-day emergency care, SDEC).
- Admit to cardiology if *red flag* cardiac features such as T-LOC during exertion, family history of sudden cardiac death, structural heart disease.
- Advise about driving regulations, e.g. if suspected seizure.

> If there is recurrent syncope, consider tilt test, Holter monitor, implantable loop recorder.

Breathlessness

> Breathlessness (dyspnoea) is a subjective sensation of awareness of rapid or difficult breathing (e.g. discomfort associated with breathing; sensation of suffocation, choking or 'air hunger'; inability to take adequate breath; rapidity of breathing or increased effort related to breathing). Dyspnoea can be acute (less than one month) or chronic (greater than one month).

Common terms associated with breathlessness include the following.

- Shortness of breath (SOB) – this is one description of dyspnoea. Sometimes SOB may be used to imply more severe dyspnoea.
- Orthopnoea – dyspnoea when lying down flat, which occurs with congestive heart failure (CHF) due to associated pulmonary oedema. You can ask how many pillows the person sleeps on to gauge how significant it is. Keep in mind that GORD or postnasal drip from allergies can also make people have to sleep upright.
- Paroxysmal nocturnal dyspnoea (PND) – refers to sudden awakening at night due to SOB. This is a more 'specific' finding with CHF, meaning not everyone with CHF has it, but if a patient does have it, then it strongly suggests CHF. Obstructive sleep apnoea, GORD, asthma or even vivid nightmares can also cause these episodes.
- Platypnoea – dyspnoea that worsens in the upright position (the opposite of orthopnoea); may be related to 'orthodeoxia' – a drop in arterial pO_2 in the upright position associated with arteriovenous malformations or other right-to-left shunts and can also be seen with advanced liver disease.
- Deconditioning – patients may have dyspnoea because of sedentary lifestyle and weight gain. This is common but you must consider other causes since deconditioning is a diagnosis of exclusion.

Dyspnoea evaluation begins by assessing the duration, quality and quantity of the symptoms. Classically, some descriptors have been associated with certain conditions.

- Rapid breathing – CHF, diabetic ketoacidosis (DKA) (Kussmaul breathing).
- Incomplete exhalation, chest tightness – asthma.
- Shallow breathing – asthma, hyperventilation, neuromuscular or chest wall disease.
- Increased work or effort of breathing – chronic obstructive pulmonary disease (COPD), interstitial lung disease (ILD), asthma, neuromuscular.
- Feeling of suffocation – COPD, CHF.
- Air hunger – COPD, CHF, pregnancy.

Timing of symptoms *may* be helpful. Is it positional (orthopnoea, platypnoea)? Is it intermittent (asthma, recurrent pulmonary emboli, cardiac ischaemia) or chronic (COPD, pulmonary fibrosis)? Do symptoms increase *after* exercise, as in exercise-induced asthma, or are they present all the time (neuromuscular, mechanical or psychological problems)?

Quantifying the dyspnoea can help you better understand its impact on your patient's activities of daily life and serve as a method of assessing improvement or progression over time or after treatment. You can ask the patient to perform a six-minute walk test (with pulse oximetry) to determine cardiopulmonary exercise tolerance.

The differential diagnosis of breathlessness is very broad and includes the following possibilities.

- Anaphylaxis.
- Aspiration pneumonitis.
- Asthma exacerbation.
- Cardiac arrhythmia.
- Cardiac tamponade.
- Chest trauma.
- CHF.
- COPD.
- DKA.
- ILD (e.g. sarcoid, idiopathic pulmonary fibrosis).
- Pleural effusion (abnormal collection of fluid in the pleural space).
- Pneumonia (including COVID-19).
- Pulmonary oedema.
- PE.
- Substance abuse (e.g. methamphetamine-associated cardiomyopathy).
- Tension pneumothorax.

ROWS (examples): cardiac tamponade, life-threatening cardiac arrhythmias, PE, tension pneumothorax.

Initial investigations include: start with basics, such as FBC looking for leucocytosis (suggesting infection) or anaemia, CRP (infection), U&E and creatinine (e.g. checking for unsuspected advanced CKD/ESRD with metabolic acidosis and fluid overload), brain natriuretic peptide (BNP, acute and/or chronic heart failure), BG (e.g. DKA), troponin (e.g. MI), D-dimer (rule out PE), TFT (exclude hypothyroidism and hyperthyroidism), infectious screen as indicated (e.g. blood cultures, COVID-19), and pregnancy test. ECG. Pulse oximetry, ABG and basic spirometry (pulmonary function test [PFT]). Chest X-ray. Exhaled nitric oxide (indication of eosinophilic inflammation in the lungs) and sputum eosinophilia is used to support the diagnosis of asthma. More advanced tests can then be ordered if still unclear (e.g. echocardiogram, bronchoscopy, CT chest, CT pulmonary angiogram, bronchoprovocation testing). The BLUE protocol (Bedside Lung Ultrasound in Emergency) presents a systematic approach to a patient with acute dyspnoea (see Figure 11.21) to help identify the underlying diagnosis using thoracic and vascular point-of-care ultrasound (POCUS).

Initial management includes the following aspects.

- First, consider *red flag* features and acute life-threatening causes (i.e. ROWS), ABCDE, optimise physiology and supportive care (oxygen therapy). Oxygen saturation targets should generally be

94–98%. In some patients with COPD and carbon dioxide retention, inspired oxygen should be titrated to achieve saturations of 88–92%.

- Identify and treat potential causes. In the BLUE protocol, POCUS profiles have been described for the main diseases (pneumonia, CHF, COPD, asthma, PE, pneumothorax), with an accuracy of >90%.
- Withdrawal of precipitating agents.
- Management of associated complications.
- Refer to appropriate team (e.g. heart failure or respiratory nurse and associated specialists).

Pleural effusions

The initial assessment depends on laboratory analysis of the fluid.

- Use Light's criteria to distinguish *exudative* (e.g. parapneumonic, TB, primary and metastatic cancer) from *transudative* (e.g. CHF, nephrotic syndrome, chronic liver disease) serous effusions. Pleural fluid is likely to be exudate if more than one of the following is present.
  o Pleural fluid protein: serum protein ratio >0.5.
  o Pleural fluid lactate dehydrogenase (LDH): serum LDH ratio >0.6.
  o Pleural fluid LDH >two-thirds of upper limit of normal serum LDH.
- Other fluids include pus, chyle (lymphatic obstruction) and blood.
- Review pleural fluid biochemistry (e.g. pH, glucose, amylase).
- Identify evidence of infection (e.g. Gram stain, culture, adenosine deaminase activity for TB).
- Look for evidence of malignancy (e.g. cytology).
- Other diagnostics as needed (e.g. pleural biopsy, POCUS, other imaging).

Heart failure

Heart failure is present when the heart is unable to pump blood forward at a sufficient rate to meet the metabolic demands of the body (i.e. *forward failure*) or can do so only if cardiac filling pressures are abnormally high, which can lead to pulmonary oedema and right heart failure (i.e. *backward failure*).

Heart failure results in a clinical syndrome of fatigue, shortness of breath and often volume overload. It may be the final and most severe manifestation of nearly every form of cardiac disease, including coronary atherosclerosis, MI, valvular diseases, hypertension, congenital heart disease and the cardiomyopathies. The number of patients with heart failure is increasing due to the ageing population and improved survival after cardiac insults such as MI. It is common to categorise heart failure patients into two general categories based on the left ventricular ejection fraction (EF).

1 Heart failure with *reduced* EF (≤40%) – HfrEF (i.e. primarily *systolic* dysfunction).
2 Heart failure with *preserved* EF (≥50%) – HfpEF (i.e. primarily *diastolic* dysfunction).

Congestive heart failure is generally the highest risk CVD state, with one-year mortality of 25–60% in New York Heart Association (NYHA) stage IV (breathlessness at rest). In addition, patients with heart failure are 6–9 times more likely to develop sudden cardiac death (SCD) than the general population.

Features	Illness script for heart failure
Epidemiological risk factors	• Increasing age, smoking, coronary artery disease (CAD), hypertension, valvular heart disease, alcoholism (including thiamine deficiency, 'wet beriberi'), infection (viral including COVID-19), diabetes, congenital heart defects, high or low haematocrit level, obstructive sleep apnoea. • Takotsubo cardiomyopathy – stress (catecholamine) related; the shape of the left ventricle resembles a Japanese octopus fishing pot, a so-called takotsubo. Also termed 'broken heart' syndrome. • Right heart failure – most often due to left heart failure. Other causes include cor pulmonale related to pulmonary vascular disease (PE, pulmonary hypertension), COPD.

Features	Illness script for heart failure
Pathophysiology	Can be either: • HfrEF: systolic dysfunction – inability of ventricle to contract effectively. Usually secondary to CAD, dilated cardiomyopathy, or • HfpEF: diastolic dysfunction – inability of ventricle to relax and fill effectively. Causes include hypertensive ventricular hypertrophy, hypertrophic obstructive cardiomyopathy (HOCM), pericardial tamponade (emergency) and amyloidosis.
Time course	• Acute, acute on chronic, or chronic. Progressive.
Key symptoms and signs	• Left heart failure hallmarks: hypotensive, narrow pulse pressure and pulsus alternans, displaced apex beat, gallop rhythm (S3), murmur of mitral regurgitation, orthopnoea, dyspnoea, PND, early inspiratory coarse or fine crackles (crepitations), pink frothy sputum. • Right heart failure hallmarks: peripheral and central oedema (lower extremities, hepatomegaly, ascites, sacral oedema), elevated jugular venous pressure (JVP), murmur of tricuspid regurgitation, gallop rhythm (S3), weight gain.
Diagnostics	• General investigations as per breathlessness discussion including troponin, BNP, U&E, creatinine, FBC, CRP, BG, TSH, lipid profile, iron panel (haemochromatosis, anaemia), COVID-19. • ECG, CXR, ABG, echocardiogram. • Non-invasive stress imaging or cardiac catheterisation is reasonable in heart failure and suspected CAD.

Treatment	Acute or acute on chronic (bi)ventricular failure.
	• ABCDE, IV access, monitor ECG for arrhythmias and treat accordingly, venous thromboembolic (VTE) prophylaxis.
	• Mnemonic – 'LMNOP'.
	   o Lasix® (trade name for furosemide: 40–80 mg IV if SBP>110 mmHg). In acute presentation, IV loop diuretic may be better than oral due to bowel oedema limiting absorption.
	   o Morphine (plus antiemetic).
	   o Nitrates (>110 mmHg systolic BP).
	   o Oxygen (non-invasive positive pressure ventilation: continuous positive airways pressure of 5–10 mmHg by a tight-fitting facemask results in more rapid clinical improvement).
	   o Positioning (sit upright). If right heart failure or PE – need high filling pressures so patient may prefer *lying flat* – do not overdiurese and may need fluid challenge.
	• Beta-blockers and ACE inhibitor/ARB should be avoided during decompensated CHF but should be restarted once patient is euvolaemic and renal function/electrolytes stable. Stop calcium channel blockers and NSAIDs where possible.
	• Correct underlying causes such as arrhythmias, myocardial ischaemia and drugs. If patient presents in fast atrial fibrillation and pulmonary oedema, consider digoxin initially until beta-blockers can be initiated and uptitrated.
	• If these measures prove ineffective, inotropic agents may be required to augment cardiac output, particularly in hypotensive patients.
	• Insertion of an intra-aortic balloon pump may be beneficial in patients with acute cardiogenic pulmonary oedema and shock.
	• Monitor progress: frequent face-to-face review, daily weights, repeat observations, labs (creatinine and U&Es) and imaging.
	• Initiate and uptitrate disease-modifying drugs. Daily antiplatelet agent and a statin are recommended if the underlying cause is CAD.
	• Cardiology and/or heart failure nurse consult.

Long-term management of CHF

- Lifestyle and other healthcare maintenance – co-morbid conditions (e.g. diabetes), and limit dietary sodium and fluid intake. Cardiac rehabilitation. Vaccinations (influenza, COVID-19).
- Diuretics (most commonly loop diuretics) – prevent volume overload.
- Start 'Core 4' drugs.
  - Bisoprolol 1.25–2.5 mg once daily (beta-blocker).
  - Dapagliflozin 10 mg once daily or similar agent (SGLT2 inhibitor).
  - Candesartan 4 mg once daily (ARB) or Entresto® 24/26 mg twice daily (angiotensin receptor–neprilysin inhibitor, ARNI).
  - Eplerenone 25 mg once daily or similar agent (mineralocorticoid antagonist).
- Monitor 'Core 4' drugs with BP, U&E and creatinine in 1–2 weeks (beware AKI and hyperkalaemia). Uptitrate as tolerated. Review dose of diuretic once euvolaemic.
- Other therapies can include digoxin, ACE inhibitor, anticoagulation.
- Consider patient prognosis and eligibility for advanced interventions.
  - Implantable cardiac defibrillator (ICD) in patients with an EF <35%.
  - Cardiac resynchronisation treatment (CRT) with biventricular pacing (wide QRS >120 milliseconds).
  - Cardiac transplantation.

Chronic obstructive pulmonary disease

COPD is the fifth most common cause of death in England and acute exacerbations present frequently to hospital; for respiratory disease in hospital, it is second only to pneumonia.

Chronic obstructive pulmonary disease is characterised by airflow obstruction. Eighty percent of COPD occurs in smokers with a 10 pack-year or more smoking history while the other 20% occurs in non-smokers with other exposures such as biomass fuels and organic/inorganic dusts. Both chronic bronchitis (productive cough for three months or more over two years) and emphysema (structural changes with destruction of lung parenchyma) may be seen in absence of airflow obstruction.

Spirometry demonstrating airflow obstruction is required for a diagnosis of COPD and is defined as a forced expiratory volume in one second (FEV_1)/forced vital capacity (FVC) ratio of <70% or below LLN (lower limit of normal), lack of which should prompt a search for alternative diagnoses that present with respiratory symptoms.

Features	Illness script for COPD
Epidemiological risk factors	• Smoking, air pollution, biomass fuels, organic/inorganic dusts. • Alpha-1 antitrypsin deficiency.
Pathophysiology	• Encompasses chronic bronchitis and emphysema (some overlap with asthma). Inflammatory – bronchial hyperresponsiveness leading to bronchoconstriction and mucus hypersecretion.
Time course	• Chronic, acute on chronic exacerbations. Progressive.
Key symptoms and signs	• Three cardinal symptoms of COPD are dyspnoea, chronic cough and sputum production. Wheezing and chest tightness are also common. • Examination – tachypnoea, cyanosis, hyperinflation, increased resonance to percussion, decreased breath sounds, wheezes, crackles and/or distant heart sounds. Use of accessory muscles. Features of CO_2 retention include venodilation, flapping tremor and altered mental status. Cachexia can occur with emphysema. Signs of right heart failure with cor pulmonale.
Diagnostics	• Investigations – ABG, FBC with differential, CRP, BNP (heart failure), COVID-19, U&E and creatinine. ECG. Sputum Gram stain and culture. • Imaging – CXR, CT chest. • Pulmonary function tests (PFT): FEV_1/FVC <70%; postbronchodilator FEV_1 determines severity. • Six-minute walk test with oximetry can aid in assessing the functional capacity of patients with cardiopulmonary disease.

Features	Illness script for COPD
Treatment	Acute exacerbations.

- ABCDE; oxygen therapy (with prescribed oxygen targets); non-invasive or invasive ventilation; inhaled or nebulised bronchodilators (i.e. beta-2-adrenergic agonists, muscarinic antagonist); oral corticosteroids; oral/IV antibiotics (procalcitonin may help guide antibiotic usage); supportive therapy including chest physiotherapy, nutritional support and VTE prophylaxis.

Chronic treatment – should be individualised and depends on severity of disease.

- Vaccines – including influenza, pneumococcal, COVID-19.
- Smoking cessation – single most important treatment strategy for COPD, prevents progression and improves mortality.
- Short- and long-acting bronchodilators. All patients with COPD should be prescribed a rescue short-acting bronchodilator for immediate symptom relief. Check inhaler technique, treatment adherence and persistence.
- Inhaled or oral corticosteroids.
- Roflumilast (oral PDE4 inhibitor) in patients with frequent exacerbations.
- Other treatments such as theophylline, diuretics (e.g. heart failure).
- Home non-invasive ventilation or oxygen therapy.
- Pulmonary rehabilitation.
- Surgical and bronchoscopic interventions.
  - Lung transplant: early referral is suggested for patients with persistent symptoms despite above measures.
  - Lung volume reduction: bronchoscopic placement of endobronchial valves to decompress diseased lung regions with air trapping.
- Palliative and end-of-life care. Anticipatory care planning.

Asthma

> Asthma is characterised by wheezing, cough and dyspnoea. Objective confirmation of airflow obstruction is required for a diagnosis of asthma given the non-specific nature of the symptom complex and risk of misdiagnosis. Broadly categorised into *allergic* asthma driven by eosinophils and immunoglobulin E (IgE) versus *neutrophilic* and *obesity*-related asthma versus *occupational* (related to workplace exposures) asthma.

Airway inflammation is the hallmark of asthma with mucus production and goblet cell hyperplasia. Symptoms are typically triggered by aeroallergens, cold air, inhaled irritants, air pollution, exercise and, less commonly, by drugs (e.g. aspirin).

Patients presenting to Acute Medicine with any of the following features should be considered unstable and may warrant admission and further escalation to critical care.

- Nocturnal symptoms interrupting sleep (usually cough and dyspnoea).
- Worsening cough.
- Increased use of beta-2-agonists (less effective and relief shorter lasting).
- Decreased efficacy of rescue medication (such as corticosteroids).
- Previous admission to hospital, particularly if it required treatment in critical care units, should be taken to indicate that the patient is prone to life-threatening episodes.

Acute management of asthma includes ABCDE; oxygen therapy (keep oxygen saturations 94–98%), nebulised bronchodilators (i.e. beta-2-agonists and ipratropium); IV/oral corticosteroids; consider IV magnesium, and oral/IV antibiotics as required. Supportive care includes rehydration and monitoring electrolytes (hypokalaemia common due to beta-2-adrenergic agonists shifting K^+ into cells). Measure ABG on admission and repeat as necessary to assess progress. A $PaCO_2$ greater than 6 kPa (45 mmHg) suggests the patient is at imminent risk of respiratory failure and so in need of mechanical ventilation. A progressive improvement in morning peak flow should be seen before discharge. Patients should normally be transferred from nebulised to inhaler therapy when peak flow approaches normal limits prior to discharge.

Patients should be discharged on inhaled and/or oral steroids and have an asthma action plan. The respiratory nurse should check inhaler technique and facilitate follow-up arrangements.

Features	Illness script for asthma
Epidemiological risk factors	• Family or personal history of atopic disease, exposure to allergens, air pollution, cold air, exercise or NSAID exposure in specific populations.
Pathophysiology	• Reversible inflammation and bronchoconstriction of the airways. Airway wall fibrosis can develop with recurrent exacerbations leading to fixed airflow obstruction.
Time course	• Acute; chronic with acute exacerbations.
Key symptoms and signs	• Patients usually present with dyspnoea and cough, worse at night. Severe and poorly controlled asthma presents with wheezing and shortness of breath. Associated symptoms and past medical history: atopy, allergies. • Physical examination – tachypnoea, hyperinflation, increased resonance to percussion, wheezes and/or distant heart sounds. Use of accessory muscles.
Diagnostics	• Spirometry: FEV_1/FVC less than lower limit of normal (LLN) that may reverse with short-acting beta-2-agonist (SABA): significant bronchodilator response (e.g. $\geq$15%) suggests reversibility of airflow obstruction (although can also be seen in COPD, cystic fibrosis). • Peak expiratory flow rate (PEFR) – useful for monitoring severity and diurnal variation. • Exhaled nitric oxide – may be elevated in allergic asthma. • Bronchoprovocation testing is considered when PFTs are normal in a patient with high clinical suspicion of asthma. In acute presentation: $PaCO_2$ greater than 6 kPa (45 mmHg) suggests the patient is at imminent risk of respiratory failure and so in need of mechanical ventilation.

Treatment	Treat bronchoconstriction and inflammation.
	• Assess symptom control, risk factors and co-morbidities.
	• Initiate and adjust treatment.
	  o Preventive inhalers: importantly, for safety, Global Initiative for Asthma (GINA) no longer recommends treatment of asthma in adults and adolescents with SABA alone, without inhaled corticosteroids (ICS). Other inhalers include long-acting beta-2 agonists (LABA) and various combinations of agent in single inhaler.
	  o Reliever inhaler for as-needed use - either low dose ICS-LABA (formoterol), ICS-SABA (albuterol) or SABA.
	  o Other treatments such as oral steroids, leukotriene antagonists.
	  o Biologic therapies: patients with persistent symptoms despite standard ICS therapies may be candidates for anti-IgE in patients with elevated IgE levels; anti-IL-4, anti-IL-5 and anti-IL-13 agents in eosinophilic asthma; and other newer biologics that appear to have an effect in absence of eosinophilia.
	  o Bronchial thermoplasty: interventional procedure that helps reduce 'abnormal' component of airway smooth muscle associated with asthma.
	  o Treat modifiable risk factors and co-morbidities.
	• Review response.
	  o Review technique, adherence.
	  o Assess symptom control again, exacerbations, side-effects.

IL, interleukin.

Obstructive and restrictive lung disease

Obstructive lung disease (e.g. COPD).

- *Disproportionate* reduction in FEV_1 compared with FVC (i.e. FEV_1/FVC ratio <0.7 or LLN).
- Normal/increased total lung capacity (air trapping).

Restrictive lung disease (e.g. ILD).

- *Proportionate* reduction in FEV_1 and FVC (i.e. FEV_1/FVC ratio normal or increased).
- Decreased total lung capacity (difficulty getting air in).

Chest pain

Chest pain is a high-volume condition, accounting for 6% of all medical admissions. The most important part of the clinical evaluation of acute chest pain is the history described by the patient.

Non-traumatic acute chest pain is one of the most common causes of emergency department visits and occurs in both inpatients and outpatients. Chest pain is most commonly thought to reflect an underlying cardiac condition, but the majority of cases are non-cardiac and not life-threatening. The primary aim is to identify acute coronary syndromes (ACS) and other life-threatening causes (e.g. aortic dissection, PE).

The differential diagnosis of acute chest pain is broad and includes the following.

- ACS.
- Aortic dissection.
- Atypical chest pain.
- Pericarditis.
- Pneumonia with pleurisy.
- Pneumothorax.
- PE.
- Reflux oesophagitis.

ROWS (examples): 'Think: 4 + 2 + 2' (see Figure 2.2).

- Cardiac *4* – ACS, aortic dissection, tamponade, takotsubo cardiomyopathy (may present with signs and symptoms of an ACS but without significant obstructive CAD).

- Pulmonary *2* – PE, tension pneumothorax.
- Oesophageal *2* - rupture, impaction.

Initial investigations include ECG and cardiac monitoring, troponin, D-dimer, coagulation studies, BG, FBC, CRP, U&E, creatinine, TFT, LFT, ABG, lipids and COVID-19. CXR. Echocardiogram.

Initial management includes the following aspects.

- First, consider *red flag* features and acute life-threatening causes (i.e. ROWS), ABCDE, optimise physiology and supportive care. Oxygen only recommended in patients with uncomplicated MI with oxygen saturation (SpO_2) <90%; hyperoxia may be harmful in such patients, presumably due to increased myocardial injury.
- Analgesia (and antiemetic).
- Identify and treat potential causes.
- Withdrawal of precipitating agents.
- Management of associated complications (e.g. CHF, shock, ventricular rupture).
- Repeat timed troponin level (timing depends on assay) if initial early test negative.
- Seek urgent cardiology input if doubt about diagnosis/management.

Acute coronary syndromes

Management of ACS (especially non-ST elevation MI and unstable angina) often requires joint working/close liaison with cardiology to provide the optimal care.

Acute coronary syndromes are a spectrum of disorders including ST elevation MI (STEMI), non-ST elevation MI (NSTEMI) and unstable angina (see Table 2.2 for representative illness script). The diagnosis is based on a history of chest pain, ECG changes and measurement of biochemical markers of cardiac damage (Figure 27.2). MI occurs due to plaque rupture, erosions and calcified nodules with thrombosis and myocardial ischaemia. A total occlusion of the coronary artery leads to STEMI, where the best treatment is an emergency percutaneous coronary intervention (Figure 27.3). A partial occlusion leads to NSTEMI/unstable angina. MI is detected by measuring increases in troponin levels as a biomarker of myocardial necrosis, while in unstable angina, troponin is not increased.

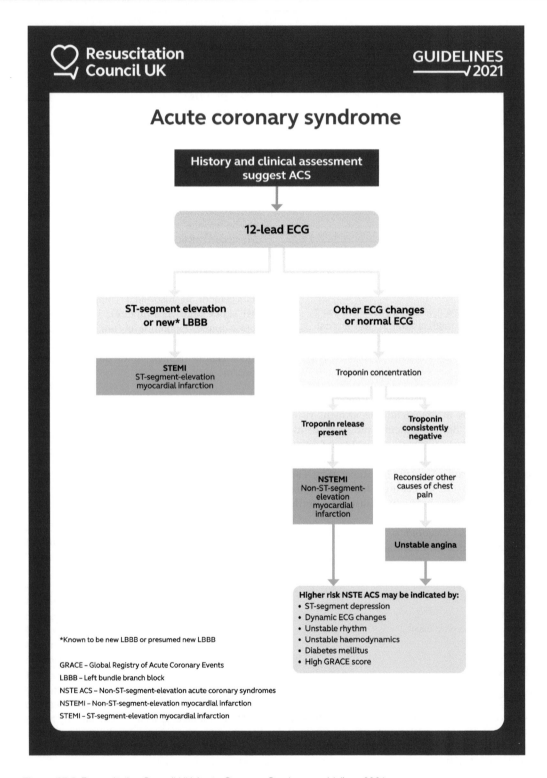

Figure 27.2 Resuscitation Council UK Acute Coronary Syndrome guidelines 2021.

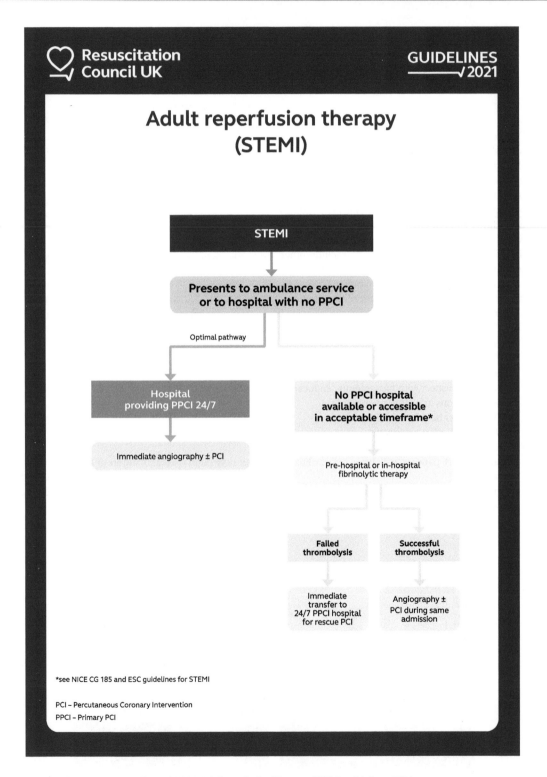

Figure 27.3 Resuscitation Council UK Adult Reperfusion Therapy STEMI guidelines 2021.

Acute pericarditis

Acute pericarditis recurs in up to 30% of patients, sometimes for years.

Diagnose pericarditis if constant, retrosternal pain with sharp, stabbing nature radiates to the arm, shoulder or trapezius ridge. Can be relieved by leaning forwards. Friction rub is best heard at left lower sternal border on inspiration or full expiration, with patient leaning forward. Characteristic ECG findings with diffuse concordant ST segment elevation, often with depression of the PR segment. Other investigations include chest X-ray, mostly to exclude other serious conditions (e.g. pneumothorax, pneumonia). Urgent echocardiogram if hypotensive, pulsus paradoxus >10 mmHg or symptoms of heart failure.

There are numerous causes, including the following.

- Infectious.
  - Viral: 20% of *all* cases (HIV work-up if risk factors).
  - Bacterial: suspect with bacteraemia, endocarditis, contiguous infection (pneumonia).
  - TB: consider based on risk factors.
  - Uraemic: check renal function.
- Autoimmune – 20–40% of systemic lupus erythematosus (SLE) patients will have pericarditis at some point.
- Acute MI and post-MI (Dressler syndrome).
- Neoplastic disease.

Management of acute pericarditis

Treat in ambulatory setting when stable, and serious causes of chest pain and moderate-severe pericardial effusion have been excluded.

- High-dose aspirin and NSAID are first-line agents for the treatment of an initial episode of viral or idiopathic pericarditis.
- Treatment with high-dose aspirin is preferred over NSAID if an acute MI is the cause of acute pericarditis because its antiplatelet effects are beneficial and because of a prevailing concern that NSAID may promote ventricular rupture by impairing myocardial scar formation.
- Colchicine has emerged as the treatment of choice for acute bouts of recurrent pericarditis and can be useful in the prevention of recurrences. Treatment duration is 3–6 months.
- Steroids should be considered only in patients who are refractory to or have contraindications for the use of all alternative agents (i.e. aspirin, NSAID, colchicine).
- Beware anticoagulants as risk of haemopericardium, especially if pericardial effusion develops or increases.

Aortic dissection

Aortic dissection is a tear in the aortic intima resulting in decreased blood flow (Figure 27.4). Can be divided into type A (ascending aorta) or type B (not involving ascending thoracic aorta).

(a)

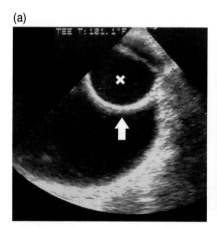

(b)

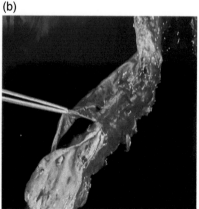

Figure 27.4 (a) Transoesophageal echo showing aortic dissection (arrow) and false lumen (cross) involving the arch of the aorta. (b) Dissecting haematoma of the descending aorta (same patient).

Features	Illness script for aortic dissection
Epidemiological risk factors	• Older age, male sex, hypertension (more common in descending aortic dissection), pre-existing aortic aneurysm, atherosclerotic vascular disease risk factors, trauma, pregnancy, and connective tissue disorders (e.g. Marfan syndrome).
Pathophysiology	• 70% are type A dissections, 30% are type B dissections. • Degenerative, traumatic tear in the aortic intima leading to blood accumulation in the aortic media which can lead to occlusion of distal arteries as it expands distal to dissection or proximal to dissection, leading to complications resulting from hypoperfusion.
Time course	• Hyperacute/acute. Progresses without intervention.
Key symptoms and signs	• Acute onset of 'tearing' anterior chest pain radiating to the back (interscapular). Presentation can be associated with signs of end-organ ischaemia presenting as an acute myocardial infarction, acute-onset heart failure, renal insufficiency, acute limb ischaemia or spinal cord ischaemia. • Physical examination – pulse pressure difference between left and right arms; inter-arm BP difference >20 mmHg, new diastolic regurgitation murmurs (aortic regurgitation) and/or distant heart sounds (cardiac tamponade); signs of end-organ damage (e.g. ischaemic stroke).

Diagnostics	• Investigations – ECG, chest X-ray (widened mediastinum), troponin, coagulation markers, type and cross-match, U&E, creatinine, LFT.
	• Imaging.
	  o Unstable patient: transoesophageal echocardiography (TOE) at bedside if immediately available, otherwise CT angiography and/or transthoracic echocardiogram.
	  o Stable patient: CT or MR angiography followed by TOE if equivocal.

Treatment	• ABCDE, analgesia (and antiemetic), supportive care. Seek expert help. • Type A – emergency stent-grafting or surgery. • Type B – BP control if no evidence of ischaemia; control heart rate (<60/min) and rapid lowering of systolic BP to at least 120 mmHg within 20 minutes with IV labetalol (or similar).

Pulmonary embolus

Features	Illness script for PE
Epidemiological risk factors	• Approximately half of all new venous thromboembolism (VTE) are diagnosed during or within three months of a hospital stay or surgical procedure. History of immobilisation, obesity (metabolic syndrome), oral contraceptive or hormone replacement, malignancy, family or personal history of VTE disease, thrombophilia. COVID-19 infection results in a hypercoagulable state.

Pathophysiology	• Virchow's triad.
	  o Vascular endothelial damage.
	  o Venous stasis.
	  o Hypercoagulability.
	• The increase in dead space (no perfusion to ventilated lung) causes an increase in alveolar–arterial (A-a) gradient and resultant hypoxaemia and pulmonary hypertension.

Time course	• Hyperacute/acute. Can deteriorate rapidly.
Key signs and symptoms	• Sudden-onset dyspnoea, pleuritic chest pain and haemoptysis. Syncope. • Physical examination – tachycardia, may have hypotension (shock), increased JVP. Evidence of deep vein thrombosis (DVT).

Features	Illness script for PE

Diagnostics	• Pretest probability of PE: Wells score.
	• Investigations – ECG (right heart strain and $S_1Q_3T_3$ pattern), ABG, FBC, CRP, coagulation markers, troponin, BNP, D-dimer, COVID-19.
	• Imaging.
	  ○ Chest X-ray.
	  ○ In hypotensive or periarrest situation: urgent POCUS or transthoracic echocardiogram to check for right heart strain and other causes such as cardiac tamponade.
	  ○ CT pulmonary angiogram (V/Q scan if pregnant). If swollen calf and high probability of DVT, Doppler USS of leg.

Treatment	• ABCDE, analgesia, supportive care (e.g. oxygen). Activate multidisciplinary PE Response Team (PERT) if available.
	• Anticoagulation with either:
	  ○ direct oral anticoagulant (DOAC): preferred. Avoid in pregnancy – use low molecular weight heparin (LMWH), or
	  ○ heparin (unfractionated heparin or LMWH) for 3–5 days while starting warfarin – bridge to warfarin (vitamin K antagonist anticoagulant).
	  ○ Duration: three months anticoagulation if transient provoking factor (extended if persistent risk factor or unprovoked).
	• <10% VTE will require thrombolysis (e.g. massive PE with haemodynamic instability, right heart strain) or interventional radiology or surgery.

Cough

Cough is a sudden voluntary or involuntary act aiming to clear the throat and airways (including any irritants or sputum). Acute cough exists for less than three weeks and is most commonly due to an acute upper respiratory tract infection. Other considerations include an acute exacerbation of underlying COPD, pneumonia and PE. Cough that has been present longer than three weeks is either subacute (3–8 weeks) or chronic (more than eight weeks). Persistent cough is most often due to asthma and COPD, GORD and postnasal drip.

The history provides important initial clues in the patient with acute, subacute or chronic cough. Cough can be life-threatening, and hence careful assessment of the patient's clinical status and use of accessory muscles of respiration, as well as the character of the cough and any associated sputum or haemoptysis, can help identify the urgency of intervention.

The differential diagnosis of cough is broad and includes the following possibilities.

• Acute bronchitis.
• Acute exacerbation of asthma or COPD (acute or chronic cough).
• Acute pulmonary oedema.
• Bronchiectasis.
• Foreign body inhalation.
• GORD (chronic cough).
• Interstitial lung disease.
• Malignancy.
• Medication induced – e.g. ACE inhibitor (up to 15% of patients).
• Postnasal drip (chronic cough).
• Pneumonia (including whooping cough, COVID-19).
• TB.

ROWS (examples): acute exacerbation of asthma or COPD, acute pulmonary oedema, foreign body inhalation, malignancy

Initial investigations include FBC, CRP, U&E, creatinine, LFT, BNP, ABG, blood cultures. Oximetry. Respiratory viral polymerase chain reaction (PCR) (including COVID-19). TB testing as indicated. Sputum cytology, Gram stain, culture and sensitivity. ECG. Imaging: CXR and cross-sectional imaging. PFTs. Exhaled nitric oxide (indication of eosinophilic inflammation in the lungs) and sputum eosinophilia are used to support the diagnosis of asthma and non-asthmatic eosinophilic bronchitis. Bronchoscopy, methacholine challenge and other tests as per suspected diagnosis.

Initial management includes the following aspects.

- Take necessary infectious disease precautions to protect yourself and others (e.g. suspected TB, COVID-19).
- First, consider *red flag* features and acute life-threatening causes (i.e. ROWS), ABCDE, optimise physiology and supportive care.
- Identify and treat potential causes.
- Withdrawal of precipitating agents (e.g. ACE inhibitor).
- Management of associated complications.

decubitus with suspected bleeding side down), obtain IV access, ensure haemodynamic stability (e.g. fluid, transfusion), and perform initial measures to control the bleeding (e.g. treat any bleeding diathesis). Intubation is usually required. Flexible bronchoscopy is the initial diagnostic procedure of choice in most patients with life-threatening haemoptysis.

Tuberculosis

Life-threatening haemoptysis (e.g. 150 ml of blood expectorated in a 24-hour period or bleeding at a rate ≥100 ml/h) can result in significant airway obstruction, significant abnormal gas exchange or haemodynamic instability. The most common causes for life-threatening haemoptysis are bronchiectasis, bronchogenic cancer, TB, trauma and fungal infections. Need urgent resuscitation (airway, blood loss), critical care and respiratory review. In 90% of patients with life-threatening haemoptysis, bleeding arises from the high-pressure bronchial circulation (compared with low-pressure pulmonary artery). Position the patient (lateral

TB is diagnosed by clinical presentation, imaging studies, molecular biologic diagnostic studies, and results of microbiological investigations.

Tuberculosis killed more than 1 billion people between 1800 and 2000. A community approach of 'search (properly), treat (effectively) and prevent (exposure)' is crucial to stopping the spread of TB. However, TB diagnostic rates have decreased whilst deaths have increased because of reduced access to care during the COVID-19 pandemic. Without an effective TB vaccine for adults, treatment is the primary form of disease control.

Features	Illness script for TB
Epidemiological risk factors	• More common in low- and middle-income countries. Risk of infection is related to duration and degree of exposure. Risk factors include social determinants of health (e.g. poverty, homelessness or living in close quarters, migrants, malnourishment), immunosuppression (HIV, transplant patients, IV drug users, medications such as tumour necrosis factor [TNF]-alpha inhibitors) and chronic disease (e.g. diabetes mellitus). More common in patient-facing healthcare workers.
Time course	Primary (acute) TB infection. • Local progression with possible disseminated (miliary) disease occurs in 5%. The other 95% of infected patients either heal or develop latent (dormant) infection. Secondary TB. • Approximately 5% of patients with latent TB can reactivate, leading to progressive secondary infection. Months to years later. Reinfection with new exposure can also occur.
Pathophysiology	• Infectious agent – *Mycobacterium tuberculosis* (MTB). Air-borne transmission. • Primary TB – most people develop immune response that limits spread of bacteria to lung (Ghon focus) and local lymph nodes, together termed a *Ghon complex*. Primary progressive disease can also occur in ~5%. • Secondary TB – progressive disease follows latent infection or reinfection. More commonly in oxygen rich upper lung lobes.

(Continued)

Features	Illness script for TB

	• Natural history of progressive pulmonary TB (primary or secondary).
	  o One-third die rapidly ('galloping consumption').
	  o One-third go into remission.
	  o One-third have progression ('consumption').
	 • Miliary TB – refers to haematogenous dissemination of the tuberculous bacilli (more common in people with HIV).

Key symptoms and signs	• Latent – asymptomatic and not contagious. Can reactivate. • Active progressive disease – fever, night sweats, weight loss, decreased appetite, lethargy, cough (especially nocturnal), dyspnoea and haemoptysis. • Examination – tachypnoea, cachexia, lymphadenopathy, pulmonary signs (including signs of pleural effusion). Evidence of extrapulmonary disease (e.g. erythema nodosum, miliary disease findings such as retinal).
Diagnostics	At least one-third to one-half of cases are not diagnosed worldwide (worsened during COVID-19 pandemic). Always check HIV status of patient with suspected TB. • *M. tuberculosis* (MTB) – unique cell wall imparts acid-fast staining characteristic. Aerobic. Culture is gold standard. • Sputum sample – microscopy, culture, molecular testing (MTB) and antibiotic resistance testing (e.g. Xpert® – tests for MTB and rifampicin resistance). • Pleural disease (occurs in up to 25%) – exudate, Ziehl–Neelsen stain, culture, pleural biopsy, adenosine deaminase level very useful (T-cell enzyme). • Imaging – CXR, classically upper lobe cavitary lung lesions. CT chest. Other imaging if extrapulmonary spread suspected (e.g. Pott's spine – combination of osteomyelitis and arthritis which involves multiple vertebrae). Prior TB exposure. • Tuberculin skin test – also termed purified protein derivative (PPD) or Mantoux test, positive if induration at 48–72 hours: >5mm: suspected TB, immunocompromised, recent contact; >10mm: endemic country, IV drug user, homeless, chronic illness; >15mm: all others. • IGRA (interferon-gamma release assay) – if patient has been infected with *M. tuberculosis*, lymphocytes in whole-blood sample should react to *in vitro* incubation with TB antigens by producing interferon-gamma; constitutes a positive test.

Treatment	Standard treatment in adults (monitor adherence with directly observed therapy).
	 • Isolate patient (air-borne precautions) with active TB until sputum negative.
	 • Multiple antituberculosis medications are needed because of the capacity of mycobacteria to develop drug resistance.
	 • Two months of daily rifampin, isoniazid, pyrazinamide and ethambutol (RIPE) followed by four months of daily isoniazid and rifampin.
	 • Extension of consolidation therapy for an additional 3–6 months may be considered in patients with extensive disease (e.g. cavities on the baseline chest film and a positive sputum culture) or extrapulmonary disease (steroids may also be used initially such as pericardium), or in those who do not have culture conversion after two months of adequate therapy, or immunosuppressed.
	
	 Drug-resistant TB (DR-TB) – consult with a specialist who is experienced in the treatment of DR-TB.
	 • Suggested by medical history such as exposure to persons with multidrug-resistant TB (MDR-TB) or results of molecular diagnostic screening test (e.g. Xpert rifampicin/MTB).
	  o MDR-TB: organism resistant to both rifampicin and isoniazid (most potent antituberculous medications).
	  o Extensively DR-TB: resistant to rifampicin, isoniazid, fluoroquinolones and at least one injectable agent.
	
	 People with HIV and TB – beware drug–drug interactions, immune reconstitution inflammatory syndromes (IRIS).

Chronic cough could be TB. Consider active TB disease in patients with cough, fever, night sweats, weight loss or fatigue in settings with a high incidence of disease, in patients without symptoms who have epidemiological risk factors such as HIV, and with suggestive chest X-ray findings. Recent upward trend in the incidence of TB in the UK, particularly in socioeconomically deprived populations (who are also more prone to serious COVID-19 infection). Refer patients to a TB specialist when concern for TB remains despite negative diagnostic test results, particularly in the absence of an alternative likely diagnosis.

Pneumonia

- Community-acquired pneumonia (CAP) refers to an acute infection of the pulmonary parenchyma acquired outside the hospital.
- Nosocomial pneumonia refers to an acute infection of the pulmonary parenchyma acquired in hospital settings and encompasses both hospital-acquired pneumonia (HAP) and ventilator-associated pneumonia (VAP). These persons are at increased risk for resistant organisms.
  - HAP refers to pneumonia acquired ≥48 hours after hospital admission.
  - VAP refers to pneumonia acquired ≥48 hours after endotracheal intubation.

Features	Illness script for CAP
Epidemiological risk factors	- Risk increases with age, recent viral upper respiratory tract infection, smoking, alcohol misuse, structural lung disease, recent hospitalisation, risk for aspiration and immunodeficiency (including asplenia).
Pathophysiology	- Infection of the lower respiratory tract with bacteria, viruses (most common) or fungi. Most common bacterial cause organism: *Streptococcus pneumoniae* (pneumococcus).
Time course	- Acute or subacute (if atypical). Progressive if untreated.
Key symptoms and signs	- Fever, productive cough, sputum, shortness of breath, tachycardia, hypoxaemia. Pleuritic chest pain if pleural involvement. Examination can include crackles (crepitations), wheezing, bronchial breathing, dullness to percussion, aegophony, increased tactile and vocal fremitus.
Diagnostics	- Infiltrate on chest X-ray (can be fooled if dry). Other imaging may be required (e.g. CT chest). Leucocytosis with left shift (primitive cell morphology). Raised inflammatory markers (e.g. CRP). Other systemic findings (e.g. abnormal LFTs) common with atypical pneumonia. Blood cultures, Gram stain and culture of sputum. COVID-19 and multiplex respiratory viruses PCR testing. Consider additional investigations depending on context (e.g. *Legionella*, HIV, fungi). - Procalcitonin helps distinguish bacterial infection from other causes of infection (e.g. COVID-19) or inflammation and may be useful for diagnosis, early discontinuation of antibiotic therapy (repeat level every 1–2 days), severity and prognosis.

Treatment	- Early antibiotic therapy (usually 5–7 days in total). Supportive care (hydration, oxygen, physiotherapy). Determine need for ventilatory support.
	- Mortality risk and site of management based on CURB-65 score and other factors (e.g. frailty, co-morbidities, homelessness): CURB-65 score (score 1 for each of the following):
	  ○ **C**onfusion of new onset
	  ○ **U**rea >7 mmol/l
	  ○ **R**espiratory rate >30/min
	  ○ **B**lood pressure <90/60 mmHg
	  ○ **65** years or older.
	Total score:
	  ○ 0–1: Low severity – outpatient treatment usual
	  ○ 2: Moderate severity – consider hospital admission or alternative site such as Acute Medicine SDEC, virtual ward or Hospital at Home service
	  ○ 3–5: High severity – admit to hospital.
	- Follow up on immunisation status for pneumococcal, influenza and COVID-19 vaccines (especially in elderly and immunocompromised).

Diarrhoea

Diarrhoea is defined as three or more unformed (loose, watery) stools (i.e. type 6 or 7 stool on the Bristol Stool Chart) in 24 hours. Acute diarrhoea is defined as less than 14 days duration. Irritable bowel disease is the most common cause of chronic diarrhoea.

Diarrhoea is traditionally classified as:

- osmotic (e.g. laxative abuse – diarrhoea stops when patient fasts)
- secretory (e.g. toxin or peptides)
- motility (e.g. irritable bowel disease or bacterial overgrowth)
- inflammatory (e.g. inflammatory bowel disease, infectious).

In adults, infectious gastroenteritis with viral organisms is the most common cause of acute diarrhoea. Other important aetiologies to consider in an acute care setting include autoimmune (e.g. immune checkpoint inhibitors), antibiotic (healthcare) associated and inflammatory colitis. Consideration of age, gender, dietary, travel, sexual (e.g. men who sleep with men with multiple sexual partners), clinical features such as presence of abdominal pain, fever, weight loss or excessive bloody diarrhoea (dysentery), recent hospitalisation, medications (including antibiotics and laxatives), immunodeficiency and surgical history (e.g. previous bowel surgery, including bariatric) is essential.

Initial and prompt management of large-volume diarrhoea is important as the risk of dehydration, AKI and haemodynamic collapse is high, especially in the frail, older person. It is also important to prevent nosocomial transmission.

Differential diagnosis is broad and includes the following.

Bloody diarrhoea	Non-bloody/watery diarrhoea
<ul><li>Amoebic or bacillary (shigellosis) dysentery</li><li>*Campylobacter* enteritis (complicated by Guillain–Barré in 1:3000)</li><li>Diverticular disease/diverticulitis</li><li>Enterohaemorrhagic *Escherichia coli* (EHEC) infection</li><li>Inflammatory bowel disease (IBD) – ulcerative colitis (UC) more common cause than Crohn's disease (CD)</li></ul>	<ul><li>Antibiotic (healthcare) associated – *Clostridioides difficile* (*C. diff*) common</li><li>Enteral nutrition</li><li>Laxatives (including abuse)</li><li>Traveller's diarrhoea</li><li>Viral gastroenteritis (e.g. norovirus)</li><li>Miscellaneous medical disorders such as thyrotoxicosis, coeliac disease, Whipple disease, chronic pancreatitis</li></ul>

ROWS (examples): antibiotic (healthcare) associated, IBD flare, diverticulitis, colorectal cancer (especially left-sided/distal).

Initial investigations include FBC, CRP, U&E, creatinine, LFT, TFT, Ca, Mg, phosphate, HIV. Stool microscopy (leucocytes, ova, cysts and parasites), culture and sensitivity. Stool viral PCR (including COVID-19). Multistep *C. diff* testing (e.g. presence and toxin production). Faecal calprotectin (IBD – note always positive result when bloody diarrhoea of *any* cause). Imaging: abdominal XR, CT abdomen and pelvis. Sigmoidoscopy and colonoscopy can aid in diagnosis (including biopsy).

Initial management includes the following aspects.

- First, consider *red flag* features and acute life-threatening causes (i.e. ROWS), ABCDE, optimise physiology and supportive care (e.g. fluid resuscitation – oral or IV, electrolyte replacement, VTE prophylaxis). Patients should not usually be kept NBM unless surgery is imminently scheduled.
- Identify and treat potential causes.
- Withdrawal of precipitating agents (e.g. laxatives; antibiotics and PPIs with *C. diff* infection).
- Management of associated complications (e.g. AKI, toxic megacolon).
- Antidiarrhoea drugs to reduce stool frequency.
- Start stool chart documenting frequency, consistency and blood, and review daily.
- Check temperature, pulse and BP every six hours.
- Check FBC, CRP, U&E, creatinine and LFT daily.

Clostridioides (formerly *Clostridium*) *difficile* is responsible for virtually all cases of pseudomembranous colitis and is implicated in 10–25% of antibiotic (healthcare)-associated diarrhoea. Previously, metronidazole was considered the reference drug to treat *C. difficile* infection, but more recently oral vancomycin and fidaxomicin have been shown to have higher cure rates. In multiple recurrences, faecal microbiota transplantation is recommended. Consider surgical intervention for fulminant infection (risk of toxic megacolon and perforation).

Crohn's disease

Features	Illness script for Crohn's disease (CD)
Epidemiological risk factors	• White ethnicity, family history and bimodal age peaks 15–40 years and 50–60 years.
Pathophysiology	• Poorly understood, characterised by transmural inflammation. • CD may involve any or all parts of the entire GI tract from mouth to peri-anal area, although it is usually seen in the terminal ileal and perianal locations. • CD is characterised by skip lesions (where normal bowel mucosa is found between diseased areas). The transmural inflammation often leads to fibrosis causing intestinal obstruction. Perforations and fistulae can also occur.
Time course	• Acute; chronic with acute flares.
Key symptoms and signs	• Patients may have cramp or constant pain. Right lower quadrant and peri-umbilical pain is common if ileitis is present. The pain may be partially relieved by defaecation. • Crohn's colitis produces diffuse abdominal pain, which may be accompanied by mucus, blood and pus in the stool. Diarrhoea (which may be bloody) is common, including at night. • Approximately 25% of patients with CD may have perianal lesions including skin tags, fistulae, abscesses, scarring or sinuses. • Physical examination may reveal a mass in the RLQ (if ileal involvement), mouth ulcers and other signs of extraintestinal features of IBD – commonly affected organs include eyes (episcleritis more common), joints (seronegative arthritis), skin (e.g. pyoderma gangrenosum) and liver (e.g. non-alcoholic fatty liver disease).
Diagnostics	• Investigations – FBC with differential, CRP, U&E, LFT, iron studies, folate, B12, Mg, Ca, phosphate. Faecal calprotectin (denotes intestinal inflammation). Stool microscopy, culture and sensitivity. Multistep *C. difficile* testing (e.g. presence and toxin production). • Anti-*Saccharomyces cerevisiae* antibodies (ASCA) and proteinase 3 (PR3) antineutrophil cytoplasmic antibody (PR3-ANCA) can help distinguish from UC. ASCA is more common in CD, while PR3-ANCA is more common in UC. • Sigmoidoscopy, ileocolonoscopy, tissue biopsy. May need small bowel capsule endoscopy. • Imaging – abdominal X-ray, CT scan of the abdomen (in acute flare).
Treatment	Acute flare (depends on the extent of involvement and disease severity) • ABCDE, NBM, IV fluids, analgesia (avoid opiates), electrolyte replacement as needed, IV corticosteroids, antibiotics (especially if infective colitis not excluded). VTE prophylaxis – prothrombotic state. • The goal is to induce remission initially with medications, followed by the administration of maintenance medications to prevent a relapse. Chronic disease • 5-Aminosalicylates. • Locally active corticosteroids (e.g. budesonide). • Systemic corticosteroids. • Thiopurines (e.g. azathioprine, mercaptopurine). • Methotrexate. • Calcineurin inhibitors (ciclosporin, tacrolimus) • Biologic therapies (e.g. TNF-alpha inhibitors, integrin receptor antagonists, IL-12/23 antagonists). New oral small molecules treatments (e.g. tofacitinib) available. Surgical therapy • Neoplastic or preneoplastic lesions (may need colonic cancer screening if long-standing Crohn's colitis); obstructing stenoses; suppurative complications; fistulating disease; and medically intractable disease.

Ulcerative colitis

Features	Illness script for UC
Epidemiological risk factors	• Usually in younger people aged 15–30. Family history. More common in Ashkenazi Jewish descent. Smoking has been shown to protect against the development of UC.
Pathophysiology	• Poorly understood, characterised by recurring episodes of inflammation limited to the mucosal layer of the colon. It commonly involves the rectum and may extend in a proximal and continuous fashion to involve other parts of the colon. • Increased risk of colon cancer.
Time course	• Acute; chronic with acute flares.
Key symptoms and signs	• Presents as chronic diarrhoea (usually bloody) with abdominal pain and weight loss. Toxic megacolon can occur with perforation. • May have signs of extraintestinal features of IBD - commonly affected organs include eyes (uveitis and iritis more common), joints (seronegative arthritis), skin (e.g. erythema nodosum) and liver/biliary system (e.g. primary sclerosing cholangitis, cholangiocarcinoma).
Diagnostics	• Investigations: FBC with differential, CRP, U&E, LFT, PR3-ANCA (~70%). Anaemia work-up as needed. Faecal calprotectin (denotes intestinal inflammation). Stool microscopy, culture and sensitivity. Multistep *C. difficile* testing (e.g. presence and toxin production). • Sigmoidoscopy, colonoscopy, tissue biopsy. • Imaging – abdominal X-ray, CT scan of the abdomen (in acute flare).
Treatment	Acute flare (depends on the extent of involvement and disease severity) • ABCDE, NBM, IV fluids, analgesia (avoid opiates), electrolyte replacement as needed, IV corticosteroids, antibiotics (especially if infective colitis not excluded). VTE prophylaxis – prothrombotic state. Inform surgeons and stoma nurse. • Severe attack passing six or more bloody bowel motions in 24 hours plus systemic features is a medical emergency (Truelove and Witt's criteria). Seek expert help. • The goal is to induce remission initially with medications, followed by the administration of maintenance medications to prevent a relapse. • In COVID-19 era – earlier use of biologicals and movement away from immunosuppression. • If findings suggestive of toxic megacolon (daily plain abdominal X-ray should be performed and toxic megacolon is indicated by a transverse colon diameter >6 cm) – urgent surgical consultation and intervention. • Rescue therapy of steroid refractory UC with ciclosporin or infliximab should be initiated after 72 hours of steroid treatment (risk-stratify using Travis criteria). Otherwise, early colectomy may be recommended. Chronic treatment: similar in principle to CD. May need colonic cancer screening depending on disease activity and duration. Surgery: unlike CD, surgery can be *curative* for GI effects of UC.

Dizziness

Dizziness is a non-specific complaint (sensation of disturbed or impaired spatial orientation without a false or distorted sense of motion) that encompasses multiple underlying causes (Table 27.3). Hence, a detailed history to establish the exact nature of the patient's symptoms and a physical examination to differentiate the underlying causes are crucial. Medication history is essential as many commonly used drugs cause orthostatic hypotension as an adverse effect. Recent head trauma, if present, should be taken seriously as the incidence of dizziness with head injury or whiplash injuries is as high as 80%.

The differential diagnosis includes the following issues.

Table 27.3 Main categories of dizziness

	Vertigo	Unsteadiness	Presyncope	Light-headedness
Frequency	(~50%)	(~15%)	(~15%)	(~10%)
Presentation	False sensation of motion, including a spinning sensation.	Patients report feeling off-balance or 'wobbly'.	Feeling of impending faintness or loss of consciousness.	Vague symptoms, related to feeling disconnected with surrounding environment.
Differentiating and associated features	Two subtypes: peripheral and central vertigo. Exacerbated by head movement. Occasionally associated with nystagmus.	The underlying causes are many, including peripheral neuropathy, cerebellar disease or Parkinsonism, among others.	Worsened by standing upright, usually present in a patient with underlying cardiovascular disease.	Usually considered with presyncope.

Vertigo.

- Acoustic neuroma.
- Benign paroxysmal positional vertigo (BPPV) – brief episodes of vertigo provoked by changes in head position.
- Ménière's disease – recurrent attacks of vertigo, fluctuating hearing loss, and tinnitus.
- Middle ear disease.
- Migraine (vestibular migraine).
- Multiple sclerosis.
- Vertebrobasilar insufficiency (brainstem ischaemia) or stroke (e.g. consider stroke in patients with new-onset acute unilateral hearing loss and vertigo).
- Vestibular neuronitis (may include tinnitus and/or hearing impairment if labyrinthitis).

Unsteadiness.

- Ataxia.
- Multisensory impairment (e.g. frailty).
- Parkinson disease
- Peripheral neuropathy.

Presyncope/lightheadedness.

- Anaemia.
- Arrhythmias – including COVID-19 and post-COVID syndrome (e.g. postural orthostatic tachycardia syndrome, POTS).
- Carotid sinus hypersensitivity.
- Epilepsy/seizure.
- Hypoxia.
- Orthostatic hypotension (e.g. drugs, hypovolaemia, autonomic dysfunction).
- Structural heart disease.
- Transient ischaemic attack (TIA).
- Vasovagal.

Non-specific dizziness.

- Hypoglycaemia.
- Normal-pressure hydrocephalus.

ROWS (examples): vertebrobasilar insufficiency (brainstem ischaemia), arrhythmias, stroke.

Initial investigations include ECG and cardiac monitoring, BG, FBC, CRP, COVID-19, echocardiogram. Imaging as per specific concern (e.g. if suspicion of vertebrobasilar insufficiency: carotid Doppler and MR angiogram of brain and neck vessels; if progressive sensorineural hearing loss, MRI to exclude acoustic neuroma). Urgent brain imaging is always indicated when acute vertigo is accompanied by other central neurological signs (such as dysphagia, dysarthria, diplopia).

Initial management includes the following aspects.

- First, consider *red flag* features and acute life-threatening causes (i.e. ROWS), ABCDE, optimise physiology and supportive care (antiemetics).
- Identify and treat potential causes.
- Withdrawal of precipitating agents. Medications review with deprescribing as needed.
- Management of associated complications (e.g. trauma following fall).
- Vital signs (including orthostatic hypotension) and neurological status assessment (e.g. evaluation of nystagmus, Dix–Hallpike manoeuvre for diagnosis of BPPV).
- Refer to ENT (e.g. audiometry) and other specialties as required.

Dizziness is discussed fully in Chapter 24.

Falls

A fall is an *unexpected* event in which the participant comes to rest on the ground, floor or lower level *without known loss of consciousness*. Each year, approximately 282 000 patient falls are reported to the National Patient Safety Agency (NPSA). Around 40–60% of falls lead to injuries (including 5% fractures).

Falls are the leading cause of injury-related admittance to hospital in the over-65s. Most falls in older people are multifactorial.

Between 30% and 40% of community-dwelling people over the age of 65 years, and 50% of those in long-term facilities, fall each year. Multiple risk factors have been identified and are characterised into *intrinsic* (e.g. lower extremity weakness, cognitive impairment, balance problems, arthritis, orthostatic hypotension, dizziness, anaemia) and *extrinsic* (e.g. medications such as psychotropic drug use, environmental factors such as loose carpets). Other factors include history of a fall and advancing age. Medication use is one of the most readily modifiable fall risks.

Differential diagnosis includes the following.

- Accidental trip including visual impairment.
- Acute illness.
- Drug related.
- Dizziness.
- Gait disturbance.
- Immobility and instability.
- Multifactorial mobility problems.
- Neuropathy.
- Normal-pressure hydrocephalus.
- Substance misuse.

ROWS (examples): Parkinson disease, alcohol abuse (risk of withdrawal).

Initial investigations include BG, FBC, CRP, U&E, creatinine, LFTs, TFTs, 25-hydroxy vitamin D. Urine dipstick, analysis of midstream specimen of urine (MSU)/catheter specimen of urine (CSU). ECG. Holter monitoring, echocardiogram and radiological studies (e.g. head injury, chest signs) are indicated only when suggested by findings on history or examination.

Immediate management includes the following steps.

- First, consider *red flag* features and acute life-threatening causes (i.e. ROWS), ABCDE, optimise physiology and supportive care. Get eyewitness account.
- Identify and treat potential causes.
- Withdrawal of precipitating agents. Medications review with deprescribing as needed.
- Management of associated complications.
- Gait assessment.
- Vital and neurological status assessment, including orthostatic hypotension.
- Assess for any sites of injury and trauma secondary to the fall. Consider osteoporosis assessment and management.
- Comprehensive geriatric assessment.
- A multidisciplinary safety assessment before discharge should be routine in patients presenting with an acute fall, or those who have had two or more falls in the last 12 months.

Falls are discussed fully in Chapter 13.

Fever

Normal body temperature is ordinarily maintained by the thermoregulatory centre of the hypothalamus despite the effects of environmental changes. Fever (or pyrexia) is an elevation of the core body temperature above the daily range for an individual. A typical working definition is a temperature of over 38 °C.

Fever, hyperthermia and hyperpyrexia are not synonymous terms.

- Differentiating between fever and a presentation of hyperthermia is usually done with a history of heat exposure or drugs that interfere with thermoregulation, such as the recreational drug 'ecstasy'.
- Hyperpyrexia (>41.0 °C) is life threatening, which can be observed in people with severe infections, drug reactions (e.g. neuroleptic malignant syndrome), acute medication cessation in people with Parkinson disease (parkinsonism–hyperpyrexia syndrome), extreme environmental temperature, but most commonly occurs in patients with intracranial pathology (impacting on hypothalamic temperature regulation).

Fever occurs most commonly as part of an acute-phase response to infection but is also seen in several non-infectious diseases such as connective tissue disease, malignancy, drug reactions, miscellaneous causes and factitious fever. Characteristic fever patterns are well reported but in most cases are more historically interesting than clinically useful. Important historical information includes the onset, magnitude and duration of fever; any associated symptoms; recent transfusion or anaesthesia; environmental exposure to very hot weather, occupation, hobbies and animal contact; sexual history; drug abuse such as ecstasy, cocaine, amphetamines and injectable agents; travel within the past year; co-morbidities; recent medication changes; recent hospitalisations; immunosuppressive states (e.g. people with HIV, transplants) or therapies including biological therapy, chemotherapy and radiotherapy; and any implanted foreign bodies such as indwelling vascular access devices, artificial heart valves or pacemakers.

Differential diagnosis is broad and includes the following examples.

- Autoimmune causes (e.g. SLE, vasculitis).
- Endocrine causes (e.g. thyroid storm).
- Fever (pyrexia) of unknown origin (FUO or PUO).
- Heat exhaustion or heat stroke.
- Infection (e.g. bacterial, viral, fungal and parasitic).
- Malignancy.
- Medication adverse drug reaction (e.g. neuroleptic malignant syndrome, serotonin syndrome, malignant hyperpyrexia).
- Transfusion reaction.

ROWS (examples): sepsis, peritonitis, meningitis, infective endocarditis, malaria, thyroid storm.

Initial investigations include the following (depending on likely underlying cause).

- Infectious cause likely – FBC, CRP/ESR, U&E, creatinine, LFTs, lactate, procalcitonin, blood cultures (×3 if concern of infective endocarditis), hepatitis screen, COVID-19, HIV test. Urinalysis/cultures. Chest X-ray. Other imaging and investigations according to history, exam and context.
- Fever in returning traveller – malaria smear (thick and thin) ×3 or rapid diagnostic tests (RDT), FBC with differential, U&E, creatinine, LFTs, blood culture. Urinalysis and culture. Stool culture and ova, cysts and parasites (if symptoms). Serology for specific viruses, hepatitis panel, sexually transmitted infection studies if high index of suspicion. Chest X-ray. Other imaging and investigations (e.g. echocardiogram, LP) according to history, exam and context.

Initial management includes the steps described below.

- First, consider *red flag* features and acute life-threatening causes (i.e. ROWS), ABCDE, optimise physiology and supportive care (e.g. antipyretics for fever relief).
- Identify and treat potential causes.
- Withdrawal of precipitating agents. Medications review with deprescribing as needed.
- Management of associated complications (e.g. rhabdomyolysis, hyperkalaemia).
- Do not start antibiotics in the *absence* of clinical evidence of bacterial infection (unless immunocompromised). If there is evidence of bacterial infection, use the local empirical antibiotic guidelines to initiate prompt effective antibiotic treatment. Take appropriate cultures prior to initiation of antibiotic therapy if possible. Document on drug chart and in medical notes: clinical indication, duration or review date, route and dose.
- Treat sepsis as per Sepsis Six care bundle.
- Empirical antibiotic (and possibly antifungal) treatment is indicated in those who are immunocompromised.
- Patients presenting with fever and a suspected temporal (giant cell) arteritis will need immediate steroids.

Assessment of FUO

Fever of unknown origin (FUO) is defined as a temperature >38.3 °C (>100.9 °F) on several separate occasions and an appropriate initial diagnostic work-up (inpatient or outpatient) does not reveal aetiology of fever.

Causes fall into four categories.

- Infections (e.g. TB, endocarditis, occult abscesses, Whipple disease, enteric fever).
- Cancer.
- Autoimmune and autoinflammatory (e.g. periodic fever syndromes) disorders.
- Miscellaneous causes.

Fever of unknown origin is not a biologically uniform phenomenon but rather a common manifestation of multiple, disparate disease processes. There are different classifications for FUO that are based on the immune status of the host, whether the patient is hospitalised, and travel history.

Fever of unknown origin in immunocompromised patients (e.g. due to HIV infection, neutropenia or medication related) is often a difficult diagnostic problem. In immunocompromised patients, many opportunistic infections, malignancies and progression

of the disease itself require effective evaluation and management.

Diagnosis of malignancy or autoimmune disorders becomes more likely as the duration of the fever increases. Unfortunately, only 50% of cases in these groups had a definitive diagnosis in a recent series. Malignancies associated with FUO typically include leukaemias and lymphomas, renal cell carcinoma and metastatic cancers. Autoimmune disorders commonly associated with unknown fever include adult-onset Still disease, polymyalgia rheumatica, temporal (giant cell) arteritis, SLE and IBD.

Other causes of FUO include medication-induced fever, hepatitis and cirrhosis, DVT, sarcoidosis, diseases of the thyroid gland and CNS disorders. Factitious fever may also be a cause.

Evaluation of FUO

- Repeat a full systematic clinical assessment.
- Basic laboratory tests should be performed and all results re-reviewed.
- Subsequent laboratory studies, including microbiological (including TB), biochemical (including TFT), immunological (including HIV test, antinuclear antibodies and extractable nuclear antigens), haematological and targeted biopsies obtained from affected areas, should be guided by any previous abnormal laboratory or clinical findings. Seek expert help.
- CT-thorax/abdomen/pelvis (CT-TAP) should be performed. Nuclear imaging should be utilised when working up a suspected infectious (e.g. osteomyelitis) or malignant source, e.g. whole-body ^{18}F-fluorodeoxyglucose positron emission tomography and CT (FDG PET/CT scan).
- Other imaging includes echocardiogram (infective endocarditis), endoscopy (e.g. IBD) and venous Doppler (DVT).
- Review all drugs: discontinue one at a time for 72 hours and then reinstate if fever persists. Factitious fever should be excluded.
- Consider trial of NSAIDs.
- Consider informing the patient that up to 50% of cases may not have a definitive diagnosis, and advise watchful waiting.

Fever in a returning traveller

Consult an infectious disease expert at an early stage for any returning traveller with unexplained fever.

Travel, especially to emerging economies, is associated with an increased risk of infection. Fever is a common symptom of illness in returning travellers; typically, about 40% will be 'tropical' (an important minority are potentially life-threatening, such as *falciparum* malaria, or are of public health importance, such as typhoid), ~35% 'cosmopolitan' and about 25% undefined or other causes. Almost all tropical infections are treatable if identified early enough.

The aim of a travel history is to assess an individual's risk of having acquired a specific infection by establishing, where possible, an epidemiological link. A detailed geographical history and the time of onset and duration of symptoms are essential. Most tropical infections become symptomatic within 21 days of exposure and most febrile returning travellers present within one month of leaving endemic areas.

The risk of acquiring specific infections varies according to destination, setting, including whether rural or urban and type of accommodation, and activities undertaken. Individuals visiting family in developing countries are at greater risk than tourists, especially for malaria, typhoid, TB, hepatitis A and E, and sexually transmitted infections. The travel history should include details of visits to game parks, farms, caves and health facilities, consumption of exotic foods, activities involving fresh or saltwater exposure, and sexual activity. A history of contact with unwell individuals can be helpful, particularly for localised epidemics (e.g. *Legionella*), emerging infections (e.g. COVID-19 and monkeypox) or risk assessment for viral haemorrhagic fever.

Patients with certain infections require source isolation (side room, gloves, apron, mask, goggles). Local hospital guidelines should be followed. Protect yourself and others (including warning lab staff of any suspicions of certain infections). It is a statutory requirement that certain infections are notified to the local health protection unit to investigate and prevent possible outbreaks.

Common travel-related diagnoses in the UK

Acute undifferentiated febrile illnesses (AUFI) are characterised by fever of less than two weeks' duration without organ-specific symptoms at the onset. These may begin with headache, chills and myalgia. Later, specific organs may be involved. AUFIs can range from mild and self-limiting disease to progressive, life-threatening illness. The mnemonic **MA-ESR** lists the five main disease groups that cause AUFI.

- **M**alaria.
- **A**rboviral infections – such as dengue, chikungunya, Zika and yellow fever.
- **E**nteric fever.
- **S**pirochaete infections – such as leptospirosis.
- **R**ickettsial infections – including typhus.

AUFIs are classified into malarial and non-malarial illnesses with the help of microscopy or rapid diagnostic tests (RDT) for malaria.

- Malaria – should be excluded in all patients with a history of fever returning from the tropics, especially sub-Saharan Africa. Most *Plasmodium falciparum* cases present within 1–3 months of returning. All febrile patients returning from malarious areas of the tropics (within a year) should have an urgent blood film (3 thin and thick films) and/or RDT for malaria performed regardless of whether or not malaria prophylaxis has been taken. If there are features of severe malaria, treat and manage as *falciparum* malaria with IV artesunate (www.britishinfectionsociety.org).
- Although there is considerable overlap, the combination of splenomegaly, hyperbilirubinaemia and thrombocytopenia suggests malaria, the main differential diagnoses being dengue fever (<10% dengue haemorrhagic fever/shock syndrome), chikungunya and enteric fever (ceftriazone drug of choice for febrile traveller from typhoid area). These are more likely than malaria in travellers from the Indian subcontinent or Asia.
- Other common causes of undifferentiated fever.
  - Katayama syndrome (acute schistosomiasis).
  - Amoebic liver abscess.
  - Brucellosis.
  - HIV.
  - Hepatitis.

Fits/seizures

Status epilepticus is a medical emergency. Status epilepticus is a seizure that lasts longer than 10 minutes or recurrent seizures without returning to a normal level of consciousness between episodes. Mortality of approximately 20%. Intervene early in the disorder, typically when seizures have persisted beyond five minutes because the risk of permanent brain damage increases with the length of attack. Management protocols divide the medical therapy for status epilepticus into three main stages (NICE 2022).

- First-line treatment – for early status epilepticus, often administered before the patient reaches the hospital, use a benzodiazepine. However, up to a third of cases are resistant to benzodiazepines.
- Second-line treatment – if status epilepticus becomes established, use any one of the available IV preparations: phenytoin/fosphenytoin (a precursor drug to phenytoin), levetiracetam or sodium valproate given by infusion, usually in the hospital.
- Third-line treatment – for refractory status epilepticus, use an anaesthetic agent such as midazolam, propofol or thiopental.

A seizure is a sudden change in behaviour caused by abnormal electrical hypersynchronisation of neuronal networks in the cerebral cortex, which gives rise to a variety of clinical manifestations. Epilepsy is the tendency to have recurrent seizures. After a first unprovoked seizure, the overall risk of recurrence may be as high as 60% (mostly within the first two years). Epilepsy is diagnosed after two unprovoked seizures that occur more than 24 hours apart or after a single event that occurs in a person who is considered to have a high risk of recurrence (>60% risk in a 10-year period).

Seizures fall into two categories: epileptic and nonepileptic. Epileptic seizures occur spontaneously and may be provoked (i.e. triggers) or unprovoked. The presentation of a seizure depends on its site of onset (generalised or focal) and pattern of spread.

- Generalised onset – the patient's symptoms or description of the seizure by a witness do not indicate an anatomical localisation of the seizure. It is thought to start within and rapidly engage bilaterally distributed cerebral networks.

- Focal (partial) onset – most new-onset seizures in adults, including tonic–clonic seizures, are of focal onset. There is clinical evidence of seizure onset localised to one part of the brain, regardless of whether it subsequently involves the remainder of the brain. The site of onset determines the features (e.g. temporal lobe epilepsy – epigastric 'rising' sensation, *déjà vu*, and smell or taste disturbance).

Causes of epileptic seizures include brain injury, stroke, brain tumours and neurological disorders. Diagnosis is clinical and informed by abnormal brain activity on an EEG. Non-epileptic seizure causes can include fever, infection, electrolyte imbalance, drug/alcohol withdrawal, psychological conditions and hypoglycaemia.

Differential diagnosis (including some triggers) for seizures is as follows.

- Alcohol and drug withdrawal.
- Arrhythmias.
- Drug intoxication.
- Eclampsia.
- Electrolyte disturbances (e.g. hypo/hypernatraemia, hypocalcaemia, hypomagnesaemia).
- Epilepsy.
- Hypoglycaemia.
- Hypotension.
- Hypoxia.
- Meningitis/encephalitis.
- Psychogenic non-epileptic seizures (pseudoseizure).
- Stroke.
- Trauma.
- Uraemia.
- Vasovagal.

ROWS (examples): status epilepticus, eclampsia, life-threatening metabolic disturbances.

Initial investigations include ECG, BG, FBC, CRP, U&E, creatinine, LFTs, Ca, Mg, ABG, toxicology, pregnancy test. Antiepileptic drug levels. Urgent neuroimaging if suspected CNS pathology. All patients who have had a suspected focal-onset seizure should undergo detailed MRI of the head. Consider LP (may need imaging first). Immune/genetic tests.

Immediate management includes the following steps.

- First, consider *red flag* features and acute life-threatening causes (i.e. ROWS), ABCDE, optimise physiology and supportive care.
- Expert history taking is essential in the diagnosis of an epileptic seizure. Telephoning or virtually contacting an eyewitness is often invaluable, and smartphone or other video recordings of patients with seizures can help in the diagnosis.

- If status epilepticus, refer to local algorithm for management. Seek urgent help.
- Identify and treat potential causes.
- Withdrawal of precipitating agents.
- Management of associated complications.
- Admit any patient with repeated seizures or significant causative factors that require inpatient management.
- Refer to neurology and arrange 'first fit' follow-up.
- If the patient is pregnant, consider eclampsia and emergency obstetrics consultation. Emergency IV magnesium and BP control.
- Prior to discharge, inform all patients of driving regulatory requirements and to avoid activities which may be dangerous if seizure reoccurs.

The medical management of epilepsy predominantly involves seizure suppression with the long-term use of oral antiepileptic medication. The aim of management is no seizures and minimal adverse effects of treatment. However, if these goals prove to be impossible, then the priority is complete control of major convulsive seizures, which are potentially dangerous because they may increase the risk of sudden unexpected death in epilepsy (SUDEP).

First-line medication for patients with:

- focal-onset seizures – either lamotrigine or levetiracetam, although other reasonable options are available
- generalised-onset seizures – often sodium valproate, except for women of childbearing potential, in whom the preferred choice is usually levetiracetam.

Fits/seizures are discussed fully in Chapter 24.

Haematemesis and melaena

Haematemesis is defined as vomiting of bright red blood or 'coffee grounds' (blood altered by gastric acid). Melaena is defined as passage of black 'tarry' stools. Both are usually indicative of bleeding from the upper GI tract (oesophagus, stomach and duodenum up to the ligament of Treitz). Patients with brisk upper GI bleed may present with haematochezia (bright red blood per rectum). However, haematochezia is more commonly associated with lower GI bleed (85%). Malaena can be caused by small bowel or right-sided colonic lesions.

The differential diagnosis includes:

- bleeding gastric or duodenal ulcers (most common cause)
- false haematemesis: epistaxis or haemoptysis
- gastric carcinoma
- gastric erosion
- GORD (reflux of gastric contents into the oesophagus or beyond into the oral cavity)
- Mallory–Weiss tear (history of vomiting or retching before the onset of haematemesis)
- oesophageal cancer
- oesophageal varices.

ROWS (examples): upper GI bleed (e.g. secondary to oesophageal varices, bleeding peptic ulcer), oesophageal cancer.

Initial investigations include FBC, CRP, U&E, creatinine, LFT, coagulation screen, group and save (and cross-match if severe bleeding). An elevated urea with normal creatinine is suggestive of upper GI bleed.

Immediate management includes the following.

- First, consider *red flag* features and acute life-threatening causes (i.e. ROWS), ABCDE, optimise physiology and supportive care (two large-bore IV cannulas and fluid resuscitation usually with crystalloids), NBM, analgesia and antiemetic. If sick, give IV PPI *pre*-endoscopy. Use acute upper GI bleeding care bundle.
- Arrest the bleeding. Identify and treat potential causes. Key decision – is it variceal or non-variceal?
  - Non-variceal: e.g. ulcers may be treated by endoscopic injection (e.g. adrenaline), thermal coagulation or mechanical treatments.
  - Variceal (~5% of acute bleeds, but 80% of mortality). Radiological and endoscopic treatments are available. Band ligation, coil and glue injection are options to cause haemostasis of the varices. Begin terlipressin (vasoconstrictor) plus antibiotics. In the event of failed banding, a transjugular intrahepatic portosystemic shunt (TIPS) procedure may be performed. Monitor for hepatic encephalopathy.
- Urgent gastroenterology consultation for OGD and intervention if:
  - variceal
  - was stable, now unstable
  - persistently unstable.
- Withdrawal of precipitating agents if safe to do so (e.g. aspirin, NSAIDs, anticoagulants). Restart antithrombotics soon after haemostasis to avoid excess CVD mortality (seek expert help).
- Management of associated complications (e.g. shock, perforation). If haemodynamically unstable and

severe ongoing bleeding, call periarrest team, gastroenterology for urgent OGD, and transfuse blood, platelets and clotting factors immediately (activate massive transfusion protocol as needed). Target haemoglobin 70–100 g/l.

- Correct coagulopathy.
  - Administer fresh frozen plasma (FFP) to patients who are actively bleeding and have an elevated prothrombin time (or international normalised ratio) or activated partial thromboplastin time >1.5 times normal. If a patient's fibrinogen level remains <1.5 g/l despite fresh frozen plasma use, administer cryoprecipitate as well.
  - In those taking warfarin and actively bleeding, administer vitamin K and prothrombin complex concentrate (PCC). You will usually need to discuss with a haematologist before PCC is made available. Similarly, those taking direct oral anticoagulants (DOACs) should also be discussed with haematology. Consider DOAC antidotes as needed.
- Calculate Glasgow-Blatchford score to assess need for admission (i.e. score 0–1 outpatient management) and timing of OGD. Assess postendoscopy Rockall score to predict risk.
  - For those with low-risk Glasgow-Blatchford scores who were discharged from ED or SDEC, liaise with endoscopy to ensure an urgent outpatient procedure is booked and the patient informed.
  - All admitted patients should have endoscopy within 24 hours.
- Prevent or promptly recognise rebleeding. Mortality rate in GI bleeding has been reported to be as high as 10%, and the risk of death is four times as high if rebleeding occurs.
  - IV or oral PPI depending on diagnosis and risk of rebleeding.
  - Tranexamic acid does not reduce death from GI bleeding and should not be used as part of a uniform approach to treat GI bleeding.
  - Treat *H. pylori*.
  - May need interventional radiology (embolisation) or surgery.
- Patients with gastric ulcers require endoscopic follow-up at eight weeks to ensure healing.

Lower GI bleed

Lower GI haemorrhage (rectal bleeding)
- Acute lower GI bleeding includes a wide clinical spectrum, ranging from minute bleeding to massive haemorrhage with haemodynamic instability.
- Lower GI bleeding is approximately one-fifth as common as upper GI bleeding.
- The most common causes of acute lower GI bleeding, resulting in significant blood loss, are colonic diverticular disease and angiodysplasia.
- Patients with severe bleeding or significant co-morbid states require rapid identification and aggressive resuscitation.
- Haemodynamically insignificant bleeding may frequently result from haemorrhoids and colonic neoplasms. Rare causes of bleeding include solitary rectal ulcer, vasculitis and endometriosis.
- Fifteen percent of patients who present with lower GI bleeding have an upper GI source following investigation.
- Colonoscopy is the mainstay of evaluation in patients in whom anorectal or upper GI causes have been ruled out. This is performed to localise the bleeding source and enable haemostasis. Endoscopic haemostasis is successful in most cases.
- Mesenteric angiography or nuclear imaging is only performed in patients in whom colonoscopy is not feasible or where there is persistent bleeding and a negative colonoscopy. The source of bleeding cannot be definitively identified in up to 25% of patients.

Headache

Headache is among the most common medical complaints. Up to 5% of attendances to emergency departments and Acute Medicine are due to headache. 'Headache' is a symptom, not a diagnosis. Headache is classified as either primary (e.g. migraine, cluster headache) or secondary to another cause (e.g. meningitis, SAH). Even in the acute setting, the majority of cases are due to primary causes. The differentiation of benign primary headaches from life-threatening headaches is crucial and time sensitive. Life-threatening pathology is rare. The role of the Acute Medicine clinician is to take a comprehensive history and complete an examination to diagnose and treat benign headache syndromes while ruling out sinister aetiologies.

Acute headache is the onset of a new headache syndrome within the last few weeks, days, hours or even minutes. Patients with headache presenting acutely do so for several reasons.

- Have experienced a severe headache, either for the first time or unlike any previous headache.
- Have worrying associated clinical features, such as fever or focal neurological signs.
- Have chronic headache syndrome and can endure it no longer.

Diagnosis of headache in the acute care setting depends primarily on the clinician taking a thorough history, supported by a focused examination. Failure to recognise *red flags* (e.g. SNOOP4) associated with headaches can result in permanent neurological deficits, visual loss and death.

The differential diagnosis includes the following possibilities.
Primary headache.

- Cluster headache.
- Migraine.
- Tension headache.

Secondary headache.

- Acute glaucoma.
- Acute posttraumatic headache.
- Arterial hypertension.
- Carbon monoxide poisoning.
- Cerebral abscess.
- Cerebral venous thrombosis – including post-COVID-19 vaccine safety signal with adenoviral-based vectors causing vaccine-induced immune thrombotic thrombocytopenia (VITT). Unusual thromboses including cerebral venous sinus thrombosis, often with severe thrombocytopenia, that becomes clinically evident 5–30 days after vaccination.
- Idiopathic intracranial hypertension (condition of raised intracranial pressure of unknown cause).
- Medication overuse – consider in anyone taking frequent analgesia for a primary headache disorder.
- Meningitis/encephalitis.
- Raised intracranial pressure (ICP).
- Sinusitis.
- SAH.
- Temporal (giant cell) arteritis.

ROWS (examples): meningitis, SAH, temporal (giant cell) arteritis, acute glaucoma, raised ICP.

Initial investigations include FBC, CRP/ESR, BG, U&E, creatinine, LFT, Ca, phosphate, coagulation studies, blood cultures, COVID-19 and HIV test.

Imaging: brain CT or MRI (plus angiography/venography) as indicated. LP (rule out space-occupying lesion first such as in focal neurology, papilloedema, reduced GCS). Further investigations depending on the findings.

- Fever, headache plus meningism (e.g. photophobia, neck stiffness) – LP (if no contraindications).
- Unilateral temporal headache plus jaw claudication – ESR/CRP, temporal artery ultrasound and temporal artery biopsy. CT aorta or PET scan: to view distribution of vasculitis if history and signs warrant.
- Thunderclap headache reaches maximum intensity within 60 seconds to five minutes. In such cases, a CT scan of the brain and LP are necessary to exclude SAH. Send CSF for usual tests plus xanthochromia.

Initial management includes the following aspects.

- First, consider *red flag* (SNOOP4) features and acute life-threatening causes (i.e. ROWS), ABCDE, optimise physiology and supportive care. Analgesia (plus antiemetics as needed).
- Identify and treat potential causes.
- If sepsis suspected (e.g. meningococcal meningitis), Sepsis Six bundle should be initiated. Early referral to critical care.
- Giant cell (temporal) arteritis – assess severity.
  - Standard presentation: prednisolone 40–60 mg PO daily.
  - Severe presentation: IV methylprednisolone 250–500 mg OD, for three consecutive days if severe presentation (e.g. blindness, transient visual loss, stroke, stenosis, aneurysm).
  - Co-prescribe PPI (e.g. omeprazole 20 mg once daily or alternative), consider bone protection long term (e.g. calcium/vitamin D).
- Withdrawal of precipitating agents. Medications review with deprescribing as needed (e.g. analgesia-related headache).
- Management of associated complications.
- Refer to neurology or neurosurgery consultation if *red flags* present (see below).
- Primary headaches, especially migraine, are common in the acute setting – it is important to diagnose and treat these.

Red flags for serious secondary headache –
SNOOP4 *mnemonic*

- **S**ystemic symptoms and signs (e.g. fever, rigors, sweats, meningism, rash, BP >180/110 mmHg, weight loss, infection, jaw claudication and temporal artery tenderness, reduced GCS, cancer, immunosuppressed,

pregnancy, obesity, recent head trauma, COVID-19 infection or recent vaccination).
- **N**eurological symptoms and signs (e.g. focal neurological deficit, meningism, visual changes including red eye).
- **O**nset sudden (e.g. thunderclap).
- **O**nset for the first time over 50 years age.
- **P**rogressive headache. May be worst ever headache.
- **P**recipitated by Valsalva manoeuvre (e.g. cough, sneeze).
- **P**ostural relationship.
- **P**apilloedema.

Headache is discussed fully in Chapter 24.

Hyperglycaemia

Hyperglycaemic crises include DKA and hyperosmolar hyperglycaemic state (HHS). DKA is composed of hyperglycaemia and ketoacidosis (although you can get euglycaemic DKA). HHS usually has more severe hyperglycaemia due to a more gradual and chronic course but no ketoacidosis (mixed presentations can occur).

Hyperglycaemia refers to high levels of BG. The most common cause is diabetes mellitus. The majority are type 2 diabetes mellitus (T2DM) (90–95%), 5–10% type 1 diabetes mellitus (T1DM), and about 2–3% have rarer types of diabetes (e.g. monogenic defects in beta-cell function or insulin action – such as types of maturity-onset diabetes of the young). Other secondary types include diseases of the exocrine pancreas (e.g. pancreatic cancer, acute and chronic pancreatitis; cystic fibrosis-related diabetes).

The differential diagnosis of hyperglycaemia includes the following.

- Diabetes mellitus (most common).
- Exogenous and endogenous steroid-induced hyperglycaemia (drug-induced common in acute care settings).
- Gestational diabetes mellitus.
- Iatrogenic (e.g. glucose-containing fluids – dextrose infusions, enteral and parenteral feeding; medications – such as immune checkpoint inhibitors that can cause acute hyperglycaemia by inducing auto-immune type 1 diabetes phenotype).

- Overcorrection of hypoglycaemia.
- Stress hyperglycaemia.

ROWS (examples): DKA, HHS, pancreatic cancer.

Investigations include BG, glycosylated haemoglobin (HbA1c), ABG/VBG, U&E, calculation of anion gap, FBC, CRP, urinalysis, serum or urine ketones, calculate or measure plasma osmolality, diabetes-specific autoantibodies. ECG. Other tests as needed (COVID-19 testing, amylase/lipase, toxicology screen).

Initial management includes the following steps.

- First, consider *red flag* features (e.g. concerns about pancreatic cancer) and acute life-threatening causes (i.e. ROWS), ABCDE, IV fluid resuscitation, electrolyte and acidosis correction (as needed), glucose-lowering therapies (usually insulin in the in-hospital setting) and general supportive care.
- Identify and treat potential causes.
- Withdrawal of precipitating agents. Medications review with deprescribing as needed.
- Management of associated complications (e.g. ACS, infection).
- Close monitoring of BG and other parameters (e.g. electrolytes, osmolality, ketones) required.
- Diabetes specialist nurse referral.
- Discharge plan regarding hyperglycaemia required (e.g. screening for complications).

Hyperglycaemia is discussed fully in Chapter 23.

Jaundice

Jaundice can both be a symptom and a sign, usually noted as yellow pigmentation of skin, sclerae and mucous membranes when bilirubin levels are >35 µmol/l. Careful attention to history and examination should guide investigations and indicate patients at risk of deteriorating or requiring specialist care.

Jaundice is due to accumulation of bilirubin in the plasma. Bilirubin can be unconjugated (water insoluble) and conjugated by hepatocytes (water soluble).

- Unconjugated hyperbilirubinaemia, usually the result of haemolysis, results in lack of bilirubin in the urine. LFTs are otherwise normal. Total bilirubin levels of >100 µmol/l are unusual (normal <18 µmol/l).
- Hyperbilirubinaemia caused by decreased uptake/conjugation by the liver (hepatocellular) or

impaired biliary drainage (cholestasis) are both associated with abnormal LFTs and dark urine. Cholestasis describes impairment in bile formation or flow which can manifest clinically with fatigue, pruritus and jaundice. Cholestasis can be due to intrahepatic and extrahepatic causes. Deep jaundice is almost always predominantly conjugated. Pale stools – biliary obstruction prevents passage of bile into the intestinal tract for deconjugation to urobilinogen, the compound responsible for the dark colour of stool.

Differential diagnosis is very broad and includes the following possibilities.
Prehepatic (unconjugated).

- Haemolysis – hereditary and acquired (e.g. sickle cell crisis, malaria, microangiopathic haemolytic anaemia, autoimmune haemolytic anaemia).

Hepatocellular (mixed).

- Acute viral hepatitis (e.g. hepatitis A–E, cytomegalovirus, Epstein–Barr virus) – chronic disease occurs in 10% patients with hepatitis B and 80% with hepatitis C.
- Alcoholic hepatitis (Glasgow Alcoholic Hepatitis Score useful).
- Autoimmune hepatitis.
- Chronic liver disease from any cause.
- Drug-induced hepatitis (e.g. paracetamol overdose, over-the-counter agents, anabolic steroids).
- Environmental toxin exposure.
- Gilbert syndrome (benign, conjugating enzyme defect affecting 2–5% of population).
- Non-alcoholic fatty liver disease (NAFLD) – non-alcoholic steatohepatitis (NASH), the progressive form of NAFLD, has superseded hepatitis C as the main cause of cirrhosis and the main reason for liver transplantation.
- Vascular (shock) liver.
- Wilson disease (inherited disorder of copper metabolism).

Posthepatic (conjugated).

- Cancer of the head of the pancreas.
- Cholangiocarcinoma.
- Drug-induced liver injury (DILI) – most common pattern (intrahepatic obstruction).
- Gallstones.
- Primary biliary cholangitis (formerly termed primary biliary cirrhosis).
- Primary sclerosing cholangitis (associated with IBD, especially ulcerative colitis).

ROWS (examples): ascending cholangitis, fulminant acute liver failure, *falciparum* malaria, pancreatic cancer, pregnancy-related (including hepatitis E).

Investigations include FBC, blood film, reticulocyte count and Coombs' test (haemolysis); ferritin (haemochromatosis); CRP (infection/inflammation); U&E and creatinine (hepatorenal, hyponatraemia); LFT, GGT; BG (hypoglycaemia can occur with liver failure); alcohol level; COVID-19, HIV, *Leptospira* tests, hepatitis serology (infective); thick and thin blood smears (malaria); TFT (e.g. thyroid storm); antinuclear anti-smooth muscle and liver-kidney microsomal antibodies (for autoimmune hepatitis), and antimitochondrial antibodies (for primary biliary cholangitis); immunoglobulins; alpha-1-antitrypsin level; caeruloplasmin (Wilson disease); alpha-fetoprotein (AFP) (hepatocellular carcinoma); PR3-ANCA (ulcerative colitis-related primary sclerosing cholangitis); prothrombin time (PT)/international normalised ratio (INR) (liver synthetic dysfunction); ABG; paracetamol level and toxicology screen (drug-related); and pregnancy test. Blood cultures. Urinalysis (presence of bilirubin), microscopy, culture and sensitivity (infection). Liver biopsy. Ascitic tap in those with ascites – white cell count and differential, culture and fluid albumin (clue to cause of ascites and diagnosis of spontaneous bacterial peritonitis), cytology (cancer) and adenosine deaminase levels (TB ascites).

Right upper quadrant USS is the initial imaging study of choice in most patients with suspected hepatobiliary disease. USS can detect stones as small as 3 mm in diameter and is highly sensitive for detecting intra- and extrahepatic biliary dilation, but not CBD stones, also known as choledocholithiasis. Doppler ultrasound abdomen (portal vein thrombosis). Other imaging includes CT abdomen, MRCP. ERCP can be both diagnostic and therapeutic (e.g. sphincterotomy). Fibroscan for NAFLD also useful.

Patterns of LFT abnormalities

Elevation in conjugated bilirubin/total bilirubin/alkaline phosphatase is greater than the relative increase in ALT/AST in conditions that cause cholestasis/extrahepatic biliary obstruction. The converse is true in hepatocellular injury.

- Severe acute liver injury (e.g. paracetamol poisoning, acute viral hepatitis, 'shock' liver, first adult acute presentation of Wilson disease or haemochromocytosis) – elevated aminotransferases (ALT, AST) >1000 IU/l.

- o ALT > AST: most common finding (A**L**T is more 'Liver' specific).
- o If **AST**>ALT (>2:1) may be related to alcohol ('**A S**cotch and **T**onic').
- Elevation of alkaline phosphatase and GGT suggests cholestasis – either intrahepatic or extrahepatic.
- Isolated GGT elevation – suggests chronic alcohol misuse.
- Decreased serum albumin and abnormal clotting factors related to liver *synthetic* functions (not just markers of damage like transaminases). Bilirubin level is also related to *excretory* functions of the liver.

Initial management includes the following.

- First, consider *red flag* features (e.g. concerns about pancreatic cancer) and acute life-threatening causes (i.e. ROWS), ABCDE and general supportive care (e.g. monitor BG).

- Identify and treat potential causes (e.g. N-acetylcysteine for paracetamol overdose and other causes of acute liver injury).
- Withdrawal of precipitating agents. Medications review with deprescribing as needed.
- Early abdominal ultrasound to define the texture of the liver; visualise any liver tumours; define the biliary tree; establish spleen size; look for ascites; establish the patency of the portal and hepatic veins and hepatic artery.
- Management of associated complications – monitor for signs of acute or chronic liver failure such as encephalopathy, coagulopathy, hypoglycaemia, hyponatraemia, cerebral oedema, metabolic acidosis, bleeding, hepatorenal syndrome. If biliary obstruction, monitor for pancreatitis, acute cholangitis.
- If sepsis suspected, Sepsis Six bundle should be initiated.
- Close monitoring required.
- Refer to hepatology for specialist input.
- Early discussion with liver transplantation centre if no evidence of extrahepatic disease and patient deteriorating (Box 27.1). The absence of existing liver disease distinguishes acute liver failure from decompensated cirrhosis or acute-on-chronic liver failure.

Box 27.1 Types of acute liver deterioration

Acute liver failure

- Sudden and rapid deterioration in liver function on a background of 'normal' liver.
- Massive liver necrosis.
- Hyperacute <7 days: e.g. paracetamol overdose (most common cause of acute liver failure).
- Acute 8–28 days: e.g. drug-induced liver injury, acute fulminant viral hepatitis.
- Subacute 4–12 weeks: e.g. seronegative hepatitis.

Decompensation of cirrhosis (10–20% in-hospital mortality)

- Deterioration in liver function in cirrhotic, that can manifest with the following.
  - o AKI/hepatorenal syndrome.
  - o Jaundice.
  - o Increasing ascites.
  - o GI bleeding.
  - o Hepatic encephalopathy.
  - o Signs of sepsis/hypovolaemia.
- Common precipitants of decompensation – infection/sepsis (e.g. spontaneous bacterial peritonitis); GI bleeding (variceal and non-variceal); alcohol-related hepatitis; acute portal vein thrombosis; development of hepatocellular carcinoma; drugs (e.g. alcohol, opiates, NSAID); ischaemic liver injury (sepsis or hypotension); constipation (encephalopathy).

Acute-on-chronic liver failure (ACLF)

- Cirrhosis with acute decompensation accompanied by organ failure(s) and high short-term mortality.

Liver cirrhosis

> Cirrhosis develops after a long period of inflammation that results in replacement of the healthy liver parenchyma with fibrotic tissue and regenerative nodules, leading to portal hypertension. The disease evolves from an asymptomatic phase (compensated cirrhosis) to a symptomatic phase (decompensated cirrhosis), the complications of which often result in hospitalisation, impaired quality of life and high mortality. Progressive portal hypertension, systemic inflammation and liver failure drive disease outcomes.

Cirrhosis is common, affecting ~1–2% of UK population. The majority are undiagnosed. Major aetiological factors are alcohol, NAFLD and viral hepatitis. Decompensated cirrhosis is a common reason for hospital admission, with ~80% of admissions due to alcohol-related liver disease.

Decompensated cirrhosis is a complex disorder affecting multiple systems and therefore requires a systematic approach to its management (use decompensated cirrhosis care bundle).

- Address underlying cause (e.g. lose weight and address cardiovascular risk factors with NAFLD).
- Every year, 1–4% of patients with cirrhosis will develop hepatocellular carcinoma. Screen every six months with USS and AFP for hepatocellular carcinoma.
- Vaccination (influenza, pneumococcal, COVID-19, hepatitis A, hepatitis B).
- Patients with cirrhosis are effectively immunosuppressed, so infections are one of the most common reasons for hepatic decompensation. External factors include the overuse of PPIs, alcohol intake, frailty, multiple antibiotic courses, and repeated hospital admissions and invasive procedures. Approximately two-thirds of patients with cirrhosis and extrahepatic organ failure have sepsis. High mortality has also been observed among patients with cirrhosis who have severe COVID-19 infection. Have a high index of suspicion for infection and low threshold for empirical broad-spectrum antibiotics or other therapies. Gram negatives and enteric bacteria most common (cirrhotics have a leaky gut). This can lead to spontaneous bacterial peritonitis (SBP), defined as a bacterial infection of the ascitic fluid, without any identifiable, intra-abdominal, surgically treatable source of infection.
  - SBP can present with abdominal pain and fever in the presence of ascites. However, it is often asymptomatic, and any patient admitted with clinically detectable ascites and decompensated liver disease should have a diagnostic ascitic tap performed on admission. SBP is confirmed by finding an ascitic fluid polymorphonuclear count of >250/mm³ (0.25×10^9/l) or positive fluid culture.
  - AKI develops in up to 40% of patients with SBP, and administration of IV albumin 1.5 g/kg on day 1 and 1 g/kg on day 3 (given as 20% human albumin solution) can significantly reduce the risk of developing hepatorenal syndrome (HRS).
- Ascites is accumulation of fluid in the abdomen due to portal hypertension. It manifests as an increase in abdominal circumference with abdominal discomfort. It is the most common complication of cirrhosis.
  - If large-volume ascites: therapeutic paracentesis or transjugular intrahepatic portosystemic shunt (TIPS, for refractory ascites). IV albumin replacement (100 ml 20% albumin for every 2.5 l drained) should be given at the time of paracentesis to reduce the risk of precipitating HRS. The patient should then be started on diuretics. Monitor for severe encephalopathy when TIPS performed (overt encephalopathy in 10–50% of patients after placement of TIPS).
  - For mild-to-moderate ascites: no added salt diet; reduce fluid intake (1.5 l/day); initiate spironolactone 50–100 mg once daily; add furosemide 40 mg if not mobilising ascites after 7–14 days. Daily weights – aim to lose 0.5–1 kg/day maximum. Can increase in a stepwise manner up to spironolactone 400 mg and furosemide 160 mg (usually maintain ratio of 100 mg spironolactone:40 mg furosemide) – very few patients tolerate this. Close monitoring of U&E until ascites controlled, and diuretics reduced.
- GI bleeding in a cirrhotic patient should be assumed to be from varices until proven otherwise and treated with terlipressin and IV antibiotics. Correct coagulopathy. Restrictive blood transfusion strategy is recommended. Urgent endoscopy should be performed. Non-selective beta-blocker (e.g. carvedilol or propranolol) for secondary prevention of variceal bleed. Antibiotics are required long term.

- Hepatic encephalopathy refers to the range of neurological abnormalities seen in patients with cirrhosis. Common findings include reversed sleep/wake cycle, personality changes and lack of awareness. Asterixis, focal neurological signs and ultimately coma can occur. It is a diagnosis of exclusion after assessing for other causes of altered mental status (e.g. CT head to exclude subdural haematoma, cerebral oedema). Serum ammonia levels do not aid the diagnosis of hepatic encephalopathy in cirrhotic patients presenting acutely. Staging of hepatic encephalopathy is via the West Haven criteria (i.e. consciousness, intellect and behaviour, neurological findings). Mainstay of treatment of acute hepatic encephalopathy involves correcting the precipitant and encouraging elimination of toxins.
  - Lactulose 20 ml three times daily (titrate dose to achieve at least two loose stools/day), via nasogastric tube if necessary.
  - The non-absorbable antibiotic rifaximin can be added if the patient fails to respond to laxatives.
- Long-term abstinence from alcohol is the most important prognostic factor in patients with alcohol-related hepatitis and every effort should be made to help patients achieve this. Specific treatment of alcohol-related hepatitis should be considered if the patient's Maddrey discriminant function, a widely used prognostic score for alcohol-related hepatitis, is >32, as this predicts an increased risk of early mortality. Prednisolone may have a modest impact on short-term mortality, but infection must be ruled out before using. If steroids are used, calculate the Day 4 Lille score to see if they are having an impact so that they can be stopped earlier to reduce risk of infection.
- AKI is common in patients with decompensated cirrhosis, with approximately 20% of patients affected. It is often multifactorial. Diuretics and nephrotoxins should be held. Other intrinsic causes of renal dysfunction should be excluded. Seek expert help.
  - HRS diagnostic criteria: 1. cirrhosis with ascites; 2. no response after two days of diuretic withdrawal and volume expansion with albumin (1 g/kg/day); 3. absence of shock; 4. no current or recent nephrotoxic drugs; 5. no macroscopic signs of structural kidney injury (e.g. no proteinuria, haematuria, normal renal USS).
  - Treatment of HRS includes vasoconstriction of systemic and splanchnic circulation to improve effective circulating volume and renal perfusion.
- Malnutrition and, consequently, sarcopenia and physical frailty parallel the severity of cirrhosis. All patients should have a nutritional assessment. Refeeding syndrome is a common complication, so phosphate, K^+ and Mg should be monitored daily. Pabrinex® (IV thiamine) should be given.
- Liver transplant is the only cure.
- Consider palliative/end-of-life referral if transplantation is not an option. Paracetamol (acetaminophen) is the safest pain reliever in patients with cirrhosis. Limit intake to <2 g/day. Avoid NSAIDs, particularly in patients with ascites. Avoid opioids, particularly in patients with hepatic encephalopathy.

Peritoneal fluid analysis is performed essentially to answer two questions.

1 What is the cause of the ascitic fluid accumulation?

2 Is the fluid infected or not (e.g. SBP)?

The single best test for determining whether ascites is due to portal hypertension is the SAAG (serum to ascites albumin gradient), which is calculated by subtracting the ascites albumin level from the serum albumin level.

- A gradient of >11 g/l is consistent with portal hypertension.
- If the SAAG is <11 g/l, another cause such as malignancy (e.g. ovarian), TB or nephrotic syndrome should be sought.

Lethargy

Lethargy is physical and/or mental exhaustion. Acute lethargy is generally <2 weeks duration. Common and often non-specific complaint. History is key to determine what is meant by the person complaining of 'lethargy' (e.g. dyspnoea, weakness, excessive sleepiness, lack of energy, general debility and any concealed concerns). Only then can a more focused assessment and specific management plan be created.

Differential diagnosis is very broad and includes the following possibilities.

- Connective tissue disorders.
- Electrolyte imbalance (e.g. hyponatraemia, hypercalcaemia).
- Haematological causes (e.g. anaemia, leukaemia).
- Infectious causes (e.g. sepsis, TB, HIV, Lyme disease, COVID-19 and post-COVID syndromes).
- Liver disease (e.g. acute or chronic hepatitis).
- Malignancy and effects of treatment and complications.

- Medication related (e.g. antidepressants, antiseizure medication).
- Metabolic causes (e.g. hypothyroidism, hyperthyroidisim, hypopituitarism, adrenal insufficiency, diabetes mellitus).
- Mood disorder (e.g. depression).
- Myalgic encephalomyelitis (or encephalopathy)/ chronic fatigue syndrome (ME/CFS).
- Renal disease (e.g. advanced CKD).
- Rheumatological (e.g. vasculitis).
- Sleep apnoea.
- Substance abuse (e.g. alcohol).

ROWS (examples): adrenal insufficiency, malignancy, sepsis, severe hyponatraemia.

Investigations include FBC, CRP, U&E, creatinine, LFT, TFT (myxoedema), BG, HbA1c, cortisol and short adrenocorticotropin hormone (ACTH) stimulation test (adrenal insufficiency), Ca, creatine kinase (muscle weakness/inflammation), COVID-19, HIV and pregnancy test. ECG (heart block or other abnormalities). Urinalysis. If dyspnoea is the primary complaint – BNP, echocardiogram and CXR (fluid overload). Oxygen saturation at rest and on exertion. Sleep apnoea studies. Other imaging as needed.

Initial management includes the following steps.

- First, consider *red flag* features and acute life-threatening causes (i.e. ROWS), ABCDE, optimise physiology and supportive care.
- Identify and treat potential causes.
- Withdrawal of precipitating agents. Trial of medicine discontinuation and restart at lower dose or alternative therapy.
- Management of associated complications.
- After appropriate investigations, diagnosis may be ME/CFS, long COVID (fatigue often accompanied by breathlessness, palpitations, chest pain and 'brain fog') or others.

> Around 2 million people in the UK were estimated to be experiencing long COVID symptoms over a four-week period ending 1st May 2022. Most common symptom was fatigue (55%).

Anaemia

> In the hospital setting, most anaemia will be related to acute and chronic blood loss, anaemia of inflammation or anaemia of kidney disease.

The normal lifespan of human erythrocytes (red blood cells) is about 120 days. Anaemia is a pathological state resulting in an insufficient number of erythrocytes to deliver oxygen to the organs and tissues. Anaemia can arise from blood loss, underproduction, destruction (acute and chronic haemolysis) or a combination of factors. Symptoms generally reflect degree and speed of onset of development, as well as the presence or absence of underlying organ or vascular disease. Other pathological states can affect anaemia.

- Erythropoietin produced by the kidneys in response to hypoxia (e.g. anaemia of kidney disease related to advanced CKD and ESRD).
- Deficiency of iron, cobalamin (B12) and folate results in decreased haemoglobin (Hgb) production.
- Chronic disease (e.g. inflammatory states such as rheumatoid arthritis and SLE; IBD; chronic infections, including TB) can lead to anaemia of inflammation. This is due to defective absorption of iron from the gut, and inadequate release of iron to erythrocyte precursors in the bone marrow (despite iron stores being preserved in marrow macrophages). This is due to increased hepcidin production (key peptide involved in iron regulation) causing ferroportin deficiency. Thus, anaemia of inflammation is primarily a disorder of iron distribution.

The severity of the anaemia can be identified by the FBC and blood film (Table 27.4). Diagnostic schemas are mental flowcharts or algorithms that allow clinicians to systematically approach a clinical problem such as anaemia, organised in a logical framework by clinically meaningful variables like size of the red blood cells, i.e. microcytic, normocytic or macrocytic, which can narrow the differential diagnosis. In addition, the reticulocyte count reflects the bone marrow response to anaemia. Patients with iron, B12 or folate deficiency or those with bone marrow problems (e.g. myelodysplasia or aplastic anaemia) will have deficient reticulocyte response. Bone marrow aspirate may be needed to clarify the diagnosis, especially if there are deficiencies in other blood lines (decreased platelets, white cells) or abnormal cells (e.g. blasts).

The differentiation and proliferation to mature blood cells from haematopoietic multipotent stem cells occurs in a tightly regulated, orderly manner.

- Bone marrow failure syndromes are characterised by the failure of haematopoiesis leading to peripheral cytopenias – anaemia, leucopenia/ neutropenia and/or thrombocytopenia. In the case of fever and neutropenia, prompt antibiotic treatment is critical as neutropenic sepsis can be life-threatening if left untreated.

Table 27.4 Basic FBC interpretation

Haemoglobin (Hgb)	• Low levels indicate an anaemia. • High levels generally indicate dehydration or true polycythaemia.
Red blood cell (RBC) count	The number of RBCs in the blood (low in anaemia and high in dehydration or polycythaemia).
Haematocrit (HCT)	The fraction (% of total blood volume) that is RBCs – low in anaemia and high in dehydration or polycythaemia. Generally, for each increase/decrease in Hgb by 10 g/l, the HCT alters by ~3% respectively.
Mean cell/corpuscular volume (MCV)	The average volume of red cells (= HCT/RBC). • High in macrocytic anaemias (e.g. B12/folate deficiency, alcoholism). • Low in microcytic anaemias (e.g. Fe deficiency, thalassaemia).
Red cell distribution width (RDW)	A measure of the range of size of red cells. • High when there are mixed populations of cell size (e.g. mixed anaemias such as B12, folate and iron deficiency due to malabsorption). • Normal RDW with anaemia suggests thalassaemia.
Platelets	Thrombocytopenia. • Decreased production (e.g. marrow suppression). • Increased destruction (e.g. autoimmune, disseminated intravascular coagulation, splenomegaly). Thrombocytosis. • Essential. • Reactive (e.g. infection, inflammation, trauma).
White cell count (WCC)	• Leucopenia (e.g. marrow disorders, drugs especially cytotoxics, infection). • Leucocytosis (e.g. infection, inflammation, malignancy). • Useful to consider the differential (i.e. which specific cells are affected).

- Acute leukemias, either myeloid (AML) or lymphoid (ALL) in origin, are aggressive clonal neoplasms in which cells lose the ability to differentiate into mature cells. Acute leukaemia should be considered in any patient with significant leucocytosis, isolated cytopenia, pancytopenia or where blasts are present on the blood film. This leads to anaemia, thrombocytopenia and functional neutropenia secondary to bone marrow replacement by abnormal clonal precursor cells. If left untreated, it is life-threatening and can lead to death within weeks. In adults, AML is more common than ALL. These disorders require urgent evaluation and treatment.
  - Patients with very high white cell counts (hyperleucocytosis) are at risk of leucostasis where the blast cell count is extremely elevated, often >100 × 10⁹/l, with microvasculature blockage causing reduced tissue perfusion. Signs and symptoms of leucostasis include shortness of breath and hypoxia, and neurological impairment such as visual disturbance, headache, dizziness, confusion and risk of intracranial haemorrhage. This

is a medical emergency and urgent treatment with leucapheresis is needed to lower the white cell count.
  - The treatment for acute promyelocytic leukaemia (APML), an aggressive subtype of AML that commonly presents with severe disseminated intravascular coagulopathy, involves all-trans-retinoic acid and is curable in 90% of patients.
- Myelodysplastic syndromes are clonal stem cell disorders with ineffective haematopoiesis leading to dysplastic, hypercellular bone marrow and peripheral blood cytopenias. They also carry the risk of progression to AML.
- Myeloproliferative neoplasms are clonal stem cell disorders characterised by proliferation of the components of the myeloid (chronic myeloid leukaemia, CML), erythroid (polycythaemia vera) and platelets (essential thrombocythaemia). Characteristic genetic changes are often seen in these conditions (e.g. *JAK2* positivity in polycythaemia vera and essential thrombocythaemia; and Philadelphia chromosome – *BCR-ABL* fusion – in CML). These genetic changes allow targeted

therapies (e.g. tyrosine kinase inhibitors bind to *BCR-ABL* oncogene and prevent downstream signalling).

Anaemia of inflammation and iron deficiency anaemia are the two most common anaemias worldwide, and they often co-exist in people who live in countries with a high prevalence of nutritional deficiencies and infections. Causes of anaemia include the following.

- Microcytic anaemia (MCV <76 fl) – iron deficiency is the most prevalent nutritional deficiency and a major precipitant of microcytic, hypochromic anaemia. Nearly 1.2 billion people suffer from iron deficiency anaemia. Iron deficiency can also be due to chronic blood loss, as well as malabsorption of iron (e.g. coeliac disease). Ferritin is an indicator of iron stores. Ferritin is an acute-phase reactant that is increased in serum during acute and chronic inflammation. Subsequently, in these inflammatory states, other measures of iron deficiency may be used (e.g. transferrin saturation <20%). Functional iron deficiency occurs with anaemia of inflammation (body iron stores adequate but cannot be released to RBC precursors in bone marrow due to hepcidin). Investigations include searching for causes of iron deficiency (e.g. blood loss, malabsorption, inflammatory states) and treating appropriately. Oral iron is the first-line treatment for iron deficiency. Newer formulations of IV iron are much safer than older formulations and should be used where oral iron is poorly tolerated or ineffective.
  - Other causes of microcytic anaemia include thalassaemia (inherited disorder of erythrocyte production). Avoid excess iron supplementation in patients with thalassaemia (risks of iron overload).
- Macrocytic anaemia (MCV >100 fl) – raises suspicion of cobalamin (B12) and/or folate deficiency. It requires prompt testing of serum B12 and folate levels. Holotranscobalamin (functional form of B12) can also be measured in situations of indeterminate or borderline B12 results. An elevated serum methylmalonic acid level reflects tissue cobalamin stores and can confirm deficiency or sufficiency in borderline cases (homocysteine is elevated in both B12 and folate deficiency). Other haematological findings in B12 deficiency include mild leucopenia, thrombocytopenia, pancytopenia and hypersegmented neutrophils. Causes of B12 deficiency include nutritional, drug induced and gastrointestinal; autoimmune pernicious anaemia (antibodies to intrinsic factor) is less common. Folate acts synergistically with B12 for its cellular function, and so

it should be checked and corrected accordingly. B12 and folate deficiency can co-exist, particularly in situations of malabsorption or severe nutritional deficiency. Treatment of B12 deficiency is generally started with oral formulation even in patients with malabsorption (parenteral can also be given). Folate is given orally. Do not treat folate deficiency until B12 deficiency has been treated or excluded, because neurological complications of B12 deficiency can continue to worsen despite improved blood findings.

- Normocytic anaemia (normal MCV) – includes patients with anaemia of inflammation. Measure B12, folate and iron studies. Treat underlying condition. Iron replacement is generally ineffective, although supplemental erythropoietin improves anaemia. For example, target haemoglobin for people with advanced CKD/ESRD receiving erythropoietin stimulating agents is 100–120 g/l (higher levels associated with worsening hypertension, and thrombotic complications).

Haemolytic anaemia is a process that occurs due to the premature destruction of red blood cells. Check blood film (red cell fragments), thick and thin blood film (malaria parasites), Coombs' test (direct antiglobulin test [DAT]), haptoglobin (decreased), LDH (increased), electrophoresis/enzymes, increased unconjugated bilirubin and reticulocyte response (increased). When further approaching haemolytic anaemia, subdividing patients into those who are 'DAT positive' (immune) or 'DAT negative' (non-immune) is a simple way to build a differential diagnosis for the haemolytic anaemia.

- Immune causes – include autoimmune haemolytic anaemia, drugs and delayed haemolytic transfusion reactions.
- Non-immune causes include:
  - congenital problems such as haemoglobinopathies (e.g. sickle cell disease), membrane problems (spherocytosis) and enzyme defects
  - acquired causes such as microangiopathic haemolytic anaemias (e.g. disseminated intravascular coagulation, haemolytic uraemic syndrome and thrombotic thrombocytopenic purpura), infections (e.g. malaria) and splenomegaly (site of erythrocyte breakdown).

Pigment gallstones (chronic haemolysis), high-output cardiac failure and VTE can occur in haemolytic states. Parvovirus B19 is cytotoxic to erythrocyte precursors, causing transient pure red cell aplasia in patients with chronic haemolysis (e.g. sickle cell disease) who can have significant anaemia.

Sickle cell disease

Sickle cell disease is a common inherited disorder prevalent in black patients and can affect nearly every organ system. Characterised by vaso-occlusive crises due to sickling of erythrocytes because of abnormal haemoglobin S that polymerises in hypoxic conditions, forming insoluble, rod-like structures that aggregate and deform the red cell membrane. This leads to acute and chronic end-organ damage (e.g. strokes, avascular necrosis, multiorgan failure). Hydroxyurea decreases acute pain events, acute chest syndrome or stroke, and prolongs survival. Life-long penicillin V and vaccination against meningococcus, pneumococcus and *Haemophilus influenzae* B aim to prevent infection with encapsulated organisms (functional asplenism). COVID-19 and annual influenza vaccination should be encouraged, and folic acid replacement.

The most common type of sickle cell crisis presents as agonising and relentless pain. The pain may be localised to a single long bone, present symmetrically in several limbs, or involve the axial skeleton (lumbar spine, ribs or pelvis). Achieving fast and adequate pain control is the priority. Supportive care includes oxygen (oxygen saturations above 94%); IV fluids if not orally maintaining adequate hydration; broad-spectrum antibiotics if signs of infection (asplenism increases susceptibility to infection with encapsulated organisms such as *Streptococcus pneumoniae* and *Haemophilus influenzae* B). Avoid transfusions in patients with sickle cell disease and uncomplicated pain crises or chronic anaemia.

Chest crisis is a life-threatening acute complication of sickle cell disease and may follow the onset of a painful crisis. Clinical markers of severity in chest crisis include rising respiratory rate, worsening hypoxia, thrombocytopenia, progressive anaemia, multilobar involvement on chest X-ray and neurological impairment.

Full top-to-toe assessment and investigation are needed when pain control allows. Urgent haematology review and early consideration of escalation to critical care.

Beware individual and structural racism and other forms of discrimination.

Vasculitis

Vasculitides are defined by inflammation of blood vessels leading to bleeding and compromise of the lumen, resulting in downstream tissue ischaemia and necrosis. In general, affected vessels vary in size, type and location in association with the specific type of vasculitis. Vasculitis may occur as a primary process or may be secondary to another underlying disease. The first consideration in classifying cases of vasculitis is the size of the major vessels involved: large, medium, or small.

- Large vessel (e.g. giant cell arteritis).
- Medium vessel (e.g. polyarteritis nodosa).
- Small vessel.
  - Antineutrophil cytoplasmic antibody (ANCA)-associated vasculitis (AAV).
  - IgA vasculitis (Henoch–Schönlein purpura).
  - Antiglomerular basement membrane disease (antibasement membrane autoantibodies with lung involvement typically cause pulmonary haemorrhage, and renal involvement causes glomerulonephritis with necrosis and crescents).

Antineutrophil cytoplasmic antibody-associated vasculitis is a small to medium vessel vasculitis associated with excess morbidity and mortality. It affects men and women from a wide age spectrum and diverse ethnic backgrounds. It is characterised by multisystem organ involvement. The most commonly affected organs include the respiratory tract, eyes, kidneys, skin and nervous system. ANCA target antigens include PR3 and myeloperoxidase (MPO), which usually correspond to cytoplasmic ANCA (cANCA) and perinuclear ANCA (pANCA), respectively. ANCA is associated with a variety of disorders.

- Granulomatosis with polyangiitis (GPA, formerly Wegener granulomatosis) – majority have PR3-ANCA. Common clinical manifestations include destructive sinonasal lesions, pulmonary nodules and glomerulonephritis.
- Microscopic polyangiitis (MPA) – majority have MPO-ANCA. Associated with rapidly progressive pauci-immune glomerulonephritis (extensive glomerular inflammation with few or no immune deposits that may result in rapid decline in renal function) and alveolar haemorrhage.

- Eosinophilic granulomatosis with polyangiitis (EGPA, Churg–Strauss) – both PR3- and MPO-ANCA types can occur. Clinical features include asthma, peripheral eosinophilia and peripheral neuropathy.
- Drug-induced ANCA-associated vasculitis – mostly MPO-ANCA.

Phenotyping patients according to ANCA type (i.e. PR3-ANCA positive or MPO-ANCA positive), rather than as GPA or MPA, may better identify homogeneous groups that share similar genetics, pathogenesis, organ involvement and response to treatment.

Disease management includes the following aspects.

- Induction – usually high-dose glucocorticoids (e.g. IV pulse methylprednisolone 500–1000 mg/day for three days) plus rituximab (preferred) or cyclophosphamide.
- Maintenance of remission. A personalised approach to maintenance of remission should be based on patient-specific (e.g. pregnancy) and disease-specific factors (e.g. renal, respiratory, upper airway involvement) versus the effects of long-term immunosuppression (e.g. opportunistic infection, malignancy risk).
- Management of associated complications.

> Fatigue is one of the major complaints related to vasculitis and negatively impacts quality of life. Fatigue can be multifactorial, including sleep disturbance and pain.

Limb pain and swelling

Patients mainly present with lower limb signs and symptoms, but upper limb presentations also occur and should be investigated and managed in a similar way.

Can be unilateral or bilateral.

- Bilateral swelling of the legs usually indicates oedema due to cardiac, renal or liver disease resulting in fluid overload. Both liver and renal disease can also lead to low albumin states with decreased osmotic pressure.
- Unilateral swelling is more likely to be due to trauma, infection, venous or lymphatic obstruction.

Differential diagnosis includes the following.

- AKI and CKD/ESRD.
- Cellulitis.

- Compartment syndrome.
- CHF.
- DVT.
- Hypoproteinaemia (e.g. liver failure, nephrotic syndrome).
- Hypothyroidism.
- Lymphoedema.
- Medications (e.g. calcium channel blockers).
- Necrotising fasciitis.
- Pelvic mass.
- Right heart failure.
- Sickle cell crisis (causes limb pain).
- Thrombophlebitis.
- Trauma.
- Venous hypertension

ROWS (examples): compartment syndrome, DVT, fluid overload, necrotising fasciitis, pelvic mass.

Investigations include FBC and film (sickle cell crisis), CRP, D-dimer, U&E, creatinine, LFT (hypoalbuminaemia), TFT (myxoedema), BG (neuropathy, nephropathy, CHF), BNP (heart failure), CK (myalgia, myositis), COVID-19 (hypercoagulable state), pregnancy test and blood culture. Urinalysis and urine ACR. X-ray of limb (history of trauma). CXR (fluid overload). Echocardiogram (heart failure, VTE). Limb venous Doppler USS. Abdominal/pelvic imaging (e.g. mass, bilateral DVT, lymphoedema).

Initial management includes the following steps.

- First, consider *red flag* features and acute life-threatening causes (i.e. ROWS), ABCDE, optimise physiology and supportive care. Analgesia.
- Identify and treat potential causes.
- Withdrawal of precipitating agents. Medications review with deprescribing as needed. Review after trial discontinuation or dose reduction.
- Management of associated complications.
- Sepsis Six care bundle if sepsis suspected.
- If compartment syndrome or necrotising fasciitis – urgent surgical review.

> *Common causes of limb pain and swelling*
>
> Lymphoedema.
>
> - Generally painless, but patients may experience a chronic dull, heavy sensation in the leg.
> - In the early stages of lymphoedema, the oedema is soft and pits easily with pressure.
> - In the chronic stages, the limb has a 'woody' texture and the tissues become indurated and fibrotic – lymphoedema is non-pitting.

Cellulitis.

- Cellulitis is an acute inflammatory condition due to spreading bacterial infection of the deep subcutaneous tissue of the skin characterised by localised pain, erythema, swelling and heat. May have systemic features (e.g. pyrexia, malaise or rigors).

DVT.

- Classic symptoms of DVT include swelling, pain and discoloration in the affected extremity.
- Examination reveals increased leg circumference and oedema.
- Can be bilateral.

Venous insufficiency.

- Following DVT, the valve leaflets are incapable of preventing retrograde flow of blood so the vein becomes rigid and thick-walled. Although veins may recanalise after an episode of thrombosis, some may remain occluded. Similar findings with varicose veins and resultant venous hypertension.
- There are often prominent varicosities, erythema, dermatitis and hyperpigmentation (due to haemosiderin deposition) along the distal aspect of the leg, and skin ulceration may occur near the medial and lateral malleoli.

Deep vein thrombosis

Thrombosis – basic terminology

- Coagulation – blood changes from liquid to blood clot (thrombus). Normally: CLOT formation = CLOT breakdown.
- Thrombosis occurs when blood clots block the blood vessels.

- Venous thromboembolism (VTE) refers to blood clots in the veins.
  - DVT occurs when a blood clot forms in a deep vein. These clots usually develop in the lower leg, thigh or pelvis, but they can also occur in the arm.
  - PE refers to when a clot breaks off and travels through the bloodstream to the lungs.
  - Other sites affected by VTE include other venous beds (e.g. hepatic, portal, splanchnic, cerebral veins).
- Arterial thrombosis refers to a blood clot in an artery. This type of blood clot can cause ACS or stroke.
- Thrombophilia – refers to increased tendency to form thromboses.
  - Acquired, usually >50 years of age.
  - Inherited, usually <50 years of age: most common is factor 5 Leiden gene mutation leading to activated protein C (APC) resistance. Antithrombin, protein C and S deficiencies (all natural anticoagulants) – affected subjects most likely to have recurrent thromboses.
  - Usually, there is a combination of several prothrombotic factors in any given individual.
  - Thrombophilia evaluation should not be performed in most patients with acute VTE. Most testing is performed after *stopping* anticoagulant if safe to do so (apart from gene mutations which can be checked at any time).
- Reduce thrombotic events by inhibiting:
  - platelet aggregation (i.e. *antiplatelet* agents)
  - coagulation (i.e. *anticoagulants*).
- Eventually, thrombus dissolution (fibrinolysis) occurs, initiated by tPA conversion of plasminogen into plasmin, which breaks down fibrin and thrombus. tPA (e.g. alteplase) can be used as a *thrombolytic* agent.

Features	Illness script for DVT
Epidemiological risk factors	• Approximately half of all new VTEs are diagnosed during or within three months of a hospital stay or surgical procedure. History of immobilisation, obesity (metabolic syndrome), oral contraceptive, malignancy, family or personal history of VTE disease, thrombophilia. COVID-19 infection results in a hypercoagulable state. • Antiphospholipid syndrome – disorder of the immune system that causes an increased risk of venous and arterial blood clots (and miscarriage in pregnancy).
Pathophysiology	• Virchow's triad: vascular endothelial damage, venous stasis and hypercoagulability. • DVT is the formation of a blood clot in a deep vein (e.g. legs, thigh, pelvis, abdomen or arm).

Features	Illness script for DVT
Time course	• Acute (chronic complications can occur).
Key symptoms and signs	• Unilateral or bilateral leg swelling, tenderness and redness or discoloration.

Diagnostics	• Calculate Wells score if suspected DVT.
	  o If ≥2, arrange compression ultrasound scan to confirm/refute diagnosis.
	  o If <2, perform D-dimer test. If negative, DVT excluded. If positive – arrange compression ultrasound scan.
	• Investigations for predisposing cause(s).

Treatment	• ABCDE, analgesia, supportive care.
	• All patients with VTE should receive anticoagulant treatment in the absence of absolute contraindications. Initial anticoagulant treatment is crucial for reducing mortality, preventing early recurrences and improving long-term outcome.
	• Anticoagulation with either:
	  o DOAC: preferred. Avoid in pregnancy – use LMWH, or
	  o heparin (unfractionated heparin or LMWH) for three days while starting warfarin – bridge to warfarin (vitamin K antagonist anticoagulant).
	  o Duration: three months if transient provoking factor (extended if persistent risk factor or unprovoked).
	• <10% VTE will require thrombolysis (e.g. massive PE, with a minority having proximal limb-threatening DVT) or interventional radiology or surgery.

Necrotising fasciitis

> Necrotising fasciitis is a life-threatening, rapidly progressive invasive soft tissue infection involving subcutaneous fat and deep fascia layers. The rapid tissue necrosis often leads to systemic sepsis, toxic shock-like syndrome and multiorgan failure. The mortality of necrotising fasciitis is reported to be 15–30%.

Necrotising fasciitis typically begins as an area of inflamed, swollen skin, with or without a history of recent local trauma. In necrotising fasciitis, pain may be disproportionately severe compared to the limited visible extent of infection. Conversely, as infection progresses, there may be new-onset local anaesthesia, presumably related to necrosis of nerve fibers. Necrotising fasciitis can be accompanied by fever and crepitus, but spontaneous drainage and pus are usually not present. As the infection progresses, bullae, petechiae, ecchymoses, purplish coloration and skin lesions resembling deep burns may develop.

Necrotising fasciitis can involve almost any part of the body (classically involving the perineum in persons with diabetes, termed Fournier gangrene), including the foot in cases with pre-existing ulcers. Scoring systems using clinical findings and blood tests, as well as CT, may aid in suspected necrotising fasciitis, but direct examination of the involved tissues is usually necessary to make a definitive diagnosis.

Treatment of necrotising fasciitis requires rapid fluid and electrolyte corrections, haemodynamic stabilisation, support for failing organ systems and appropriate parenteral antibiotic therapy. In general, consider broad-spectrum agents, such as piperacillin-tazobactam, or carbapenems, often with concomitant clindamycin, or vancomycin if methicillin-resistant *Staphylococcus aureus* (MRSA) is suspected. In addition, early aggressive surgical debridement (often repeated to ensure all necrotic tissue has been removed) is usually necessary.

Joint swelling

Limb pain and swelling can also be caused by acute joint swelling. Swelling may arise from periarticular structures (e.g. bursitis) or the joint itself. Prosthetic joint swelling is especially worrisome.

Differential diagnosis includes the following possibilities.

- Bone cancer and metastatic disease.
- Bleeding into joint (haemarthrosis).
- Crystal arthropathy (calcium pyrophosphate disease – pseudogout; or gout).
- Inflammatory monoarthritis or part of polyarthritis (e.g. osteoarthritis, rheumatoid arthritis, seronegative arthritis).
- Reactive arthritis (recent gastrointestinal or genitourinary infection).

- Septic arthritis (haematogenous spread or local infection).
- Trauma.

ROWS (examples): septic arthritis, bone cancer or metastatic deposits, trauma.

Investigations include FBC, CRP, U&E, creatinine, coagulation studies, TFT, LFT, Ca, urate, anticyclic citrullinated protein antibody (rheumatoid arthritis), rheumatoid factor, ANA and extractable nuclear antigens, autoantibodies, BG and blood culture. If other infective cause is suspected, perform appropriate tests (e.g. parvovirus, COVID-19, TB, Lyme disease, gonococcal). X-ray of joint. Joint aspiration with microscopy (including birefringence and Gram stain), culture and sensitivity. Imaging – consider joint ultrasound and MRI.

Initial management includes the following.

- First, consider *red flag* features and acute life-threatening causes (i.e. ROWS), ABCDE, optimise physiology and supportive care. Sepsis Six care bundle if sepsis suspected.
- Analgesia.
- Identify and treat potential causes. If an effusion is present, aspirate the joint where possible and send sample for urgent analysis. Macroscopic appearance coupled with microscopy, Gram stain and culture will help confirm (or exclude) infection. Polarised light microscopy should be used to detect crystals of uric acid or pyrophosphate. The exclusion of infection will permit local steroid injection. If aspirate looks infected, seek possible bacterial source by taking appropriate culture samples (e.g. blood, MSU, urethral swab). Do not give the antibiotic by injection into the *joint*.
- Withdrawal of precipitating agents (e.g. agents that predispose to gout). Medications review with deprescribing as needed.
- Management of associated complications.
- The joint(s) should be immobilised when inflamed; start rehabilitation as soon as symptoms have resolved. If diagnosis unclear or if septic arthritis is diagnosed, seek urgent advice from the rheumatology or orthopaedic team.

Rheumatoid arthritis

- Idiopathic, autoreactive, small joint symmetrical polyarthritis resulting in synovitis, cartilage damage, bone erosions, loss of function of joint(s), as well as other features (e.g. pain, swollen joints, early morning stiffness and stiffness after rest, fatigue and other systemic features, and decreased quality of life).

- Diagnosis is based on pattern recognition, supported by positive anticyclic citrullinated protein antibody and rheumatoid factor, and imaging including joint ultrasound which confirms synovial thickening and hyperaemia on colour Doppler.
- Treatment – induce remission: analgesia, NSAIDs, step-down oral steroids, steroid joint injections (as needed), and methotrexate as anchor disease-modifying antirheumatic drugs (DMARDs). Review patient regularly and modify dose(s). Remission defined using Clinical Disease Activity Index (i.e. 'Treat to target'). If not at target, consider:
  - other synthetic DMARDs (e.g. sulfasalazine, hydroxychloroquine)
  - biological therapies: cytokine-directed (e.g. anti-IL-6 blockers, TNF-alpha antagonists); T-cell co-stimulation antagonists; and B-cell antagonists (rituximab)
  - targeted synthetic DMARDs: cell signalling inhibitors (Janus kinase inhibitor).
- Treatment – maintenance phase.
- Supportive – lose weight if obese, smoking cessation, improve mental health. If infection – hold DMARDs and biologicals and treat infection (may need stress-dose steroid). Restart DMARDS and biologicals on recovery.

Palliative and end-of-life care

Palliative and end-of-life care is provided by health and social care professionals to those living with and dying from any advanced, progressive incurable condition.

Palliative care is defined as the active holistic care of individuals across *all* ages with serious health-related suffering due to severe illness and especially of those near the end of life. It aims to improve the quality of life of patients, their families and caregivers at every stage of the disease process from diagnosis onwards. Palliative care focuses on the person, *not* the disease. An important consideration is providing relief from pain (i.e. 'total pain' management including physical, psychological, social and spiritual factors) and other symptoms (www.palliativecareguidelines.scot.nhs.uk/). Seek expert help from palliative care team and agree who patient is going to follow up with (and who is responsible for what) and contact details.

End-of-life care

> One in three adults admitted to hospital through the acute take and 80% of care home residents are in their last year of life. Nearly half of all deaths in England occur in hospital.

The definition of the end of life (EOL) is not confined to people identified as imminently dying, but also includes those who may be in their final weeks, months or year of life. Patients who die from all but sudden causes, including those who die from dementia and frailty, heart failure, COPD, cancer, liver or renal failure as well as other causes, may have a recognisable EOL care phase. One of the most challenging aspects of the COVID-19 pandemic involved palliative and EOL care of many people affected by this infection and related complications.

It can be difficult to deliver high-quality EOL care in busy, high-turnover, Acute Medicine care environments. Identifying that someone is approaching EOL is often challenging in acute settings, where active treatment is the default course of action. Offering quality time to discuss future care options can also be difficult. Time-pressured physicians understandably may not be able to broach the topic in an ambulatory setting, and there is little privacy on a ward. Confidence among doctors at all levels is another barrier. As a result, people with long-term, end-stage conditions with limited reversibility are often admitted repeatedly to hospital despite their best interests.

Advance care planning and early introduction of palliative care can improve the patient's quality of life and mood, reduce aggressive care at the end of life, reduce emergency hospital admissions and even extend life expectancy of certain groups.

End-of-life care for patients should be individualised and those caring for them should recognise that every patient will have different priorities for how their EOL care is managed. Patients' choices are supported when there is excellent holistic care, and sensitive and honest communication with patients, families and between all members of staff and the teams caring for them in different settings. Conversations should not just centre on *withholding* specific treatments, such as cardiopulmonary resuscitation (CPR), but rather discussion about the patient's illness and what will or will not be helpful moving forward. Talking about care planning using the six-step REDMAP (**R**eady, **E**xpect, **D**iagnosis, **M**atters, **A**ctions, **P**lan) framework is useful for initiating and structuring anticipatory care planning discussions (www.spict.org.uk/red-map/).

End-of-life care should include the following aspects.
- Use clear language and avoid euphemisms.
- An explanation to the patient that they may be in the last year of life, with limited reversibility of their underlying condition.
- Review of *current* treatment and care, based on patient goals.
- Agreement with the patient on goals for *future* care, focusing on what can be done to support the patient to live well, but also on those interventions that are no longer helpful for that person; this may also include discussions about discharge to another care setting, and a plan for future deteriorations and whether these should result in readmission to hospital.
- All discussions and treatment plans should be documented clearly in the medical notes with a treatment escalation plan (TEP), including do not attempt CPR (DNACPR) order. The Resuscitation Council UK's ReSPECT (Recommended Summary Plan for Emergency Care and Treatment) process can be used to support conversations and documentation.
- Advance care planning enables those close to the patient and professionals to follow a patient's previously expressed wishes regarding their care and treatment (including preferred place of care and death), should they lose capacity in the future.
- In the last days to weeks of life, the focus of care should be *comfort* based. Unhelpful investigations and ineffective treatments should be avoided or discontinued where the burdens outweigh the benefits. Medications to relieve pain, nausea, dyspnoea, agitation or troublesome respiratory secretions should be prescribed in anticipation (i.e. *anticipatory care*).
- An individual plan of care for the *dying* person includes early recognition, sensitive communication, agreement regarding food, drink and hydration, symptom control (e.g. pain relief), and psychological, social and spiritual support, and is co-ordinated and delivered with compassion.
- Regular review and monitoring of the dying person's clinical condition, the goals of and responses to care, and the family's/carer's concerns are of paramount importance.
- Facilitate a peaceful death in the patient's preferred place by arranging *rapid transfer home* if desired.

Setting a ceiling of treatment is based on the likelihood that the intervention will achieve the intended outcome, that that outcome is acceptable to the patient and the patient feels the burden of treatment is worthwhile. This needs to be discussed sensitively with the patient and their loved ones to avoid misunderstandings. Key points to consider when discussing ceilings of treatment include the following.

- Health professionals should be prepared for anger/upset/questions. These are usually not aimed *directly* at you, but you may have to absorb these emotions and react professionally, even if they are upsetting/difficult at the time.
- All efforts should be made to '*de-escalate*' confrontational situations to maintain a patient/professional or carer/professional relationship wherever possible.
- Patients or those close to them may request a 'second opinion' – this should be facilitated wherever possible.

Palpitations

Palpitations are described as an unpleasant awareness of the heartbeat. Often described as a feeling of 'fluttering' in the chest. Cardiac arrythmias can be divided into:

- tachycardia – defined as abnormal heart rhythms with a ventricular rate of 100 or more beats per minute, frequently symptomatic. Can be wide complex (QRS >120 milliseconds) or narrow complex
- bradycardia – seek underlying cause (e.g. hypothyroidism, cardiac medications).

Differential diagnosis of tachycardia includes the following.

- Atrial arrhythmias (atrial fibrillation, atrial flutter, atrial tachycardia).
- Cardiac ectopics (premature atrial or ventricular extrasystoles).
- Paroxysmal supraventricular tachycardia.
- Sinus tachycardia (anxiety/emotional stress; caffeine, nicotine, alcohol).
- Ventricular tachycardia.

Differential diagnosis of bradycardia includes the following.

- Sick sinus syndrome.
- Intermittent or permanent AV block.

ROWS (examples): ventricular tachycardia/fibrillation, atrial fibrillation, complete heart block.

Investigations include urgent 12-lead ECG, cardiac telemetry or exercise ECG, followed by ambulatory ECG monitoring if negative findings. FBC, U&E, creatinine, TFT, BG, troponin, COVID-19, pregnancy test, Ca, Mg. Urine/serum metanephrines (phaeochromocytoma). Echocardiogram. Consider coronary angiography.

Initial management includes the following steps.

- First, consider *red flag* features and acute life-threatening causes (i.e. ROWS), ABCDE, optimise physiology and supportive care. Refer to emergency management of tachycardia (see Figure 6.1) and bradycardia (see Figure 6.2) guidelines.
- The key to diagnosis lies in capturing the cardiac rhythm during symptoms.
- Identify and treat potential causes.
  - Do not forget non-cardiac causes of palpitations (e.g. thyroid disease).
  - Palpitations are common in COVID-19 infection and post-COVID syndromes (e.g. inappropriate sinus tachycardia, POTS).
- Withdrawal of precipitating agents. Medications review with deprescribing as needed.
- Management of associated complications.
- Refer to cardiology if *red flags* present or for further evaluation and management.

Atrial fibrillation (AF)

Atrial fibrillation is the most common cardiac dysrhythmia and affects 1 million people in the UK. The prevalence increases with age, such that it is 1–2% in the under-65s and 8–11% in the over-85s. Older age (and prevalence of COPD) are associated with a higher hospital admission rate.

Atrial fibrillation is a supraventricular arrhythmia due to unco-ordinated atrial contraction, leading to irregular heart rhythm and a rapid ventricular response. Complications include VTE disease (including stroke) and acute heart failure.

The natural history of AF is variable but tends to progress from paroxysmal to persistent over time and depends on control of underlying co-morbid conditions.

- Paroxysmal (episodes terminate spontaneously or after targeted intervention within seven days).
- Persistent (lasting more than seven days).
- Permanent (does not terminate despite intervention, or when the patient and clinician decide not to pursue any attempt to restore normal rhythm).

Features	Illness script for AF
Epidemiological risk factors	• Increasing age. Common co-morbidities include hypertension, coronary artery disease (CAD), obesity and other features of metabolic syndrome, and obstructive sleep apnoea. Other causes include alcohol, heart failure, valvular heart disease, hyperthyroidism.
Pathophysiology	• Supraventricular arrhythmia. Exact mechanisms not fully understood but suggested mechanisms include proinflammatory state (as part of metabolic syndrome) and altered electrical activity within the atrial myocardium, resulting in arrhythmogenic activity.
Time course	• Acute onset. Time course: paroxysmal, persistent or chronic (permanent).
Key symptoms and signs	• Most patients are asymptomatic. Most common symptoms include palpitations, dyspnoea, exercise intolerance, presyncope symptoms and syncope. • Physical examination – bradycardia, normal rate, or tachycardia with irregularly irregular heart rhythm. May have features of VTE disease (e.g. acute stroke).
Diagnostics	• ECG – ambulatory ECG monitoring may be needed for paroxysmal AF. • Investigations – search for reversible causes (e.g. thyroid disease, alcohol excess, CAD). • Imaging – echocardiogram.

Treatment	Focuses on four main pillars.
	1 Efforts to correct risk factors, lifestyle interventions and co-morbidities (e.g. obesity, sleep apnoea, diabetes, hypertension, heart failure, CAD, smoking cessation and alcohol abstinence/reduction).
	2 Rate control strategies – beta-blockers or calcium channel blockers generally first line, also consider amiodarone or digoxin.
	3 Rhythm control strategies.
	  ○ Patients with ongoing AF at the time of initial evaluation, and with very slow or rapid ventricular rates (typically <40 bpm and >150 bpm), evidence of haemodynamic instability, severe symptoms or decompensated heart failure should be referred for stabilisation and possible electrical cardioversion.
	  ○ In case of unknown duration of AF and no haemodynamic instability, electrical or pharmacological cardioversion should be preceded by echocardiogram to rule out intracardiac thrombus or anticoagulation for at least four weeks.
	  ○ Patients are required to be on anticoagulation for at least four weeks after cardioversion to reduce the risk of thromboembolism.
	  ○ Invasive strategies (e.g. catheter ablation) can also be considered.
	4 Reduction of stroke risk.
	  ○ Prevention of thromboembolic complications with anticoagulation: according to CHA_2DS_2VASc score (risk of thromboembolism) and ORBIT bleeding prediction tool (absolute risk of bleeding). NICE (2021) – ORBIT tool is preferred to HAS-BLED score.
	  ○ DOACs should be used in preference to warfarin for most patients; the choice of DOAC depends on patient preference and clinical indication.

Poisoning

Accidental and intentional poisoning remains a major cause of morbidity and mortality world-wide. Poisoning is an important public health issue in the UK, with approximately 160000 presentations occurring annually because of poisoning, which may include self-harm, accidental exposures, medication errors and drug misuse. Many more patients are managed in the community.

Although the management is largely supportive, a knowledge of the constellation of signs and symptoms that constitute specific poisonings, referred to as *toxidromes*, may enable early empirical decontamination, antidote administration, enhanced elimination and supportive care, and may also predict the clinical course.

A poison is a substance that through its chemical action usually kills, injures or impairs an organism. Poisoning occurs when a poison interferes with normal body functions after it is swallowed, inhaled, injected or absorbed. It is important to note that drug poisoning can produce a wide range of symptoms and clinical findings and may occur in isolation or with other pathology (e.g. trauma, infection). Presentation depends upon type and quantity of agent, whether the exposure is acute, staggered or chronic, baseline medications and health status of the patient (e.g. liver or kidney disease), and whether the exposure involves a single agent or multiple (including alcohol). Initial management is primarily focused on pattern recognition (i.e. *toxidromes*) and acute stabilisation.

Differential diagnosis includes various toxidrome features (e.g. opioid, cholinergic, anticholinergic, stimulant, sedative, serotonin, cannabinoid, dissociative, inhalant abuse).

ROWS (examples): respiratory depression, cardiac arrhythmias, seizures, caustic ingestion.

Investigations include FBC, BG, U&E, creatinine, LFT, ABG, alcohol level, toxicology screen (e.g. paracetamol or salicylates), pregnancy test. ECG and cardiac monitoring. Imaging if signs of injury or other diagnosis possible (e.g. other cause of altered GCS, aspiration).

Initial management includes the following steps.

- First, protect yourself and others (e.g. fentanyl exposure, used needles, agitation and violence), consider acute life-threatening causes (i.e. ROWS), supportive care (e.g. seizures, hypoglycaemia, hyper/hypothermia, arrhythmias and other abnormalities).
- ABCDEFGH approach.
  - ○ **A**irway.
  - ○ **B**reathing.
  - ○ **C**irculation: cardiac monitoring critical and serial ECGs with particular emphasis on arrhythmias, PR, QRS and QT intervals.
  - ○ **D**isability (conscious level): GCS or ACVPU – if low, give 'coma cocktail'; **D**econtamination (if applicable).
  - ○ **E**xposure, **E**xamination and **E**valuation; **E**mergency Antidote.
  - ○ **DEFGH**: '**D**on't **E**ver **F**orget **G**lucose and **H**eroin (opioids)' if comatose.
- Withdrawal of precipitating agents (e.g. remove transdermal fentanyl patch). Medications review with deprescribing as needed.
- Management of associated complications.

You can consider calling dedicated toxicologists such as the National Poisons Information Service (NPIS), to discuss unexplained toxidromes, polypharmacy overdoses or poisoning with uncommon toxins, as well as subsequent possible management strategies.

Poisoning is discussed fully in Chapter 21.

Rash

The integumentary system is the largest organ of the body (weighs ~4–5 kg) and consists of the skin and related appendages (i.e. hair, nails, glands, mucous membranes). The skin separates the body from the surrounding environment. It is composed of the epidermis and dermis overlying subcutaneous tissue, and related skin appendages. Skin diseases are very common, affecting up to a third of the population at any one time. The skin is intimately linked to other organ systems of the body, therefore systemic disease may also affect the skin (e.g. jaundice). Skin disease can also be local. Skin diseases have serious impacts on life, including the '5 Ds'.

- **D**iscomfort
- **D**isfigurement
- **D**epression
- **D**isablement
- **D**eath

The skin serves multiple functions that are crucial to health, quality of life and survival (as can be seen with skin failure, e.g. burn victims, erythroderma).

- Barrier to harmful exogenous substances, pathogens and radiation.
- Barrier to loss or absorption of water, electrolytes and other molecules.
- Sensory organ (also protects against physical injury).
- Regulates body temperature.
- Peripheral outpost of immune system.
- Vitamin D production by absorbing UVB.

- Wound healing.
- Shock absorption – strong, yet elastic and compliant covering.
- Appearance – psychological and cosmetic importance such as hair, nails, tan, tattoos, skin piercings.
- Organ of sexual attraction and social interaction.
- Facilitates administration of certain drugs (e.g. testosterone, GTN, fentanyl).
- Repairs injury.

A rash is a 'breaking out' (or becoming visible) of abnormal skin changes (e.g. colour, appearance, texture). Evaluation of a rash involves a detailed history and physical exam, taking the patient's general medical history into account. Rashes can be associated with itching, pain, blisters, urticaria and other features. The clinical appearance of a rash, a thorough history and some knowledge of pathology of common conditions are necessary to make an accurate dermatological diagnosis ('pattern recognition'). Certain rashes follow a typical pattern anatomically and can aid the diagnosis. Other rashes are important markers of systemic disease and must be recognised in acute medical presentations.

Emergency dermatology refers to rapidly progressive skin conditions and some that are potentially life-threatening.

Differential diagnosis is broad and includes the following possibilities.

- Allergic causes – urticaria (swelling involving the superficial dermis, raising the epidermis), angiooedema (deeper swelling involving the dermis and subcutaneous tissues, swelling of tongue and lips). Anaphylaxis can present initially with urticaria and angioedema. Atopic dermatitis is a common itchy skin condition.
- Associated with systemic disease – erythema nodosum (hypersensitivity response to a variety of stimuli leading to discrete tender nodules, especially on the shins), dermatitis herpetiformis (coeliac disease), pyoderma gangrenosum (e.g. IBD).
- Autoimmune (with blisters) such as bullous pemphigoid (autoantibodies against antigens between the epidermis and dermis causing a subepidermal split in the skin leading to tense, fluid-filled bullae on an erythematous base), pemphigus vulgaris (autoantibodies against antigens within the epidermis causing an intraepidermal split in the skin

leading to flaccid, easily ruptured blisters forming erosions and crusts).
- Drug eruptions – approximately 3% of all patients admitted to hospital have a drug eruption due to adverse drug reaction.
- Erythroderma (erythematous exfoliative dermatitis involving 90% or more of the cutaneous surface).
- Infectious causes – cellulitis, erysipelas, erythema migrans, viral exanthems, varicella zoster, herpes zoster, petechial rash of meningococcal meningitis (can progress to non-blanching purpuric rash).
- Leg ulcers are often a mixture of arterial, venous and/or neuropathic components.
- Purpura (including vasculitis with 'palpable purpura') – caused by leaking of blood from intravascular space. Can be related to underlying bleeding tendency.
- Psoriasis (papulosquamous eruption).
- Stevens–Johnson syndrome (SJS, mucocutaneous necrosis with at least two mucosal sites involved; affects <10% body surface), and toxic epidermal necrolysis (TEN, extensive skin and mucosal necrosis accompanied by systemic toxicity; affects >30% skin surface).

ROWS (examples): anaphylaxis, erythroderma, SJS/TEN, malignant melanoma.

Initial management includes the following steps.

- First, consider *red flag* features and acute life-threatening causes (i.e. ROWS), ABCDE, optimise physiology and supportive care (e.g. wound care, fluid and electrolyte replacement, nutritional support, temperature management, pain control and treatment of infections if present).
- The key to diagnosis lies in detailed dermatological and general history taking and examination which provide important diagnostic clues in the assessment of skin problems. Appropriate investigations can help 'rule in' or 'rule out' diagnosis. Describe the morphology (structure) of lesions (an area of altered skin) and eruptions (rash) on patients, using correct dermatological language to aid communication and diagnosis. Learn to apply this approach to any skin presentation. The usual framework is as follows.
  - Dermatological history. If the lesion is pigmented, remember the dermatological version of **ABCDE** (the presence of any of these features increases the likelihood of melanoma): **A**symmetry (one half of mole does not match the other half); irregular **B**order; Two or more **C**olours within the lesion; **D**iameter >6mm; **E**volving symptoms (e.g. bleeding, itching), Elevation or Enlargement.

○ Skin examination: well-lit room, hand-held light, ruler, dermatoscope. There are four important principles in performing a good examination of the skin: inspect, describe, palpate and systematic check (Box 27.2).
○ Dermatological investigations.
○ Other investigations as needed.
- Identify and treat potential causes.
- Withdrawal of precipitating agents. Medications review with deprescribing as needed.
- Management of associated complications.
- Refer to dermatology if *red flags* present or for further evaluation and management.

Distribution – the pattern of spread of skin lesions

- Generalised – all over the body.
- Widespread – extensive.
- Localised – restricted to one area of skin only.
- Symmetrical – one side mirrors the other.
- Flexural – on the flexor surfaces or body folds (i.e. groin, neck, behind ears, popliteal and antecubital fossa).
- Extensor – on the extensor surfaces of knees, elbows, shins.

- Intertriginous – in an area where two skin areas may touch or rub together.
- Köebner phenomenon – linear lesion arising at site of trauma.
- Palmoplantar – on the palm of the hand or bottom of the foot.
- Periungual/subungual – around or under a fingernail or toenail.
- Photosensitive – affects sun-exposed areas such as face, neck and back of hands.
- Pressure areas – sacrum, buttocks, ankles, heels.
- Dermatomal – area of skin supplied by a single spinal nerve.

Erythroderma

Erythematous dermatitis involving 90% or more of the cutaneous surface. Associated with extensive desquamation in some cases, which may develop as a result of primary dermatitis.

- Causes – idiopathic, drug allergy, lymphoma/leukaemia, atopic dermatitis, psoriasis, contact dermatitis, seborrhoeic dermatitis (order of decreasing prevalence).

Box 27.2 Four important principles in performing a good examination of the skin

INSPECT
- General observation.
- Site and number of lesion(s).
  ○ Primary lesion(s): directly associated with disease process and is described with established dermatological terminology (e.g. macule, papule).
  ○ Secondary lesion(s): lesions that evolve from primary lesions usually due to scratching or infection (e.g. scale, crust).
  ○ If multiple, pattern of distribution (where lesions are localised) and configuration (how lesions are locally grouped or 'organised').

DESCRIBE
For individual lesions – SCAM.
- **S**ize (the widest diameter), **S**hape.
- **C**olour.
- **A**ssociated secondary change.
- **M**orphology, **M**argin (border) – well defined (e.g. psoriasis) or ill-defined (e.g. eczema).

PALPATE
- Surface, consistency, mobility, tenderness and temperature.

SYSTEMATIC CHECK
- Examine the nails, scalp, hair and mucous membranes.
- General examination of *all* systems.

- Pathophysiology – the erythema is due to an increased skin blood perfusion from dilation of the dermal capillaries. This results in temperature dysregulation and possible cardiac failure. Basal metabolic rate rises to compensate for heat loss, with fluid loss increasing in proportion to this.
- Clinical presentation – the situation is like that observed in patients following burns – negative nitrogen balance characterised by oedema, hypoalbuminaemia and loss of muscle mass.
- Treatment includes the following aspects.
  - Discontinue all unnecessary medications.
  - Monitor/control fluid intake.
  - Monitor body temperature.
  - Institute systemic antibiotics if signs of secondary infection.
  - Antihistamines reduce pruritus (itchiness).
- Prognosis – depends on underlying aetiology. Overall mortality 20–40%.

Toxic epidermal necrolysis (TEN)

Acute severe bullous cutaneous disease characterised by extensive areas of skin necrosis. Most commonly drug induced (95%). Clinical presentation: acute phase – persistent fevers, generalised epidermal sloughing and mucous membrane involvement which can become denuded (loss of epidermis), including buccal, nasal, pharyngeal, tracheobronchial, oesophageal, perineal, urethral and anal mucosa. Prognosis: 10–70% mortality.

If a patient presents with symptoms of a viral illness and an atypical skin rash, think of COVID-19. However, monkeypox can also cause a characteristic rash on the body, often on the face, arms and hands, and systemic features such as fever, headache, muscle aches, backache, swollen lymph nodes, chills and exhaustion. During the monkeypox outbreak, some patients have developed a rash or lesions around the genitals or anus before any other symptoms, and some have not developed flu-like symptoms at all. For both COVID-19 and monkeypox, personal protective equipment (PPE) should be worn.

Scabies is common in overcrowding (e.g. homeless shelters) and in institutions. Look out for and treat secondary bacterial infection to prevent acute and chronic complications of *Streptococcus* or *Staphylococcus*.

Vomiting and nausea

Nausea is an unpleasant sensation of being about to vomit. Vomiting is the forceful expulsion of gastric contents via the oesophagus and is usually preceded by nausea. Nausea and vomiting in acute illness can be caused by stimulation of the:

- GI tract
- chemoreceptor trigger zone and 'vomiting centre' in the brainstem (e.g. opioid-induced nausea)
- vestibular system.

Nausea is a common symptom and when accompanied by vomiting, is usually self-limiting. Although there are numerous causes, originating from peripheral (GI or inner ear) or central stimuli, the history should identify the cause in most cases. Consideration of amount, frequency, nature, timing and associated symptoms (weight loss, fevers, headache and abdominal pain) can help narrow the differential diagnosis. This will allow a more tailored approach to antiemetic therapy. Different antiemetics or combinations which act at different sites can be used prophylactically (e.g. postoperatively, chemotherapy) or if the symptoms are persistent or severe. Accurate assessment of fluid status is crucial to prevent clinical deterioration and electrolyte disturbance.

Differential diagnosis is very broad and includes the following.

- ACS.
- Acute gastroenteritis – most common cause of acute (i.e. ≤10 days) nausea and vomiting.
- Acute viral labyrinthitis (associated with vertigo, tinnitus, nystagmus and hearing loss).
- Addison disease.
- Bowel obstruction – small and large bowel.
- Cannabis hyperemesis syndrome.
- Diabetic gastroparesis – can be related to autonomic neuropathy, hyperglycaemia (including DKA) and glucagon-like peptide (GLP)-1 receptor agonists.
- Drug induced (overdose, excessive alcohol, opioids, chemotherapy).
- Functional – including eating disorders.
- Headaches – migraine, raised intracranial pressure.
- Hypercalcaemic crisis.

- Intra-abdominal inflammatory causes – acute appendicitis, pancreatitis, peptic ulcer, gastritis, cholecystitis, IBD.
- Malignancy.
- Pregnancy – including hyperemesis gravidarum.
- Postoperative.
- Renal colic.
- Severe CKD and ESRD.
- Toxin-mediated food poisoning.
- Vestibular neuronitis.

ROWS (examples): ACS, Addison disease, bowel obstruction, oesophageal perforation, acute pancreatitis.

Initial investigations include FBC, CRP, BG, TFT, Ca, Mg, phosphate, U&E, creatinine, LFT, coeliac screen, amylase and lipase. Toxicology screen. ECG. Urinalysis and culture if considering renal calculi/pyelonephritis. Pregnancy test in women of child-bearing age. Abdominal X-ray, CT or USS in select cases. Other imaging as per clinical reasoning (e.g. *red flag* headache features requiring CT head). Upper GI endoscopy as needed. Consider ENT investigations.

Initial management includes the following steps.

- First, consider *red flag* features and acute life-threatening causes (i.e. ROWS), ABCDE, keep NBM and supportive care (e.g. fluid resuscitation, electrolyte replacement, nutritional support including vitamin replacement and monitor for refeeding syndrome). Analgesics as required.
- Identify and treat potential causes.
- Antiemetic ladder of agents which can be given orally or parenterally (e.g. metoclopramide or cyclizine first; then prochlorperazine; 5-HT3 receptor antagonists; through to haloperidol or dexamethasone, depending on patient factors, severity and aetiology of nausea and vomiting). Combinations of drugs which act at different sites are particularly effective.
- In oncology and palliative care patients, consider reversible factors such as excess opioid therapy, constipation, electrolyte abnormalities and raised intracranial pressure.
- Withdrawal of precipitating agents (e.g. NSAIDs, alcohol, cannabis use). Medications review with deprescribing as needed.
- Management of associated complications.
  - Aspiration.
  - Oesophageal rupture.
  - Haematemesis (Mallory–Weiss oesophageal tears).
  - Nutritional deficiencies and hypokalaemic metabolic alkalosis (chronic vomiting).

> **Nausea and vomiting red flags**
> - Anaemia or haematemesis occurring in patients with foregut malignancy.
> - Significant weight loss (>5%).
> - Dysphagia.
> Generally, alarm features predicate an urgent gastroscopy with or without cross-sectional imaging.

Weakness and paralysis

Weakness refers to reduction of muscle power. Paralysis refers to a reduction in muscle strength with limited range of voluntary movement. May be focal or generalised. Paralysis can be spastic or flaccid, referring to underlying upper and lower motor neurone lesions respectively.

- Lower motor neurone lesions are associated with hypotonia, hyporeflexia and fasciculations, and their respective origins of pathology are attributed to the nerve roots, peripheral nerves or neuromuscular junctions.
- Upper motor neurone lesions are associated with rigidity, spasticity and hyperreflexia, and their respective origins of pathology involve the brain or spinal cord.

Knowledge of the type of paralysis presented can help narrow the differential diagnosis and further plans of management.

Differential diagnosis is very broad and includes the following possibilities.

- Acute stroke, including TIA.
- Space-occupying lesions.
- Cervical myelopathy.
- Functional aetiology.
- Guillain–Barré syndrome.
- Lambert Eaton myasthenic syndrome and other paraneoplastic syndromes.
- Multiple sclerosis.
- Myasthenia gravis.
- Motor neurone disease.
- Poisoning: organophosphate.
- Spinal cord compression.
- Transient following focal seizure (Todd paralysis).

ROWS (examples).

- Unilateral weakness – ischaemic stroke, intracerebral hemorrhage, SAH.

- Bilateral weakness – brainstem stroke, spinal cord compression, Guillain–Barré syndrome, myasthenia gravis, organophosphate poisoning, botulism.

Initial investigations include FBC, CRP, BG, U&E, creatinine, Ca, phosphate, CK, TFT, vitamin B12 and D level, HIV test. Autoantibodies (e.g. anti-acetylcholine receptor, voltage-gated calcium channels) as needed. CT or MRI brain, CT or MR angiogram, MRI spine, nerve conduction study electromyography. Muscle channelopathy tests as needed (Box 27.3).

Initial management includes the following steps.

- First, consider *red flag* features and acute life-threatening causes (i.e. ROWS), ABCDE and supportive care (e.g. FVC monitoring for ventilation).
- Identify and treat potential causes (e.g. stroke).
- Withdrawal of precipitating agents. Medications review with deprescribing as needed.
- Management of associated complications.
- Close monitoring required.
- Neurology or stroke consult.

Weakness and paralysis (and acute stroke) are discussed fully in Chapter 24.

Box 27.3 Channelopathies

Channelopathies refer to disorders resulting from defective ion channel functioning and include neurological (e.g. headache, epilepsy), cardiovascular (e.g. causing arrhythmia or sudden cardiac death - such as long QT and Brugada syndromes), and muscle disorders.

Muscle channelopathies:
Rare neuromuscular diseases that cause symptoms of episodic muscle weakness/paralysis (e.g. periodic paralyses) or cause difficulty in relaxing muscles (myotonia).

Periodic paralyses (PPs) are autosomal dominantly inherited channelopathies that manifest as abnormal, often potassium-sensitive, muscle membrane excitability leading to episodic flaccid paralysis. PP is classified as *hypokalaemic* when episodes occur in association with low potassium levels or *hyperkalaemic* when episodes can be induced by elevated potassium.

Thyrotoxic periodic paralysis (TPP) is a rare complication of thyrotoxicosis characterised by acute, reversible episodes of muscle weakness and hypokalaemia. TPP is often precipitated by heavy exercise or high-carbohydrate meals and is most commonly described in Asian men.

Early treatment of PP (as well as treating thyrotoxicosis in TPP) is necessary to avoid reversible but potentially life-threatening complications, such as cardiac arrhythmias and respiratory failure.

Index

4AT tool, 155–156
5 Ds, 426

A

ABCDE *see* Airway, Breathing, Circulation, Disability and Exposure
ABCDEFGH approach, 224, 426
abdominal pain, 367–376
  biliary causes, 371–373
  intestinal ischaemia, 373–374
  peptic ulcers, 374–375
abdominal ultrasound, 127–131
  free fluid in abdomen, 129
  limitations and pitfalls, 129–130
  normal anatomy, 129
  paracentesis, 129
  technique, 127–129
acid–base disorder, 62–63
acidosis, 62–63
ACS *see* acute coronary syndrome
acute back pain, 376–378
acute coronary syndrome (ACS), 79, 81–82
  illness script, 16
  pregnant patients, 181
  presentations, 389–391
acute fluid loss, 56–58
acute intoxication, alcohol, 231–232
acute kidney injury (AKI)
  perioperative medicine, 173–174
  presentation, 378–380
acute liver failure, paracetamol overdose, 227–229
acute medical emergencies, 50
  see also acutely unwell patients; medical emergencies
acute medical take, 138–143

clinical decision making, 141–142
  debriefing, 142–143
  handover, 142
  roles and responsibilities, 139
acute medical units (AMUs), 3–6, 87
acute myocardial infarction, 81–82
acute pancreatitis, 372–373
acute pericarditis, 392
acute respiratory distress syndrome (ARDS), 89–90
acute withdrawal, alcohol, 233–234
acutely unwell patients, 50–64
  active bleeding, 58–60
  airway assessment, 55
  blood transfusions, 57–58, 60
  circulatory status, 56–60
  clinical reasoning, 21
  definitive diagnosis, 61–64
  disability, 61
  early warning scores, 51–53
  exposure, 61
  history, 62
  immediate assessment, 53–54
  investigations, 62–63
  massive haemorrhage, 58–60
  physical examination, 62
  recognition, 51–53
  transfusions, 57–58
  ward selection, 55
ACVPU tool *see* Alert, Confusion, responsive to Voice, Pain, or Unresponsive
Addisonian crisis, 170
adjustment disorder, 341
administration, insulin, 277–278, 280–281
admission avoidance, 104–105, 108–109
admissions
  Criteria to Reside tool, 109
  critical care, 88

adolescents and young adults (AYAs), 194–196
ADR *see* adverse drug reactions
adrenal disorders, 268–273
  Cushing syndrome, 269
  incidentalomas, 270
  insufficiency, 170, 269, 270–273
  perioperative medicine, 170
  phaeochromocytoma, 269
advanced life support (ALS), 72–78
adverse drug reactions (ADR), 42–46
  anticancer therapeutics, 360–361
  classification, 44–45
  common causes, 43–44
  definitions, 42–43
  management, 45–46
  modified SNAP regimen, 229
  risk factors, 43
adverse events
  definition, 32
  Swiss cheese model, 32
AEC *see* ambulatory emergency care
AF *see* atrial fibrillation
aggressive behaviour, 347–349
airway assessment and management, 55
  cardiac arrest, 75–77
  post-resuscitation, 84
Airway, Breathing, Circulation, Disability and Exposure (ABCDE) approach, 21
AKI *see* acute kidney injury
alcohol misuse, 231–234
  CAGE questionnaire screening, 234
  clinical presentations, 232
  intoxication, 231–232
  malnutrition, 243–244
  perioperative medicine, 166–167
  withdrawal, 233–234

Alert, Confusion, responsive to Voice, Pain, or Unresponsive (ACVPU) tool, 61, 302
alkalosis, 62–63
alkyl nitrates, 236–237
ALS *see* advanced life support
Alzheimer's disease, 153
ambulatory emergency care (AEC), 100
ambulatory settings, 6, 100–103
amiodarone, 66, 79
amiodarone-induced thyrotoxicosis, 263
amphetamines, 237
AMUs *see* acute medical units
anaemia, 415–418
    bone marrow failure syndromes, 415–417
    diagnosis, 415–416
    haemolytic, 417
    inflammatory, 417
    macrocytic, 417
    microcytic, 417
    normocytic, 417
    perioperative medicine, 172
    sickle cell disease, 418
analgesia
    perioperative, 174–175
    pregnant patients, 192
anaphylaxis, 42, 66, 69–71
ANCA *see* antineutrophil cytoplasmic antibody
anorexia nervosa, 343–345
antiarrhhythmic drugs, 79, 192, 263
anticholinergic toxidrome, 227
anticoagulants
    bleeding, 60
    perioperative, 171, 172–173
    pregnant patients, 184, 192
    reversal, 173
anticonvulsants, 318–319
antidiuretic hormone, 253, 255–256, 258
antidotes
    poisoned patients, 225–227
    recreational drugs, 235
antiemetics, 187, 192
antiepileptic agents, pregnant patients, 192
antihypertensives, 98, 188–189, 192
antimicrobial stewardship, 49

antineutrophil cytoplasmic antibody (ANCA)-associated vasculitis, 418–419
antipsychotics, 345–346
antiretroviral therapy (ART), 217–219
anxiety-related disorders, 337
aortic dissection, 392–393
ARDS *see* acute respiratory distress syndrome
Argyll Robertson pupil, 306
arrhythmias, 66–68
    perioperative medicine, 164
    pregnant patients, 182
ART *see* antiretroviral therapy
arterial blood gas (ABG), 56
ascending cholangitis, 371
assessment, 38–39
    acute kidney injury, 174
    adrenal insufficiency, 270–272
    airway status, 55
    alcohol overuse, 232
    anorexia nervosa, 343–345
    breathing status, 55–56
    circulation, 56–60
    coma, 302
    cranial nerves, 303–304
    delirium, 155
    deteriorating patients, 53–64
    diabetes mellitus, 273–276
    disability, 61
    epilepsy, 317–318
    exposure, 61
    fever of unknown origin, 404
    gait, 305
    hyponatraemia, 254–255
    meningitis, 328
    mental state, 302
    muscle weakness, 303–304
    neurological, 301–306
    rashes, 427–428
    self-harm and suicide, 338–339
    sensory, 304–305
    speech, 302–303
    thyroid disorders, 259–261
    see also diagnosis
asthma
    perioperative medicine, 165
    pregnant patients, 178
    presentation, 387–389
asylum seekers, 204–207
ataxia, 312
ataxic gait, 305

atrial fibrillation (AF), 66–67, 171, 424–425
atropine, 66
AYAs *see* adolescents and young adults

B

B-mode *see* brightness mode
back pain, 376–378
bacterial meningitis, 327–329
basal insulin, 277, 278
basic life support (BLS), 72–73
Bedside Lung Ultrasound in Emergency (BLUE) protocol, 127
Bell's palsy, 310
benign paroxysmal positioning vertigo, 311
best practice, prescribing, 47–49
bias, 18–21
    clinical decision making, 141–142, 200
    mitigation, 20–21
bile ducts, gallstones, 371
bilevel positive airway pressure (BiPAP), 89
biliary colic, 371
bilirubin, 410–414
biomarkers, liver injury, 229
BiPAP *see* bilevel positive airway pressure
bipolar affective disorder, 346
bitemporal hemianopia, 307
blackout, 382
    see also collapse
bladder volume, ultrasound, 132–133
blood pressure, hypertensive emergencies, 97–99
blood transfusions, 57–58, 60
bloody diarrhoea, 398
BLS *see* basic life support
BLUE protocol *see* Bedside Lung Ultrasound in Emergency
board round checklist, 111
body fluid compartments, 252
body mass index (BMI), 295–296
body packers, 240
body temperature
    fever, 403–405
bone disorders, metabolic, 264–268

bone marrow failure syndromes, 415–417
bone metastases, 362
bone mineral density, scans, 150
bradycardia, 66, 68
brain tumors, 331, 361
breathing assessment and management, 55–56
breathlessness
  asthma, 387–389
  COPD, 386–387
  heart failure, 384–385
  pregnant patients, 178–179
  presentations, 382–389
brightness mode (B-mode), ultrasound, 118–119
bronchodilators, pregnant patients, 192
bulbar palsy, 311
bulimia nervosa, 343–345

C

C-ABCDE approach, 53–61
  airway, 55
  breathing, 55–56
  circulation, 56–60
  disability, 61
  exposure, 61
calcium channel blockers (CCB), overdose, 225
calcium metabolism, 263–268
  hypercalcaemia, 267–268
  hypocalcaemia, 264–267
Calgary-Cambridge Guide, 30
cancer, 351–364
  best practice, 363
  bone metastases, 361
  brain metastases, 361
  diagnosis, 363
  fluid collection, 361
  hypercalcaemia, 267, 356–357
  initial management, 354–356
  late effects, 363
  LGBTQ+ patients, 213
  metastatic, 361–362
  multiple myeloma, 359
  neuroendocrine tumours, 361–362
  paraneoplastic syndromes, 362
  thromboses, 361
  thyroid, 259
  see also oncology

CAP *see* community-acquired pneumonia
capabilities in practice (CiPs), 23–26
  see also generic capabilities
capacity, mental illness, 340, 349
carbon monoxide (CO), 222–223
cardiac arrest, 71–72
  advanced life support, 72–78
  basic life support, 72
  cause unknown, 84
  postresuscitation care, 82–84
  prior symptoms, 51, 65–71
  reversible causes, 78–79
  specific causes, 79–82
  withdrawal of treatment, 84–85
cardiac disease
  pregnant patients, 187–188
cardiac tamponade, 79, 82
cardiopulmonary resuscitation (CPR), 72–78
cardiovascular disease (CVD)
  chronic kidney disease, 292
  diabetes, 279, 288–295
  glucose-lowering therapies, 279
care levels, 87
cauda equina syndrome (CES), 377–378
CCB *see* calcium channel blockers
cellulitis, 420
cerebellopontine angle lesions, 310
cerebrovenous sinus thrombosis (CVST), 322
CES *see* cauda equina syndrome
CFS *see* clinical frailty scale
CGA *see* comprehensive geriatric assessment
CGM *see* continuous glucose monitoring
challenges in acute medicine, 7–8
challenging behaviour, 199
chemsex, 236
chest compressions, 72
chest pain, 389–394
  acute coronary syndromes, 389–391
  acute pericarditis, 392
  aortic dissection, 392–393
  pneumonia, 397
  pregnant patients, 179–181
  pulmonary embolus, 393–394
cholecystitis, 371
choledocholithiasis, 371

cholinergic toxidrome, 227
chronic kidney disease (CKD), 292–293, 378, 380–382
chronic liver disease, 166
chronic obstructive pulmonary disease (COPD), 56, 165, 386–387
chronic respiratory failure, 56
Churg-Strauss syndrome, 419
CiPs *see* capabilities in practice
circulatory assessment and management, 56–60, 162–165
circulatory support
  critical/enhanced care, 90
  post-resuscitation, 84
cirrhosis, liver, 413–414
classification
  adverse drug reactions, 44–45
  diabetes mellitus, 274–276
  diarrhoea, 398
  shock, 57
  stroke, 319–320
  thyroid disorders, 260
clinical decision making, acute medical take, 141–142
clinical documentation, 30–31
clinical frailty scale (CFS), 64, 157–158
clinical neurology
  basic, 300–306
  see also neurological disorders
clinical practice, ethics and legal issues, 27–28
clinical reasoning, 12–21
  acutely unwell patients, 21
  data gathering, 14
  decision making, 18–19
  diagnostic errors, 19–21
  illness scripts, 15–18
  problem representation, 14–15
clinical risk management, 33
clinical teaching, 37–38
clinical toxicology, 221–222
clinical trials, 34–37
clinician burnout, 26
Clostridioides difficile, 398
clozapine, 345–346
cluster headache, 314
CO *see* carbon monoxide
coaching, 39
cocaine, 237–238
cognitive autopsy, 21
cognitive biases, 18–19

cognitive function, post-
  resuscitation, 84
collapse, 186–187, 382
collapse query cause, 152
coma, 61, 302
Coma Cocktail, 224
common presentations, 7, 367–431
  abdominal pain, 367–376
  acute kidney injury, 378–380
  back pain, 376–378
  blackout, 382
  breathlessness, 382–389
  chest pain, 389–394
  chronic kidney disease, 378,
    380–382
  collapse, 382
  confusion, 378
  cough, 394–397
  delirium, 378
  diarrhoea, 398–400
  dizziness, 400–402
  end-of-life care, 422–423
  falls, 402–403
  fever, 403–405
  fits, 406–407
  haematemesis, 407–408
  hyperglycaemia, 410
  jaundice, 410–414
  lethargy, 414–419
  limb pain and swelling, 419–422
  medical emergencies, 51
  melaena, 407–408
  nausea, 429–430
  palliative care, 422–423
  palpitations, 424–425
  paralysis, 430–431
  poisoning, 425–426
  rash, 426–427
  seizures, 406–407
  travel-related, 405
  vomiting, 429–430
  weakness, 430–431
communication, 9, 28–30
  debriefing, 142–143
  handovers, 142
  skills, 29–30
  in teams, 29
community mental health
  services, 350
community-acquired pneumonia
  (CAP), 397
compartments, body fluids, 252
complex partial-onset seizures,
  315–316

comprehensive geriatric
  assessment (CGA), 158
confusion, 378
  see also delirium
consent, 28
  learning disabilities, 199–200
  mental illness, 340, 349
  self-harm and suicide, 340
consultations
  Calgary-Cambridge Guide, 30
  neurological, 301–302
continuous glucose monitoring
  (CGM), 276–277
continuous positive airway
  pressure (CPAP), 89
contraindications, positive
  pressure respiratory
  support, 89
COPD *see* chronic obstructive
  pulmonary disease
coronary artery disease (CAD)
  diabetes, 294
  perioperative medicine,
    163–164
coronary thrombosis, 79, 81–82
cortisol deficiency, 248–249
cough, 394–397
  tuberculosis, 395–397
COVID-19, 8–9
  cancer patients, 364
  critical/enhanced care, 92,
    95–97
  diabetic patients, 285–286
  long, 92
  multisystem complications, 97
  palliative care, 97
  pregnant patients, 179
  rash, 429
CPAP *see* continuous positive
  airway pressure
cranial nerves
  disorders, 306–311
  examination, 303–304
Criteria to Reside tool, 109
critical care, 86–99
  acute respiratory distress
    syndrome, 89–90
  admission, 88
  circulatory support, 90
  COVID-19, 92, 95–97
  daily assessment, 90
  FASTHUGS BID approach, 91
  general patient management,
    90–92

hypertension, 97–99
malnutrition, 91–92
monitoring, 90
multidisciplinary meetings, 92
neurological support, 90
outreach, 88
post-ICU, 92
refeeding syndrome, 92
renal support, 90
respiratory support, 88–91
sepsis, 92–95
withdrawal of treatment, 92
see also enhanced care
Crohn's disease, 399
CSF *see* cerebrospinal fluid
cultural literacy, 25–26
Cushing syndrome, 269
CVD *see* cardiovascular
  disease
CVST *see* cerebrovenous sinus
  thrombosis
cyanide exposure, 223

D

D-mode *see* Doppler mode
daily assessment, critical/
  enhanced care, 90
DAPT *see* dual antiplatelet
  therapy
data
  care improvement, 37
  gathering, 13–14
  research, 34–37
de-escalation, 348–349
debriefing, 142–143
decision making, 18–19
  see also diagnosis
decontamination, poisoning,
  224–225
deep vein thrombosis (DVT)
  illness script, 420–421
  pregnant patients, 198
  presentation, 420
  ultrasound, 134–137
defibrillation, 72–75
deficiencies, early warning scores,
  52–53
delirium
  assessment, 155–156
  management, 155–157
  older people, 154–157
  perioperative medicine, 171

delirium (*cont'd*)
  PINCH ME, 171
  presentation, 378
  prevention, 157
delirium tremens (DTs), 233
dementia
  older people, 153–154
  perioperative medicine, 171
dementia with Lewy bodies,
  153–154
demyelinating diseases,
  325–327
depressive disorder, 337
DI *see* diabetes insipidus
diabetes insipidus (DI), 258
diabetes mellitus, 246, 273–295
  acute complications, 281–288
  acutely unwell patients, 277
  cardiovascular disease, 279,
    288–295
  classification, 274–276
  complications, 274, 281–295
  coronary artery disease, 294
  COVID-19, 285–286
  diagnosis, 273–276
  discharge planning, 295
  foot ulcers, 288–291
  glucose-lowering therapies, 278
  glycaemic control, 276–277
  heart failure, 295
  hyperglycaemia, 279–281,
    284–288
  hyperosmolar hyperglycaemic
    state, 284–285, 286–288
  hypoglycaemia, 281–284
  incretins, 280
  macrovascular complications,
    293–295
  microvascular complications,
    277, 291–293
  perioperative medicine,
    167–170
  pregnant patients, 191
  prevalence in hospital
    populations, 246
  renal disorders, 292–293
  retinopathy, 293
  stroke, 294–295
  time in range, 277
  treatment, 277–281
diabetic foot ulcers, 288–291
diabetic ketoacidosis (DKA),
  284–288
diabetic neuropathy, 291–292

diagnosis, 18–21
  acute kidney injury, 174
  adrenal insufficiency, 270–272
  alcohol overuse, 232
  breathing status, 55–56
  cancer, 363
  cardiac tamponade, 82
  circulatory status, 56–60
  coronary thrombosis, 81
  deep vein thrombosis, 135
  delirium, 155
  dementia, 153–154
  diabetes mellitus, 273–276
  diabetic foot ulcers, 289
  differential, 13, 17–18
  epilepsy, 317
  errors, 19–21
  fever of unknown origin, 404
  final, 13
  free fluid in abdomen, 129
  Guillain–Barré syndrome, 329
  headaches in pregnancy, 185
  hydronephrosis, 131–132
  hypercalcaemia, 267–268
  hyperemesis gravidarum,
    183, 185
  hypocalcaemia, 265–266
  hypoglycaemia, 282
  hyponatraemia, 253–256
  hypopituitarism, 250
  interstitial syndrome, 125
  intracranial tumors, 331
  medical emergencies, 61–64
  multiple sclerosis, 326
  myasthenia gravis, 329–330
  neurological, 301–306
  osteoporosis, 150
  pituitary apoplexy, 251
  pleural effusion, 124–125
  pneumonia, 125–126
  pneumothorax, 123–124
  pre-eclampsia, 189
  pulmonary embolus, 81
  rashes, 427–428
  schemas, 14
  stroke, 320–322
  syndrome of inappropriate
    antidiuretic hormone, 255–256
  tension pneumothorax, 82
  thyroid disorders, 259–261
  toxin ingestion, 82
  upper airway obstruction, 55
  working, 13
  see also assessment

diagnostic momentum, 141
diagnostic schemas, 14
diagnostic testing, 13
diarrhoea, 398–400
differential diagnosis, 13, 17–18
  diabetes mellitus, 275–276
  epilepsy, 316–317
  headaches in pregnancy, 185
  jaundice, 411
  kidney injuries, 378–379
direct oral anticoagulants,
  perioperative, 173
disability, assessment, 61
discharge
  best practice, 110–112
  board round checklist, 111
  Criteria to Reside tool, 109
  diabetic patients, 295
  hospital at home, 105
  learning disabilities, 200
  planning, 107–112
  SAFER patient flow bundle, 110
  safety, 111
  self-, against medical advice,
    111–112
  self-harm and suicide, 339–340
diversity, 24–26
diverticulitis, 370–371
dizziness, 400–402
DNACPR *see* do not attempt
  cardiopulmonary
  resuscitation
do not attempt cardiopulmonary
  resuscitation (DNACPR),
  78, 84
documentation, 30–31
Doppler mode (D-mode),
  ultrasound, 119
dosing
  anticonvulsants, 318
  insulin, 278
DoTS classification, 45
drug allergy, 42–43
drug misuse, 234–245
  antidotes, 235
  body packers, 240
  general management, 241–243
  intravenous, 240
  malnutrition, 243–245
  special circumstances, 240–241
  toxidromes, 242
  see also specific substances. . .
drug toxicity, 42
drug-induced parkinsonism, 323

drugs, cardiac arrest, 77–78
DTs *see* delirium tremens
dual antiplatelet therapy (DAPT), 163–164
dual process theory, 18–19
DVT *see* deep vein thrombosis
dying patients, 64
dyspnoea, 382–389
   see also breathlessness

E

early warning scores, 51–53
eating disorders, 343–345
EBM *see* evidence-based medicine
ECG *see* electrocardiograms
eclampsia, 186, 189
ED *see* emergency department
education, 10–11
EEG *see* electroencephalograms
electrocardiograms (ECG)
   acute coronary syndrome, 81–82
   arrythmias, 66, 77
   cardiac tamponade, 82
   pregnant patients, 181
electroencephalograms (EEG), 306
   epilepsy, 317
   post-resuscitation, 84
electrolyte solutions, 57
elimination, poisons, 225
emergency department (ED), 4
end-of-life care, 422–423
endocrinology, 245–298
   Addisonian crisis, 170
   adrenal disorders, 170, 268–273
   basics, 246–247
   calcium metabolism, 263–268
   cortisol deficiency, 248–249
   Cushing syndrome, 269
   diabetes insipidus, 258
   diabetes mellitus, 167–170, 191, 246, 273–295
   fluid balance, 251–258
   hypercalcaemia, 267–268
   hyperglycaemia, 279–281, 284–288
   hypernatraemia, 257–258
   hypocalcaemia, 264–267
   hypoglycaemia, 281–284
   hyponatraemia, 252, 253–257
   hypopituitarism, 249–250

hypothalmic-pituitary disorders, 248–251
   incidentalomas, 270
   inherited metabolic disorders, 297–298
   laboratory testing, 247–248
   myxoedema coma, 262–263
   obesity, 295–297
   perioperative medicine, 167–170
   phaeochromocytoma, 269
   pituitary apoplexy, 251
   pituitary tumours, 250–251
   SIADH, 253, 255–256, 258
   sodium balance, 251, 253–258
   thyroid disease, 258–263
enhanced care, 86–99
   acute respiratory distress syndrome, 89–90
   circulatory support, 90
   COVID-19, 92, 95–97
   daily assessment, 90
   definition, 87
   FASTHUGS BID approach, 91
   general patient management, 90–92
   hypertension, 97–99
   malnutrition, 91–92
   monitoring, 90
   multidisciplinary meetings, 92
   neurological support, 90
   outreach, 88
   post-ICU, 92
   refeeding syndrome, 92
   renal support, 90
   respiratory support, 88–91
   sepsis, 92–95
   withdrawal of treatment, 92
   see also critical care
enteral nutrition, 91
entrustable professional activities (EPAs), 22, 23–24
EPAs *see* entrustable professional activities
epilepsy, 315–319
   anticonvulsants, 318–319
   assessment, 317–318
   causes, 315
   diagnosis, 317
   differential diagnosis, 316–317
   management, 318–319
   perioperative medicine, 171
   presentation, 406–407
   seizures, 315–316

equity, 24–26
errors
   diagnostic, 19–21
   insulin dosing, 48
   prescription, 46–47
erythroderma, 428–429
ethics, clinical practice, 27–28
euthyroid-sick syndrome, 259
evaluation
   breathlessness, 383–384
   clinical studies, 36–37
   see also assessment; diagnosis
evidence-based medicine (EBM), 35
examination
   drug misuse, 241–243
   neurological, 303–305
   see also assessment; diagnosis
exposure
   assessment, 61
   carbon monoxide, 222–223
   cyanide, 223
   organophosphates, 227
   see also toxicology

F

facial nerve disorders, 310
falls, 152, 402–403
FASTHUGS BID approach, 91
FBC *see* full blood count
feet, diabetic ulcers, 288–291
fever, 403–405
   returning travellers, 404–405
   unknown origin, 404
fever of unknown origin (FUO), 404
FiO_2 *see* inspired oxygen concentration
fits, 406–407
   see also seizures
fluid balance, 251–258
   hypernatraemia, 257–258
   hyponatraemia, 252, 253–257
   sodium homeostasis, 253
fluid loss, 56–58
fluids, cardiac arrest, 77–78
focused abdominal ultrasound, 127–131
   free fluid in abdomen, 129
   limitations and pitfalls, 129–130
   normal anatomy, 129
   paracentesis, 129
   technique, 127–129

focused renal ultrasound, 131–134
  bladder volume, 132–133
  hydronephrosis, 131–132
  limitations and pitfalls, 133–134
  normal anatomy, 131
  technique, 131
folate deficiency, 244
four Hs, 79
four Ts, 79
frailty
  assessment, 64, 148–149,
    157–158
  concepts, 148–149
  delirium, 154–157
  dementia, 153–154
  falls, 152
  incontinence, 153
  multimorbidity, 151
  polypharmacy, 151–152
  sarcopenia, 148–149
  syndromes, 150–157
free fluid, in abdomen,
    ultrasound, 129
frontotemporal dementia, 153
full blood count (FBC), 416
functional disorders,
    neurological, 333
FUO *see* fever of unknown origin

G

gait, examination, 305
gallstones, 371
gamma-butyrolactone (GBL), 235
gamma-hydroxybutyrate
    (GHB), 235
gastroenterology
  diarrhoea, 398–400
  haematemesis, 407–408
  lower gastrointestinal
    bleeding, 408
  melaena, 407–408
  nausea and vomiting, 429–430
  perioperative, 166
  symptoms with alarm features,
    375
GBL *see* gamma-butyrolactone
GCA *see* giant cell arteritis
GCS *see* Glasgow Coma Scale
generalised seizures, 316
generic capabilities, 22–39
  burnout, 26
  communication, 28–30

consultations, 30
entrustable professional
    activities, 23–24
ethics, 27–28
legal, 28
NHS organizational/
    management systems, 26–27
patient safety, 31–33
professionalism, 30–31
quality improvement, 33–34
research, 34–37
supervision, 37–39
teaching, 37–38
geriatric medicine
  5 Ms, 149
  best practice, 158–159
  delirium, 154–157
  dementia, 153–154
  falls, 152
  frailty assessment, 148–149,
    157–158
  incontinence, 153
  multimorbidity, 151
  osteoporosis, 149–151
  polypharmacy, 151–152
  sarcopenia, 148–149
Getting It Right First Time
    (GIRFT) report, 10, 11
GHB *see* gamma-hydroxybutyrate
giant cell arteritis (GCA), 314–315
GIRFT *see* Getting It Right First
    Time
Glasgow Coma Scale (GCS),
    61, 302
GLP *see* glucagon-like peptide
glucagon-like peptide (GLP)-1
    receptor agonist, 278, 280
glucocorticoids, 269
glucose-lowering therapies,
    167–169, 278, 284, 292
glycaemic control, 276–277
Graves' disease, 259
Guillain–Barré syndrome, 329
gym drugs, 241
gypsies, 207–208

H

H@H *see* hospital at home
haematemesis, 407–408
haematology, perioperative,
    172–173
haemolytic anemia, 417

haemorrhagic stroke, 320–322
HALT *see* hungry, angry, late, tired
handover, acute medical take, 142
Hashimoto thyroiditis, 259
HCM *see* hypercalcaemia of
    malignancy
HDU *see* high-dependency units
head injury, 249, 331–333
headache, 312–315
  cluster-type, 314
  common presentations,
    408–410
  giant cell arteritis, 314–315
  idiopathic intracranial
    hypertension, 315
  medication overuse, 314
  migraine, 313–314
  posttraumatic, 314
  pregnant patients, 183–186
  SNOOP4, 409–410
  tension-related, 313
  trigeminal neuralgia, 314
health inequity, 25–26
health needs
  learning disabilities, 198
  LGBTQ+ patients, 211–213
heart failure
  diabetes, 295
  perioperative medicine, 164
  presentation, 384–386
hemiplegia, 311
hemiplegic gait, 305
heparin
  perioperative, 172–173
  pregnant patients, 190
hepatic disease
  perioperative medicine, 166
  presentation, 410–414
  see also liver
hepatic encephalopathy, 414
heroin, 239
heuristics, 18
hierarchy of evidence, 35–36
high-dependency units (HDU),
    admissions, 87, 88
high-dose insulin euglycaemic
    therapy, 225
hip fractures, 150
history, 62
  epilepsy, 317
  neurological, 302
  poisoned patients, 225–227
HIV *see* human immunodeficiency
    virus

homelessness, 202–205
homonymous hemianopia, 307–309
hospital at home (H@H), 6–7, 104–106
  blood tests, 105
  early discharge, 105
  imaging, 105–106
  indications, 105
  multidisciplinary teams, 106
  oxygen therapy, 106
  parenteral therapy, 106
  primary care teams, 106
  specialist investigations, 106
hot clinics see rapid access clinics
human factors, 33
human immunodeficiency virus (HIV), 215–220
  best practice, 219–220
  course of infection, 216
  IRIS, 217
  management, 217–219
  opportunistic infections, 216–218
  transmission, 216
hungry, angry, late, tired (HALT), 19, 20
hydronephrosis, ultrasound, 131–132
hypercalcaemia, 267–268
hypercalcaemia of malignancy (HCM), 267, 356–357
hypercapnic respiratory failure, 56
hyperemesis gravidarum, 182–185
hyperglycaemia, 279–281, 284–288, 410
hyperkalaemia, 80
hyperlactaemia, 57
hypernatraemia, 257–258
hyperosmolar hyperglycaemic state (HHS), 284–285, 286–288
hyperparathyroidism, 264
hypertension
  critical/enhanced care, 97–99
  perioperative medicine, 164, 165–166
  pregnant patients, 188–189
hyperthermia, 79, 81
hyperthyroidism, 259
  classification, 260
  investigation, 260–261
  perioperative medicine, 170
  thyroid storm, 261–262

hypertonic saline, 256–257
hypocalcaemia, 264–267
  diagnosis, 265–266
hypoglycaemia, 281–284
hypokalaemia, 79–80, 244
hyponatraemia, 252, 253–257
  diagnosis, 253–256
  pregnant patients, 191
  SIADH, 253, 255–256
  treatment, 256–257
hypoparathyroidism, 264
hypopituitarism, 249–250
hypothalmic-pituitary disorders, 248–251
  cortisol deficiency, 248–249
  diabetes insipidus, 258
  hypopituitarism, 249–250
  pituitary apoplexy, 251
  pituitary tumours, 250–251
hypothermia, 79, 80–81
hypothyroidism, 259
  classification, 260
  investigation, 260–261
  myxoedema coma, 262–263
  perioperative medicine, 170
hypovolaemia, 57, 79, 90
hypoxaemia, 88–89
hypoxia, 79

I

ICIs see immune checkpoint inhibitors
ICU see intensive care unit
idiopathic intracranial hypertension, 185, 315
illness scripts, 15–18
  acute pancreatitis, 372–373
  aortic dissection, 393
  asthma, 388
  atrial fibrillation, 425
  cholecystitis, 371
  community-acquired pneumonia, 397
  COPD, 386–387
  Crohn's disease, 399
  deep vein thrombosis, 420–421
  diverticulitis, 370–371
  heart failure, 384–385
  oncology, 353
  peptic ulcers, 374–375
  pulmonary embolus, 393–394
  renal calculi, 375–376

  small bowel obstruction, 370
  tuberculosis, 395–396
  ulcerative colitis, 400
IM see intramuscular
imaging
  abdominal, 369
  epilepsy, 318
  home care, 105–106
  neurological, 305–306, 318
  point-of-care ultrasound, 113–137
IMDs see inherited metabolic disorders
immune checkpoint inhibitors (ICIs), 249
immune reconstitution inflammatory syndrome (IRIS), 219
immune-related adverse events 360
immune-related endocrine events 249
immunosuppression, perioperative, 174–175
immunotherapy, complications, 360–361
implicit bias, 141
in-hospital cardiac arrest
  epidemiololgy, 71–72
  postresuscitation care, 82–84
  resuscitation, 72–78
  reversible causes, 78–79
  specific causes, 79–82
  stopping resuscitation, 78, 84–85
inclusion health, 24–26, 201–208
  best practice, 208
  criminal justice services, 207
  gypsies and travellers, 207–208
  homelessness, 202–205
  migration-related concerns, 204–207
  principles, 202
  sex workers, 207
incontinence, older people, 153
incretins, 280
indications
  hospital at home, 105
  learning disabilities, 198
  respiratory support, 89
  same-day emergency care, 101, 103
inequities, 25–26

infectious diseases
  contamination, 220
  diabetic foot ulcers, 290
  human immunodeficiency
    virus, 215–220
  meningitis, 327–329
  neurological disorders, 327–329
inherited metabolic disorders
  (IMDs), 297–298
inpatient management
  Parkinson disease, 325
  see also admissions
inspired oxygen concentration
  (FiO$_2$), 56
insulin
  basic prescribing, 280–281
  dosing, 278
  medication errors, 48
  perioperative medicine,
    167–170
  type 1 diabetes, 277–278, 281
  type 2 diabetes, 280–281
intensive care units (ICU)
  admissions, 63–64, 84, 87, 88
  discharge, 92
  post-resuscitation, 84
interface medicine, 6
internal medicine, 4–5
internal water balance, 252
internally displaced people,
  204–207
interstitial syndrome,
  ultrasound, 125
intestinal ischaemia, 373–374
intoxication, alcohol, 231–232
intracerebral haemorrhage,
  320–322
intracranial tumours, 331
intravenous (IV) access, 56–58
intravenous (IV) drug misuse, 240
intravenous (IV) fluids
  at home, 106
  hypercalcaemia of
    malignancy, 356
  hyperemesis gravidarum, 184
  hypertonic saline, 256–257
intravenous (IV) resuscitation,
  57–58
  cardiac arrest, 77–78
intubation, 56
invasive ventilation, 89
investigations
  medical emergencies, 62–63
  see also assessment; diagnosis

Ipswich touch test, 289
IRIS *see* immune reconstitution
  inflammatory syndrome
iron deficiency, 244
ischaemic colitis, 373–374
ischaemic heart disease,
  perioperative medicine,
  163–164
IV *see* intravenous

J

jaundice, 410–414
joint swelling, 421–422

K

Kernig's sign, 328
ketamine, 240
kidneys
  diabetic complications, 292–293
  glucose homeostasis, 280
knowledge, psychomotor skills
  and attitudes (KSA), 22–39
  entrustable professional
    activities, 22, 23–26
  see also generic capabilities
KSA *see* knowledge, psychomotor
  skills and attitudes

L

laboratory tests
  drug screening, 243
  endocrine, 247–248
large vessel occlusion, 321
leadership, 9, 27
  styles, 27
learning disabilities, 197–200
  best practice, 198–200
  consent, 199–200
  everyday effects, 197–198
  health needs, 198
  indicators, 198
left upper quadrant (LUQ),
  abdominal ultrasound,
  128–130
left ventricular ejection
  fraction, 66
legal issues, clinical practice,
  27–28

length of stays, reduction, 108
Lesbian, gay, bisexual,
  transgender, queer or
  questioning, and others
  (LGBTQ+), 209–214
  best practice, 213–214
  cancer, 213
  gender identities, 210–211
  health needs, 211–213
  infections, 213
  medical definitions, 210
  medical transitioning, 212–213
  sexual orientation, 211
lethargy, 414–419
levels of care, 87
levodopa, 324
Lewy body dementias, 153–154
liason psychiatry, 349–350
light-headedness, 401–402
limb pain and swelling, 419–422
lithium, 346
liver cirrhosis, 413–414
liver disease
  acute deterioration, 412
  non-alcoholic fatty, 296–297
  perioperative medicine, 166
liver function
  biomarkers, 229
  jaundice, 410–414
  paracetamol overdose, 227–229
  pregnant patients, 191
LMWH *see* low molecular weight
  heparin
long COVID, 92
long-term sequelae, head injury,
  332–333
lorazepam, 318
low molecular weight heparin
  (LMWH), pregnant
  patients, 190
lower gastrointestinal
  bleeding, 408
LP *see* lumbar puncture
LSD *see* lysergic acid diethylamide
lumbar puncture (LP), 306
lungs
  interstitial syndrome, 125
  normal sonographic
    presentation, 121–123
  pleural effusion, 124–125
  pneumonia, 125–126
  pneumothorax, 123–124
  thoracentesis, 126
LUQ *see* left upper quadrant

lymphoedema, 419
lysergic acid diethylamide
(LSD), 240

M

M-mode see motion mode
macrocytic anemia, 417
macrovascular complications,
diabetes, 293–295
magic mushrooms, 240
magnesium levels, 244
malnutrition, 91–92
drug and alcohol misuse,
243–244
perioperative medicine, 167
management
acute alcohol withdrawal,
233–234
acute medical takes, 138–143
acute respiratory distress
syndrome, 90
acute thrombosis in
pregnancy, 190
adrenal insufficiency, 272–273
adverse drug reactions, 45–46
carbon monoxide exposure, 223
COVID-19, 95–97
delirium, 155–157
diabetes mellitus, 277–281
diabetic foot ulcers, 289–291
diabetic ketoacidosis, 286–288
drug misuse, 241–243
epilepsy, 318–319
Guillain–Barré syndrome, 329
head injury, 332
headaches, pregnancy, 185
human immunodeficiency
virus, 217–219
hyper/hypokalaemia, 80
hyper/hypothermia, 81
hypercalcaemia, 268
hypercalcaemia of malignancy,
356–357
hyperemesis gravidarum, 184
hyperglycaemia, 279–281
hypernatraemia, 257–258
hyperosmolar hyperglycaemic
state, 286–288
hypertensive emergencies,
97–99
hypocalcaemia, 266–267
hypoglycaemia, 282–284

hypopituitarism, 250
intracranial tumors, 331
ischaemic heart disease,
163–164
jaundice, 412
massive haemorrhage, 58–60
medically unexplained physical
symptoms, 342–343
meningitis, 328
metastatic spinal cord
compression, 357
motor neurone disease,
330–331
multiple sclerosis, 326–327
myasthenia gravis, 330
neutropenic sepsis, 359
obesity, 296–297
opioid withdrawal, 239–240
osteoporosis, 151
paracetamol overdose, 228–229
Parkinson disease, 324–325
poisoned patients, 223–229
schizophrenia, 345–346
self-harm, 338–340
sepsis/septic shock, 94–95
shock, 56–58
stroke, 320–322
transfusions, 57–58
tumour lysis syndrome,
357–359
ward selection, 55
MAP see mean arterial pressure
marijuana, 235
massive haemorrhage, 58–60
MDMA, 237
MDT see multidisciplinary teams
mean arterial pressure (MAP),
57, 71
mechanical ventilation, 56
medical emergencies
active bleeding, 58–60
airway status, 55
blood transfusions, 57–58, 60
C-ABCDE approach, 53–61
circulatory status, 56–60
definitive diagnosis, 61–64
disability, 61
early warning scores, 51–53
exposure, 61
history, 62
immediate assessment, 53–54
investigations, 62–63
massive haemorrhage, 58–60
physical examination, 62

recognition, 51–53
transfusions, 57–58
ward selection, 55
medical history, poisoned
patients, 225–227
medical registrars, 138–143
acute take shifts, 140
clinical decision making,
141–142
debriefing, 142–143
handover, 142
night working, 140–141
roles and responsibilities, 139
Medical Research Council scale,
muscle weakness, 303
medically unexplained physical
symptoms, 341–343
medication errors, 46–47
medication overuse
headache, 314
medication safety, 41–42
melaena, 407–408
Ménière's disease, 310
meningiomas, 331
meningitis, 185, 327–329
aetiology, 327
diagnosis, 328
management, 328
tuberculous, 328–329
Mental Capacity Act (2005),
199–200, 340
mental health, 335–350
adjustment disorder, 341
aggressive behaviour, 347–349
anxiety-related disorders, 337
bipolar affective disorder, 346
bulimia nervosa, 343–345
capacity, 340, 349
depressive disorder, 337
eating disorders, 343–345
health services, 349–350
LGBTQ+ patients, 212
medically unexplained physical
symptoms, 341–343
mood disorders, 336–337
personality disorders, 346–347
physical illness, 336
poisoned patients, 225
posttraumatic stress
disorder, 341
pregnant patients, 191
schizophrenia, 345–346
self-harm, 337–340
severe illnesses, 345–346

mental health (*cont'd*)
  stress, 340–341
  suicidal thoughts, 337–340
  trauma, 340–341
Mental Health Act (MHA), 349
mental state examination, 302
mentoring, 39
meta-analysis, 36–37
metabolic bone diseases, 264–268
metabolic disorders
  inherited, 297–298
  see also hormonal disorders
metabolic emergencies, pregnant
    patients, 191
metacognition, 20
metastatic cancer, 361–362
metastatic spinal cord
    compression (MSCC), 357
metformin, 278, 292
methadone, 239
MEWS *see* Maternity Early
    Warning Score
MHA *see* Mental Health Act
microcytic anemia, 417
microvascular complications
  diabetes, 277, 291–293
  time in range, 277
migraine, 313–314
migration-related concerns,
    204–207
Miller's pyramid, 23
mini-mental test, 302
Maternity Early Warning Score
    (MEWS), 177
modified SNAP regimen, 229
monitoring
  critical/enhanced care, 90
  glycaemic control, 276–277
monoamine oxidase B inhibitors,
    324–325
monoplegia, 311
mood disorders, 336–337
morphine, 239
motion mode (M-mode),
    ultrasound, 118–119
motor limb examination, 303–304
motor neurone disease, 330–331
motor pathways, 300
MS *see* multiple sclerosis
MSCC *see* metastatic spinal cord
    compression
multidisciplinary teams (MDT)
  critical/enhanced care, 92
  discharge planning, 110–111

home care, 106
surgery decision-making,
    161–162
multimorbidity, 151
multiple myeloma, 359
multiple sclerosis (MS), 325–327
  aetiology, 325
  clinical features, 326
  diagnosis, 326
  management, 326–327
  prognosis, 327
  relapses, 327
  types, 326
multisystem complications,
    COVID-19, 97
muscle diseases, 333
muscle weakness, 303–304
myasthenia gravis, 329–330
myocardial infarction (MI) *see*
    acute myocardial infarction
myocardial ischaemia, 66
myopathy, neurological, 333
myxoedema coma, 262–263

N

N-acetylcysteine (NAC), 228–229
NAC *see* N-acetylcysteine
NAFLD *see* non-alcoholic fatty
    liver disease
narcolepsy, 334
National Early Warning Score
    (NEWS2), 51–52
nausea, 182–185, 429–430
necrotising fasciitis, 421
needlestick contamination, 220
nerve conduction studies, 306
neuroanatomy, 300
neuroendocrine tumours,
    361–362
neurological disorders, 299–334
  anatomy, 300
  ataxia, 312
  basic clinical practice, 300–306
  Bell's palsy, 310
  benign paroxysmal positioning
    vertigo, 311
  bulbar palsy, 311
  central nervous system
    infections, 327–328
  cerebrovenous sinus
    thrombosis, 322
  coma, 302

common patterns, 311–312
consultations, 301–302
cranial nerves, 303–304,
    306–311
diagnosis, 301–306
epilepsy, 315–319
facial nerve, 310
functional, 333
gait examination, 305
Guillain–Barré syndrome, 329
headache, 312–315, 408–410
hemiplegia, 311
infections, 327–329
intracerebral haemorrhage,
    320–322
intracranial tumours, 331
lumbar puncture, 306
Ménière's disease, 310
meningitis, 327–329
mental state assessment, 302
monoplegia, 311
motor limb examination,
    303–304
motor neurone disease,
    330–331
motor pathways, 300
multiple sclerosis, 325–327
muscle diseases, 333
myasthenia gravis, 329–330
optic atrophy, 309
optic nerve, 306–309
papilloedema, 309
Parkinson disease, 153–154,
    170, 305, 322–325
peripheral neuropathy, 312
pseudobulbar palsy, 311
pupil abnormalities, 306–307
quadriparesis, 311
radiology, 305–306
sensory examination, 304–305
sensory pathways, 300–301
spastic paraparesis, 311
speech assessment, 302–303
stroke, 310, 319–322
subarachnoid haemorrhage,
    320–322
traumatic brain injury, 249,
    331–333
tuberculous meningitis,
    328–329
vestibulocochlear nerve,
    310–311
visual field effects, 307–309
Wilson disease, 323–324

neurological patterns, 311–312
neuropathy, diabetic, 291–292
neurophysiological
    assessment, 306
neutropenic sepsis, 359
NEWS2 *see* National Early
    Warning Score
NHS organizational/management
    systems, 26–27
nitrous oxide, 236
NIV *see* non-invasive ventilation
non-alcoholic fatty liver disease
    (NAFLD), 296–297
non-bloody diarrhoea, 398
non-epileptic attack disorder,
    316–317
non-invasive ventilation (NIV),
    56, 89
non-ST elevation myocardial
    infarction (NSTEMI), 81–82,
    163–164, 389
non-steroidal anti-inflammatory
    drugs (NSAIDs), 47, 174
non-thyroidal illness, 259
normal anatomical findings
    focused abdominal
        ultrasound, 129
    focused renal ultrasound, 131
    thoracic ultrasound, 120–123
normocytic anemia, 417
novel highs, 235–236
NRTIs *see* nucleoside reverse
    transcriptase inhibitors
NSAIDs *see*
    non-steroidal anti-
    inflammatories
NSTEMI *see* non-ST elevation
    myocardial infarction
nucleoside reverse transcriptase
    inhibitors (NRTIs), 217

O

obesity
    cardiopulmonary
        resuscitation, 78
    hormonal disorders, 295–297
obesity hypoventilation
    syndrome, 165
obstructive sleep apnoea, 165
oncology, 351–364
    best practice, 363
    bone metastases, 362

brain metastases, 361
diagnosis, 363
emergencies, 355, 356–359
fluid collection, 361
hypercalcaemia of malignancy,
    356–357
initial management, 354–356
late effects, 363
metastatic spinal cord
    compression, 357
metastatic spread patterns, 352
neuroendocrine tumours,
    361–362
neutropenic sepsis, 359
paraneoplastic syndromes, 362
superior vena cava
    obstruction, 359
therapy complications, 360–361
thromboses, 361
tumour lysis syndrome,
    357–359
opiates, 174–175, 239
opioids, 239
opportunistic infections, human
    immunodeficiency virus,
    216–218
optic nerve disorders, 306–309
organisation, same-day
    emergency care, 101–102
organophosphate poisoning, 227
osteoporosis, 149–151, 264
out-of-hospital cardiac arrest, 71
outreach, critical care, 88
overdose
    calcium channel blockers, 225
    paracetamol, 227–229
    see also toxicology
oxygen therapy, 56, 88–89, 106

P

pacemakers, perioperative
    medicine, 165
palliative care, 97, 422–423
palpitations, pregnant patients,
    181–182
pancreatitis, 372–373
papilloedema, 309
paracentesis, ultrasound-
    guided, 129
paracetamol overdose, 227–229
paralysis, 430–431
paraneoplastic syndromes, 362

parathyroid hormone, 264–268
parenteral nutrition, 91
parenteral therapy
    at home, 106
    see also intravenous. . .
Parkinson disease dementia,
    153–154
Parkinson disease, 322–325
    aetiology, 323
    clinical features, 323
    differential diagnosis, 323
    gait, 305
    management, 324–325
    perioperative medicine, 170
    prognosis, 325
Parkinson Plus syndromes, 323
partial-onset seizures, 315–316
patient safety incidents, 31–33
patient-centred shared decision
    making, 13
PCI *see* percutaneous coronary
    intervention
PE *see* pulmonary embolus
pedagogy, 37–38
PEEP *see* positive end-expiratory
    pressure
peptic ulcers, 374–375
percutaneous coronary
    intervention (PCI), 79
peri-arrest care, 65–71
    anaphylaxis, 66, 69–71
    arrhythmias, 66–68
pericarditis, 392
perioperative medicine, 160–175
    alcohol misuse, 166–167
    analgesia, 174–175
    cardiac issues, 162–165
    decision making, 161–162
    endocrinology, 167–170
    gastrointestinal issues, 166
    haematology, 172–173
    immunosuppression, 174–175
    neurology, 170–171
    nutrition, 167
    outcome improvement, 162
    physician roles, 160
    renal support, 173–174
    respiratory issues, 165–166
peripartum cardiomyopathy, 188
peripheral artery disease, 288–291
peripheral nervous system, 300
peripheral neuropathy, 312
peripheral oxygen saturation,
    55–56

permanent pacemakers,
perioperative medicine, 165
personality disorders, 346–347
pH, 62–63
phaeochromocytoma, 269
pharmacovigilance, 42–46
phenytoin, 318
phosphate levels, 244
physical examination, 14
physiology, pregnancy, 177, 187
PICO tool, 35
PINCH ME mnemonic, 171
pituitary apoplexy, 251
pituitary tumours, 250–251, 331
planning, discharge, 107–112
pleural effusion, ultrasound,
124–125
pleuritic chest pain, pregnant
patients, 181
pneumonia, 125–126, 397
pneumothorax, ultrasound,
123–124
POC see point-of-care
POCUS see point-of-care
ultrasound
point-of-care (POC) testing,
endocrine, 248
point-of-care ultrasound
(POCUS), 79, 113–137
artifacts, 115–116
bladder volume, 132–133
BLUE protocol, 127
deep vein thrombosis, 134–137
focused abdominal, 127–131
focused renal, 131–134
free fluid in abdomen, 129
hydronephrosis, 131–132
image optimisation, 119–120
image production, 117–118
interstitial syndrome, 125
paracentesis, 129
physics of, 114–115
pleural effusion, 124–125
pneumonia, 125–126
pneumothorax, 123–124
preparation, 120
probes, 116–117
procedural guidance, 136
resolution, 118–120
scanning modes, 118–119
scanning planes, 118
thoracentesis, 126
thoracic, 120–127
poison, definition, 222

poisoned patients, 221–229
ABCDEFGH approach, 224
alcohol, 231–234
antidotes, 225–227
carbon monoxide, 222–223
cardiac arrest, 79, 82
Coma Cocktail, 224
cyanide, 223
decontamination, 224–225
elimination, 225
general management
principles, 223–227
medical history, 225–227
paracetamol overdose, 227–229
presentation, 425–426
psychiatry review, 225
recreational drugs, 234–241
RRSIDEAD approach, 224
toxicological definitions, 222
toxidromes, 224, 227
poisoning, cardiac arrest, 79, 82
polypharmacy, older people,
151–152
positive end-expiratory pressure
(PEEP), 56
posterior reversible
encephalopathy
syndrome 185
postresuscitation care, 72, 82–84
posttraumatic headache, 314
posttraumatic stress disorder
(PTSD), 341
pre-eclampsia, 185, 189
pre-syncope, 401–402
pregnancy testing, 176
Pregnancy-Unique Quantification
of Emesis (PUQE) index, 183
pregnant patients, 176–193
arrhythmias, 182
breathlessness, 178–179
cardiac disease, 187–188
chest pain, 179–181
collapse, 186–187
COVID-19, 179
eclampsia, 186, 189
headache, 183–186
hypertension, 188–189
liver function, 191
mental health crises, 191
metabolic emergencies, 191
MEWS, 177
nausea and vomiting, 182–185
palpitations, 181–182
physiological changes, 177, 187

pre-eclampsia, 185, 189
prescriptions, 191–192
pulmonary embolism, 179,
189–191
radiological investigations,
177–178
resuscitation, 192
sepsis, 187
venous thromboembolism,
189–191
preparation
acute medical take, 139–140
ultrasound, 120
prescribing, 40–49
adverse drug reactions, 42–46
antimicrobial stewardship, 49
best practice, 47–49
errors, 46–47
insulin, 280–281
pharmacovigilance, 42–46
polypharmacy, 151–152
pregnant patients, 191–192
rational, 41
safety, 41–42
prevention
delirium, 157
secondary stroke, 321–322
primary headache, 409
primary hyperparathyroidism,
264, 267
probes, ultrasound, 116–117
problem lists, 13
problem representation, 13, 14–15
procedural guidance,
ultrasound, 136
professionalism, 30–31
prolactinomas, 251
proteinuria, pregnant
patients, 189
pseudobulbar palsy, 311
psychiatric disorders
poisoned patients, 225
pregnant patients, 191
PTSD see posttraumatic stress
disorder
pulmonary embolus (PE), 78, 81
illness script, 393–394
pregnant patients, 179,
189–191, 198
pulmonary oedema, pregnant
patients, 178–179
pulseless electrical activity, 71, 81
pulsus paradoxus, 82
pupil abnormalities, 306–307

PUQE index *see* Pregnancy-
   Unique Quantification of
   Emesis

Q

qSOFA *see* quick SOFA
quadriparesis, 311
quality improvement, 33–34
quick SOFA (qSOFA) scores, 932

R

race, 25–26
radiation doses, fetal/
   maternal, 178
radiology
   neurological, 305–306
   pregnant patients, 177–178
RAPD *see* relative afferent
   pupillary defect
rapid access (hot) clinics, 6
rashes, 426–429
rational decision making, 19
rational prescribing, 41
rationality failure, 19
Realistic Medicine 7-Steps
   approach, 152
reasonable adjustments, 199
recreational drugs, 234–245
   antidotes, 235
   body packers, 240
   CAGE questionnaire
      screening, 234
   generic management, 241–243
   intravenous administration, 240
   screening, 243
   special circumstances, 240–241
   toxidromes, 242
   see also specific substances...
recruitment, 9
red flags, 13
reduction, length of stay, 108
refeeding syndrome, 92
refractory anaphylaxis, 70
refractory hypotension, 225
refugees, 204–207
refusal of treatment,
   self-harm, 340
relative afferent pupillary defect
   (RAPD), 306
renal calculi/colic, 375–376

renal support, 90
   perioperative, 173–174
renal transplants, 174
renal ultrasound, 131–134
   bladder volume, 132–133
   hydronephrosis, 131–132
   limitations and pitfalls, 133–134
   normal anatomy, 131
   technique, 131
rescue breaths, 72
research trials, 34–37
respiratory acidosis, 56
respiratory arrest, 75–77
respiratory failure, 56
respiratory support, 88–91
   cardiac arrest, 75–77
   oxygen therapy, 56, 88–89
   perioperative, 165–166
   post-resuscitation, 84
responsibilities, medical
   registrars, 139
restraint, 349
resuscitation, 65–85
   advanced life support, 72–78
   anaphylaxis, 66, 69–71
   arrhythmias, 66–68
   basic life support, 72–73
   cardiac arrest, 71–72
   cardiac tamponade, 79, 82
   coronary thrombosis, 79,
      81–82
   four Hs, 79
   four Ts, 79
   hyper/hypokalaemia, 79–80
   hyper/hypothermia, 80–81
   maternal, 192
   obesity, 78
   peri-arrest, 65–71
   postresuscitation care, 82–84
   pulmonary embolus, 78, 81
   reversible causes, 78–79
   sepsis, 71, 79
   specific causes, 79–82
   tension pneumothroax, 79, 82
   toxic agents, 79, 82
   withdrawal of treatment, 78,
      84–85
retention, 9
retinopathy, diabetic, 293
return of spontaneous circulation
   (ROSC), 71–72, 77, 82–84
returning travellers, fever, 404–405
reverberation artifacts, 116
reversal, anticoagulants, 173

reversible causes, cardiac arrest,
   78–79
rheumatoid arthritis, 422
right upper quadrant (RUQ),
   abdominal ultrasound,
   128–130
risk factors
   adverse drug reactions, 43
   aggressive behaviour, 348
   diabetic foot ulcers, 289
   stroke, 320
   sudden unexpected death in
      epilepsy, 187
risk management
   clinical, 33
   self-harm and suicide, 339
roles, medical registrars, 139
ROSC *see* return of spontaneous
   circulation
ROWS *see* rule out worst-case
   scenarios
RRSIDEAD approach, 224
rule out worst-case scenarios
   (ROWS), 13, 17
RUQ *see* right upper quadrant

S

safeguarding, learning
   disabilities, 200
SAFER patient flow bundle, 110
safety, 31–33
   antimicrobial stewardship, 49
   discharge, 111
   medication, 41–42
   prescribing, 40–49
SAH *see* subarachnoid
   haemorrhage
saline, hypertonic, 256–257
SAM *see* Society of Acute
   Medicine
same-day emergency care
   (SDEC), 4, 5–6, 100–103
   benefits, 102
   organisation, 101–102
   patient selection, 103
   principles, 101–102
sarcopenia, 148–149
SBARR *see* situation, background,
   assessment,
   recommendation and
   readback system
scabies, 429

schizophrenia, 345–346
Screening Tool of Older Persons' Prescriptions (STOPP), 48
Screening Tool to Alert to Right Treatment (START), 48
SDEC *see* same-day emergency care
secondary headache, 409
secondary hyperparathyroidism, 264
secondary prevention, stroke, 321–322
sedative toxidrome, 227
sedatives, 238–239, 349
seizures, 406–407
  epileptic, 315–316
  pregnant patients, 186–187
self-discharge against medical advice, 111–112
self-harm, 337–340
semantic qualifiers, 15
sensory examination, 304–305
sepsis
  critical/enhanced care, 92–95
  definition, 92–93
  during cardiac arrest, 79
  management, 94–95
  neutropenic, 359
  pregnant patients, 187
  resuscitation, 71, 79
  screening, 93
  Six care bundle, 94, 187
septic shock, 71, 93–95
serious adverse drug reactions, 42
severe hypoglycaemia, 283–284
severe hyponatraemia, 254
severe mental illness, 345–346
sex workers, 207
SGLT2 *see* sodium glucose co-transporter-2
shared decision-making, surgery, 161–162
shock, 56–58, 66
SIADH *see* syndrome of inappropriate antidiuretic hormone
sickle cell disease, 418
side effects, 42
simple partial-onset seizures, 315
situation, background, assessment, recommendation and readback (SBARR) system, 29, 54

situational awareness, 54
sleep, night working, 140–141
small bowel obstruction, 370
SNAP regimen, 229
SNOOP4, 409–410
Society of Acute Medicine (SAM), 4
SOCRATES, 368
sodium balance, 251, 253–258
  homeostatic control, 253
  hypernatraemia, 257–258
  hyponatraemia, 252, 253–257
sodium glucose co-transporter-2 (SGLT2) inhibitors, 278, 280
somatic neuropathy, diabetic, 291–292
spastic gait, 305
spastic paraparesis, 311
speech assessment, 302–303
spice, 236
ST elevation myocardial infarction (STEMI), 81–82, 389, 391
START *see* Screening Tool to Alert to Right Treatment
status epilepticus, 318
STEMI *see* ST elevation myocardial infarction
steppage gait, 305
steroids
  complications, 360
  hypercalcaemia of malignancy, 356
  perioperative medicine, 174
  pregnant patients, 192
Stevens–Johnson syndrome, 43
stimulant toxidrome, 227
stimulants, 237–238
STOPP *see* Screening Tool of Older Persons' Prescriptions
stress
  and coping resources, 339
  psychological reactions, 340–341
stroke, 319–322
  cerebral circulation, 319–320
  clinical patterns, 320
  definitions, 319
  diabetes, 294–295
  facial nerve disorders, 310
  haemorrhagic, 320–322
  management, 320–322
  perioperative medicine, 171
  prognosis, 322
  risk factors, 320

secondary prevention, 321–322
types, 319
styles of leadership, 27
subarachnoid haemorrhage (SAH), 320–322
substance abuse, 230–244
  alcohol, 231–234
  antidotes, 235
  body packers, 240
  CAGE questionnaire screening, 234
  generic management, 241–243
  intravenous administration, 240
  laboratory tests, 243
  LGBTQ+ people, 212
  malnutrition, 243–244
  management, 241–243
  recreational drugs, 234–241
  toxidromes, 242
  see also specific substances. . .
sudden unexpected death in epilepsy (SUDEP), 187, 319
SUDEP *see* sudden unexpected death in epilepsy
suidical thoughts, 337–340
sulfonylureas, 278, 284
superior vena cava obstruction, 359
supervision, 37–39
surgery
  decision to operate, 161–162
  Parkinson disease, 325
  perioperative medicine, 160–175
  risk assessment, 161–162
Swiss cheese model, 32
sympathomimetic toxidrome, 227
syncope, 66, 382
  pregnant patients, 186–187
  vs epilepsy, 316
syndrome of inappropriate antidiuretic hormone (SIADH), 253, 255–256, 258
synthetic highs, 235–236
systems thinking, 32–33, 141

T

T-LOC *see* transient loss of consciousness
T1DM *see* type 1 diabetes
T2DM *see* type 2 diabetes
tachycardia, 66–67

TALK debriefing, 143
tamponade, 79, 82
targeted temperature
    management, 84
teaching, 37–38
teams, communication, 29
telemedicine, 6–7
temperature
    fever, 403–405
    normal, 403
temporal arteritis *see* giant cell
    arteritis
tension headache, 313
tension pneumothorax, 79, 82
therapeutic reasoning, 13
thiamine (B1) deficiency, 154,
    233, 243
Think, Do framework, 20
thoracentesis, ultrasound-
    guided, 126
thoracic ultrasound, 120–127
    clinical protocol, 127
    interstitial syndrome, 125
    limitations and pitfalls,
        126–127
    normal anatomical findings,
        120–123
    pleural effusion, 124–125
    pneumonia, 125–126
    pneumothorax, 123–124
    technique, 120
    thoracentesis, 126
thrombocytopenia, 60, 172
thrombolytics, 78
thromboprophylaxis, 184
thrombosis
    cancer-related, 361
    cardiac arrest, 79
    deep vein, 134–137, 198,
        420–421
thyroid cancer, 259
thyroid disorders, 258–263
    amiodarone-related, 263
    classification, 260
    clinical features, 259–260
    myxoedema coma, 262–263
    perioperative medicine, 170
    thyroid storm, 261–262
    treatment, 261–263
thyroid storm, 261–262
thyroiditis, 259
thyrotoxicosis, 260
    amiodarone-induced, 263
    thyroid storm, 261–262

TIA *see* transient ischaemic
    episode
time management, 26
tonic-clonic status epilepticus, 318
toxic epidermal necrolysis, 429
toxicity, 222
toxicology, 221–229
    ABCDEFGH approach, 224
    antidotes, 225–227
    carbon monoxide, 222–223
    cardiac arrest, 79, 82
    Coma Cocktail, 224
    cyanide, 223
    decontamination, 224–225
    definitions, 222
    elimination, 225
    general management
        principles, 223–227
    medical history, 225–227
    paracetamol overdose,
        227–229
    psychiatry review, 225
    recreational drugs, 235–241
    RRSIDEAD approach, 224
    time course, 222
    toxidromes, 224, 227
toxidromes, 224, 227, 242
toxin, definition, 222
trafficking victims, 204–207
transfusions, 57–58, 60
transient ischaemic attack (TIA)
    definition, 319
    diabetes, 294–295
    surgical considerations, 171
transient loss of consciousness
    (T-LOC), 382
    see also syncope
traumatic brain injury, 249,
    331–333
travel-related diagnoses, 405
travellers, 207–208
treatment, thyroid disorders,
    261–263
trigeminal neuralgia, 314
tuberculosis, 395–397
tuberculous meningitis,
    328–329
tumour lysis syndrome,
    357–359
tumours, intracranial, 331
type 1 diabetes (T1DM), 274,
    277–278, 281
type 2 diabetes (T2DM), 274–275,
    278–279, 280–281, 284

U

UAO *see* upper airway obstruction
ulcerative colitis, 400
ultrasound
    artifacts, 115–116
    bladder volume, 132–133
    BLUE protocol, 127
    deep vein thrombosis, 134–137
    focused abdominal, 127–131
    focused renal, 131–134
    free fluid in abdomen, 129
    hydronephrosis, 131–132
    image optimisation, 119–120
    image production, 117–118
    interstitial syndrome, 125
    paracentesis, 129
    physics of, 114–115
    pleural effusion, 124–125
    pneumonia, 125–126
    pneumothorax, 123–124
    preparation, 120
    probes, 116–117
    procedural guidance, 136
    resolution, 118–120
    scanning modes, 118–119
    scanning planes, 118
    thoracentesis, 126
    thoracic, 120–127
undocumented migrants,
    204–207
unsteadyness, 401–402
updated Beers criteria, 48
upper airway obstruction (UAO),
    55, 178

V

vascular dementia, 153
vascular parkinsonism, 323
vasculitis, 418–419
vasopressor drugs, 77
venous insufficiency, 420
venous thromboembolism (VTE),
    79, 173, 189–191
ventilation, 56
    cardiac arrest, 75–77
    critical/enhanced care, 88–91
    oxygen therapy, 56, 88–89
    post-resuscitation, 84
ventricular fibrillation (VF), 77
ventricular tachycardia (VT),
    66–67, 77

vertebral compression fractures, 150
vertigo, 401–402
vestibulocochlear nerve disorders, 310–311
viral meningitis, 327–329
virtual wards, 7
visual field disorders, 307–309
vitamin D deficiency, 244, 264
vomiting, 182–185, 429–430
VT *see* ventricular tachcardia
VTE *see* venous thromboembolism
vulnerable migrants, 204–207

W

waddling gait, 305
ward selection, 55
warfarin, 172–173
water balance, 252–253
   see also fluid balance
watery diarrhoea, 398
waveform capnography, 77
weakness, 430–431
weight loss, 296–297
Wernicke encephalopathy, 233
Wernicke–Korsakoff syndrome, 154, 233

Wilson disease, 323–324
withdrawal
   alcohol, 233–234
   opioids, 239
   resuscitation, 78, 84–85
workplace-based assessments (WPBAs), 38–39
WPBAs *see* workplace-based assessments

Y

young adults, 194–196